Extreme IR

Ziv J Haskal

Editor

Extreme IR

Extraordinary Cases in Interventional Radiology and Endovascular Therapies

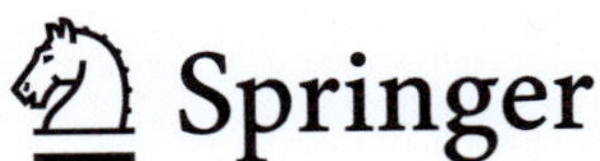
Springer

Editor
Ziv J Haskal, MD
Department of Radiology and Medical Imaging
Interventional Division, University of Virginia
Charlottesville, VA, USA

ISBN 978-3-031-24253-3   ISBN 978-3-031-24251-9   (eBook)
https://doi.org/10.1007/978-3-031-24251-9

Foreword

There's a reason everyone does what they do. Whether it is money, lifestyle, social status, career advancement, prestige, family connection, service to society, aptitude, or a combination of motivating factors, each of us tries to choose the perfectly matched vocation that is calling our name.

So, when IR calls, what do we hear? The potential for direct patient contact while dealing with a wide range of diseases; the opportunity to develop and apply new technologies in a variety of high impact procedures that deliver clear patient benefits; the chance to collaborate with clinicians across the full spectrum of medical specialties, and an impactful career that uses image-guided minimally invasive therapies to provide solutions to problems and benefits to patients with less risk, cost, and recovery time.

It sounds great to a first-year medical student.

And it is.

After all, who's got it better than us?

No one!

If it weren't for the tribal nature of medical politics and the in-bred stodginess of the medical specialty establishment, IRs would be rightfully viewed as the Kings and Queens of Medicine. We consistently challenge the status and question the quo. Indeed, questioning staid ideas is one dimension of what makes IR so enthralling and creatively intense.

When IR calls however, external validation is not what we are responding to. What makes IR the perfect fit for us on a daily basis?

It is the cases. The more complex the anatomy, the more complicated the challenge, the more we appreciate IR and what we do. IR is essentially a case-based or procedurally centered vocation. Not to discount by any measure our patient care responsibilities, but this specialty was built on cases. IRs live for the case planning—developing the precise procedural strategy, detailing the tactical elements one by one to advance the procedure, selecting the ideal catheters and devices to successfully achieve the goal and importantly, considering the contingencies available when the initial technical steps are not feasible or unsuccessful.

When things go well, to an IR's ears it is musical. And during the handful of signature cases, an IR encounters in his/her career, when the impossible becomes possible and the insurmountable anatomical or technical challenge is somehow met, it transcends lyrical—it is magical. When, as an IR, you experience this feeling, you remember the call and understand why you could not resist.

Extreme IR is a collection of those special cases that describe the beauty and wonder of IR better than any words. Undoubtedly, with each case you will viscerally sense the emotions—the agony and the ecstasy—experienced by the interventionalist as they approach and attempt to tackle an extreme IR challenge.

"Call me Ishmael." In this volume, Ziv Haskal, has compiled the best of the best extreme IR cases. I know you will enjoy vicariously the thrills encountered by the contributing IR Ahabs as they describe the perils and uncertainties of facing a formidable challenge and no matter what the stage of your career, I am confident you will hear the IR call.

The University of Arizona
Tucson, AZ, USA
Michael D. Dake

Introduction

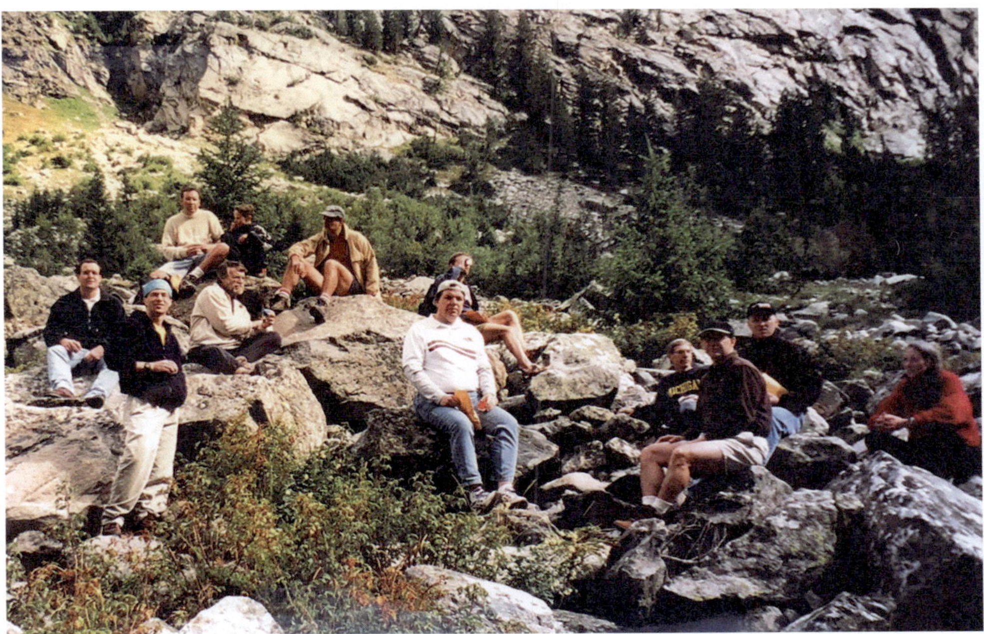

The Hike to CME. Some of the original 1998 Extreme IR course participants, stopping for lecture on the Cascade Canyon Trail, Grand Teton National Park. That's me on the far left, wearing the blue bandanna.

Innovation often grows from years of methodical, grinding work built around a thread of an idea. Sometimes, though, it can occur in a day, or in the moment, in considering an extraordinary problem, or reacting to an unanticipated event while treating a patient. And sometimes that Eureka idea may lay in waiting for decades until reawoken with fresh eyes and empowering technology–witness TIPS. We recognize both within ourselves and our specialties.

The alpinist's drive to climb a new route has driven interventional radiology and endovascular work since its early days and drives us still. Perhaps it is the medical form of Type 2 fun: difficult and uncertain while we are amidst but satisfying and sometimes spectacular in reflection afterwards.

We dream of world-changing advances, but rally around the individual for showing us avenues into the new, elevated by their success, or hard lessons, and providing us new "angles" we can use for our future patients. While we drive our field forward by the hard work of data, signal, and proof, there is no denying that flame that brought us into this specialty—and certainly sustains me after 30 years. As one of my mentors, Prof Ernie Ring said during my fellowship: "You need one good case every few months to keep you going."

In 1998, I held the first Extreme IR course in Jackson Hole WY. We had lectures in the mornings and adventures thereafter, from rock climbing and rafting, to the daylong "Hike to

CME" to Lake Solitude. And for the brave (or foolhardy), a brief swim in its icy waters, surrounded by a rim of snow. The transplant intervention lecture was given on the rocks, 2 h in, with 35 mm slides and viewers, cliffs behind us, moose, stream, and the Grand Teton in front. This course morphed into one of the more popular events at the Society of Interventional Radiology annual meeting, where my friend and colleague (MDD) and I host 40+ faculty in rapid presentations of extraordinary successes and crashing failures in a 4–5 h breakneck session. These events have been mimicked, under various names worldwide—imitation is the most sincere form of flattery. I translated those events into the Extreme IR manuscripts during my terms as Editor in Chief of the JVIR. But I rarely published more than one case per issue. And thus, comes this first book of Extreme IR and Endovascular cases.

I trust you enjoy, share, and inspire others with your own extremity.

Interventional Division   Ziv J Haskal, MD
Department of Radiology and Medical Imaging
University of Virginia School of Medicine
Charlottesville, VA, USA

Contents

Contributors

Osman Ahmed Department of Vascular and Interventional Radiology, University of Chicago Medical Center, Chicago, IL, USA

Rakesh S. Ahuja Department of Vascular and Interventional Radiology, Boston Children's Hospital, Boston, MA, USA

R. Torrance Andrews Department of Interventional Radiology, Swedish Medical Center, First Hill Campus, Seattle, WA, USA

John F. Angle Department of Radiology and Medical Imaging, UVA Health, Charlottesville, VA, USA

Shafkat Anwar Department of Pediatrics and Radiology, Center for Advanced 3D+ Technologies, University of California San Francisco, San Francisco, CA, USA

Mohammad Arabi Medical Imaging Department, King Abdulaziz Medical City, Ministry of National Guard Health Affairs, Riyadh, Saudi Arabia

Vascular Interventional Radiology, Medical Imaging Department, King Abdulaziz Medical City, National Guard Health Affairs, Riyadh, Saudi Arabia

Yasuaki Arai, MD, FSIR, FCIRSE Department of Diagnostic Radiology, National Cancer Center, Tokyo, Japan

Meena Archie Department of Vascular Surgery, Providence St. Joseph Hospital, Orange, CA, USA

Bulent Arslan Vascular and Interventional Service Line, Rush University Medical Center, Chicago, IL, USA

Eli Atar Department of Radiology, Rabin Medical Center, Petah Tikva, Israel

Carlos Eduardo Baccin Department of Interventional Neuroradiology, Hospital Israelita Albert Einstein, São Paulo, São Paulo, Brazil

Thomas Barge Department of Radiology, John Radcliffe Hospital, Oxford, UK

William Behl University of Virginia Health System, Charlottesville, VA, USA

Elliot Berger College of Osteopathic Medicine, Des Moines University, Des Moines, IA, USA

Zachary T. Berman Department of Radiology, University of California, San Deigo, CA, USA

Tiago Bilhim, MD, PhD, EBIR-ES, FSIR, FCIRSE Department of Interventional Radiology, Curry Cabral Hospital, Centro Hospitalar Universitário de Lisboa Central (CHULC), Lisbon, Portugal

Zaeem Billah Department of Vascular and Interventional Radiology, Kaiser Permanente Los Angeles Medical Center, Los Angeles, CA, USA

Christoph A. Binkert Institute of Radiology and Nuclear Medicine, Kantonsspital Winterthur, Winterthur, Switzerland

Justin E. Bird Department of Orthopaedic Oncology, UTMD Anderson Cancer Center, Houston, TX, USA

Elias Brountzos 2nd Department of Radiology, Medical School National and Kapodistrian University of Athens, General University Hospital Attikon, Haidari, Greece

Daniel B. Brown Department of Radiology, Vanderbilt University Medical Center, Nashville, TN, USA

Elchanan Bruckheimer Department of Pediatric Cardiology, Schneider Children's Medical Center, Petah Tikva, Israel

Michael J. Bunker Center for Advanced 3D+ Technologies, University of California San Francisco, San Francisco, CA, USA

Matthew R. Callstrom Department of Radiology, Mayo Clinic, Rochester, MN, USA

Leigh Casadaban University of Colorado Anschutz Medical Campus, Aurora, CO, USA

Roberto Luigi Cazzato Department of Interventional Radiology, University Hospital of Strasbourg, Strasbourg, France

Hélène Cebula Department of Neurosurgery, University Hospital of Strasbourg, Strasbourg, France

Victor Chao Department of Cardiothoracic Surgery, National Heart Centre Singapore, Singapore, Singapore

Tze Tec Chong Department of Vascular Surgery, Singapore General Hospital, Singapore, Singapore

Timothy W. I. Clark Department of Radiology, Section of Interventional Radiology, University of Pennsylvania Perelman School of Medicine, Philadelphia, PA, USA

Aenov Cohen Department of Radiology, Rabin Medical Center and Schneider Children's Medical Center, Petah Tikva, Israel

Clayton W. Commander Department of Radiology, University of North Carolina School of Medicine, Chapel Hill, NC, USA

Miles B. Conrad Department of Radiology and Biomedical Imaging, University of California, San Francisco, San Francisco, CA, USA

Benjamin Contrella Allegheny Health Network, Pittsburgh, PA, USA

Jacob Cynamon Department of Radiology, Montefiore Medical Center, Bronx, NY, USA

Christian Debry Department of Head and Neck Surgery, University Hospital of Strasbourg, Strasbourg, France

Chadi Diab Department of Radiology, University of Kentucky, College of Medicine, Lexington, KY, USA

Athanasios Diamantopoulos Department of Interventional Radiology, Guy's and St. Thomas' NHS Foundation Trust, London, UK

School of Biomedical Engineering and Imaging Sciences, Faculty of Life Sciences and Medicine, Kings College London, London, UK

Bart Dolmatch Department of Interventional Radiology, The Palo Alto Medical Foundation, Mountain View, CA, USA

John R. Dryden Department of Radiology/Radiological Sciences, Uniformed Services University of the Health Sciences, Bethesda, MD, USA

Patrick W. Eiken Department of Radiology, Mayo Clinic, Rochester, MN, USA

Aaron Fischman Department of Interventional Radiology, Mount Sinai Hospital, New York, NY, USA

Brian Funaki Department of Radiology, University of Chicago, Chicago, IL, USA

Roberto Galuppo Department of Radiology, University of Kentucky, College of Medicine, Lexington, KY, USA

Ripal T. Gandhi Department of Interventional Radiology, Miami Cardiac and Vascular Institute, Baptist Health South Florida, Miami, FL, USA

Afshin Gangi Department of Interventional Radiology, University Hospital of Strasbourg, Strasbourg, France

Gaurav Dilip Gangwani Department of Interventional Radiology, Bhaktivedanta Hospital and Research Institute, Thane, Maharashtra, India

Jared Gans Envision Healthcare, Fort Lauderdale, FL, USA

R. Garcia-Monaco Department of Vascular and Interventional Radiology, Hospital Italiano de Buenos Aires, Ciudad de Buenos Aires, Argentina

Julien Garnon Department of Interventional Radiology, University Hospital of Strasbourg, Strasbourg, France

M. Gonsalves Department of Interventional Radiology, St. George's University Hospitals NHS Foundation Trust, London, UK

Allen R. Goode Department of Radiology and Medical Imaging, University of Virginia Health System, Charlottesville, VA, USA

Sebouh Gueyikian Department of Interventional Radiology, Northshore University Healthcare System, Evanston, IL, USA

Zachary Haber Department of Interventional Radiology, University of California, Los Angeles, CA, USA

Adnan Hadziomerovic Department of Medical Imaging, The Ottawa Hospital-University of Ottawa, Ottawa, ON, Canada

Ziv J Haskal Department of Radiology and Medical Imaging, Interventional Division, University of Virginia, Charlottesville, VA, USA

Paul Haste Department of Radiology and Imaging Sciences, Indiana University School of Medicine, Indianapolis, IN, USA

Matthew Henry Medical College of Wisconsin, Milwaukee, WI, USA

Glenn Hoots Department of Radiology, Tampa General Hospital, Florida Interventional Specialists, University of South Florida, Tampa, FL, USA

Jeffrey Hull Department of Interventional Radiology, Richmond Vascular Center, North Chesterfield, VA, USA

Eddie Hyatt UT Southwestern Medical Center, Dallas, TX, USA

Masanori Inoue Department of Radiology, Keio University School of Medicine, Tokyo, Japan

Maxim Itkin Division of Interventional Radiology, Department of Radiology, Hospital of the University of Pennsylvania, Penn Medicine, Philadelphia, PA, USA

Masahiro Jinzaki Department of Radiology, Keio University School of Medicine, Tokyo, Japan

Kaj H. Johansen Department of Interventional Radiology, Swedish Medical Center, First Hill Campus, Seattle, WA, USA

Sanjeeva Kalva Department of Radiology, Massachusetts General Hospital, Boston, MA, USA

Kartik Kansagra Department of Vascular and Interventional Radiology, Kaiser Permanente Los Angeles Medical Center, Los Angeles, CA, USA

Baljendra Kapoor Cleveland Clinic, Cleveland, OH, USA

Dimitrios Karnabatidis Department of Interventional Radiology, Patras University Hospital, Patras, Greece

Interventional Radiology, Patras University Hospital, Patras, Greece

Konstantinos Katsanos Department of Interventional Radiology, Patras University Hospital, Patras, Greece

Hooman Khabiri Section of Interventional Radiology, Washington DC VA Medical Center, Washington, DC, USA

Minhaj S. Khaja Department of Vascular and Interventional Radiology, University of Virginia Health, Charlottesville, VA, USA

Bhavraj Khalsa Department of Interventional Radiology, Providence St. Joseph Hospital, Orange, CA, USA

Dhara Kinariwala Department of Radiology and Medical Imaging, University of Virginia, Charlottesville, VA, USA

Panagiotis M. Kitrou Department of Interventional Radiology, Patras University Hospital, Patras, Greece

Maureen P. Kohi Department of Radiology, University of North Carolina School of Medicine, Chapel Hill, NC, USA

Marc C. Kryger Department of Radiology and Medical Imaging, University of Virginia Health System, Charlottesville, VA, USA

Abhishek Kumar Division of Vascular and Interventional Radiology, Department of Radiology, Rutgers—New Jersey Medical School, Newark, NJ, USA

A. Nicholas Kurup Department of Radiology, Mayo Clinic, Rochester, MN, USA

Justin Kwan Department of Diagnostic and Interventional Radiology, Tan Tock Seng Hospital, Singapore, Singapore

Janesh Lakhoo Department of Radiology, Vanderbilt University Medical Center, Nashville, TN, USA

Jeffery Leef Department of Vascular and Interventional Radiology, University of Chicago Medical Center, Chicago, IL, USA

Lawrence Lin Division of Vascular and Interventional Radiology, Department of Radiology, Medical College of Wisconsin, Milwaukee, WI, USA

R. Peter Lokken Department of Radiology and Biomedical Imaging, University of California, San Francisco, San Francisco, CA, USA

Robert Lookstein Department of Interventional Radiology, Mount Sinai Hospital, New York, NY, USA

Jorge E. Lopera Department of Radiology, UT Health San Antonio, San Antonio, TX, USA

Mina S. Makary Division of Vascular and Interventional Radiology, Department of Radiology, The Ohio State University Wexner Medical Center, Columbus, OH, USA

Michael Markovitz Department of Radiology, University of South Florida, Tampa, FL, USA

John Matson Department of Radiology and Medical Imaging, University of Virginia Health System, Charlottesville, VA, USA

Alan Matsumoto Department of Radiology and Medical Imaging, University of Virginia Health System, Charlottesville, VA, USA

Monica M. Matsumoto Division of Interventional Radiology, Department of Radiology, Hospital of the University of Pennsylvania, Penn Medicine, Philadelphia, PA, USA

Keshav Menon UT Southwestern Medical Center, Dallas, TX, USA

Robert Morgan Department of Interventional Radiology, St George's University Hospital, London, UK

Cardiovascular Clinical Academic Group, Molecular and Clinical Sciences Research Institute, St. George's, University of London and St. George's University Hospitals NHS Foundation Trust, London, UK

John M. Moriarty Division of Vascular and Interventional Radiology, Department of Radiology, UCLA Medical Center, Los Angeles, CA, USA

Ryan D. Murray Department of Interventional Radiology, University of Texas MD Anderson Cancer Center, Houston, TX, USA

Abdul Rehman Mustafa College of Medicine, Alfaisal University, Riyadh, Saudi Arabia

Alfaisal University College of Medicine, Riyadh, Saudi Arabia

Seishi Nakatsuka Department of Radiology, Keio University School of Medicine, Tokyo, Japan

Ray Norby Department of Radiology & Medical Imaging, University of Virginia, Charlottesville, VA, USA

Romman Nourzaei Department of Interventional Radiology, Guy's and St. Thomas' NHS Foundation Trust, London, UK

Scott Olson Department of Neurosurgery and Radiology, University of California, San Diego, La Jolla, CA, USA

Murat Osman Vascular and Interventional Service Line, Rush University Medical Center, Chicago, IL, USA

Keigo Osuga Department of Diagnostic Radiology, Osaka Medical and Pharmaceutical University, Takatsuki, Osaka, Japan

Merve Ozen Department of Radiology, University of Kentucky, College of Medicine, Lexington, KY, USA

Siddharth A. Padia Division of Interventional Radiology, Department of Radiology, David Geffen School of Medicine at University of California, Los Angeles, CA, USA

Auh Whan Park Department of Radiology, University of Texas Southwestern, Dallas, TX, USA

Ahmad Parvinian Department of Radiology, Mayo Clinic, Rochester, MN, USA

Kyle Pate Department of Interventional Radiology, MedStar Georgetown University Hospital, Washington, DC, USA

Rahul S. Patel Department of Radiology, Mount Sinai Medical Center, New York, NY, USA

Ricardo Paz-Fumagalli Division of Interventional Radiology, Mayo Clinic Florida, Jacksonville, FL, USA

O. Peralta Department of Vascular and Interventional Radiology, Hospital Italiano de Buenos Aires, Ciudad de Buenos Aires, Argentina

Jillian Plonsker Department of Neurological Surgery, University of California, San Diego, La Jolla, CA, USA

Raghuram Posham Department of Interventional Radiology, Mount Sinai Hospital, New York, NY, USA

Austin J. Pourmoussa Department of Interventional Radiology, Miami Cardiac and Vascular Institute, Baptist Health South Florida, Miami, FL, USA

François Proust Department of Neurosurgery, University Hospital of Strasbourg, Strasbourg, France

Uei Pua Department of Diagnostic Radiology, Tan Tock Seng Hospital, Singapore, Singapore

Sundeep Punamiya Department of Diagnostic and Interventional Radiology, Tan Tock Seng Hospital, Singapore, Singapore

Maximilian Pyko Department of Radiology and Imaging Sciences, Indiana University School of Medicine, Indianapolis, IN, USA

M. Rabellino Department of Vascular and Interventional Radiology, Hospital Italiano de Buenos Aires, Ciudad de Buenos Aires, Argentina

Mona Ranade Department of Interventional Radiology, University of California, Los Angeles, CA, USA

Lakshmi Ratnam Department of Interventional Radiology, St George's University Hospital, London, UK

Cardiovascular Clinical Academic Group, Molecular and Clinical Sciences Research Institute, St. George's, University of London and St George's University Hospitals NHS Foundation Trust, London, UK

Mahmood Razavi Department of Interventional Radiology, Providence St. Joseph Hospital, Orange, CA, USA

Howard M. Richard III Division of Interventional Radiology, Department of Diagnostic Imaging, University of Maryland School, Baltimore, MD, USA

William S. Rilling Division of Vascular and Interventional Radiology, Department of Radiology, Medical College of Wisconsin, Milwaukee, WI, USA

Charles Ritchie Division of Interventional Radiology, Mayo Clinic Florida, Jacksonville, FL, USA

Thoedore F. Saad Department of Nephrology, Nephrology Associates, P.A., Christiana Care Health System, Newark, DE, USA

Saher Sabri Department of Interventional Radiology, MedStar Georgetown University Hospital, Washington, DC, USA

David R. Santiago-Dieppa Department of Neurosurgery, University of California, San Deigo, CA, USA

Jeffrey Savin Department of Diagnostic Radiology, Beaumont Health, Royal Oak, MI, USA

Michael Savin Department of Diagnostic Radiology, Section of Interventional Radiology, Oakland University William Beaumont School of Medicine, Royal Oak, MI, USA

Malay B. Shah Department of Surgery, University of Kentucky, College of Medicine, Lexington, KY, USA

Raja Shaikh Department of Vascular and Interventional Radiology, Boston Children's Hospital, Boston, MA, USA

Daniel Sheeran Department of Radiology, University of Virginia, Charlottesville, VA, USA

Ji Hoon Shin Department of Radiology, University of Ulsan, Asan Medical Center, Seoul, South Korea

Tyler Lee Smith Department of Radiology and Medical Imaging, University of Virginia Health System, Charlottesville, VA, USA

Amanda Smolock Division of Vascular and Interventional Radiology, Department of Radiology, Medical College of Wisconsin, Milwaukee, WI, USA

Caleb Solivio California University of Science and Medicine, Riverside, CA, USA

Miyuki Sone, MD Department of Diagnostic Radiology, National Cancer Center, Tokyo, Japan

Duncan Stevens Department of Radiology, Oakland University William Beaumont School of Medicine, Royal Oak, MI, USA

Shunsuke Sugawara, MD Department of Diagnostic Radiology, National Cancer Center, Tokyo, Japan

Dylan Suttle Greensboro Radiology, Greensboro, NC, USA

Daniel Y. Sze Division of Interventional Radiology, Stanford University, Stanford, CA, USA

Alda L. Tam Department of Interventional Radiology, University of Texas MD Anderson Cancer Center, Houston, TX, USA

Kaishu Tanaka Department of Diagnostic and Interventional Radiology, Osaka University Graduate School of Medicine, Suita, Osaka, Japan

Rafael Trindade Tatit Department of Medicine, Faculdade Israelita de Ciências da Saúde Albert Einstein, São Paulo, São Paulo, Brazil

Kiang Hiong Tay Department of Vascular and Interventional Radiology, Singapore General Hospital, Singapore, Singapore

Seth Toomay UT Southwestern Medical Center, Dallas, TX, USA

Hideyuki Torikai Department of Radiology and Medical Imaging, University of Virginia Health System, Charlottesville, VA, USA

Beau B. Toskich Division of Interventional Radiology, Mayo Clinic Florida, Jacksonville, FL, USA

Margaret C. Tracci University of Virginia Health System, Charlottesville, VA, USA

Raman Uberoi Department of Radiology, John Radcliffe Hospital, Oxford, UK

Ethan Ungchusri Department of Radiology, University of Chicago Medical Center, Chicago, IL, USA

Geogy Vatakencherry Department of Vascular and Interventional Radiology, Kaiser Permanente Los Angeles Medical Center, Los Angeles, CA, USA

Luke Wilkins University of Virginia Health System, Charlottesville, VA, USA

David M. Williams Department of Vascular and Interventional Radiology, Frankel Cardiovascular Center, Michigan Medicine, University of Michigan, Ann Arbor, MI, USA

George R. Wong Department of Radiology, University of North Carolina School of Medicine, Chapel Hill, NC, USA

Jason K. Wong Department of Radiology, Foothills Medical Centre, Cumming School of Medicine, University of Calgary, Calgary, AB, Canada

Steven Yevich Department of Interventional Radiology, MD Anderson Cancer Center, Houston, TX, USA

David J. S. Zucker Division of Vascular and Interventional Radiology, Department of Radiology, UCLA Medical Center, Los Angeles, CA, USA

Part I

Arteries: Thoracic and Abdominal Aorta and Iliac Arteries

Percutaneous Trans-Atrial Embolization of an Ascending Aortic Pseudoaneurysm

David J. S. Zucker and John M. Moriarty

A 58-year-old female with history of systemic lupus erythematosus, autoimmune hemolytic anemia, breast cancer status post mastectomy, chemotherapy, thoracic radiation therapy, and Marfan syndrome status post Bentall procedure and single-vessel CABG in 1999 presented for management of a slowly growing pseudoaneurysm of the ascending aorta. She was considered high risk for redo surgery due to her comorbidities and history of radiation. At the time of intervention, the pseudoaneurysm measured 4.2 × 2.3 cm (Fig. 1.1).

After induction of general anesthesia and selective intubation with single left lung ventilation, a 19-gauge coaxial needle was placed through the right chest wall and across the right atrium into the pseudoaneurysm sac under intermittent CT guidance (Fig. 1.1). A 0.014″ Transend® wire (Stryker Neurovascular, Fremont, CA) was passed into the sac, followed by a straight Renegade® STC microcatheter (Fig. 1.1c) (Boston Scientific, Marlborough, MA).

The patient was transferred to the angiography suite. The pseudoaneurysm sac was embolized to stasis using Interlock coils (Boston Scientific) under transesophageal echocardiography (TEE) and fluoroscopic guidance. Completion aortography demonstrated complete thrombosis of the pseudoaneurysm (Fig. 1.2). The transthoracic needle was withdrawn under fluoroscopic guidance with no post-procedure pericardial effusion on TEE.

The patient was discharged without complication to skilled nursing facility 2 days post-procedure. One-year follow-up shows no further PsA growth and no complications of the trans-atrial route.

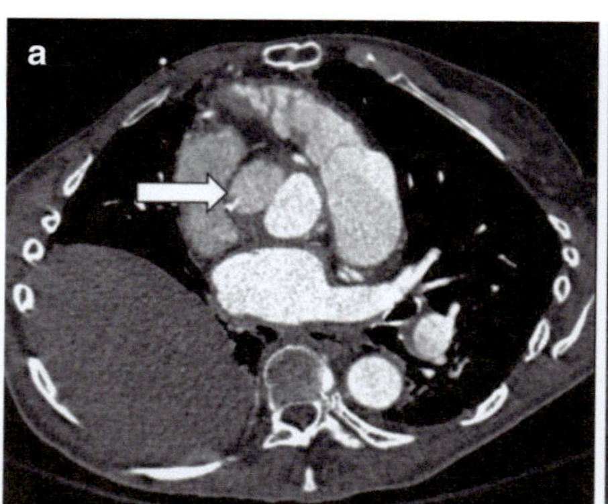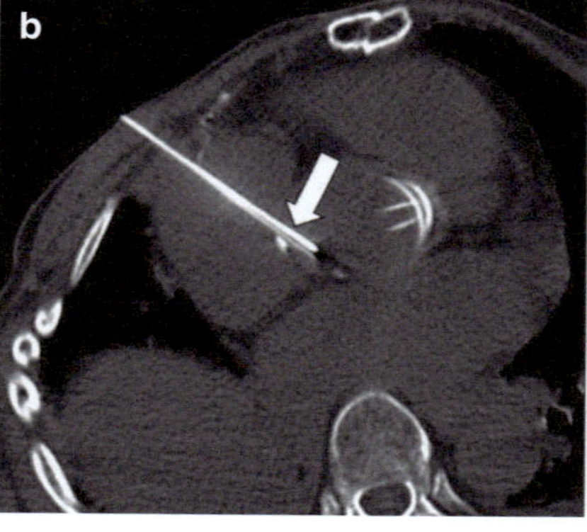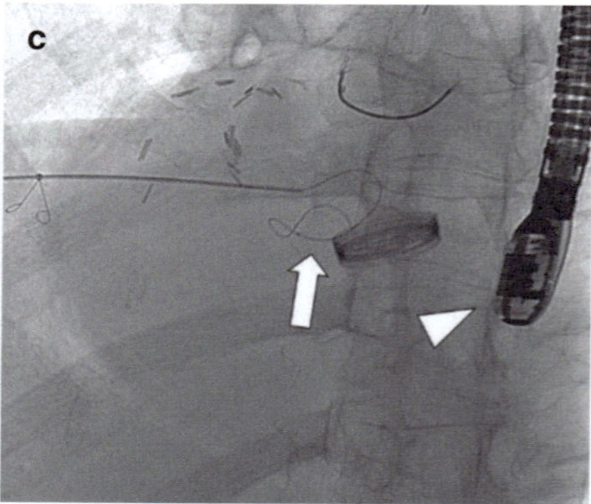

Fig. 1.1 Transthoracic, trans-atrial access of the ascending aortic pseudoaneurysm. (**a**) Multiplanar reformatted image from a pre-procedural CTA of the chest demonstrates a pseudoaneurysm (arrow) arising from the ascending aorta. (**b**) The 19-gauge needle (arrow) traverses the right atrium with the tip positioned within the pseudoaneurysm. Single-lung ventilation allowed avoidance of the right pleural space. (**c**) Microcatheter and microwire (arrow) were passed through the access needle under CT guidance. A transesophageal ultrasound probe (arrowhead) was used for additional guidance

D. J. S. Zucker · J. M. Moriarty (✉)
Division of Vascular and Interventional Radiology, Department of Radiology, UCLA Medical Center, Los Angeles, CA, USA
e-mail: JMoriarty@mednet.ucla.edu

Fig. 1.2 Embolization. (**a**) Grayscale and color Doppler transesophageal echocardiographic image of the ascending aortic pseudoaneurysm (arrows) demonstrating the presence of flow. (**b**) Color Doppler image of the pseudoaneurysm (arrow) after embolization. Echogenic embolic material is present without color flow. (**c**) Aortogram demonstrates embolic coils in the pseudoaneurysm (arrow) with no opacification of the sac

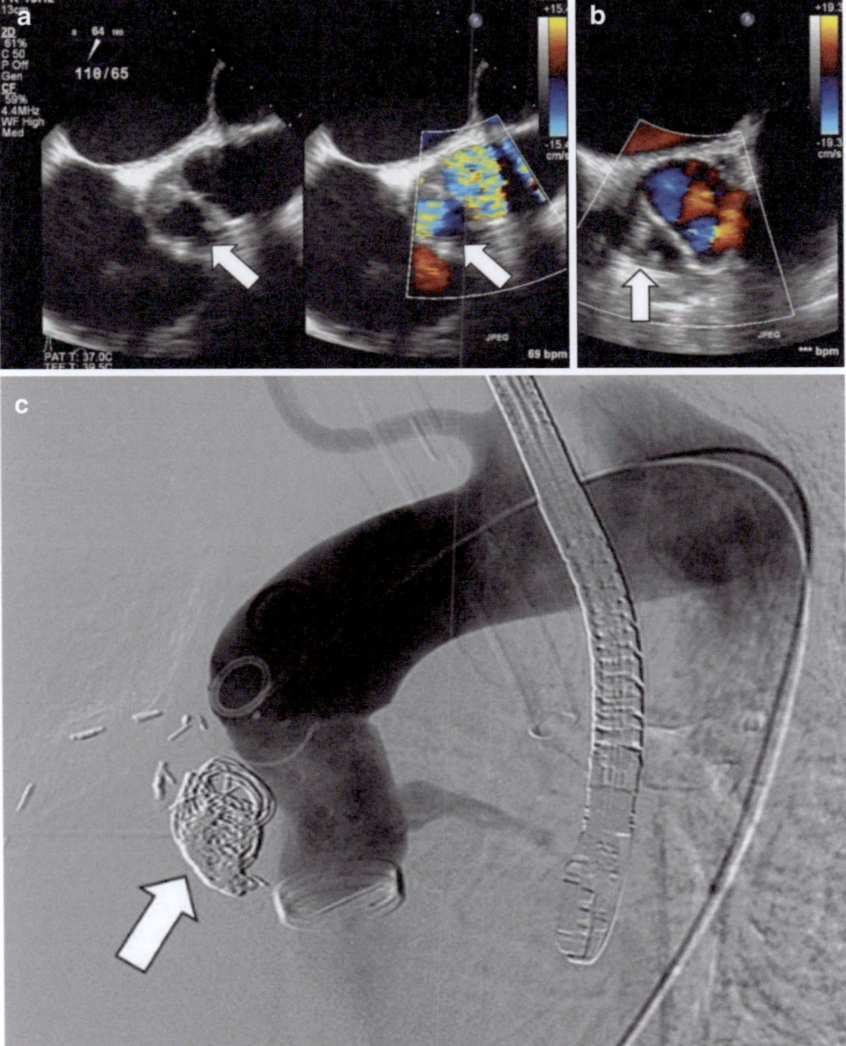

Complete Endovascular Arch Repair for Type A Aortic Dissection

Ray Norby, Minhaj S. Khaja, and David M. Williams

A 73-year-old female presented to an outside hospital with acute chest pain and confusion. CTA demonstrated a Type A aortic dissection (TAAD) (Fig. 2.1), and she was transferred to a tertiary care center.

Due to significant medical comorbidities, she was deemed unsuitable for open repair, and Interventional Radiology (IR) was consulted for thoracic endovascular aortic repair (TEVAR). Prior to TEVAR, vascular surgeons performed partial supra-aortic debranching, with right common carotid to left subclavian artery bypass and left common carotid artery transposition onto the bypass.

Using four accesses, the bilateral common femoral arteries, right common femoral vein, and right brachial artery, an endovascular total aortic arch repair was successfully performed using the Gore Ascending Stent Graft (Fig. 2.2) and Thoracic Branch Endoprosthesis [1, 2] (Fig. 2.3a) with side-branch component placed in the innominate artery (Fig. 2.3b). See Fig. 2.4 for completion aortograms.

She initially recovered well, and CTA on postoperative day 3 demonstrated good stent position and patent branch vessels (Fig. 2.4b). Unfortunately after 2 weeks, she developed GI bleeding, complicated by carotid-subclavian graft occlusion and cerebral infarctions after anticoagulation/antiplatelet therapy was held. Her healthcare was changed to supportive care only, and she died shortly thereafter.

Endovascular treatment of aortic pathology has come a long way since the pioneering work of Drs. Volodos, Parodi, and Dake in the late 1980s and early 1990s [3], with TEVAR of the arch and ascending aorta considered the final frontier of endovascular aortic therapy [4]. Current FDA-sponsored device trials are ongoing [1, 2], and TEVAR represents a viable treatment option for high-risk TAAD patients who are unable to undergo open repair [4].

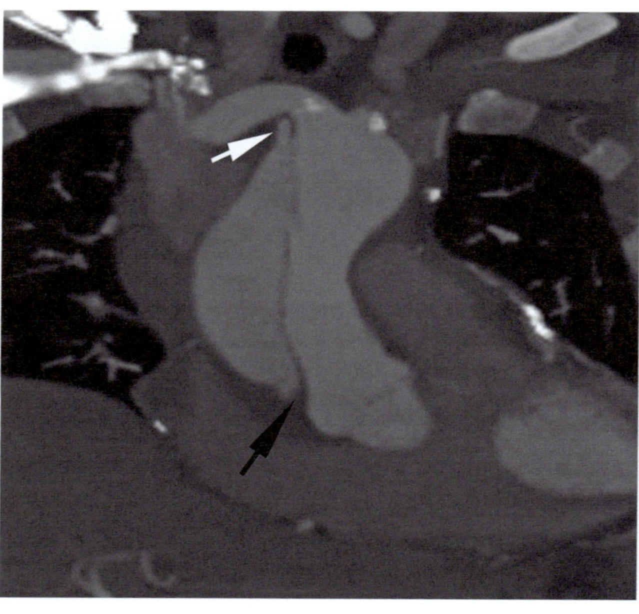

Fig. 2.1 Coronal CTA chest maximum intensity projection (MIP) demonstrates a Type A aortic dissection beginning at the base of the innominate artery (white arrow) and extending retrograde to the sinotubular junction (black arrow). The dissection extends antegrade through the aortic arch and terminates in the proximal descending aorta (not shown)

R. Norby
Department of Radiology & Medical Imaging, University of Virginia, Charlottesville, VA, USA
e-mail: rgn2zb@virginia.edu

M. S. Khaja (✉)
Department of Vascular and Interventional Radiology, University of Virginia Health, Charlottesville, VA, USA

D. M. Williams
Department of Vascular and Interventional Radiology, Frankel Cardiovascular Center, Michigan Medicine, University of Michigan, Ann Arbor, MI, USA
e-mail: davidwms@med.umich.edu

Z. J. Haskal (ed.), *Extreme IR*, https://doi.org/10.1007/978-3-031-24251-9_2

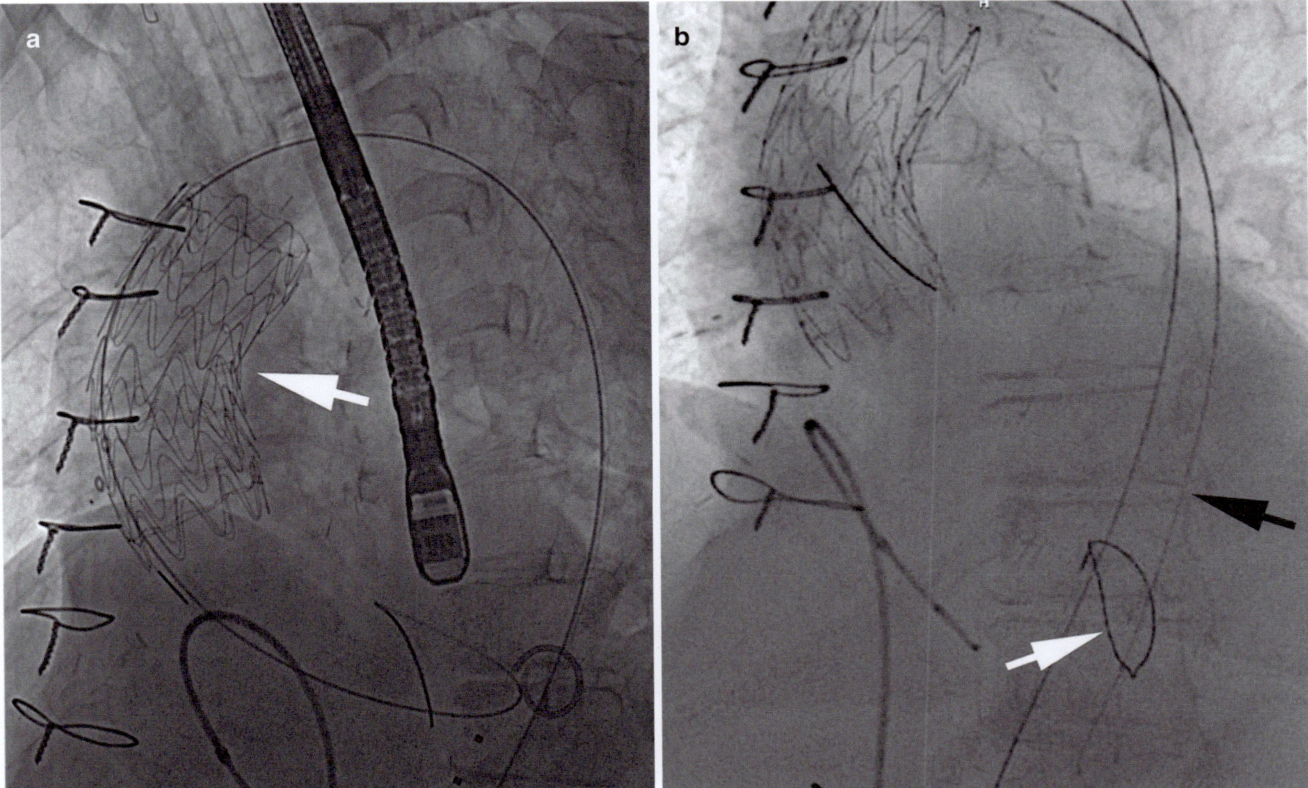

Fig. 2.2 (**a**) Successful deployment of the ascending aortic TEVAR component (white arrow) during rapid ventricular pacing. (**b**) Transfemoral loop snare (white arrow) being used to capture a guide-wire (black arrow) from a right brachial access, establishing through and through access

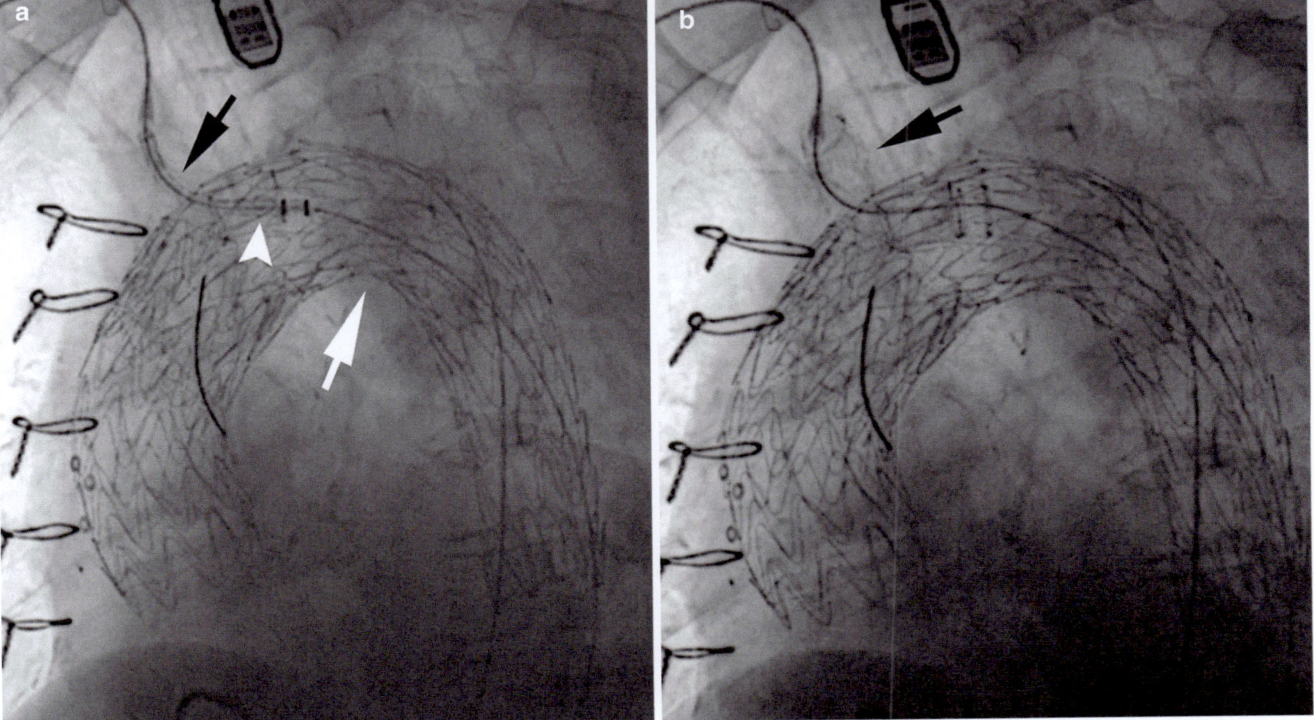

Fig. 2.3 (**a**) Successful deployment of the endograft side-branch aortic component (white arrow) with alignment of the innominate portal (white arrowhead) and innominate branch component (black arrow) through the portal. (**b**) Post deployment image of the innominate branch component (black arrow)

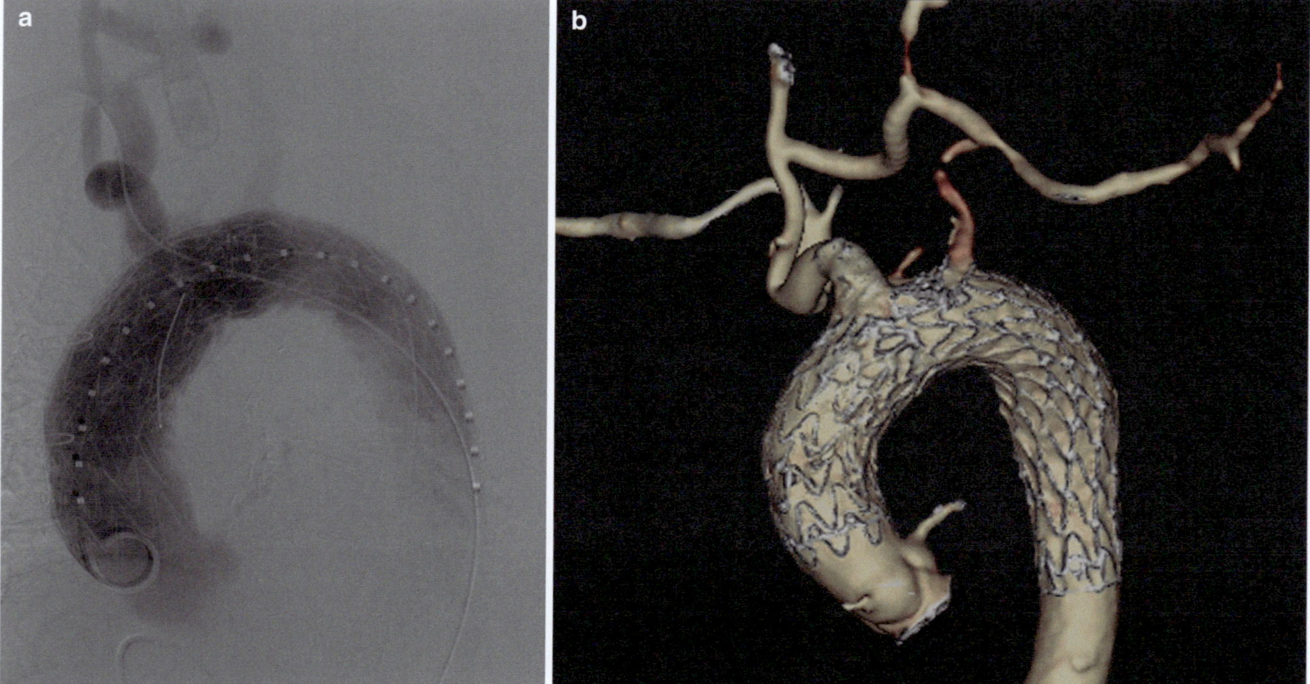

Fig. 2.4 (**a**) Completion aortogram demonstrates complete aortic arch reconstruction with patent innominate branch component and excluded native origins of the left subclavian and common carotid arteries. (**b**) 3D volume rendered image from CTA obtained on postoperative day 3 demonstrates unchanged stent positioning and patency of the side-branch component and all branch vessels

Bibliography

1. Patel HJ, Dake MD, Bavaria JE, Singh MJ, Filinger M, Fischbein MP, Williams DM, Matsumura JS, Oderich G. Branched endovascular therapy of the distal aortic arch: preliminary results of the feasibility multicenter trial of the gore thoracic branch endoprosthesis. Ann Thorac Surg. 2016;102:1190–8.
2. Dake MD, Bavaria JE, Singh MJ, Oderich G, Filinger M, Fischbein MP, Matsumura JS, Patel HJ. Management of arch aneurysms with a single-branch thoracic endograft in zone 0. JTCVS Tech. 2021;7:1–6.
3. Ivancev K, Vogelzang R. A 35 year history of stent grafting, and how EVAR conquered the world. Eur J Vasc Endovasc Surg. 2020;59:685–94.
4. Ahmed Y, Houben IB, Figueroa CA, Burris NS, Williams DM, Moll FL, Patel HJ, van Herwaarden JA. Endovascular ascending aortic repair in type a dissection: a systematic review. J Card Surg. 2021;36:268–79.

COVID Aortic Clot

Geogy Vatakencherry, Kartik Kansagra, Zaeem Billah,
and Caleb Solivio

A 47-year-old female with COVID pneumonia presented to the emergency department with abdominal pain and findings of peritonitis. CT imaging demonstrated bilateral renal infarcts, occlusion of the superior mesenteric artery (SMA), and supraceliac aortic thrombus with clinical concern for acute mesenteric ischemia (Figs. 3.1 and 3.2). The extent of thrombus was felt to preclude surgery. She was referred for endovascular visceral revascularization.

In the interventional suite, right groin access was pre-closed in anticipation of large bore access. Aortography showed extensive SMA thrombus (Fig. 3.3). Aspiration thrombectomy of the proximal SMA using a CAT8 catheter (Penumbra Inc., California), was followed by aspiration of multiple second and third order branches using an ACE64 catheter. Once SMA flow was established, we continued with an endovascular approach, rather than surgical aortic embolectomy because of her worsening status. Given the size of thrombus, the sheath was upsized to a 16 Fr and a T16 FlowTriever (Inari Medical) was used to successfully perform aortic thrombectomy (Fig. 3.4). A 10 mm × 37 mm Express LD stent (Boston Scientific) was deployed across the pre-existing calcific aortic stenosis (Fig. 3.5). The procedure was complicated by a repeat SMA embolus; this was successfully aspirated using the CAT8 catheter (Figs. 3.6 and 3.7).

At completion, she remained intubated and sedated for exploratory laparotomy, and later underwent abdominal surgeries and bowel resections; with 110 cm of viable bowel remaining (Fig. 3.8). In January 2021, she was discharged to a skilled nursing facility before returning home to her family

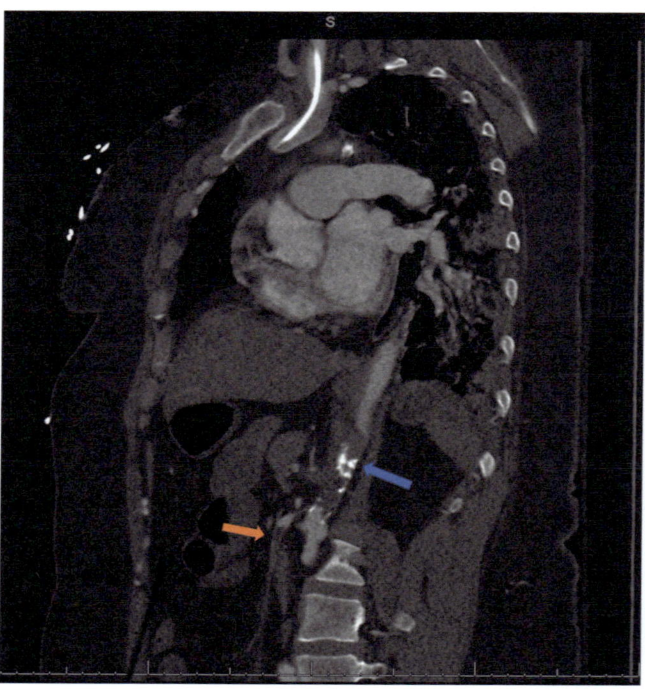

Fig. 3.1 Curved reformat of preoperative CTA shows the long segment SMA clot (orange arrow) and the aortic thrombus (blue arrow). Lungs also show changes consistent with known diagnosis of COVID pneumonia

in March 2021. After 4 months with her family, she was hospitalized for anemia and ultimately passed.

G. Vatakencherry (✉) · K. Kansagra · Z. Billah
Department of Vascular and Interventional Radiology, Kaiser
Permanente Los Angeles Medical Center, Los Angeles, CA, USA
e-mail: George.G.Vatakencherry@kp.org;
Kartik.Kansagra@kp.org; Zaeem.M.Billah@kp.org

C. Solivio
California University of Science and Medicine,
Colton, CA, USA
e-mail: SolivioC@cusm.org

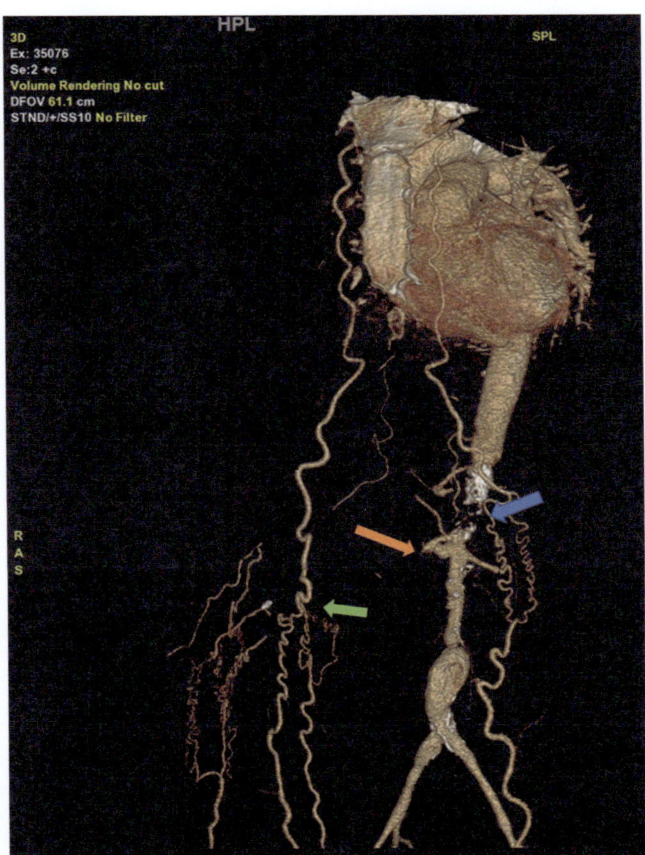

Fig. 3.2 3D volume rendering of preoperative CTA shows discontinuity of the aorta due to thrombus (blue arrow) as well as lack of SMA branches (orange arrow) due to thrombus. Given suspicion of acute insult on underlying aortitis and aortic stenosis, patient had developed extensive superior to inferior epigastric collateral vessels (green arrow)

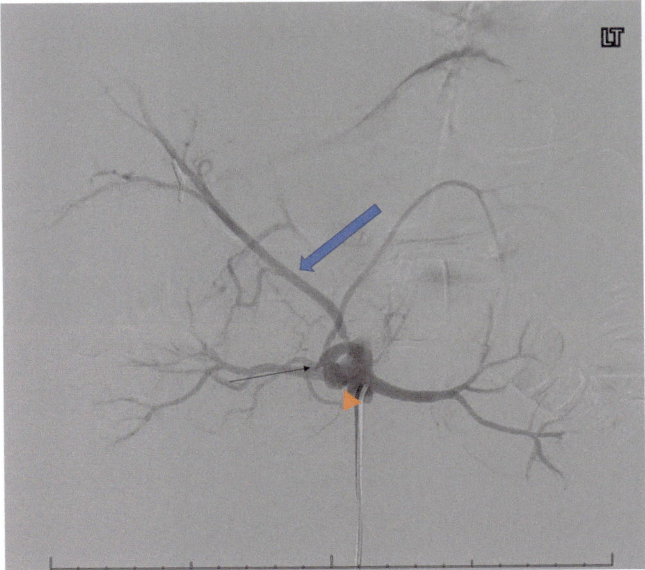

Fig. 3.3 Infrarenal aortogram shows variant anatomy with a replaced right hepatic artery (blue arrow) and proximal SMA thrombus (black arrow). Patient also had a proximal right renal aneurysm (orange arrowhead)

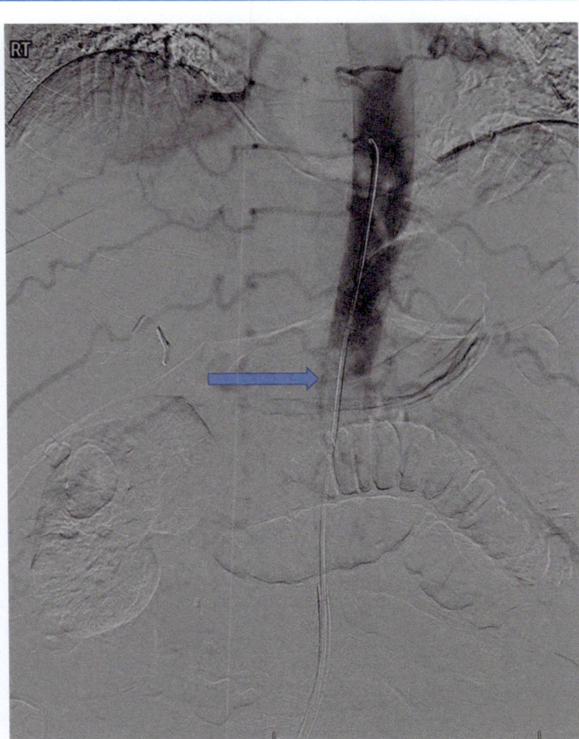

Fig. 3.4 Thoracic aortogram demonstrating focal aortic occlusion due to luminal thrombus (blue arrow)

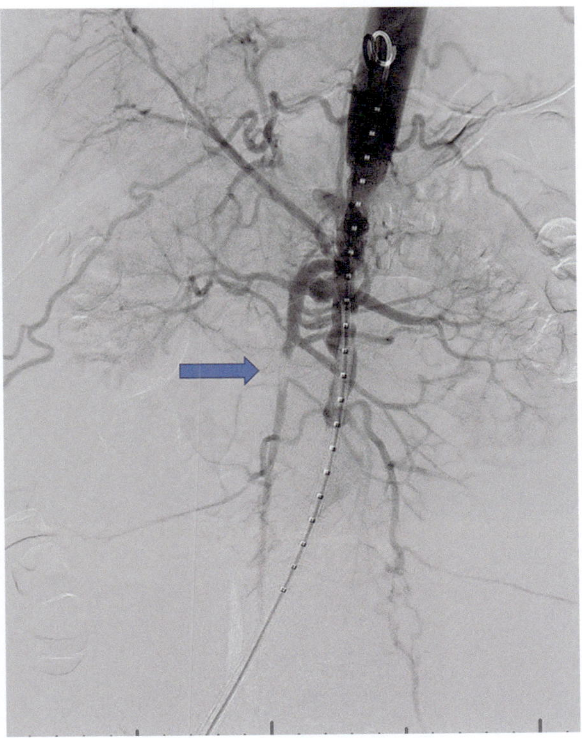

Fig. 3.5 Post-thoraco-aortic thrombectomy and stent deployment shows successful revascularization. Note new embolus in SMA which was subsequently successfully removed with repeat thrombectomy (blue arrow)

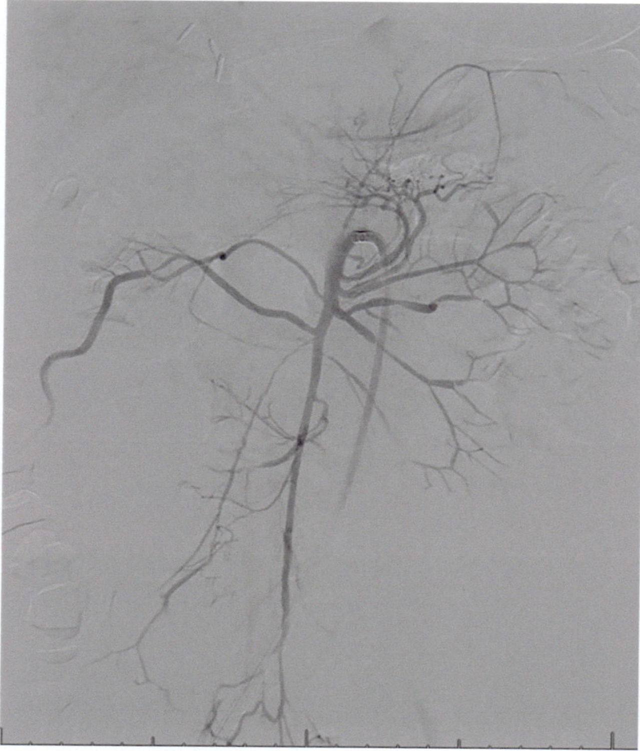

Fig. 3.6 Post-revascularization shows markedly improved flow in the SMA

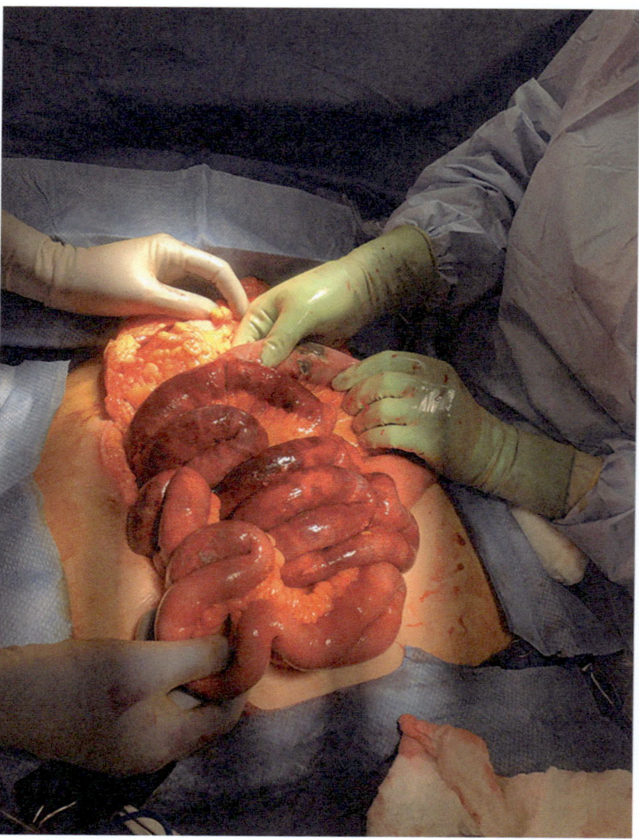

Fig. 3.8 Gross post-operative image showing extent of necrotic bowel taken during first bowel resection on 11/20/2020. The patient had 110 cm of viable bowel left

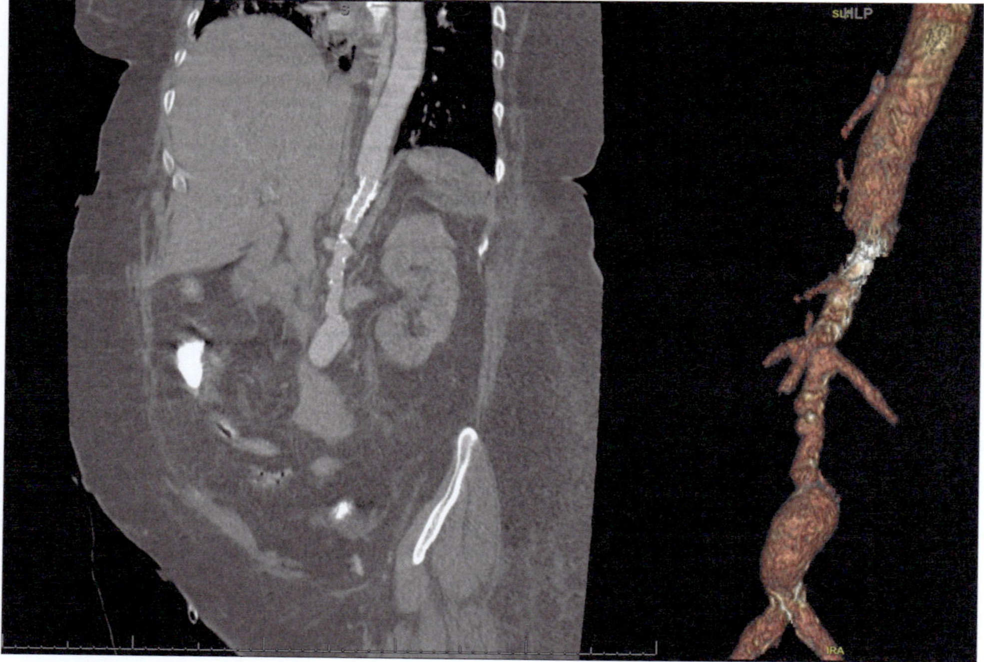

Fig. 3.7 Post-stenting CT curved reformat and 3D volume rendering show patent stent with preserved distal aortoiliac flow. Note distal areas of alternating stenosis and aneurysmal dilation from underling aortitis

Transcaval Endoleak Repair Complicated by Onyx Leak into the IVC and Heart

Eddie Hyatt, Keshav Menon, Seth Toomay, and Sanjeeva Kalva

A 75-year-old man with an enlarging abdominal aortic aneurysm (AAA) following endovascular aneurysm repair (EVAR) was found to have a Type II endoleak on follow-up computed tomography angiography (CTA) (Fig. 4.1). Using a transcaval approach, the aneurysm sac was accessed via the inferior vena cava (IVC) using a Rosh-Uchida needle under fluoroscopic and intravascular ultrasound (IVUS) guidance. Ethylene vinyl alcohol liquid embolic (Onyx®) was instilled into the sac via a microcatheter placed through a 5 F Kumpe catheter (Fig. 4.2). After embolization, as the microcatheter and base catheter were retracted into the IVC, Onyx® spilled into the IVC and became attached to the IVUS probe and guidewire (Fig. 4.3).

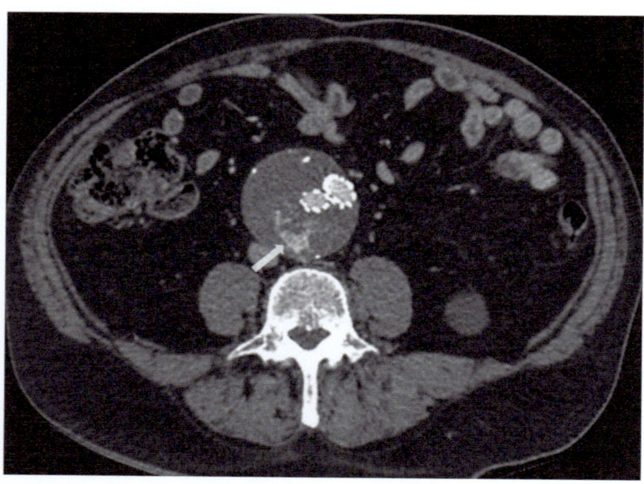

Fig. 4.1 Axial computed tomography angiography (CTA) through the lower abdomen shows an abdominal aortic aneurysm with a Type II endoleak (white arrow) arising from an adjacent lumbar artery

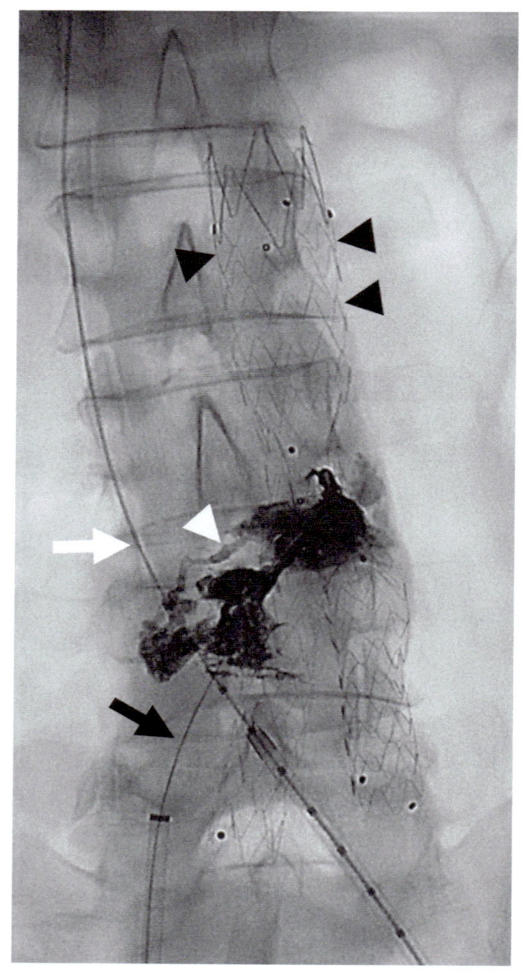

Fig. 4.2 Fluoroscopic image obtained during the embolization procedure showing ethylene vinyl alcohol liquid embolic (Onyx®) administration via the microcatheter (black arrow). Guidewire and intravascular ultrasound probe (white arrow) within the IVC inserted through the left common iliac vein. Aortic stent graft (black arrowheads). Onyx® within the excluded aneurysm sac (white arrowhead)

E. Hyatt · K. Menon · S. Toomay
UT Southwestern Medical Center, Dallas, TX, USA
e-mail: Seth.Toomay@UTSouthwestern.edu

S. Kalva (✉)
Department of Radiology, Massachusetts General Hospital, Boston, MA, USA
e-mail: SKALVA@PARTNERS.ORG

An IVC filter was immediately placed via the right internal jugular vein to prevent an Onyx® pulmonary embolus (PE). Various snares, a retrieval cone, endobronchial forceps, and several rounds of IVC filter placement and retrieval were required to meticulously remove the embolic material (Fig. 4.4). A larger piece of the Onyx® traveled to the heart (Fig. 4.5), but was eventually snared and safely removed. At the conclusion of the procedure only a few tiny pieces of embolic material had embolized to the pulmonary arteries (Figs. 4.5 and 4.6). Completion venogram demonstrated a patent IVC (Fig. 4.7). He was admitted overnight for observation and was discharged home the following day. The AAA was stable in size at 1-year follow-up CTA imaging.

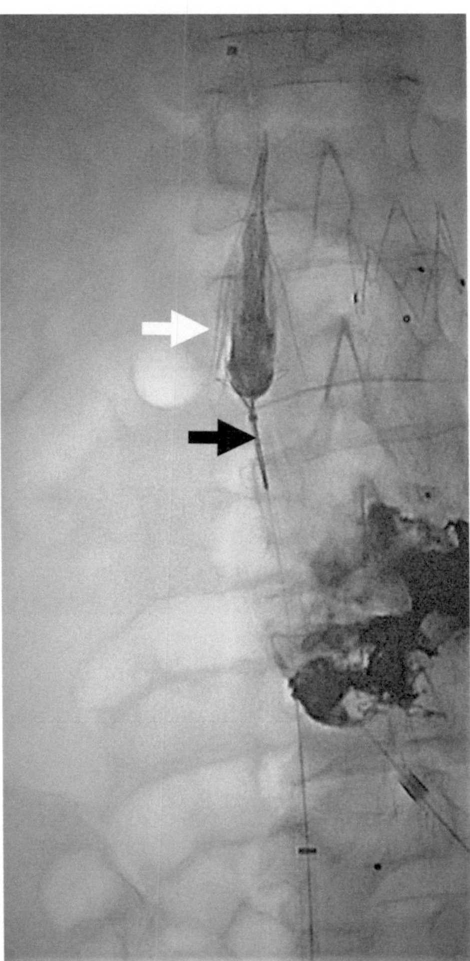

Fig. 4.4 Fluoroscopic image with the newly placed IVC filter (white arrow). A snare has grasped the large embolus within the IVC (black arrow)

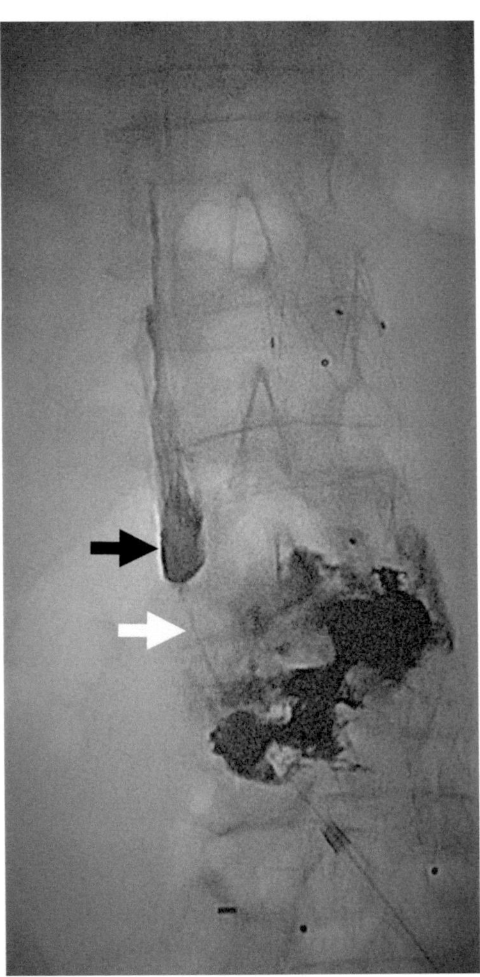

Fig. 4.3 Fluoroscopic image shows the Onyx® embolus within the IVC (black arrow) attached to the adjacent guidewire (white arrow)

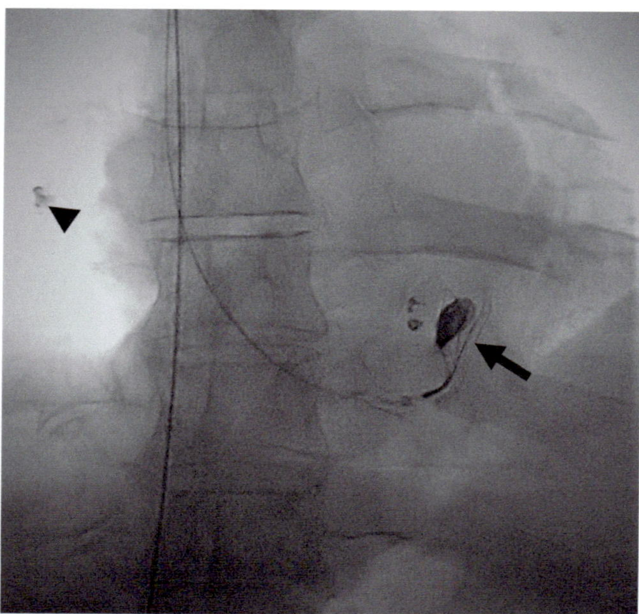

Fig. 4.5 Fluoroscopic image over the lower chest shows a snare being used to grasp a portion of the Onyx®, which had embolized to the right ventricle (arrow). A few tiny pieces of embolic material can be seen in the pulmonary arteries (arrowhead)

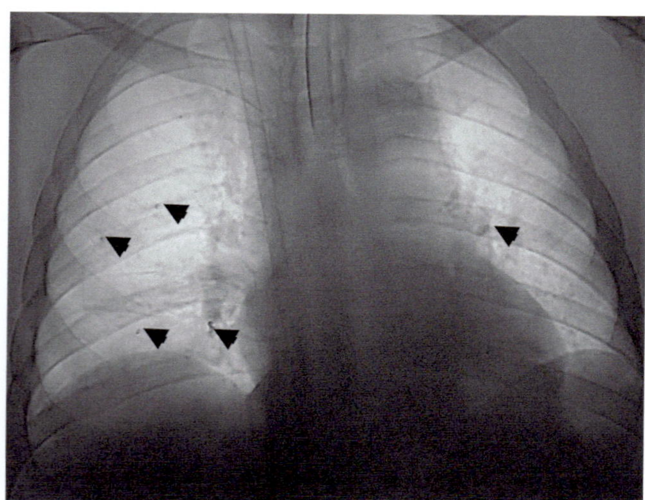

Fig. 4.6 Fluoroscopic image of the chest with tiny fragments of embolic material seen in the pulmonary arteries (arrowheads)

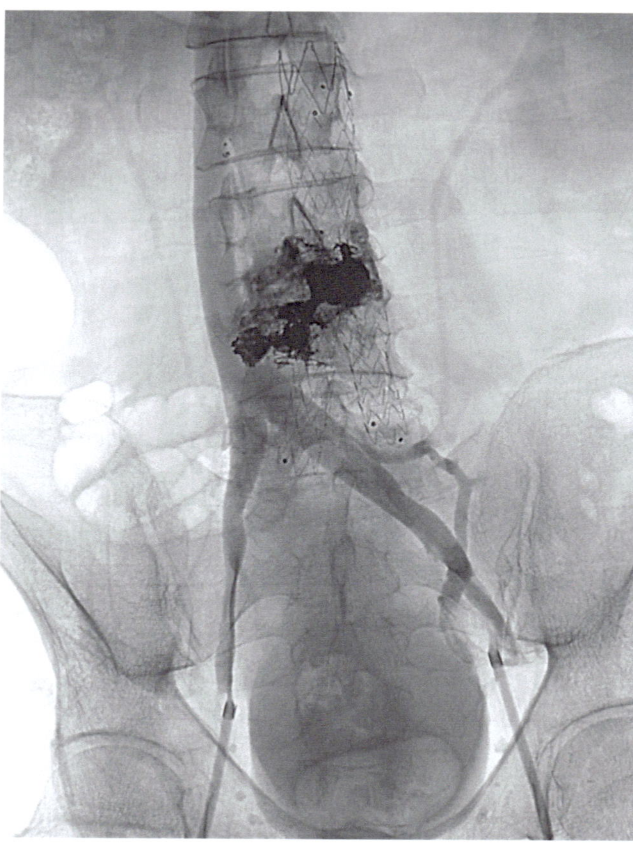

Fig. 4.7 Venogram through the common femoral vein sheaths demonstrates a patent IVC

Failed Endovascular Repair of Mycotic Aortic Arch Aneurysm Using the Atrial Septal Defect Occluder

5

Kiang Hiong Tay [iD], Tze Tec Chong, and Victor Chao

A 56-year-old man with hypertension, ischemic heart disease, and end-stage renal failure presented with a 6.5 cm mycotic aortic arch aneurysm. The aneurysm arose from a 12 mm aortic wall defect between the origins of the left common carotid artery (LCCA) and left subclavian artery (LSA) (Fig. 5.1). The patient was unfit for open surgical repair hence endovascular treatment was adopted. The plan was to close the aortic defect with a 12 mm atrial septal defect occluder (ASDO), inspired by two prior case reports [1, 2]. The ASDO was successfully deployed but it failed to seal the aneurysm (Fig. 5.2a). Thoracic endovascular aortic repair (TEVAR) with deployment of a Cook TX2 36 × 150 mm stent graft distal to the right innominate artery as well as insertion of an LCCA chimney (10 × 38 mm Atrium V12 covered stent) were performed next but failed to exclude the aneurysm due to proximal gutter leak (Fig. 5.2b). Embolization of the proximal LSA with a 12 mm Amplatzer AVP 2 plug was performed but in the process, the ASDO was dislodged and fell into the mycotic aneurysm sac (Fig. 5.3), likely due to breaking down of the friable aortic wall in the setting of an infected aneurysm. The endoleak persisted and the mycotic aneurysm continued to enlarge post op. The patient eventually succumbed on the 24th post op day.

The outcome for this patient may have been different if TEVAR was performed with a right innominate artery chimney, carotid–carotid bypass, deploying the aortic stent graft from the ascending aorta to the descending aorta (normal to normal aorta) and plugging the LSA.

K. H. Tay (✉)
Department of Vascular and Interventional Radiology, Singapore General Hospital, Singapore, Singapore
e-mail: tay.kiang.hiong@singhealth.com.sg

T. T. Chong
Department of Vascular Surgery, Singapore General Hospital, Singapore, Singapore
e-mail: chong.tze.tec@singhealth.com.sg

V. Chao
Department of Cardiothoracic Surgery, National Heart Centre Singapore, Singapore, Singapore
e-mail: victor.chao.t.t@singhealth.com.sg

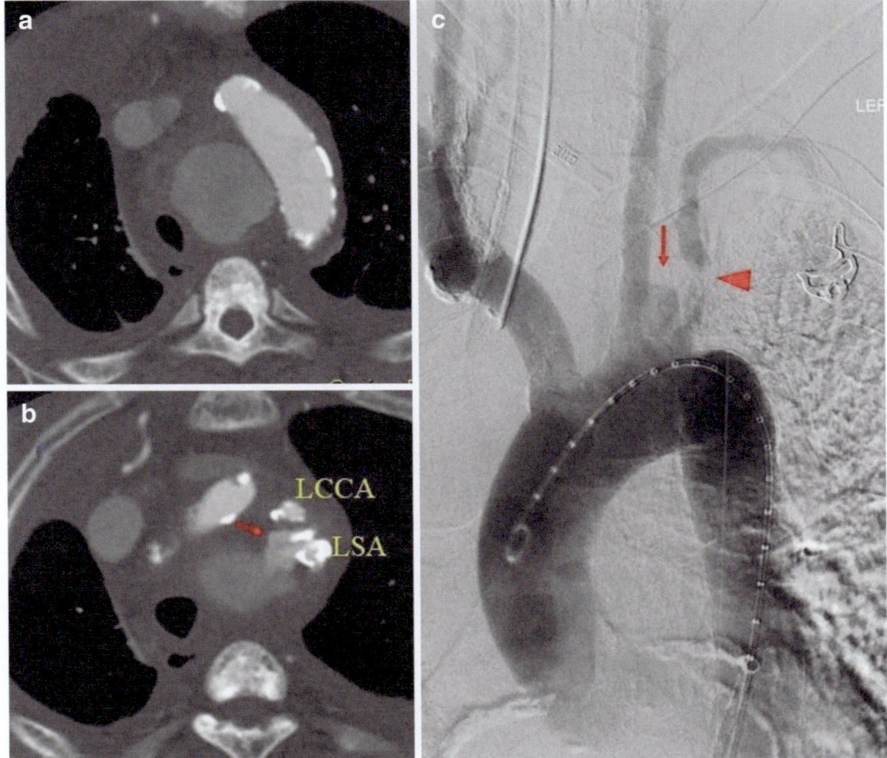

Fig. 5.1 CT angiogram in axial plane (**a**, **b**) showing a mycotic aortic arch aneurysm arising from an aortic wall defect (red arrow) between the origins of the left common carotid artery (LCCA) and left subclavian artery (LSA). Catheter arch aortogram in LAO 40 projection (**c**) confirming the location of the aortic defect between the LCCA and LSA. There was also a severe stenosis in the proximal LSA (arrow head) (**c**)

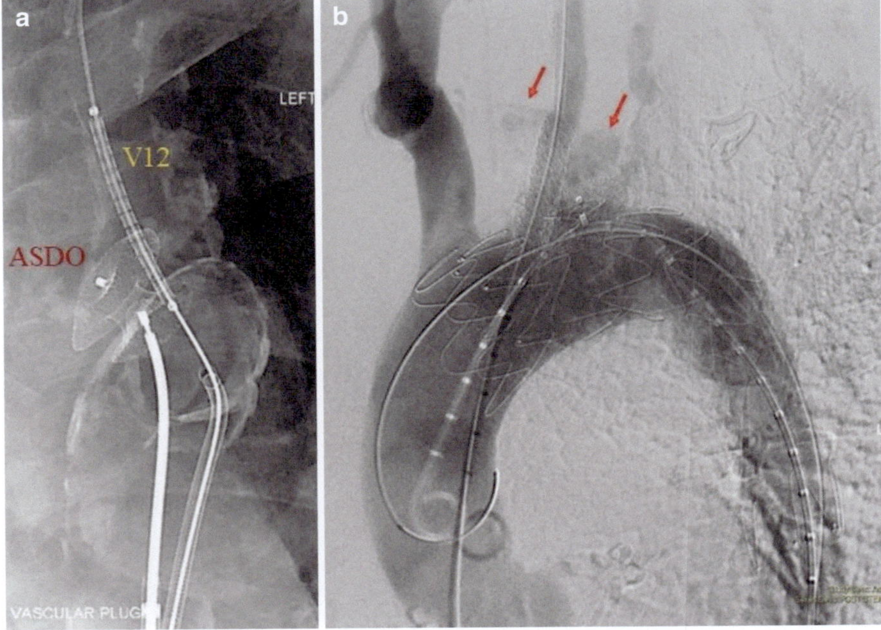

Fig. 5.2 Deployment of atrial septal occluder (ASDO) was performed in RAO 15 projection (**a**). An Advanta V12 covered stent (V12) was prophylactically positioned within the left common carotid artery (LCCA) in case the ASDO obstructs and restricts flow in the LCCA. The densely calcified aortic wall made it easy to deploy the ASDO such that the discs were positioned one on each side of the calcified aortic wall. Unfortunately, the ASDO failed to seal the mycotic aneurysm. Thoracic endovascular aortic repair (TEVAR) with Cook TX2 36 × 150 mm stent graft and LCCA chimney using the 10 × 38 mm V12 covered stent were performed next. Post chimney TEVAR angiogram showed persistent filling of the mycotic aneurysm (arrows), likely from proximal gutter leak (**b**)

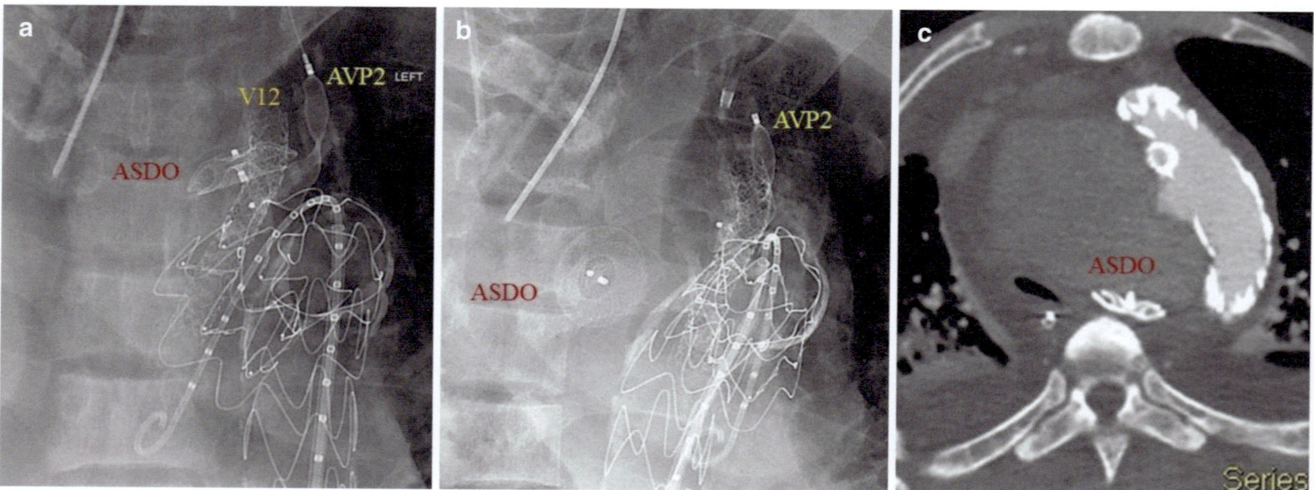

Fig. 5.3 As the aortic defect was near the origin of the left subclavian artery (LSA), embolization of the proximal LSA was performed with a 12 mm Amplatzer AVP 2 plug (AVP2) to prevent retrograde filling of the aneurysm via the LSA. The atrial septal defect occluder (ASDO) was dislodged during deployment of the AVP2 (**a**) and the ASDO migrated into the aneurysm sac (**b**). The left common carotid artery chimney (V12) was in stable position. Post op CT angiogram showed persistent filling and enlargement of the mycotic aneurysm. The dislodged ASDO was seen within the mycotic aneurysm (**c**)

Bibliography

1. Bashir F, Quaife R, Carroll JD. Percutaneous closure of ascending aortic pseudoaneurysm using Amplatzer septal occluder device: the first clinical case report and literature review. Catheter Cardiovasc Interv. 2005;65(4):547–51. https://doi.org/10.1002/ccd.20422.

2. Chang G, Chen W, Yin H, Li Z, Li X, Wang S. Endovascular repair of an aortic arch pseudoaneurysm by an atrial septal defect occluder combined with a chimney stent. J Vasc Surg. 2013;57(6):1657–60. https://doi.org/10.1016/j.jvs.2012.10.095.

Kiang Hiong Tay , Tze Tec Chong, and Victor Chao

A 84-year-old man with hypertension, diabetes mellitus, ischemic heart disease, and previous endovascular repair of abdominal aortic aneurysm presented with an enlarging atherosclerotic aneurysm of the left subclavian artery (LSA) (Fig. 6.1a). The plan was for endovascular repair using the COOK custom made fenestrated aortic arch stent graft with a fenestration for the LSA and scallop for the left common carotid artery (LCCA). During the procedure, there was inadvertent premature unsheathing of the fenestrated arch stent graft resulting in the leading edge of the partially deployed stent graft being stuck in the aneurysmal LSA (Fig. 6.1b, c).

The stent graft delivery catheter could not be advanced forward as a result. Attempts to resheath the exposed stent segment were not successful. The situation was salvaged with introducing a gooseneck snare from the femoral approach and snaring the nose cone of the stent graft delivery catheter from below to disengage the exposed stent from the LSA aneurysm which allowed forward advancement of the delivery catheter to align the fenestration with the LSA origin (Fig. 6.2). Fortunately, the procedure was successfully completed (Fig. 6.3) without causing a stroke despite the extensive manipulation around the vicinity of the arch vessels.

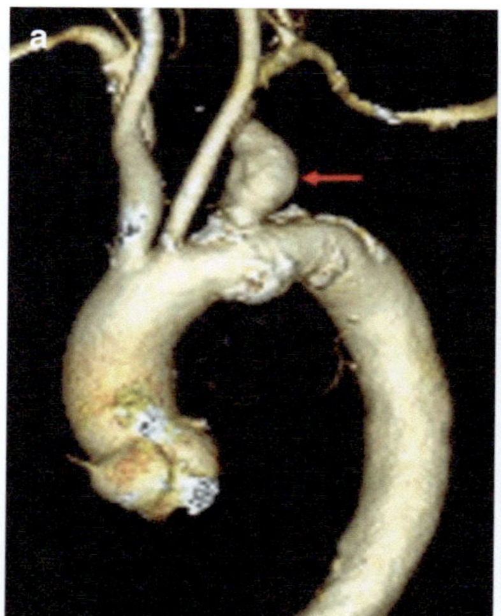
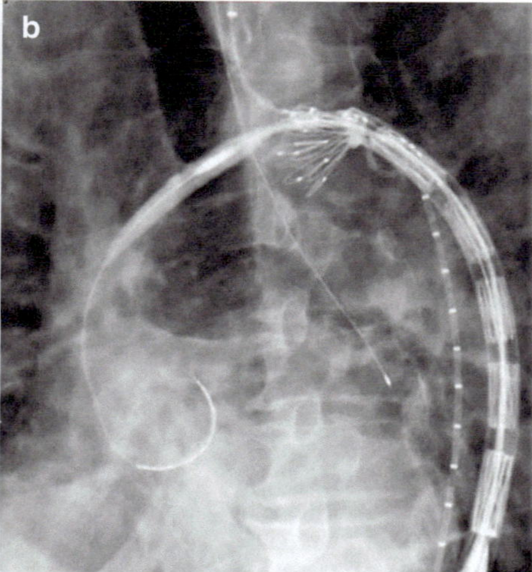
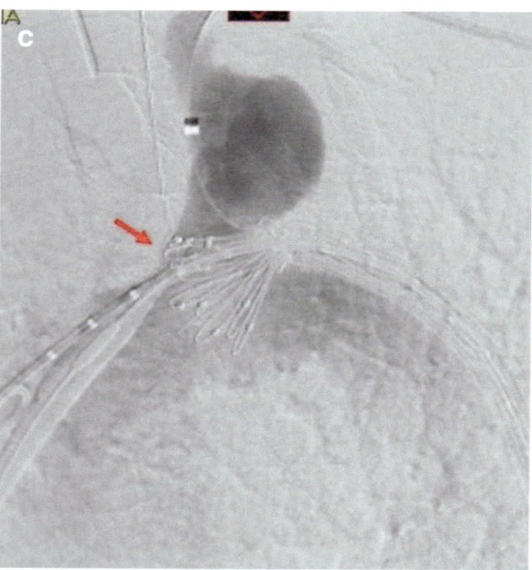

Fig. 6.1 (**a**) 3D CT angiogram using volume rendering technique (VRT) showing the proximal left subclavian artery (LSA) aneurysm (arrow). (**b**) Fluoroscopy image during endovascular repair with COOK custom-made fenestrated aortic arch stent graft showing inadvertent premature unsheathing of the stent graft delivery catheter with partial deployment of the proximal stent. (**c**) Angiogram via the left brachial sheath showing the leading edge of the partially deployed stent stuck in LSA aneurysm (arrow) which prevented forward advancement of the delivery catheter to align the LSA fenestration with the origin of the LSA

K. H. Tay (✉)
Department of Vascular and Interventional Radiology,
Singapore General Hospital, Singapore, Singapore
e-mail: tay.kiang.hiong@singhealth.com.sg

T. T. Chong
Department of Vascular Surgery, Singapore General Hospital,
Singapore, Singapore
e-mail: chong.tze.tec@singhealth.com.sg

V. Chao
Department of Cardiothoracic Surgery, National Heart Centre
Singapore, Singapore, Singapore
e-mail: victor.chao.t.t@singhealth.com.sg

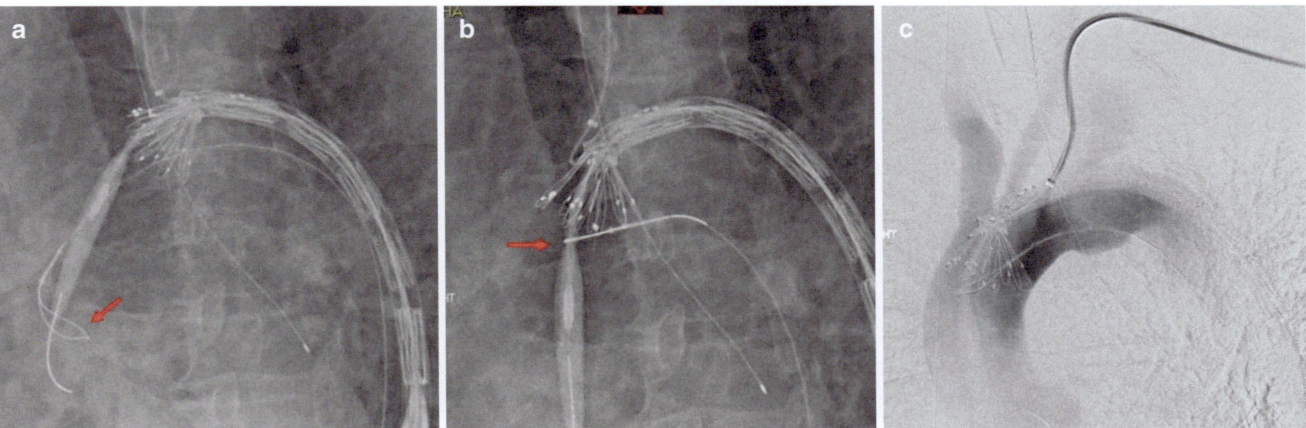

Fig. 6.2 (**a**) A 20 mm goose neck snare was introduced from the femoral approach to loop around the nose cone of the stent graft delivery catheter (arrow). (**b**) The goose neck snare was manipulated to the base of the nose cone just proximal to the partially deployed stent graft (arrow) and downward traction was applied to the snare to deflect the delivery catheter inferiorly so as to disengage the deployed stent out of the LSA aneurysm to allow forward advancement of the delivery catheter to align the aortic stent graft fenestration with the origin of the LSA. (**c**) Angiogram via the left brachial sheath confirmed successful disengagement and advancement of the delivery catheter

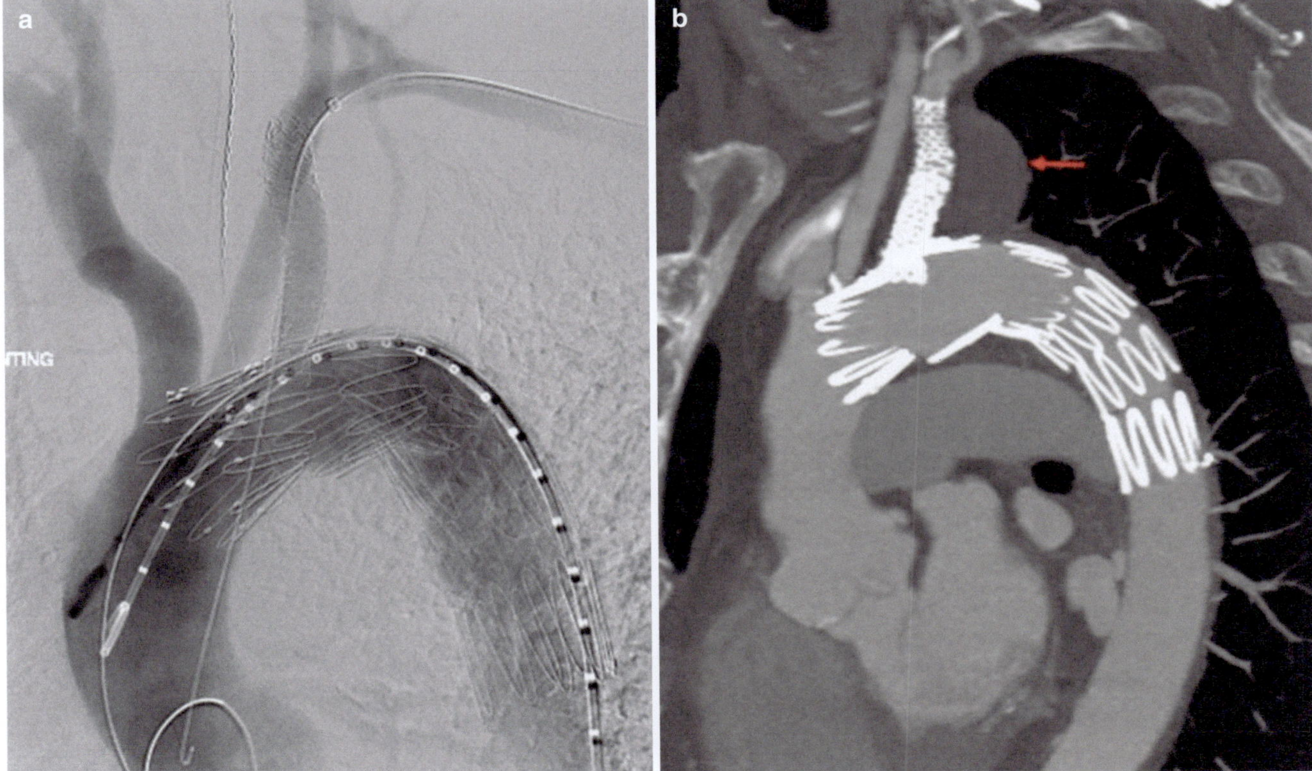

Fig. 6.3 (**a**) The fenestrated stent graft was fully deployed and an 8 × 37 mm Begraft was deployed into the proximal LSA and across the stent graft fenestration. Another 8 × 37 mm Begraft was deployed proximally to fully exclude the LSA aneurysm. Completion aortogram showed good results. (**b**) The 6-month post op CT angiogram in sagittal oblique plane showed that the LSA aneurysm (arrow) had thrombosed and reduced in size with no evidence of endoleak

"Mind the Gap": Bridging the Branched Graft Disconnect

Adnan Hadziomerovic

A 76-year-old man underwent endovascular treatment of a thoracoabdominal aortic aneurysm using a custom aortic 4-branch endograft (Cook Medical, Bloomington, Indiana). The "cuffs" were extended into their corresponding branches using overlapping self-expandable stent grafts (Fluency, Bard, Tempe, Arizona). He presented 5 years later with symptoms of mesenteric ischemia, including a 10-kg weight loss. CTA (Fig. 7.1) showed a disconnection at the SMA branch with an over-riding stent and type 3 endoleak into the aneurysm sac.

Using a left brachial access, a 7 Fr 70-cm long sheath (Ansel 1, Cook) was advanced into the aortic stent graft. 5 Fr 100-cm long angled KMP and RIM catheters (Cook) and an angled 0.035-inch hydrophilic wire were used to exit through the SMA branch, create a loop in the sac and enter into the floating Fluency stent graft (Fig. 7.2). A 12-mm × 4-cm balloon (Mustang, Boston Scientific, Marlborough, Massachusetts) matching the diameter of the Fluency stent was advanced and inflated in the stent, anchoring the system. The balloon/wire were pulled back to straighten the loop (Fig. 7.3). Balloon dilatation at the junction allowed for wire exchange to a 260-cm 0.035-inch Amplatz Super Stiff wire (Boston Scientific) and advancement of the sheath into the Fluency stent graft while the balloon was being deflated. The gap was bridged using a 9-mm × 59-mm balloon-expandable stent graft (Advanta V12, Atrium Medical Corporation, Hudson, New Hampshire) distally dilated to 12 mm. Final angiogram (Fig. 7.4) confirmed patency of the SMA with no further flow into the aneurysm sac. At 33-month follow-up patient remained asymptomatic with CTA (Fig. 7.5) showing a patent SMA and no endoleak.

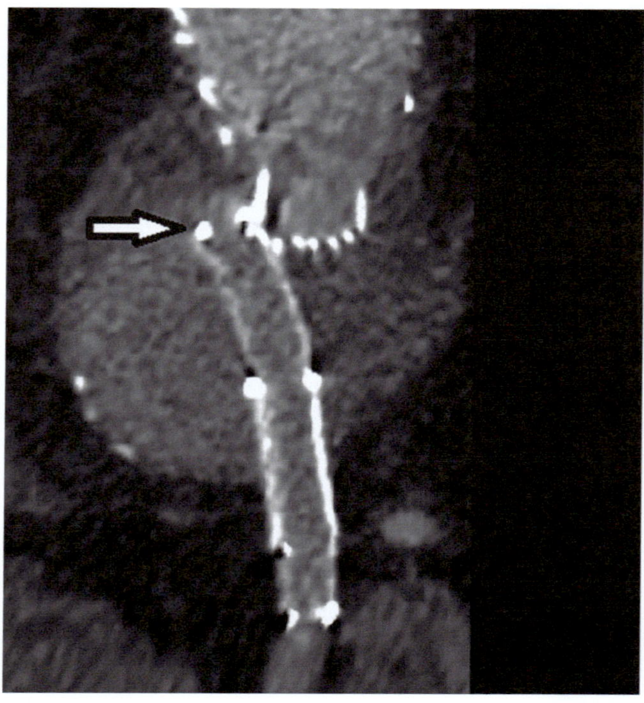

Fig. 7.1 Reconstructed CTA demonstrating disconnected stent graft (arrow) and large type 3 endoleak into the aneurysm sac

A. Hadziomerovic (✉)
Department of Medical Imaging, The Ottawa Hospital-University of Ottawa, Ottawa, ON, Canada
e-mail: ahadziomerovic@toh.ca

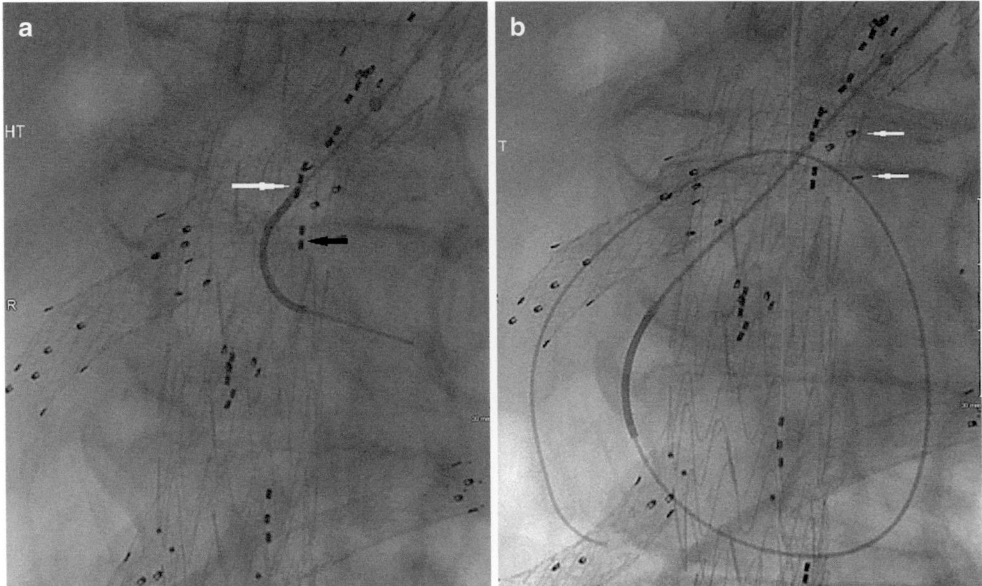

Fig. 7.2 (**a**) Diagnostic catheter was advanced through the branch identified by three proximal (white arrow) and two distal (black arrow) markers. (**b**) Wire loop created in the aneurysm sac facilitated catheterization though the proximal ostium of the Fluency stent (white arrows) into the SMA

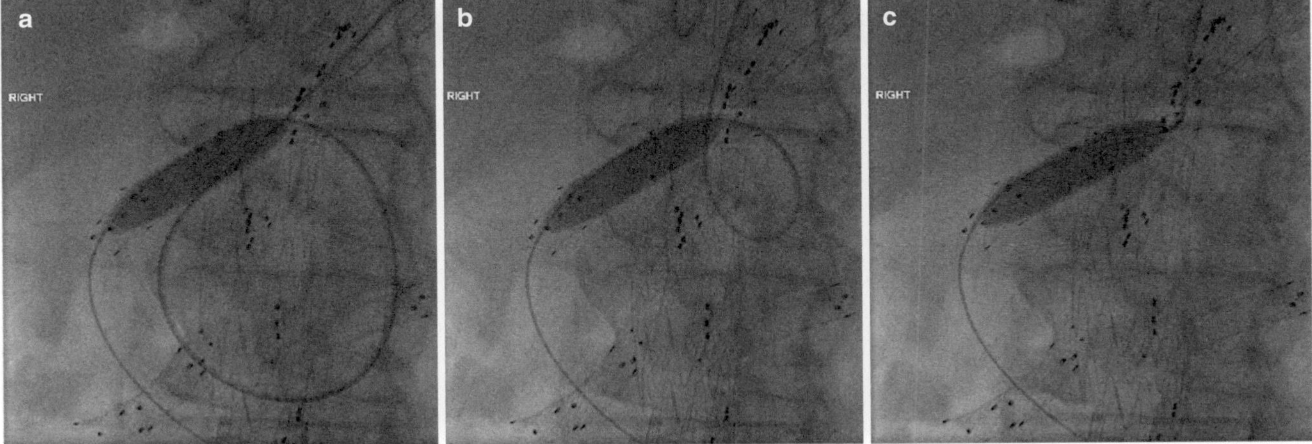

Fig. 7.3 A 12-mm balloon was inflated in the Fluency stent graft (**a**) allowing for straightening of the loop (**b**, **c**)

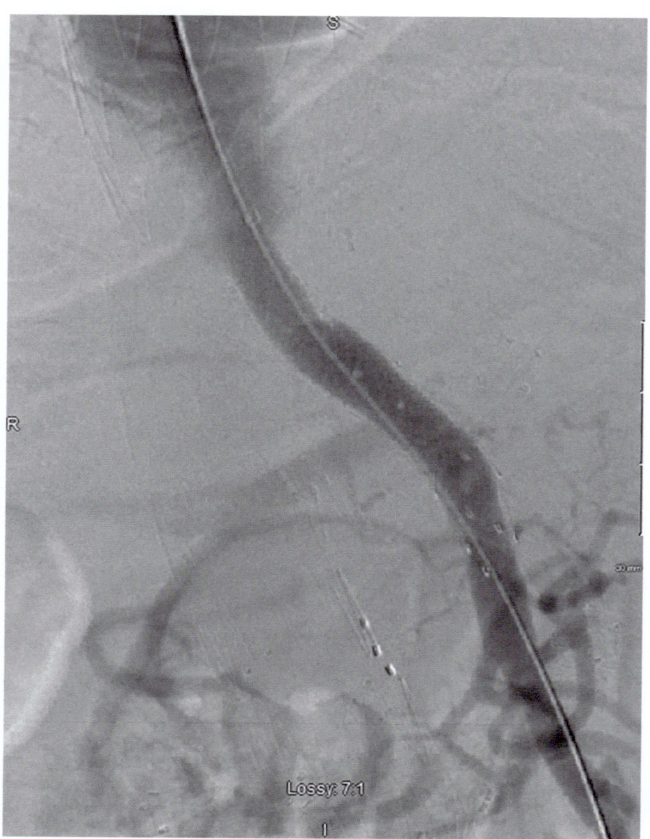

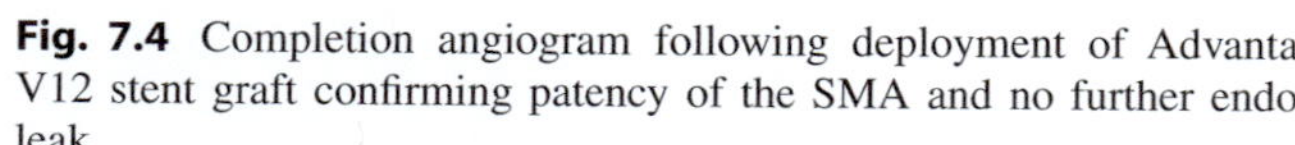

Fig. 7.4 Completion angiogram following deployment of Advanta V12 stent graft confirming patency of the SMA and no further endo leak

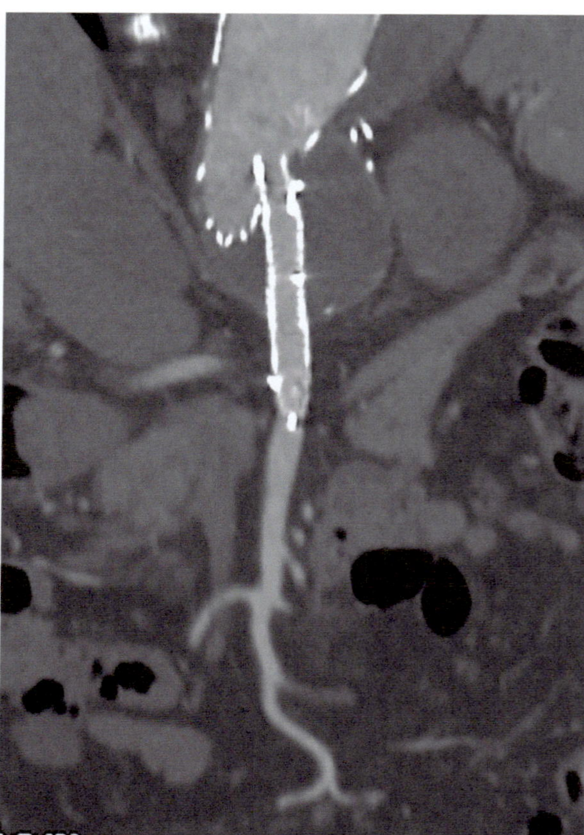

Fig. 7.5 Reconstructed CTA at 33 months shows in line flow into the SMA

Percutaneous Iliac Artery Type II Endoleak Embolization Complicated by Active Extravasation

Howard M. Richard III

A 79-year-old male underwent endograft treatment of a 6.2 cm × 6.9 cm diameter right iliac artery aneurysm. Thereafter, an endoleak was treated with an Amplatzer plug. Following a decrease in size, the aneurysm grew to 8 × 7.1 cm diameter.

Using a combined CT and fluoroscopy suite, a 4 French 11 cm sheath and a 4 French angled catheter were placed directly into the aneurysm sac through a transabdominal approach (Fig. 8.1) [1]. Angiography was performed to define any outflow. During catheter manipulation, the 4 French sheath inadvertently backed out of the aneurysm leaving the 4 French Kumpe catheter alone within the aneurysm sac. Angiography demonstrated an increasing amount of contrast overlying the pelvis (Fig. 8.2) and active extravasation was confirmed by immediate repeat pelvic CT. This confirmed a large amount intra-pelvic extravasation (Fig. 8.3). The patient became hemodynamically unstable and was resuscitated with normal saline boluses and emergency blood transfusion.

In parallel to the resuscitation, the 4 French sheath was exchanged for a 5 French 25 cm sheath, advanced into the aneurysm sac. The aneurysm sac was rapidly embolized with 130 Nester coils (Cook Medical, Inc) and 5000 units of thrombin. The thrombin-soaked Nester coils were injected into the aneurysm with a 1 mL syringe at a rate greater than four coils per minute. The patient's hemodynamic status improved. Distal aortic and pelvic angiography confirmed that the extravasation had ceased; both the catheter and sheath were removed. He was admitted for observation. He received a total of two units of blood. Daily pelvic ultrasound demonstrated aneurysm stability and he was discharged on the third post-embolization day. One-month follow-up ultrasound demonstrated a 9 cm aneurysm without Doppler flow. At 1-year follow-up, the endoleak recurred. A CT scan scout image demonstrated the right iliac artery aneurysm sac and coils (Fig. 8.4). A third embolization procedure, of the anterior and posterior internal iliac artery outflow, was successful. Eight-year follow-up confirmed durable control of the 4.1 cm aneurysm.

When performing direct sac embolization, it is imperative to maintain constant control to prevent inadvertent retraction of the "base" entry catheter. This phenomenon may be a greater risk when working under pure CT guidance or in a non-orthogonal, i.e., down the gun-barrel fluoroscopic view.

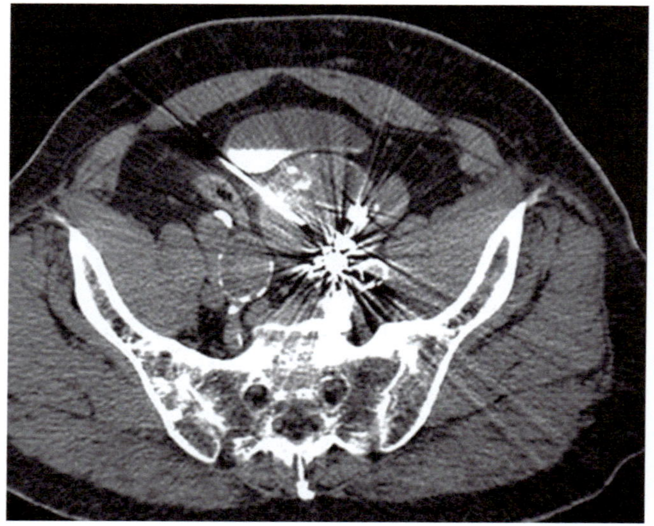

Fig. 8.1 CT guided transabdominal aneurysm sac puncture

H. M. Richard III (✉)
Division of Interventional Radiology, Department of Diagnostic Imaging, University of Maryland School, Baltimore, MD, USA
e-mail: HRICHARD@umm.edu

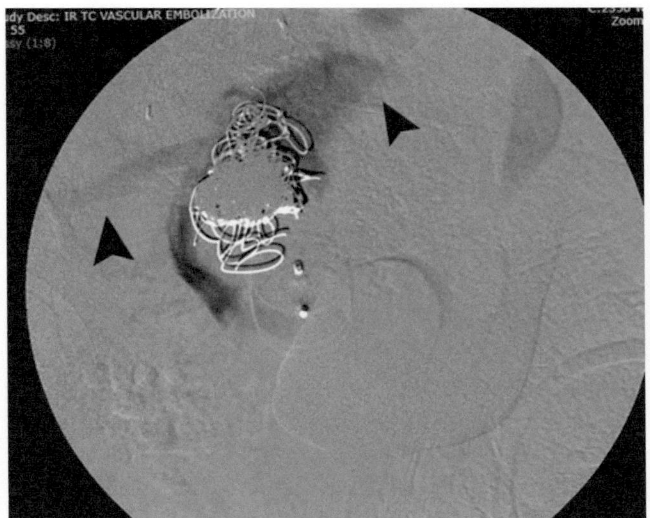

Fig. 8.2 Digital subtracted angiography demonstrates contrast medial and lateral to the aneurysm (arrowheads). Coils and Amplatzer plug were placed at the time of prior interventions

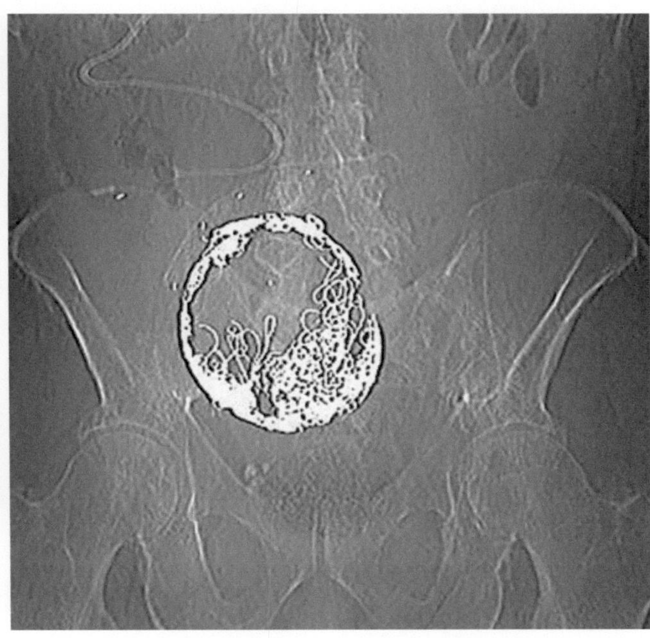

Fig. 8.4 Follow up CT scout image demonstrates coils within the aneurysm sac

Bibliography

1. Zener R, Oreopoulos G, Beecroft R, Rajan DK, Jaskolka J, Tan KT. Transabdominal direct sac puncture embolization of type II endoleaks after endovascular abdominal aortic aneurysm repair. J Vasc Interv Radiol. 2018;29(8):1167–73.

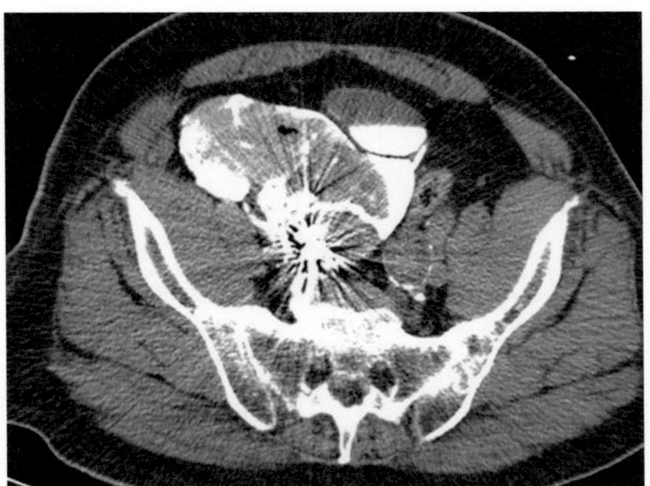

Fig. 8.3 CT scan demonstrates active contrast extravasation and hematoma in the pelvis

"One Way In": Percutaneous Transarterial Embolization of a Persistent Iliac Aneurysm

Brian Funaki

A 67-year-old man who had undergone endovascular aortic stent graft repair for bilateral common iliac and left internal iliac aneurysms had continued perfusion of the left internal iliac aneurysm; it enlarged further by 1.2 cm over the course of 9 months (Fig. 9.1). The left internal iliac aneurysm had been partly embolized with coils, then covered with the left limb of the stent graft at the time of initial repair, precluding subsequent arterial access (Fig. 9.2).

Using CT guidance, the aneurysm sac was punctured with a 21-gauge needle directed into the perfused cavity (Fig. 9.3a). Upon obtaining blood return, 20 microcoils (Nestors, Cook, Bloomington, IN) were deployed through the puncture needle into the aneurysm (Fig. 9.3b). Despite this, continued back-bleeding through the needle occurred (Fig. 9.4). The patient was moved to the IR suite and the needle exchanged for a 5 F dilator. An angiogram showed multiple feeding arteries and a larger than expected residual cavity (Fig. 9.5). Multiple feeding branches were then catheterized using a microcatheter advanced co-axially through 5 F dilator and embolized with microcoils (Nestors, Cook) until hemostasis was achieved (Fig. 9.6). At 2 years follow-up, CT showed no further perfusion and no further growth of the aneurysm (Fig. 9.7).

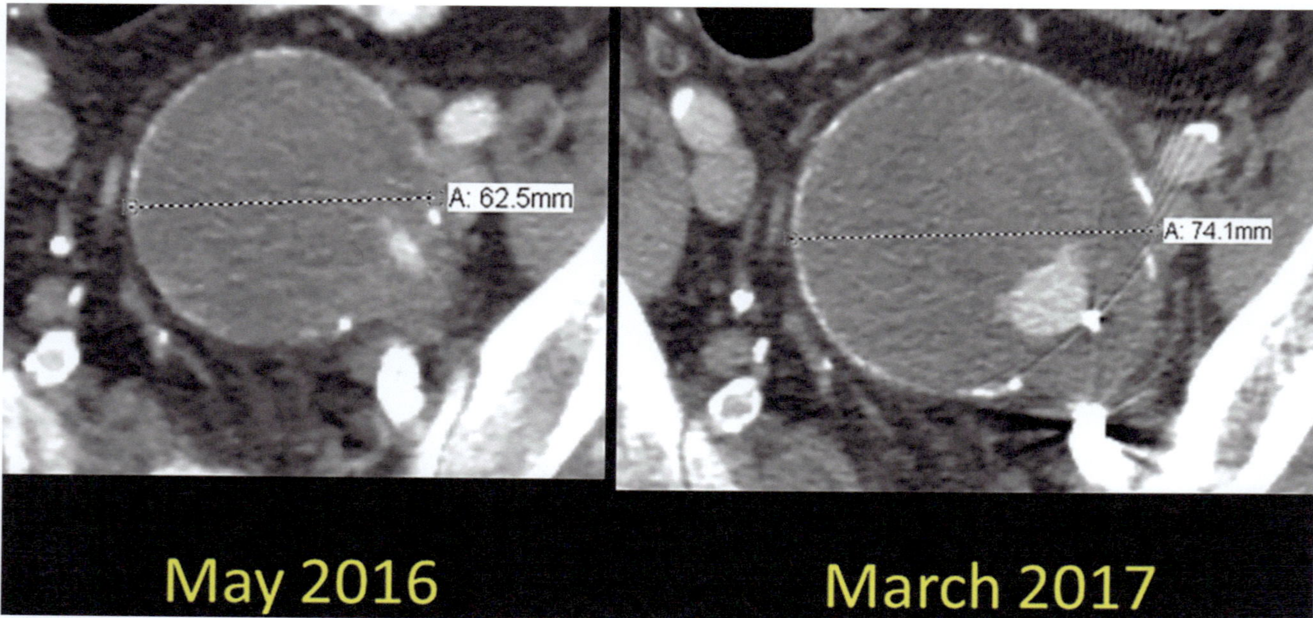

Fig. 9.1 CT images showing enlargement of left internal iliac artery aneurysm

B. Funaki (✉)
Department of Radiology, University of Chicago,
Chicago, IL, USA
e-mail: bfunaki@bsd.uchicago.edu

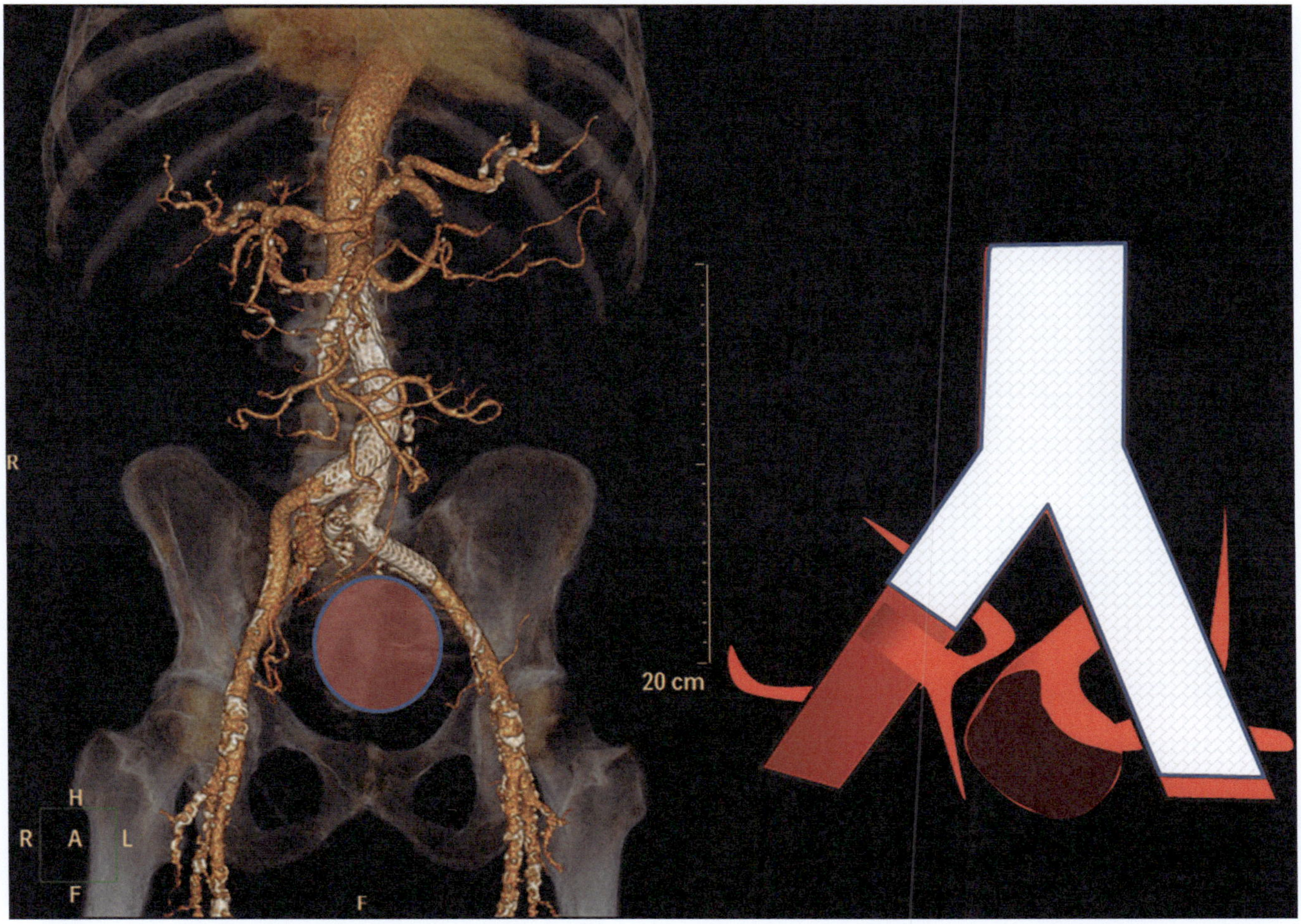

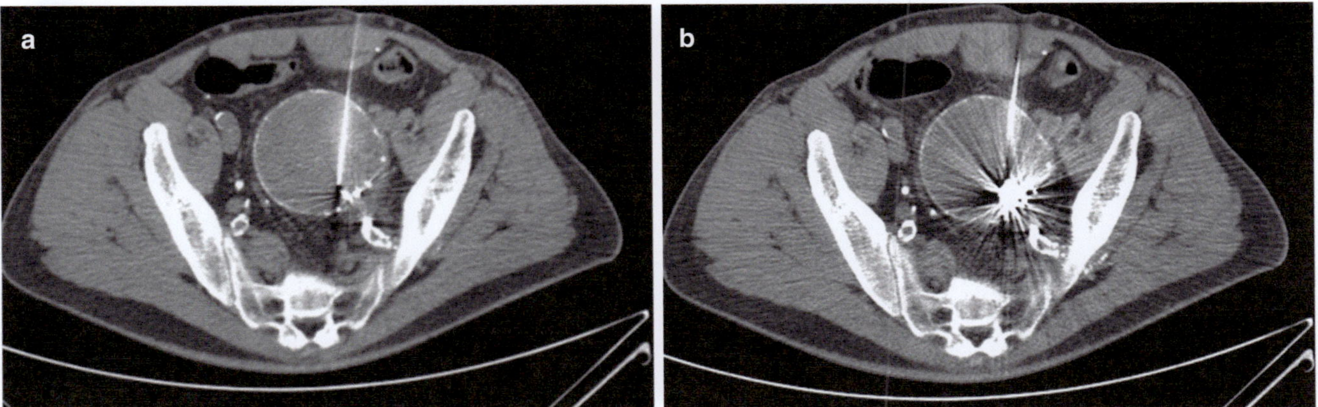

Fig. 9.2 CT reconstruction and illustration of left internal iliac artery aneurysm

Fig. 9.3 (**a**) Axial CT image shows needle puncture of left hypogastric artery aneurysm. (**b**) Axial CT image demonstrates multiple deployed coils in perfused portion of aneurysm

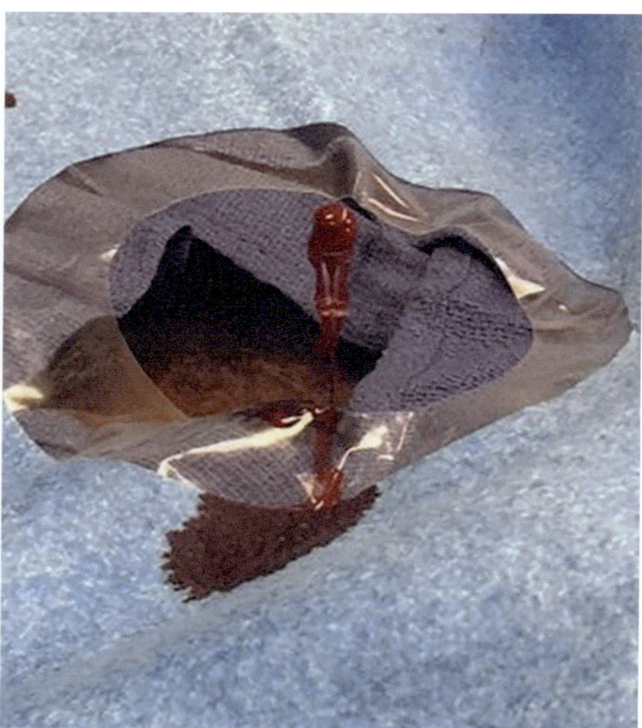

Fig. 9.4 Photograph shows continued backbleeding through needle

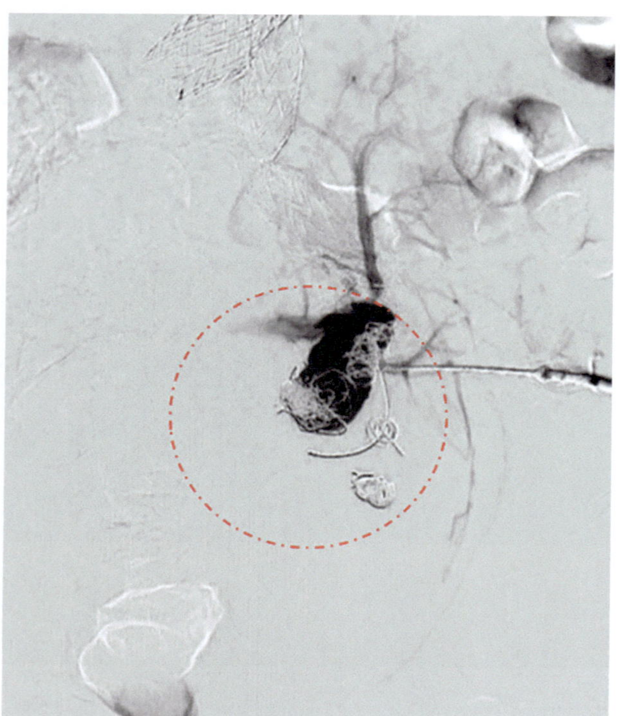

Fig. 9.5 Angiogram obtained via the puncture needle shows multiple feeding arteries (red dotted line shows overall size of aneurysm sac)

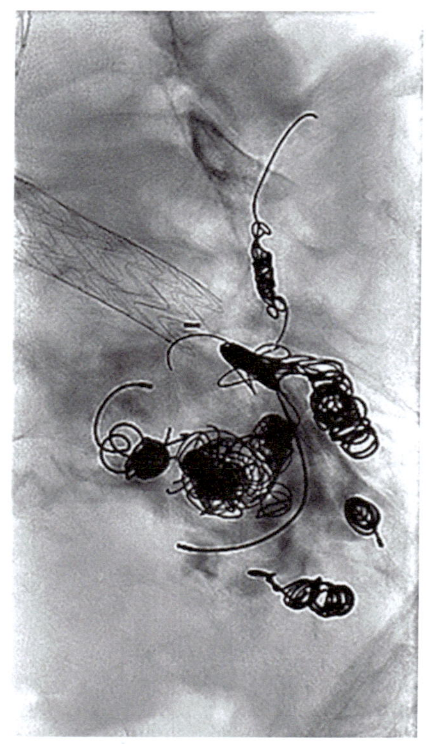

Fig. 9.6 Final fluoroscopic image showing coil embolization of perfused cavity and multiple feeding arteries

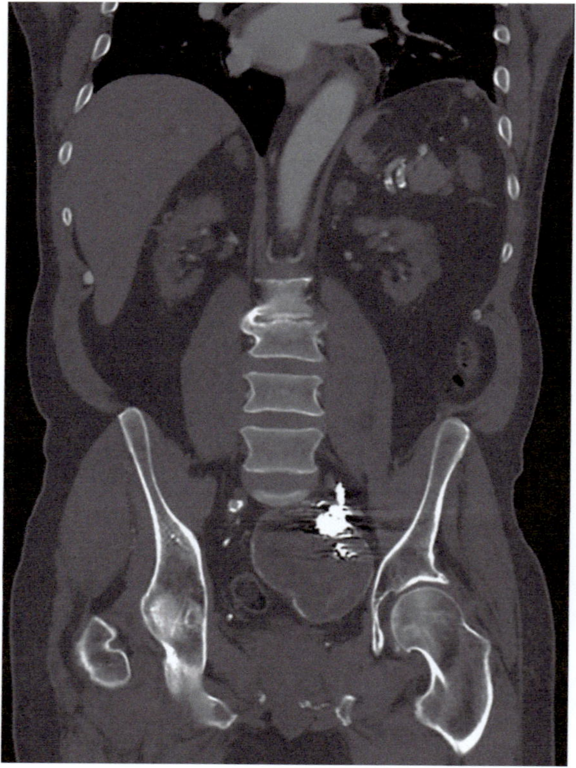

Fig. 9.7 Coronal reformatted CT showing embolized nidus with no residual perfusion of aneurysm

Percutaneous Ilio-Femoral Arterial Bypass

Bulent Arslan

A 42-year-old male presented with toe pain, and purulent toe wound and claudication. He had undergone multiple surgeries after a pelvic gunshot wound 15 years earlier.

Computed tomography (CT) and catheter angiography showed a failed fem-fem bypass graft, occlusion of left common and external iliac arteries, and reconstitution of the left common femoral artery (Fig. 10.1a, b).

Using a right proximal SFA approach, an 8.5 Fr Aptus steerable sheath (Medtronic) was advanced into occluded left common iliac artery (Fig. 10.1c); the left common femoral artery was inaccessible due to extensive surgical scarring. The back-end of an HydroST 0.014 wire (Cook) and a Quickcross catheter (Merit Medical) were used to reach the external iliac artery (EIA) level (Fig. 10.1d). The back-end of a −0.035″ Glidewire (Boston Scientific) was advanced from the contralateral approach to reach the same level (Fig. 10.2a).

Cone beam CT showed the ureter to lie between the two wires, thus the contralateral sheath was advanced further to the mid left EIA. At that level, a 30 mm Ensnare (Merit) deployed. A second steerable sheath was advanced from left SFA approach and through this sheath, a transseptal needle (Cook) was advanced into the snare after confirming its position by orthogonal fluoroscopy (Fig. 10.2b, c) and cone beam CT. Through the transseptal needle a 0.014″ HydroST guidewire was grasped and externalized (Fig. 10.2e). Two 8 × 15 and 8 × 10 Viabahn stent grafts (W.L Gore) were deployed and dilated (Fig. 10.3a–c). Suture mediated closure of the SFA was performed. Patient was placed on Clopidogrel 75 mg and Aspirin 81 mg for 1 month, followed by Aspirin indefinitely.

At 1 month, CTA demonstrated a patent iliofemoral system (Fig. 10.3d, e). The patient maintained his newly palpable distal pulses and wound showed interim healing.

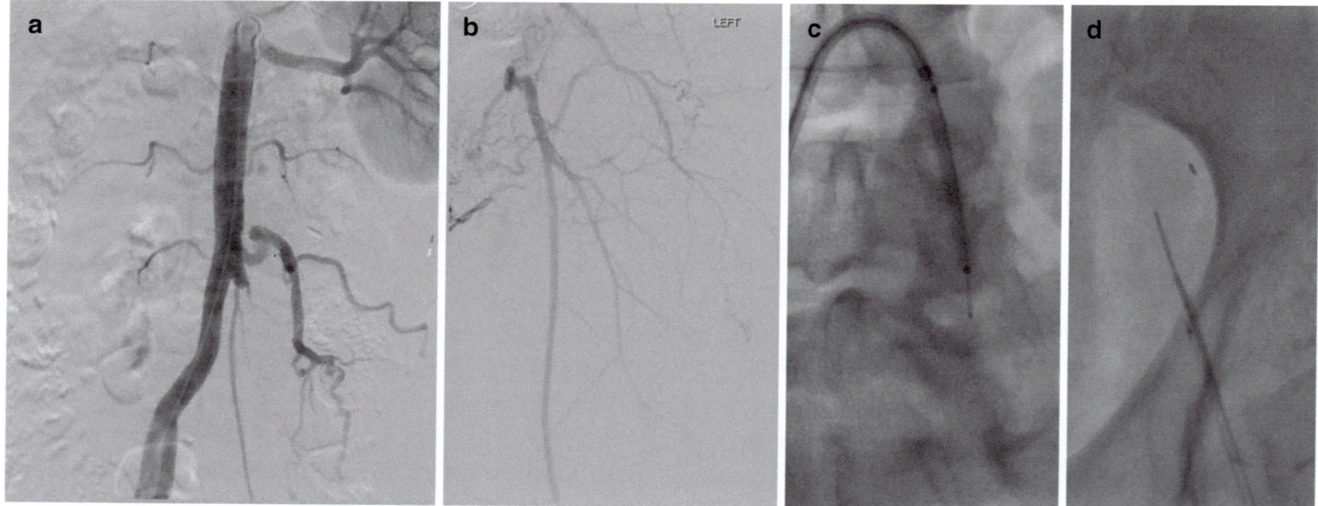

Fig. 10.1 (**a**) Aortogram demonstrates the occluded left common iliac artery with a short stump. (**b**) Reconstitution at the proximal left common femoral artery through collaterals. (**c**) Advancement of the contralateral balloon-assisted steerable sheath with sharp recanalization using back-end of a 0.035″ hydrophilic wire. (**d**) Sharp recanalization using back-end of a 0.014″ guidewire through the triaxial system

B. Arslan (✉)
Vascular and Interventional Service Line, Rush University Medical Center, Chicago, IL, USA
e-mail: BULENT_ARSLAN@rush.edu

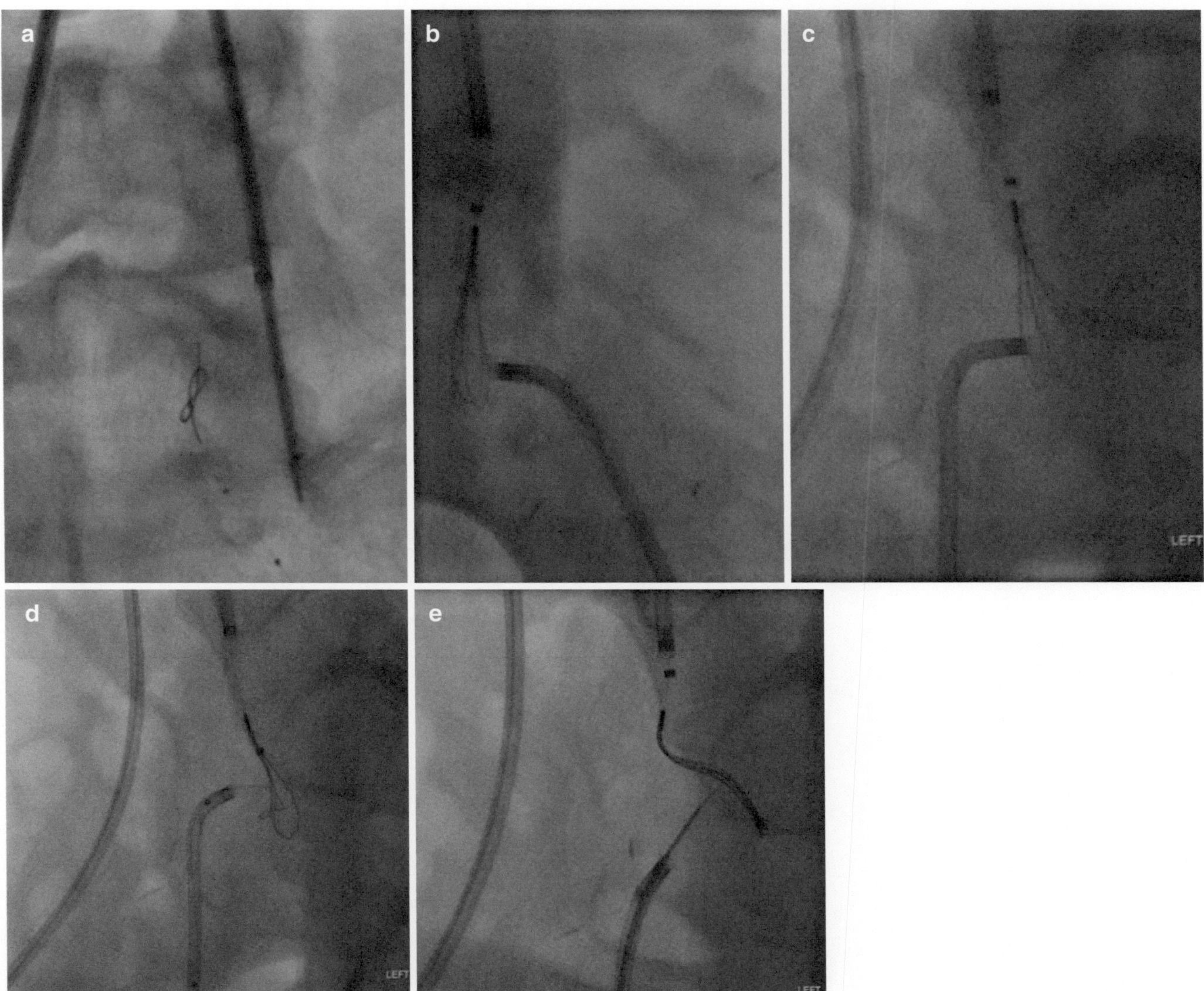

Fig. 10.2 (**a**) The contralateral steerable sheath and triaxial retrograde access are at the same level but actually distant from each other. (**b**, **c**) The retrograde steerable sheath faces towards the up-and-over Ensnare, seen in different obliquities (**d**) Failed attempt to use the back-end of a 0.014″ wire to connect into snare (**e**) Successful attempt to advance through the snare with a transseptal needle

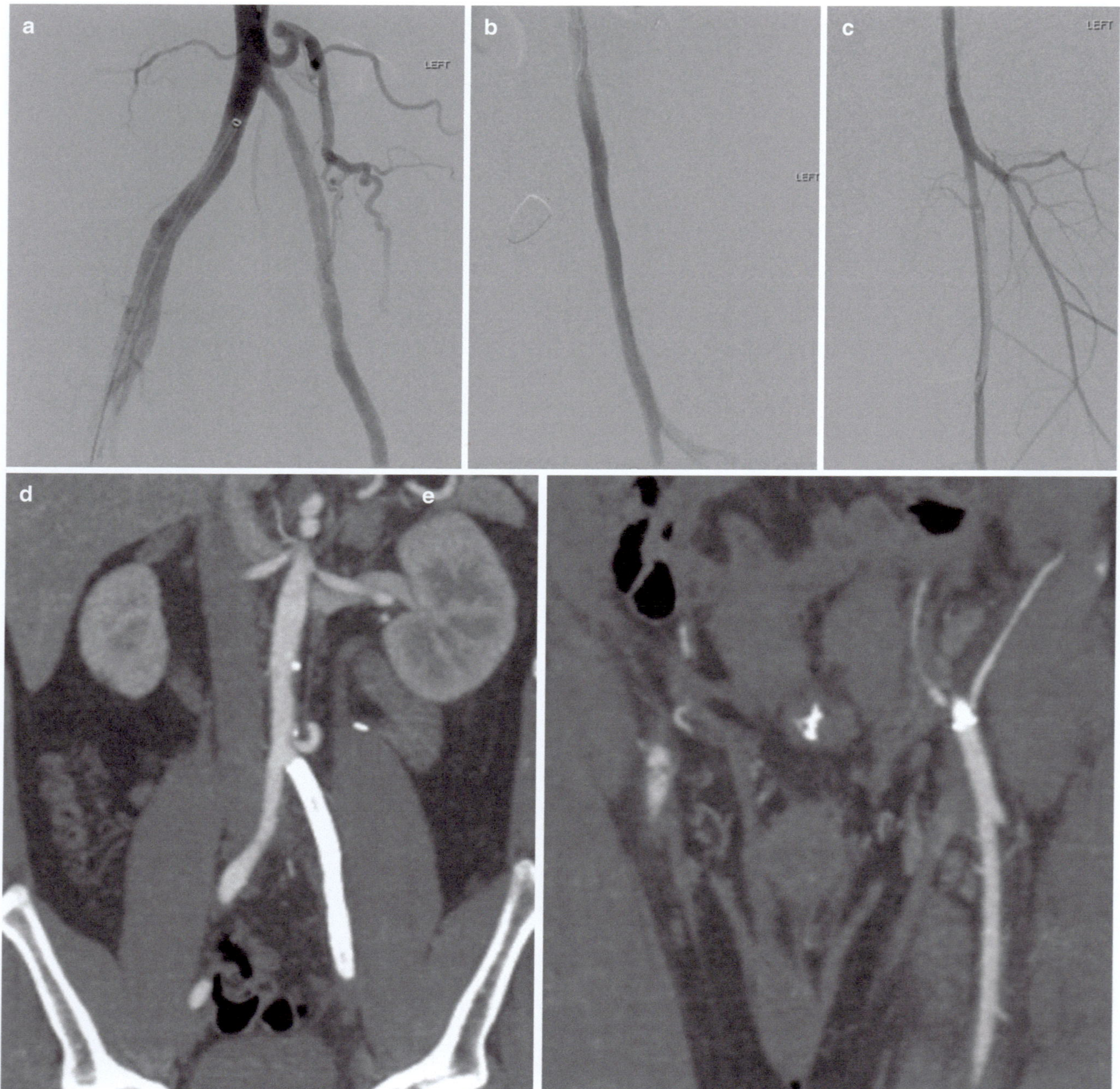

Fig. 10.3 Digital subtraction angiography after placement of the 8 mm Viabahn stent grafts spanning the left common iliac artery stump to proximal left common femoral artery (**a**–**c**); Follow-up CTA in 1 month demonstrates patency (**d**, **e**)

Branched Arterial Reconstruction and Recanalization of Occluded Right Lower Extremity Stents and Giant Femoral Anastomotic Pseudo Aneurysm in an Aortobifemoral Graft Patient

Murat Osman and Bulent Arslan

A 74-year-old male with a history of hypertension, surgical bypass for coronary artery disease and remote aorto-bifemoral bypass presented with lifestyle limiting right > left claudication and enlarging 1-year-old right common femoral artery (CFA) 8 × 8 × 11 cm anastomotic pseudoaneurysm. His bilateral superficial femoral artery (SFA) stents were occluded. The plan was to recanalize the occluded right fem-oropopliteal segments and connect the deep femoral artery (DFA) and SFA to an iliac branch endoprosthesis (IBE) (W.L. Gore and Associates, Flagstaff, AZ); which would be deployed into the right limb of the aorto-bifemoral graft.

Pre-procedural computed tomographic angiography (CTA) (Fig. 11.1) and catheter angiography demonstrated the known right CFA pseudoaneurysm at the aorto-bifem

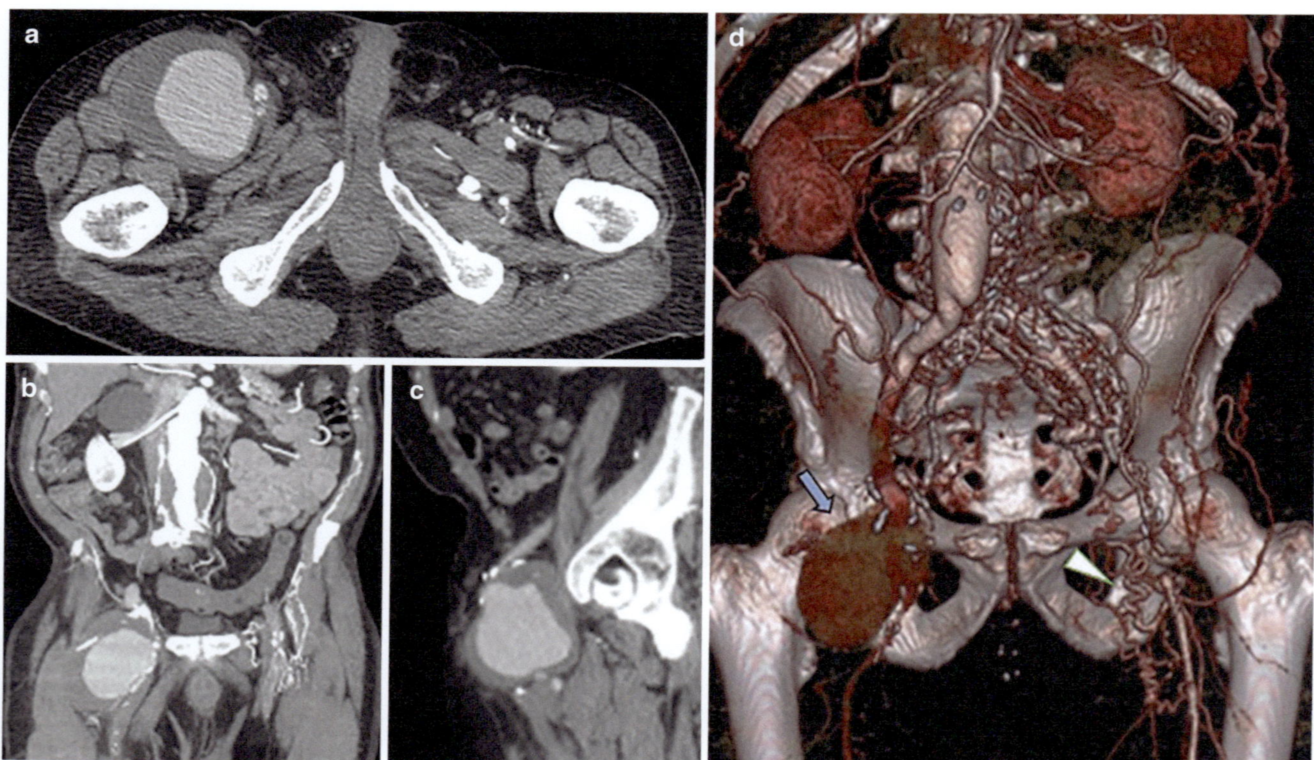

Fig. 11.1 Pre-procedure axial (**a**), coronal (**b**), sagittal (**c**), and 3D reconstruction (**d**) CTA of the abdomen and pelvis demonstrate a wide-neck 8 × 8 × 11 cm right CFA pseudoaneurysm (arrow) at the distal site of the existing aortobifemoral bypass graft. Note the long segment occlusion of the left external and common iliac arteries, with collateral reconstitution of the SFA (arrowhead)

M. Osman · B. Arslan (✉)
Vascular and Interventional Service Line, Rush University Medical Center, Chicago, IL, USA
e-mail: BULENT_ARSLAN@rush.edu

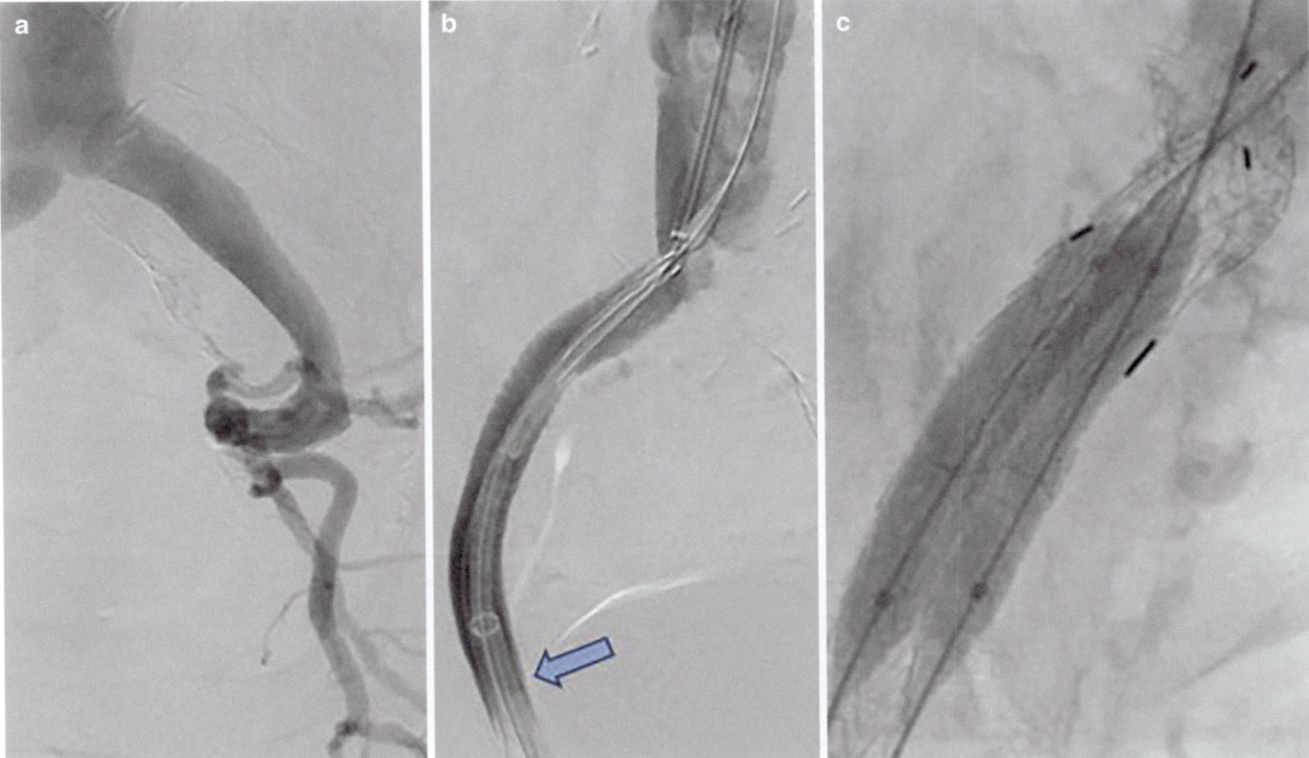

Fig. 11.2 Sequential fluoroscopic images demonstrate exclusion of the right CFA pseudoaneurysm. (**a**) Aortography shows the known occlusion of the left iliac graft component. Multiple attempts to recanalize the occluded left limb of the aortobifemoral graft and native left EIA were unsuccessful. Panels (**b**, pre) and (**c**, post) show deployment of the 23 × 10 × 10 mm IBE through the 16Fr Gore DrySeal Flex sheath (blue arrow), which was apposed to the pre-existing surgical graft with kissing balloon angioplasty

anastomosis and occlusion of the right SFA, left limb of the graft (Fig. 11.2a), external iliac artery (EIA), common iliac artery (CIA), and femoropopliteal segments. The anterior tibial (AT) artery provided the single distal right runoff.

Eight French left axillary and 16 Fr right retrograde groin-level graft access were obtained. The IBE was deployed aortobifemoral graft limb (Fig. 11.2b, c). A pedal approach (through Dorsalis Pedis) was used to recanalize the occluded femoropopliteal segment. The existing occluded SFA stent was traversed through a subintimal plane and an exchange length 0.035″ hydrophilic guidewire (Glidewire, Terumo, Japan) was advanced to the pseudoaneurysm (Fig. 11.3a, b).

An Ensnare (Merit Medical, Utah) was used to grasp the wire (Fig. 11.3d) and draw it into the IBE limb, through the axillary access. The IBE device limbs were extended into the recanalized SFA and to the DFA with Viabahn stent-grafts (Fig. 11.4). VBX balloon expandable stent-grafts (W.L. Gore) were used to securely bridge the Viabahns and each limb of the IBE. At the end of the procedura, the 16 French graft access was simply removed as there was no flow outside the new stent grafts. Follow-up CTA at 2 months demonstrated patent flow through newly constructed system, no flow to the pseudoaneurysm, and patent continuous inflow to his right foot (Fig. 11.5).

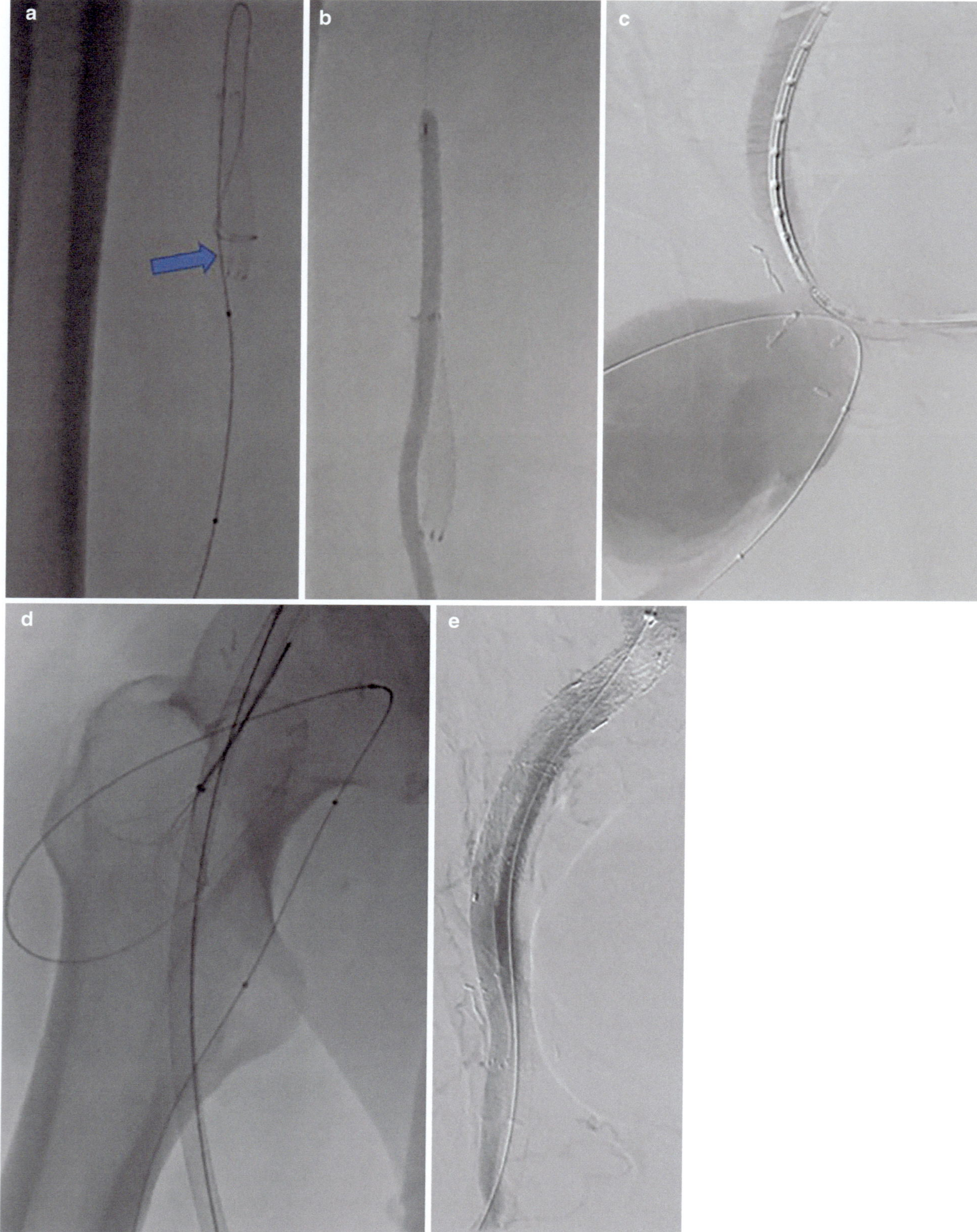

Fig. 11.3 Retrograde access and SAFARI prior to exclusion of R CFA aneurysm. (**a**, **b**) The pre-existing occluded right SFA stent was traversed through a subintimal approach. (**c**) Retrograde catheterization of the distal graft through the right anterior tibial artery demonstrates the wide-neck right CFA pseudoaneurysm. (**d**) A snare was used to obtain through and through access and the DFA and SFA were stented across the pseudoaneurysm. (**e**) Post-stent angiography demonstrates the patent IBE-stent construct with no residual filling of the pseudoaneurysm

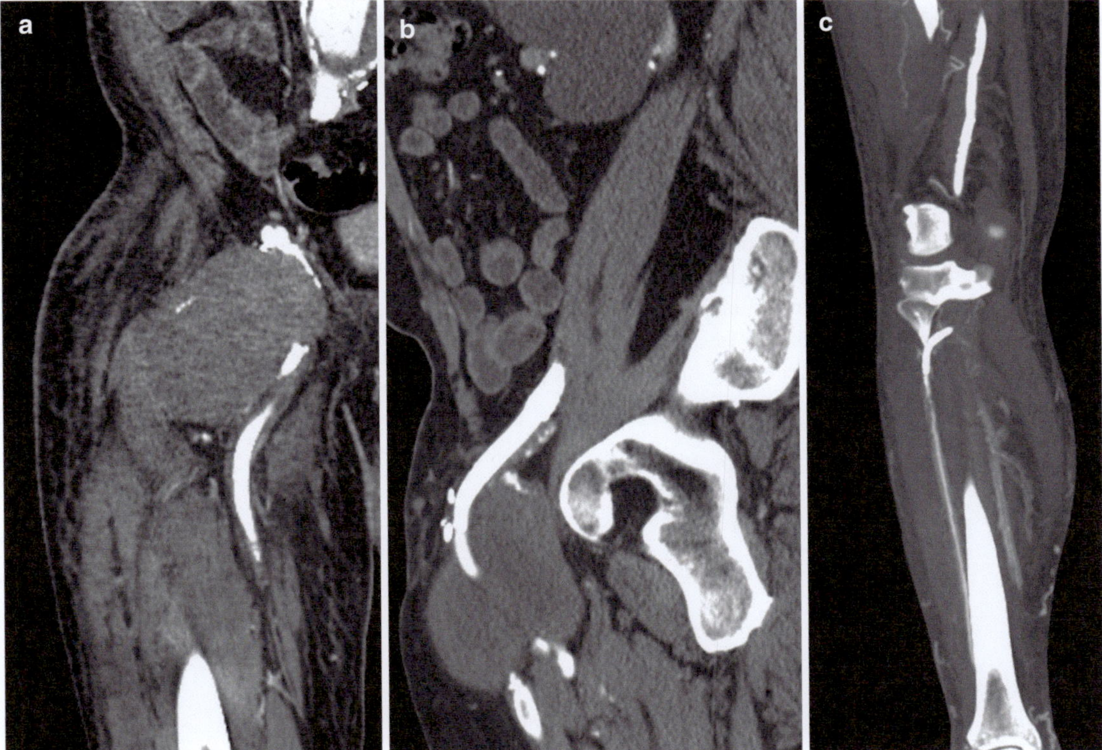

Fig. 11.4 Recanalization of the right lower extremity. Following exclusion of R CFA pseudoaneurysm, additional Viabahn stent-grafts were placed to extend the previously placed pelvic and CFA (**a**, **b**). Fluoroscopic images demonstrate drug-eluting balloon dilation of the distal SFA and proximal AT (**c**) and placement of a drug-eluting coronary stent (blue arrow) spanning the right AT to distal popliteal artery with improvement of flow into the AT (**d**)

Fig. 11.5 Two-month follow-up CT angiography in coronal (**a**) sagittal (**b**) planes demonstrate exclusion of the right CFA pseudoaneurysm and patent stents spanning the right CIA to SFA. 3-D reconstruction of aorto-bifemoral graft and IBE-stent construct (**c**) demonstrates patency of the distal SFA-popliteal stent and continuous 1-vessel runoff to the foot

Managing Complex Iatrogenic Guidewire Dissection and a Damaged Stent

Austin J. Pourmoussa and Ripal T. Gandhi

A 74-year-old male with a history of diabetes and coronary disease presented with left buttock and thigh claudication. Angiography demonstrated high grade stenosis at the origin of both the left external iliac and hypogastric arteries (Fig. 12.1). A self-expanding bare metal stent was placed in the left external iliac artery (Fig. 12.2), followed by a balloon-expandable stent in the left hypogastric artery, through the interstices of the previously placed stent (Fig. 12.3). Subsequent angiography demonstrated a high grade flow-limiting dissection of the distal left external iliac artery (Fig. 12.4).

The left common femoral artery (CFA) was accessed under sonographic guidance and the dissection was addressed with a self-expanding stent (Fig. 12.5). After deployment of the stent, the distal end of the stent was inadvertently damaged and compressed by advancement of the common femoral sheath (CFA) without its internal dilator (Fig. 12.6). The damaged stent was successfully traversed with a guidewire using a contralateral crossover approach and the stenosis within the stented area was treated with a self-expanding covered stent (Fig. 12.7), with a good angiographic result (Fig. 12.8).

The iatrogenic dissection of the left external iliac artery was likely secondary to guidewire trauma. This complication can be prevented by being aware of the location of the guidewire tip at all times.

The access site in the CFA was extremely close to the newly deployed stent which resulted in damaging the stent. The sheath should be advanced over a dilator under fluoroscopy in this situation, to avoid injuring or invaginating a self-expanding laser-cut nitinol stent. Accessing of the CFA at a more caudal position or using the proximal superficial femoral artery might have allowed for additional safety.

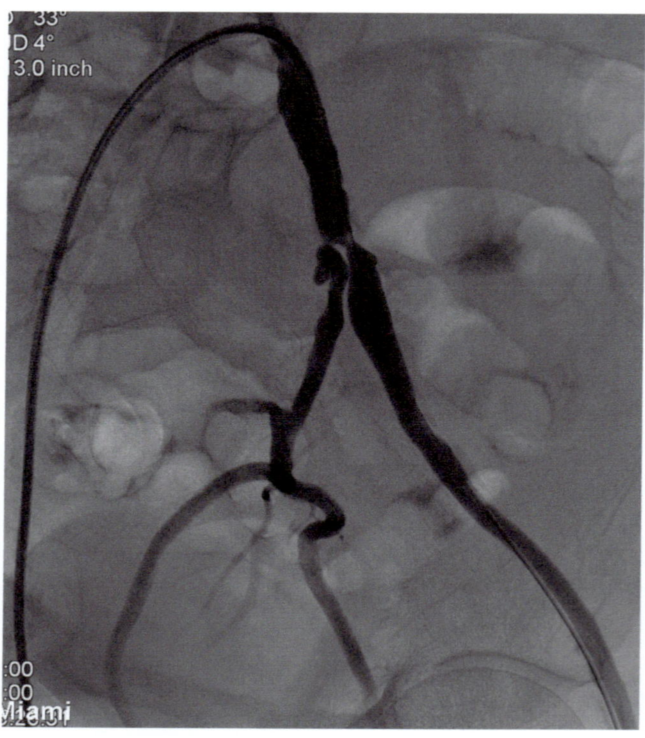

Fig. 12.1 Angiography of the left common iliac artery demonstrates high grade stenosis at the origin of both the left external iliac and left hypogastric arteries

A. J. Pourmoussa · R. T. Gandhi (✉)
Department of Interventional Radiology, Miami Cardiac and Vascular Institute, Baptist Health South Florida, Miami, FL, USA
e-mail: gandhi@baptisthealth.net

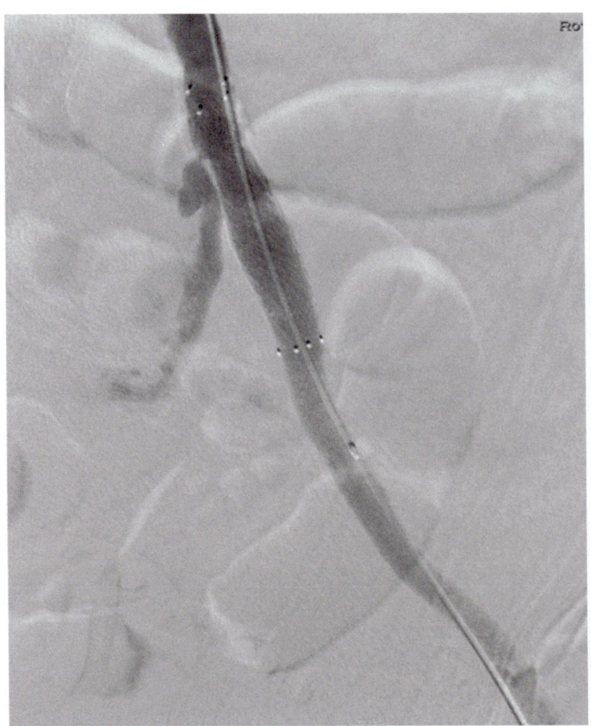

Fig. 12.2 A self-expanding bare metal stent placed to treat left external iliac artery stenosis

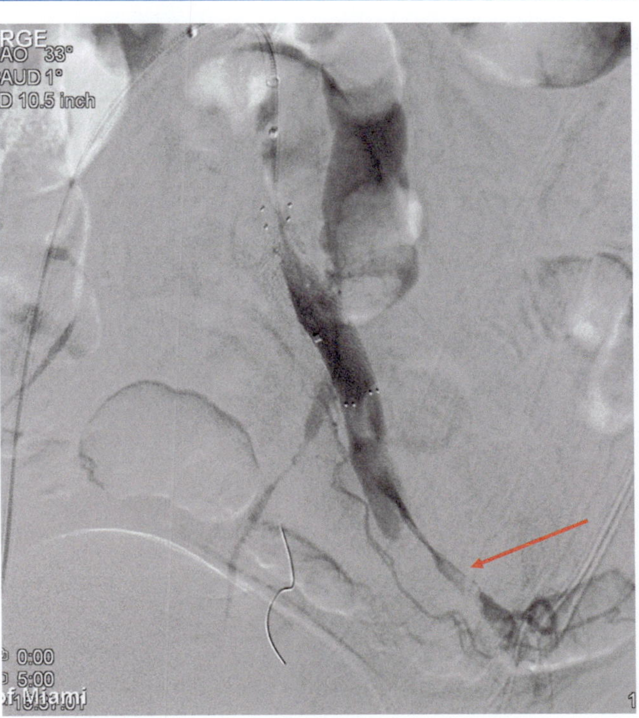

Fig. 12.4 Subsequent angiogram demonstrated a high grade flow-limiting dissection (red arrow) in the distal left external iliac artery

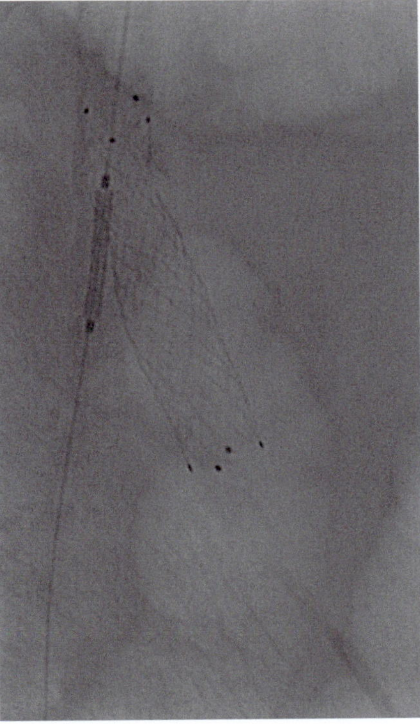

Fig. 12.3 A catheter and guidewire were placed through the interstices of the previously placed stent and a balloon expandable stent was deployed in the left hypogastric artery at its origin

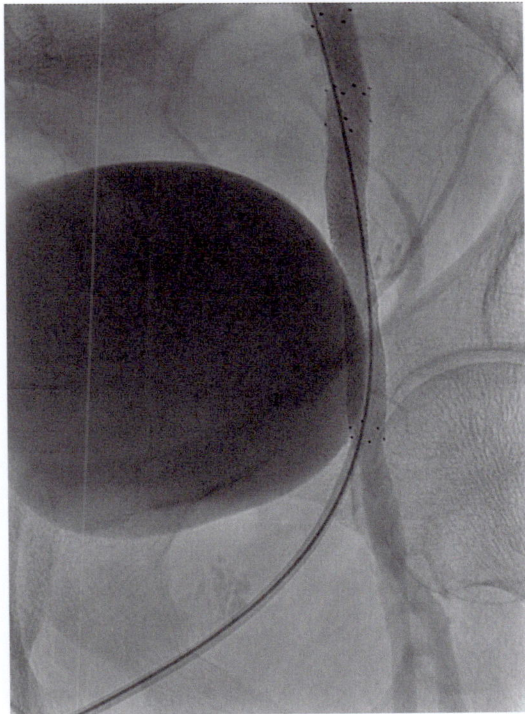

Fig. 12.5 The left common femoral artery was accessed under ultrasound guidance and the flow-limiting dissection was successfully treated with a self-expanding stent

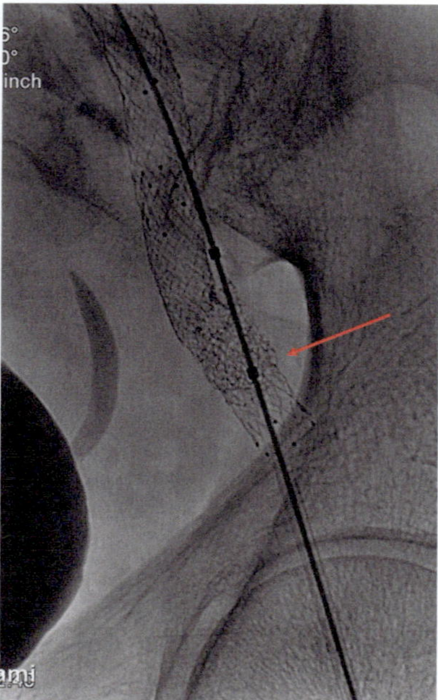

Fig. 12.6 After deployment of the stent, the distal end of the stent was inadvertently damaged and compressed (red arrow) by advancement of the left common femoral sheath without the dilator

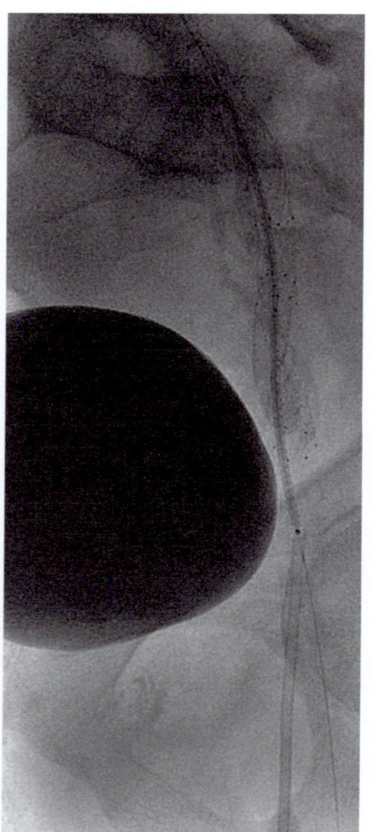

Fig. 12.7 The lumen of the damaged stent was successfully traversed with a guidewire from a crossover approach and the stenosis within the stented area was treated with a self-expanding covered stent

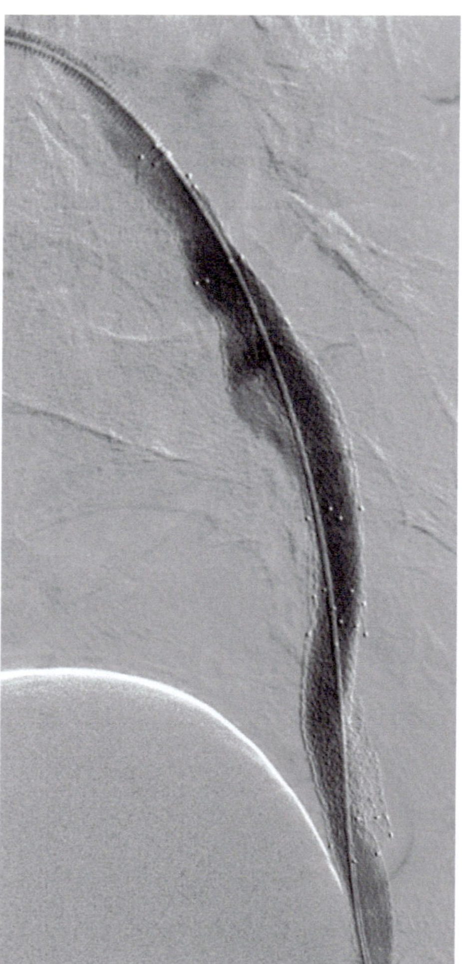

Fig. 12.8 Marked improvement in blood flow and no translesional residual pressure gradient

Part II

Arteries: Peripheral Vessels and Branches

Retrograde Puncture of the Profunda Femoris Artery to Facilitate Treatment of Critical Limb Ischemia

Bhavraj Khalsa, Meena Archie, and Mahmood Razavi

An 85-year-old female with chronic-limb threatening ischemia presented with severe worsening of right lower extremity rest pain. She had a history of chronically occluded right femoropopliteal stents and severe tibial occlusive disease with an ABI of 0.4.

Her right femoral pulse was nonpalpable; CT angiography demonstrated acute thrombosis of her right external iliac artery (EIA) and common femoral artery (CFA) (Fig. 13.1). The patient underwent a right iliofemoral endarterectomy with patch angioplasty, right EIA thrombectomy, and stent placement with restoration of a palpable femoral pulse thereafter.

On post-operative day 1, she lost her femoral pulse. Angiography demonstrated rethrombosis of the right EIA and CFA in addition to the profunda femoris artery (PFA) (Figs. 13.2 and 13.3).

Through a 6F sheath, thrombectomy of the right EIA and CFA was performed using a 6F Jeti device; however, flow was unable to be restored due to the occluded outflow. Antegrade recanalization of the occluded PFA origin was unsuccessful despite multiple attempts.

Percutaneous retrograde access of the PFA was performed under fluoroscopic guidance (Fig. 13.4) with successful recanalization of the occluded PFA origin, establishment of contralateral through-and-through access, angioplasty, and aspiration thrombectomy (6F Jeti) of the PFA (Fig. 13.5), and stenting of the right EIA (6 mm Viabahn) and CFA (6.5 mm Supera) with restoration of antegrade flow to the right lower extremity (Fig. 13.6).

The patient was able to avoid an above knee amputation and was discharged to home on comfort care.

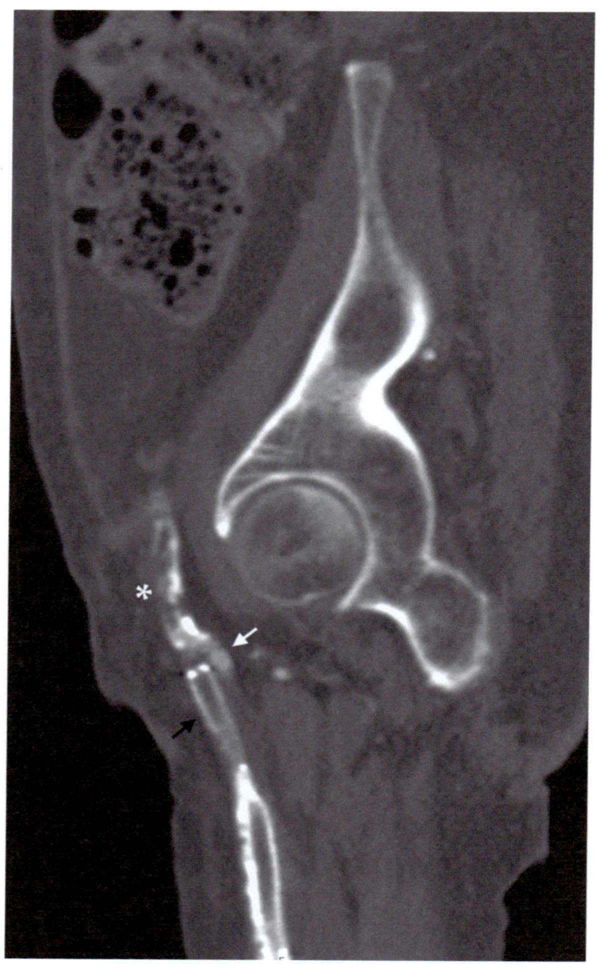

Fig. 13.1 Sagittal CT image through the level of the right CFA demonstrates calcified plaque at the CFA and PFA origin, occluded CFA and chronically occluded SFA stents. Common femoral artery (CFA, white asterix), profunda femoris artery (PFA, white arrow), superficial femoral artery (SFA, black arrow)

B. Khalsa (✉) · M. Razavi
Department of Interventional Radiology, Providence St. Joseph Hospital, Orange, CA, USA
e-mail: khalsa@visoc.org; mrazavi@razavimd.com

M. Archie
Department of Vascular Surgery, Providence St. Joseph Hospital, Orange, CA, USA
e-mail: marchie@visoc.org

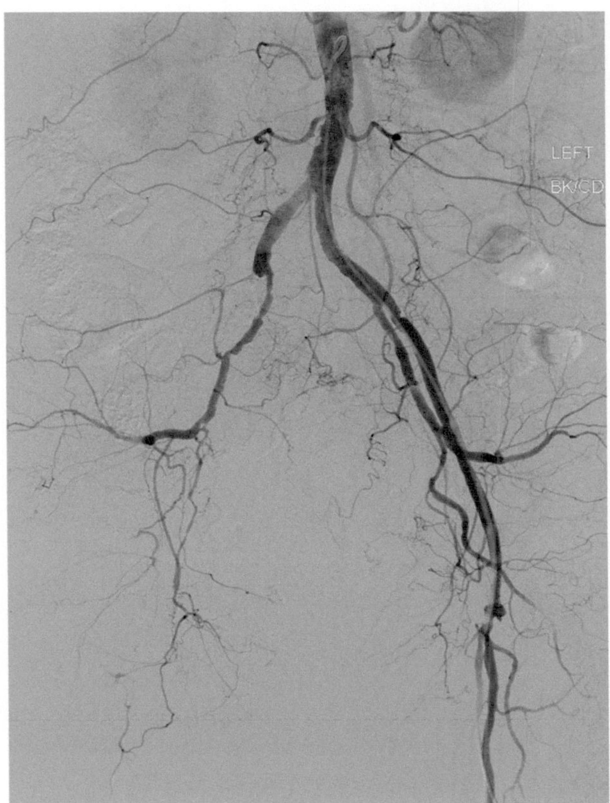

Fig. 13.2 Distal abdominal aortogram and pelvic arteriogram demonstrates occluded right EIA, CFA and PFA with minimal distal reconstitution. External iliac artery (EIA), common femoral artery (CFA), profunda femoris artery (PFA)

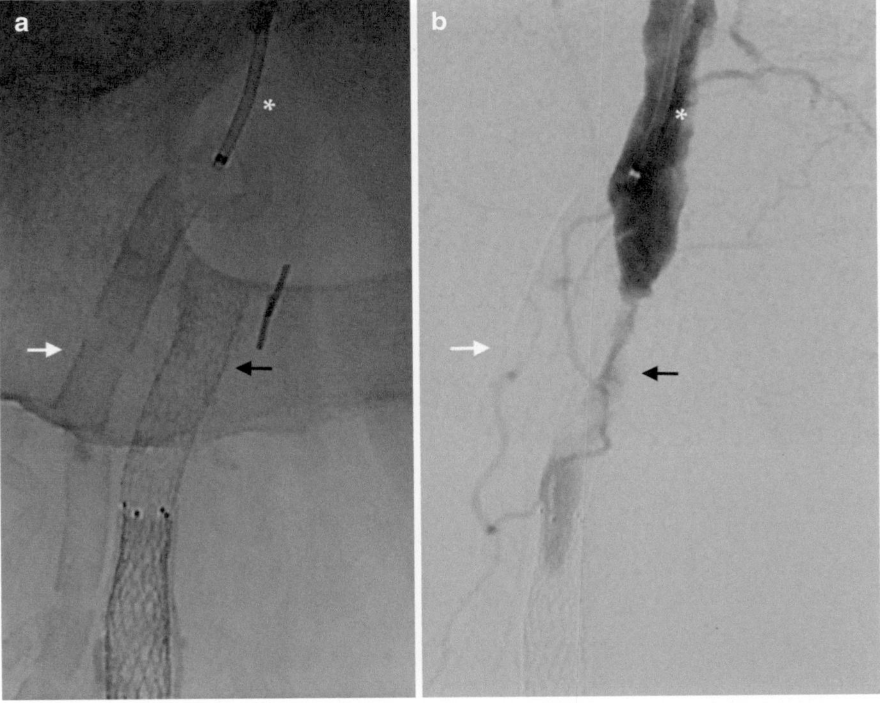

Fig. 13.3 Native image at the level of the right CFA demonstrates severely calcified arteries with previously placed SFA stents (**a**). Digital subtraction angiogram (DSA) demonstrates occluded PFA and SFA (**b**). Common femoral artery (CFA, white asterix), profunda femoris artery (PFA, white arrow), superficial femoral artery (SFA, black arrow)

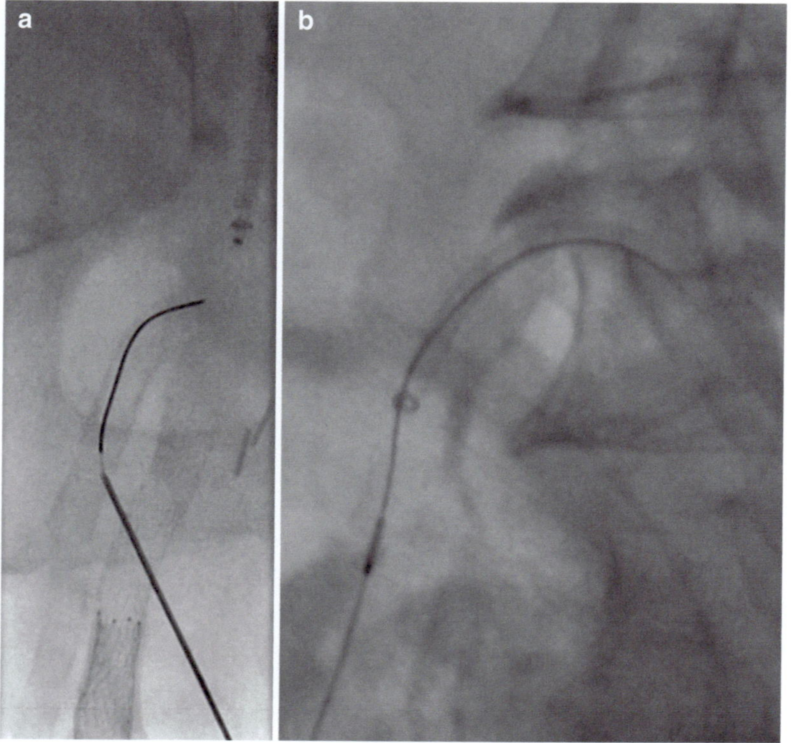

Fig. 13.4 Fluoroscopic-guided percutaneous retrograde access of the right PFA enables successful recanalization across the occluded origin (**a**). Through-and-through access is established by navigating the microwire into the sheath (**b**) and externalizing via the contralateral femoral access site. Profunda femoris artery (PFA)

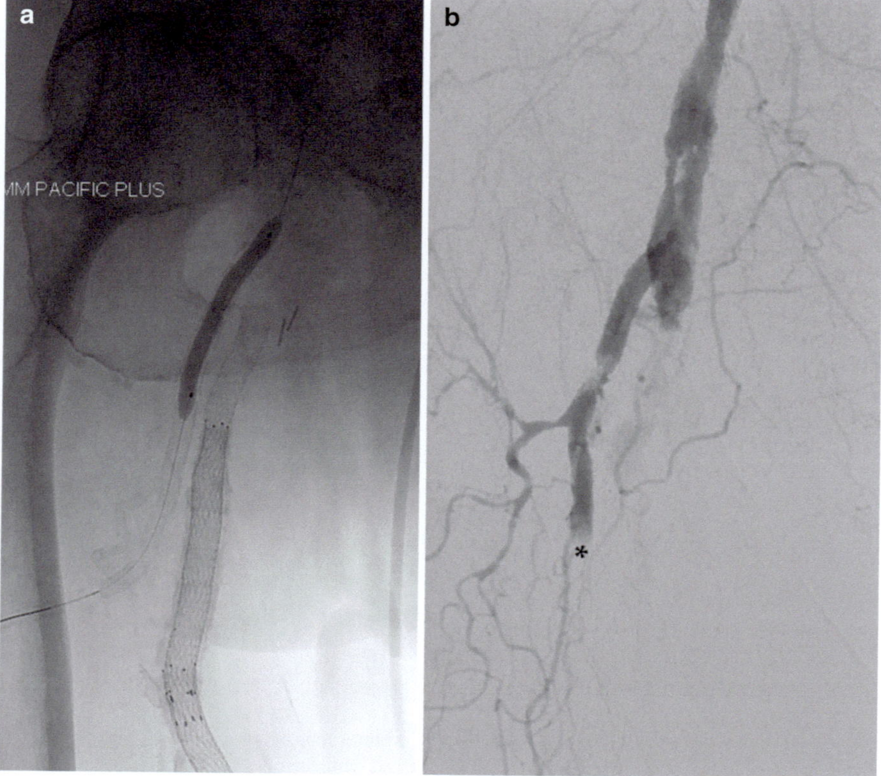

Fig. 13.5 Angioplasty of the right PFA (**a**) followed by arteriogram (**b**) demonstrates flow into the previously occluded artery, however, with distal thrombus (black asterix). Profunda femoris artery (PFA)

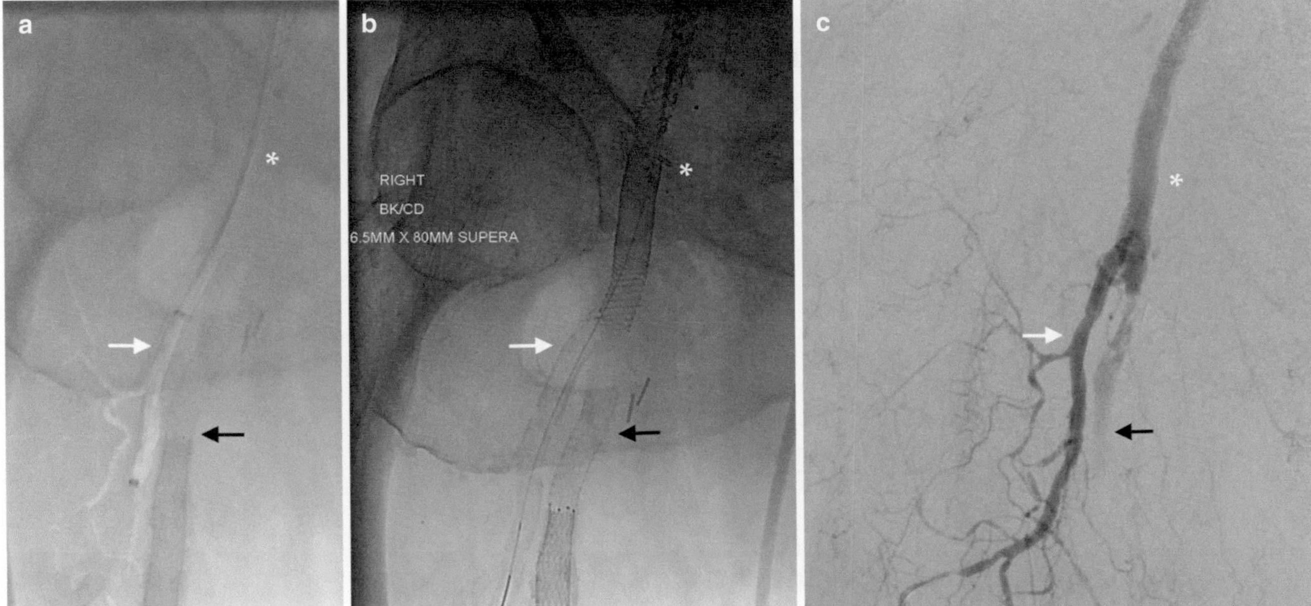

Fig. 13.6 DSA roadmap image demonstrates aspiration thrombectomy of the right PFA and its second order branches (**a**), followed by stenting of the right EIA and CFA (**b**). Final DSA arteriogram through the level of the right CFA (**c**) demonstrates patent iliofemoral segment into the PFA (chronically occluded SFA stents) with brisk washout on delayed images. External iliac artery (EIA), common femoral artery (CFA, white asterix), profunda femoris artery (PFA, white arrow), superficial femoral artery (SFA, black arrow)

Endovascular Recanalization and Stenting of Chronic Superficial Artery Occlusion through the Dorsalis Pedis Artery

Timothy W. I. Clark

A 76-year-old male was presented with lifestyle-disabling right calf claudication. His past medical history included coronary artery disease, prior bilateral iliac stent placement, and a remote history of stroke. His physical exam and pulse volume recordings were consistent with chronic superficial femoral artery (SFA) occlusion.

Endovascular recanalization of his flush occlusion of his right SFA from an antegrade approach was unsuccessful (Fig. 14.1). Therefore, the dorsalis pedis artery was accessed with ultrasound and a five French sheath placed (Fig. 14.2). The distal cap of the femoropopliteal occlusion was entered with a hydrophilic catheter and guidewire using subintimal technique and this combination traversed to the level of the SFA origin. Conventional techniques at lumen re-entry were unsuccessful. Using an Outback LTD device (Cordis, Miami Lakes, FL) true-lumen guidewire re-entry into the common femoral artery (CFA) was successfully achieved through a combination of fluoroscopic and sonographic guidance to orient the direction of the Outback needle toward the CFA lumen (Fig. 14.3a–c). Angioplasty was performed throughout the SFA using a 6 mm balloon followed by placement of two 6 mm × 150 mm nitinol stents, subsequently dilated with the 6 mm balloon. Post-procedure arteriograms showed widely patent runoff to the foot (Fig. 14.4a, b). The dorsalis pedis sheath was removed and hemostasis achieved with a VasoStat device (Forge Medical, Bethlehem, PA).

The patient had complete resolution of claudication symptoms. Over the next 6 years, he returned on two occasions for angioplasty of in-stent restenosis. Serial Duplex ultrasound examinations showed a widely patent dorsalis pedis artery (Fig. 14.5).

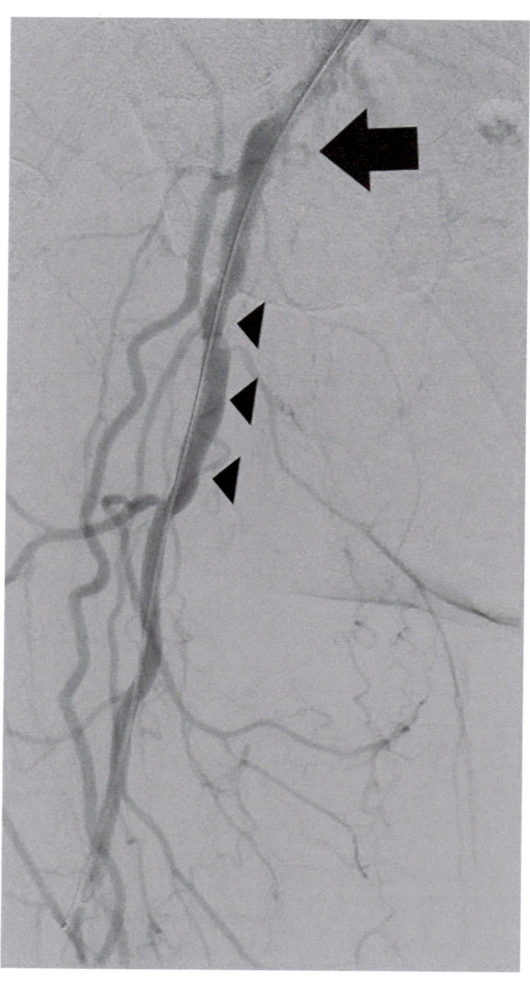

Fig. 14.1 Digitally subtracted angiogram showing flush occlusion at the origin (arrow) of the right superficial femoral artery and patent profunda femoris artery (arrowheads). Antegrade attempts at recanalization were unsuccessful

T. W. I. Clark (✉)
Department of Radiology, Section of Interventional Radiology, University of Pennsylvania Perelman School of Medicine, Philadelphia, PA, USA
e-mail: Timothy.Clark@uphs.upenn.edu; timothy.clark@pennmedicine.upenn.edu

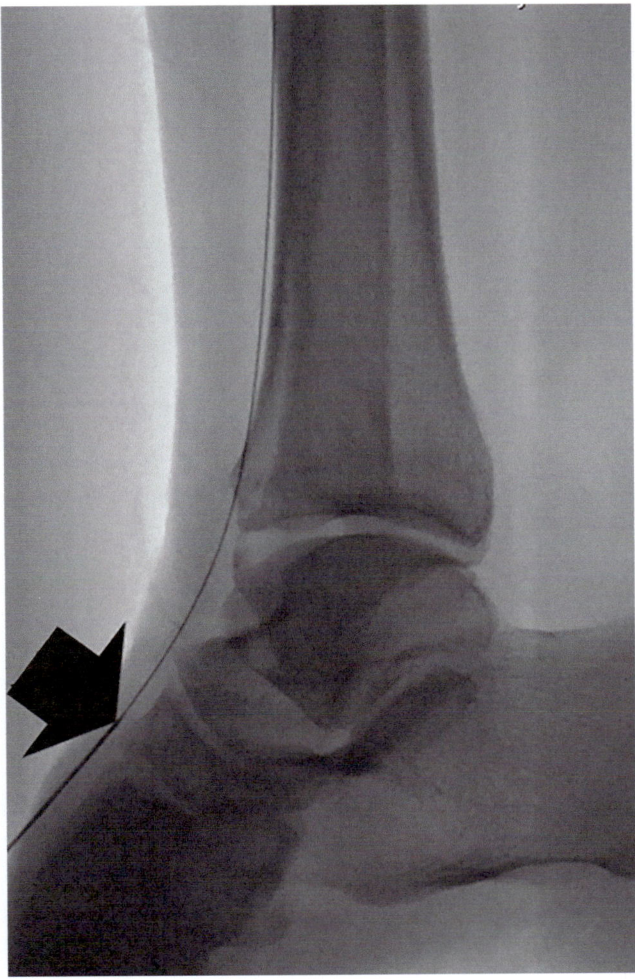

Fig. 14.2 Fluoroscopic view showing site of micropuncture access (arrow) of the dorsalis pedis artery prior to five French sheath placement

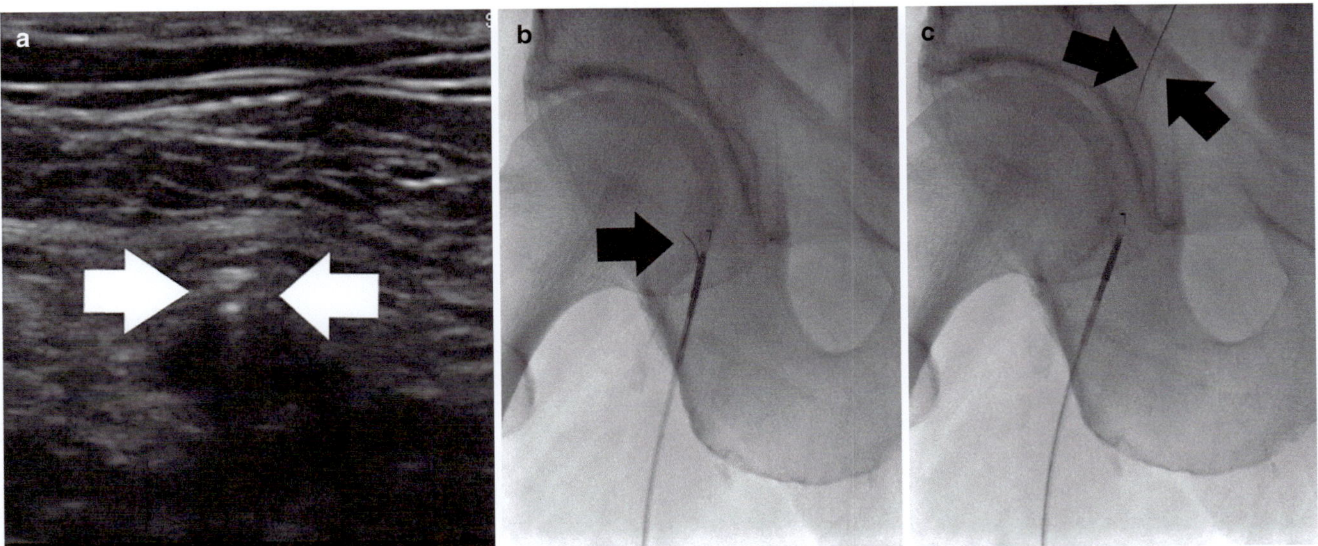

Fig. 14.3 (**a**) Ultrasound showing anterior orientation of Outback device (arrows) prior to needle re-entry. (**b**) Oblique fluoroscopic view during advancement of Outback needle (arrow) into common femoral artery lumen. (**c**) Guidewire advanced through common femoral artery into external iliac artery (arrows)

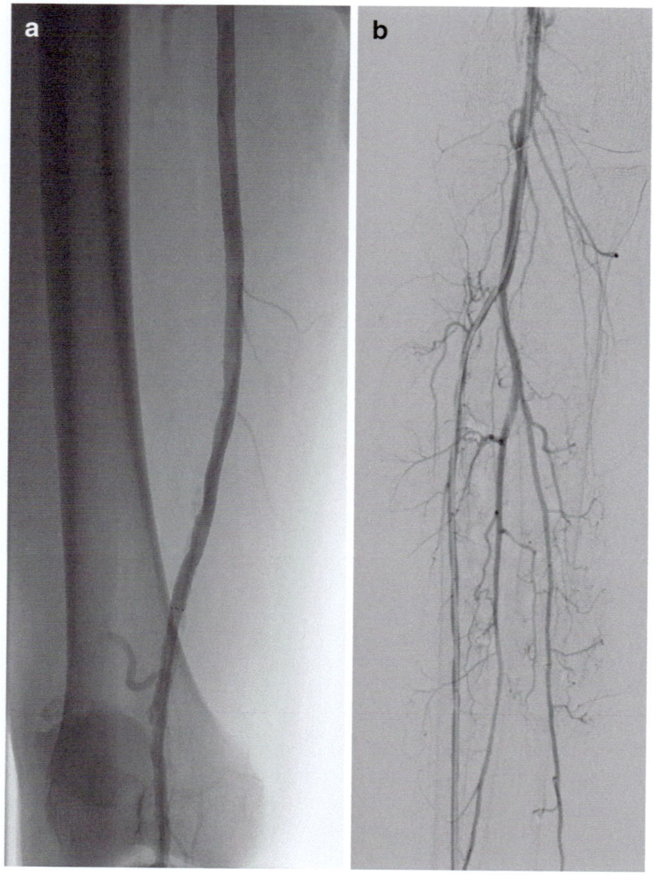

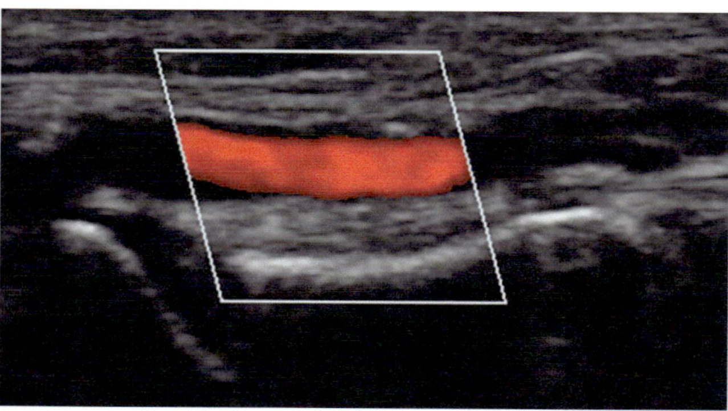

Fig. 14.5 Color duplex ultrasound of dorsalis pedis artery at site of prior access 3 months following recanalization procedure

Bibliography

1. Vance AZ, Leung DA, Clark TWI. Tips for pedal access: technical evolution and review. J Cardiovasc Surg. 2018;59:685–91.

Fig. 14.4 (**a**) Angiogram post recanalization showing widely patent superficial femoral artery and popliteal artery. (**b**) Digitally subtracted angiogram showing widely patent below-knee runoff

Deep Venous Arterialization with Ellipsys Side-to-Side Anastomosis

Jeffrey Hull

Deep Venous Arterialization (DVA) involves arterial to venous fistula creation with reversal of venous flow to treat no option critical limb ischemia. The earliest attempts at DVA were described in a 1912 case review where surgical arteriovenous fistula and spontaneous venous valve failure salvaged 30% of limbs treated [1]. Modern surgical DVA has utilized the most distal patent artery anastomosed to a bypass conduit or deep vein (with valvulotomy) to direct flow to veins in the foot and have achieved a pooled 75% limb salvage rate at 1 year in a meta-analysis [2]. Percutaneous DVA has reported similar results using stent grafts as an end-to-end arterial venous anastomosis and then as the conduit to the posterior tibial vein at the ankle [3]. This approach was associated with a high rate of conduit thrombosis of 68% at a mean of 2.6 months.

In this case, percutaneous DVA was performed in a 63-year-old Caucasian man with diabetic neuropathy, and non-healing wound over his first metatarsal bone (Fig. 15.1). The plantar wound and osteomyelitis persisted despite prior anterior tibial artery angioplasty that improved TBI to 0.23, intravenous and chronic oral antibiotics, and regular wound therapy.

A proximal side-to-side anastomosis was created with the Ellipsys vascular access catheter using a hybrid conduit of stent graft and in situ autologous vein (Figs. 15.2, 15.3, 15.4, and 15.5). The side-to-side anastomosis avoided stent graft occlusion of the distal arterial flow (Fig. 15.4). The DVA remained patent for 7 months until below knee amputation was required to treat unresolved osteomyelitis (Fig. 15.6). The Ellipsys system is approved for intentional creation of percutaneous arteriovenous fistulae for hemodialysis access. This case demonstrates its new use for DVA for the treatment of critical limb ischemia.

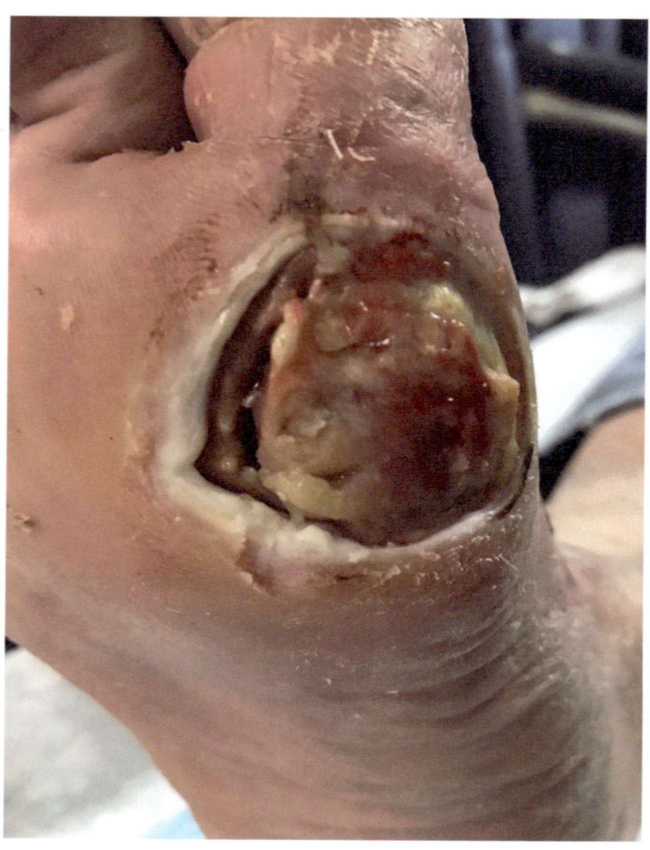

Fig. 15.1 Non-healing wound over first metatarsal head WIfI 232 stage 4 with unresolved ulceration and osteomyelitis despite maximal medical treatment with wound care and intravenous antibiotics

J. Hull (✉)
Department of Interventional Radiology, Richmond Vascular Center, North Chesterfield, VA, USA

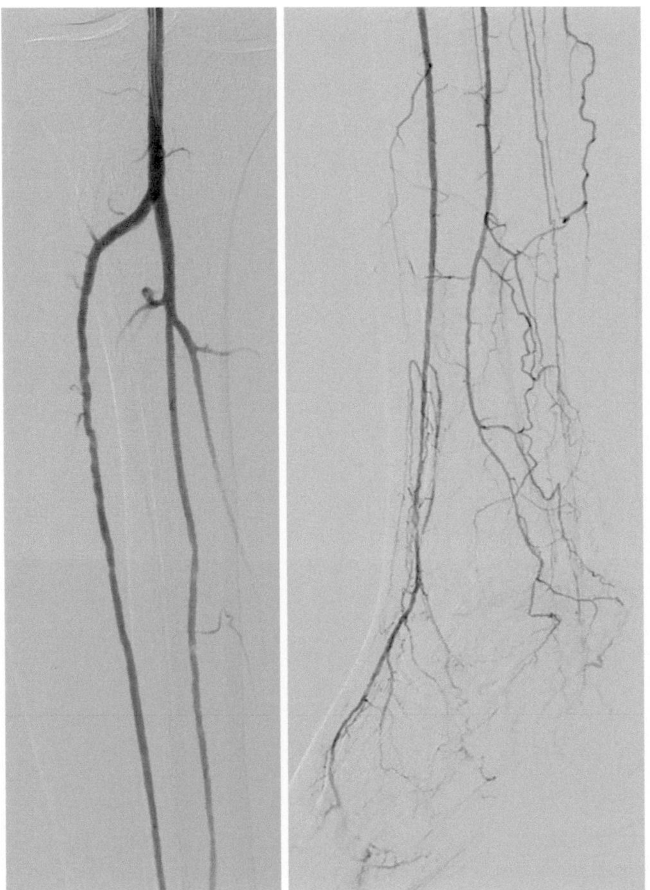

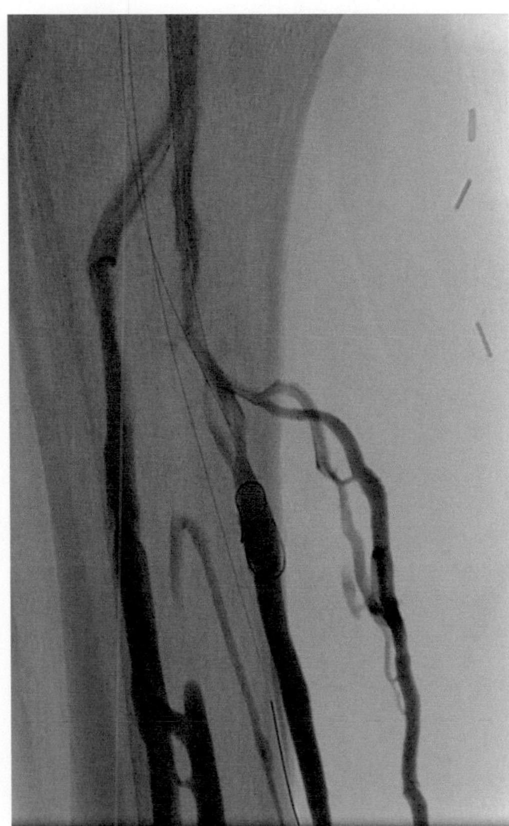

Fig. 15.3 Venogram after crossing from tibial peroneal artery to posterior tibial vein with Pioneer Plus catheter (Phillips)

Fig. 15.2 Angiogram demonstrates GLASS stage III with grade 0 femoral popliteal flow, grade 4 infra-popliteal flow to the target posterior tibial artery, and a P1 Pedal arch with occlusion of posterior tibial artery and lateral plantar artery [1]. The distal anterior tibial artery was previously balloon dilated without clinical improvement. The posterior tibial and plantar artery failed recanalization

Fig. 15.4 Tissue-fused anastomosis between tibial peroneal artery and posterior tibial vein was performed with Ellipsys catheter (Avenu Medical, San Juan Capistrano, CA). The length of the Ellipsys catheter required percutaneous access to the posterior tibial vein through the calf. This access was covered with 5 by 100 mm Viabahn stent for hemostasis (Gore, Flagstaff, AZ). A 16 mm Amplatzer plug was placed in the proximal posterior tibial vein. The distal posterior tibial vein was in spasm that was treated with valvulotomy (Lemaitre Vascular) and 5 mm balloon dilation to provide flow to the ankle

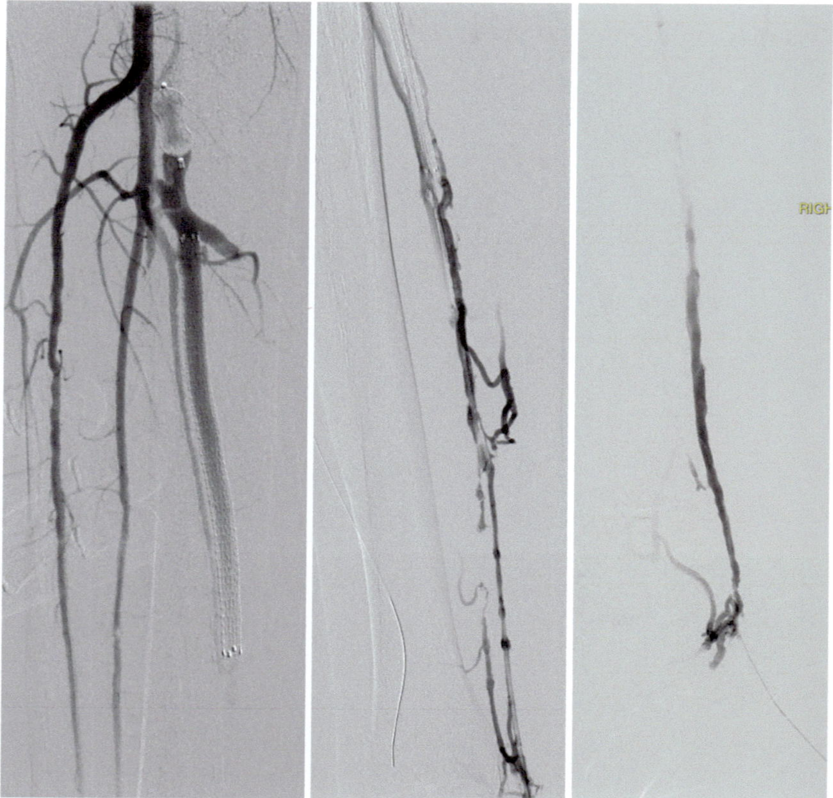

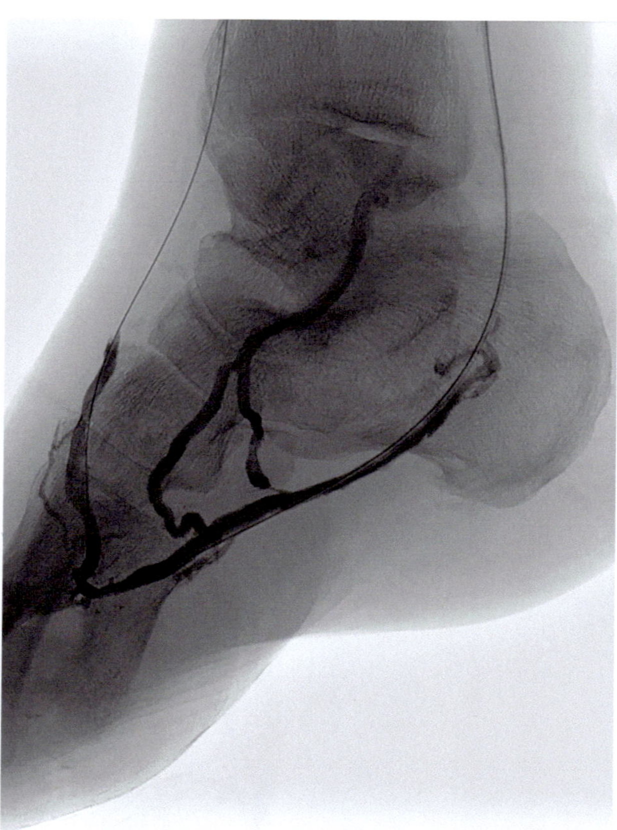

Fig. 15.5 Flow into the plantar vein was established with A. retrograde access to the posterior tibial vein with navigation through the perforating vein to the dorsalis pedal vein. The posterior tibial veins were treated with the Flex Vessel Prep (Venture Med Group) and balloon dilation. Valvulotomy and balloon dilation are considered essential to success of DAV

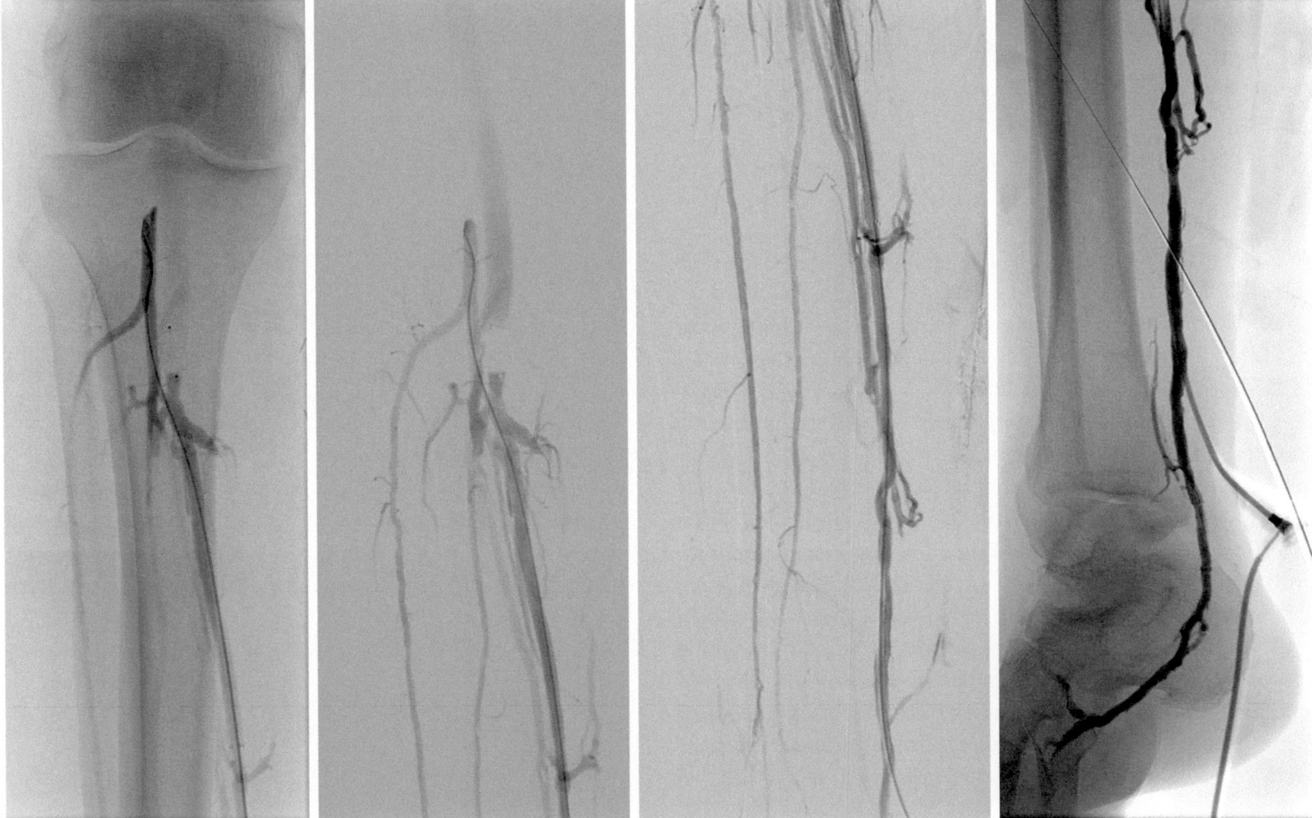

Fig. 15.6 Follow-up venogram at 4 weeks prior to foot surgery demonstrating patent DVA to the plantar vein of the foot. Doppler ultrasound image demonstrated flow volume of 400 mL/min in the posterior tibial vein at the ankle

Bibliography

1. Bernheim BM. Arteriovenous anastomosis-reversal of the circulation-as a preventive of gangrene of the extremities: review of the literature and report of six additional cases. Ann Surg. 1912;55:195–207.
2. Schreve MA, Vos CG, Vahl AC, et al. Venous arterialisation for salvage of critically Ischaemic limbs: a systematic review and meta-analysis. Eur J Vasc Endovasc Surg. 2017;53:387–402.
3. Schmidt A, Schreve MA, Huizing E, et al. Midterm outcomes of percutaneous deep venous arterialization with a dedicated system for patients with no-option chronic limb-threatening ischemia: the ALPS multicenter study. J Endovasc Ther. 2020;27(4):152660282092217.

Shooting Your Way Out: Endovascular Arterial Bypass Via Gunsight

16

Marc C. Kryger, Benjamin Contrella, and Luke Wilkins

A 64-year-old woman presented with a history of bilateral calf claudication. Noninvasive vascular imaging, including a CTA, demonstrated chronic total occlusions of both superficial femoral arteries (SFA).

Endovascular revascularization was undertaken. Percutaneous left brachial access allowed advancement of a sheath to the left common femoral artery (CFA) and angiography reaffirmed the SFA occlusion (Fig. 16.1). Percutaneous access to the left dorsalis pedis (DP) artery allowed creation of a subintimal plane to bypass the SFA lumen up to the femoral head to the same level as the brachial access wire. Despite multiple attempts, through-and-through wire access could not be achieved from either retrograde or antegrade approaches. Separate snare catheters were then advanced from the brachial and DP accesses (Fig. 16.2), and a coaxial plane established through which a micropuncture set was used to obtain through-and-through wire access via a "Gunsight" approach (Fig. 16.3).

The tract was dilated with a 2 mm diameter × 60 mm length angioplasty balloon. The post-angioplasty arteriogram demonstrated a left groin pseudoaneurysm. A 5 × 50 mm Viabahn stent was deployed; the post-stent arteriogram demonstrated persistent perfusion of the pseudoaneurysm (Fig. 16.4). Because of the inability to advance additional stents into the subintimal tract or across the pseudoaneurysm, an additional antegrade left CFA access was used to advance a braided sheath into the distal SFA. The subintimal tract was then stented from distal to proximal, above the level of the pseudoaneurysm, and serial angioplasty performed. Follow-up angiogram showed a patent subintimal conduit (Figs. 16.5 and 16.6) with exclusion of the left groin pseudoaneurysm (Fig. 16.7). The stent and vessel remained patent at 12-month follow-up imaging.

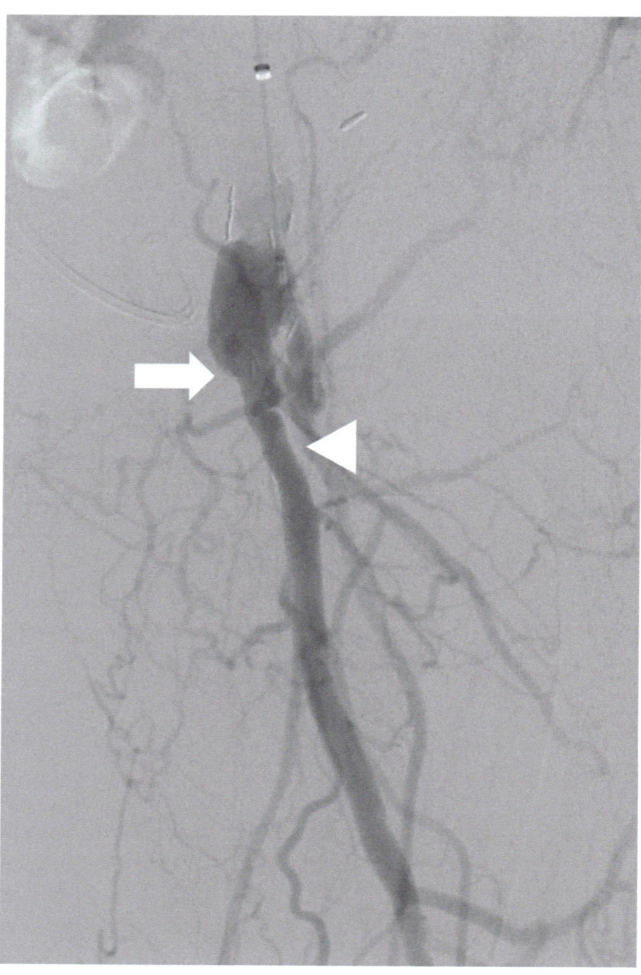

Fig. 16.1 Complete left SFA occlusion (white arrow). Profunda femoris artery (white arrowhead)

M. C. Kryger (✉)
Department of Radiology and Medical Imaging, University of Virginia Health System, Charlottesville, VA, USA
e-mail: MK9ZV@hscmail.mcc.virginia.edu

L. Wilkins
University of Virginia Health System, Charlottesville, VA, USA
e-mail: LRW6N@hscmail.mcc.virginia.edu

B. Contrella
Allegheny Health Network, Pittsburgh, PA, USA

© The Author(s), under exclusive license to Springer Nature Switzerland AG 2023
Z. J. Haskal (ed.), *Extreme IR*, https://doi.org/10.1007/978-3-031-24251-9_16

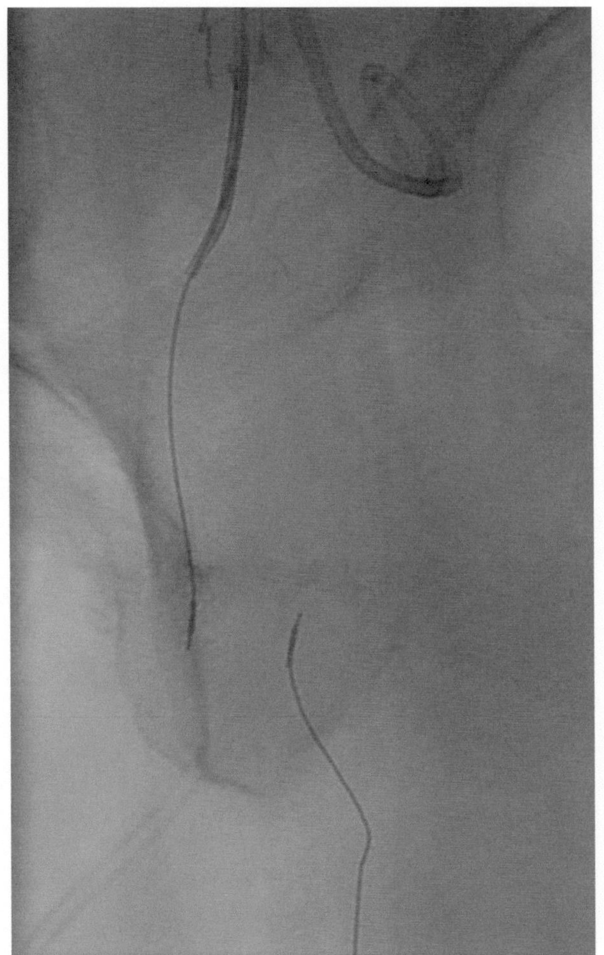

Fig. 16.2 Superior and inferior approach snare loops

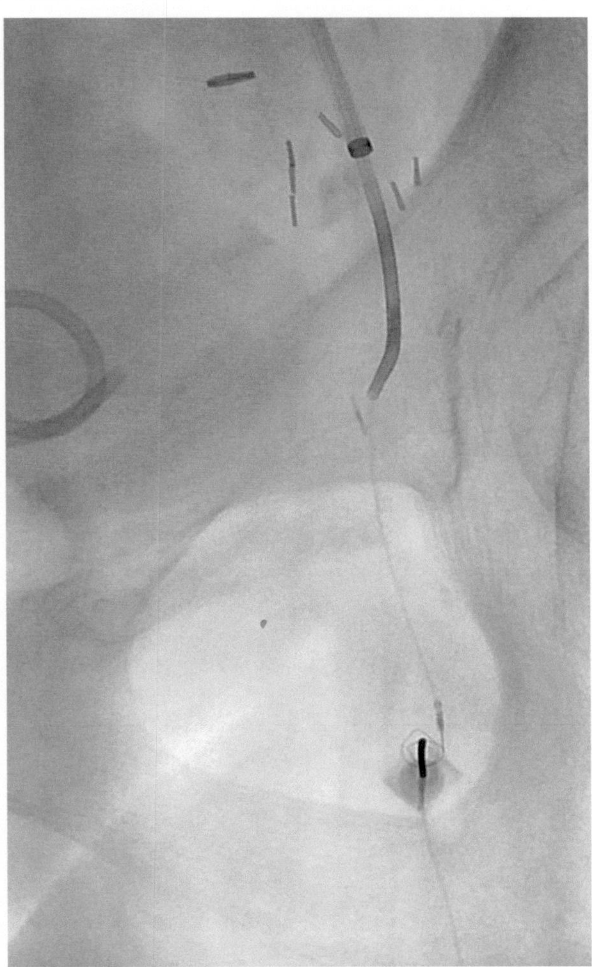

Fig. 16.3 Coaxial needle access through superior and inferior snare loops

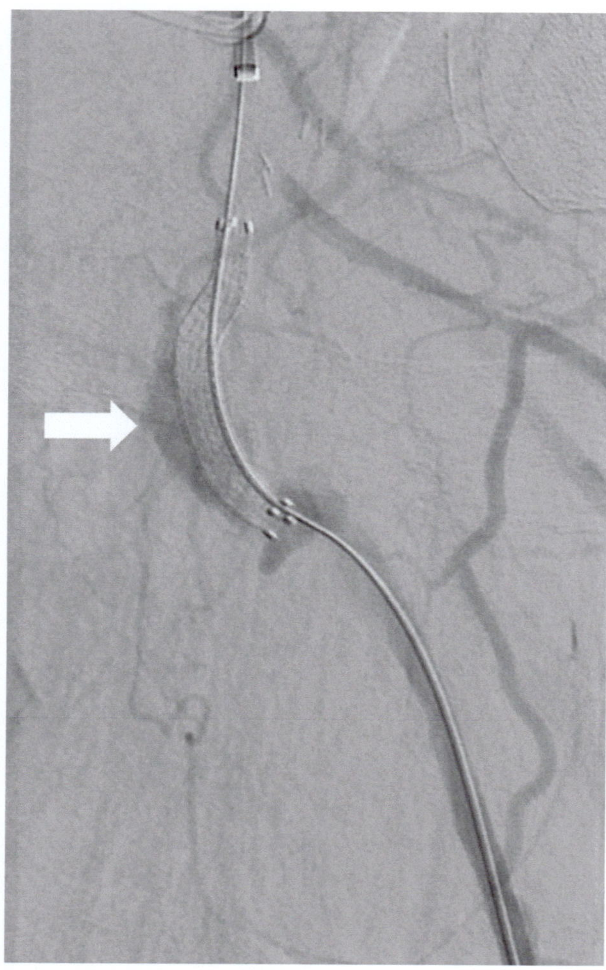

Fig. 16.4 Pseudoaneurysm (white arrow) status post initial placement of Viabahn stent

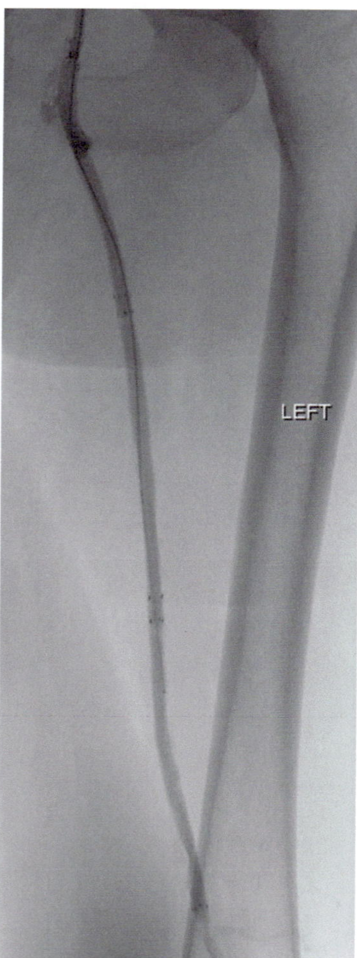

Fig. 16.5 Status post stenting and angioplasty of the subintimal conduit. Proximal pseudoaneurysm is still visible

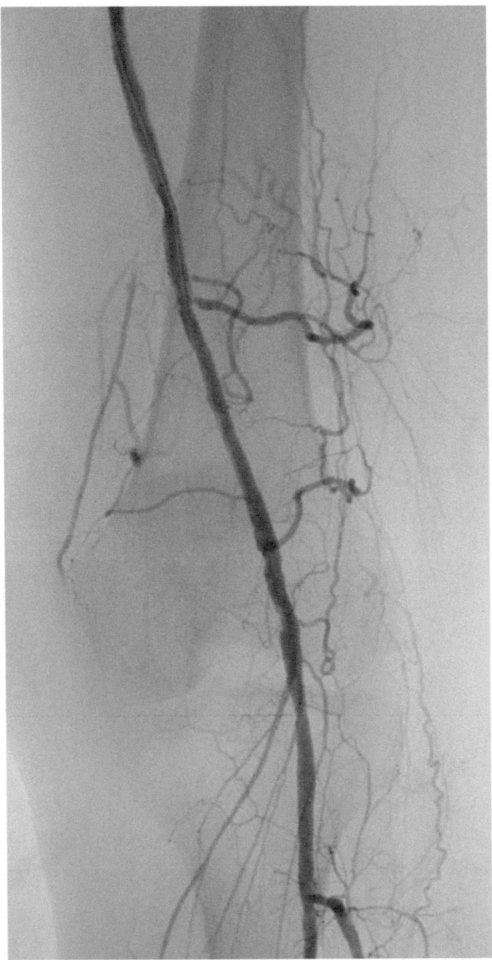

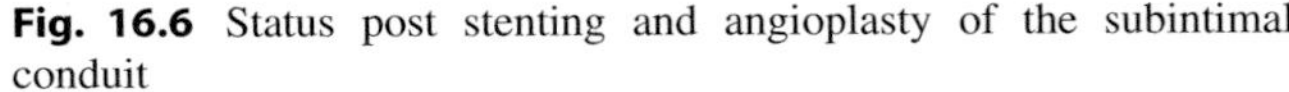

Fig. 16.6 Status post stenting and angioplasty of the subintimal conduit

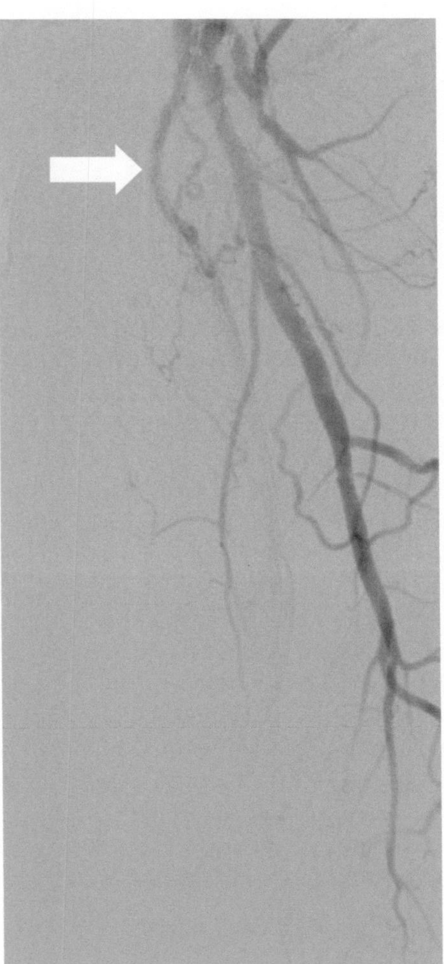

Fig. 16.7 Exclusion of previous left SFA pseudoaneurysm (white arrow)

Unconventional Endovascular Salvage of an Iatrogenic Dissecting Fusiform Long Segment SFA Aneurysm

Gaurav Dilip Gangwani

A 50-year-old male patient with 20 years of uncontrolled diabetes and tobacco use presented with severe rest pain in his right thigh and foot; his visual analogue scale pain score was 9/10. He had undergone multiple prior endovascular interventions for severe bilateral life-limiting claudication at another institute; among these were bilateral common iliac arterial stents 8 years ago, and right superficial femoral artery (SFA) stent placement 5 months earlier with E-Luminex 6 mm × 120 mm bare stents for a long segmental SFA occlusion. He provided a vague history of a proximal SFA pseudoaneurysm 1 month after stent placement, which was reportedly treated with ultrasound-guided compression.

After excluding infectious causes, the working diagnosis for his sonographic findings (Fig. 17.1) was fusiform dissecting SFA aneurysm—likely due to subintimal deployment of the self-expandable metallic stent without adequate proximal and distal coverage of proximal entry zone or distal exit zone. The patient refused the options of surgical femoral-popliteal bypass (with ligation of proximal and distal aneurysm neck). Accordingly endovascular intervention was planned.

Access site choice was a challenge due to bilateral iliac stents, the relatively large introducer profile for stent grafts and "short" proximal deployment zone required to prevent jailing of profunda femoris artery but nevertheless yield proximal neck sealing. Thus an 8-French ipsilateral retrograde popliteal arterial access (Fig. 17.2) was used to deploy two overlapping SFA stent grafts [6 × 100 mm and 6 × 80 mm Fluency, BD, Germany] (Fig. 17.3) resulting in complete aneurysmal occlusion; this was confirmed on final femoral angiography (See Fig. 17.4). Interim sonographic follow-up at 6 weeks and 3 months affirmed continued aneurysm occlusion and thrombosis. The patient was relieved of rest pain for 6 months after which he developed an unrelated burn injury and secondary necrotizing fasciitis requiring a below knee amputation.

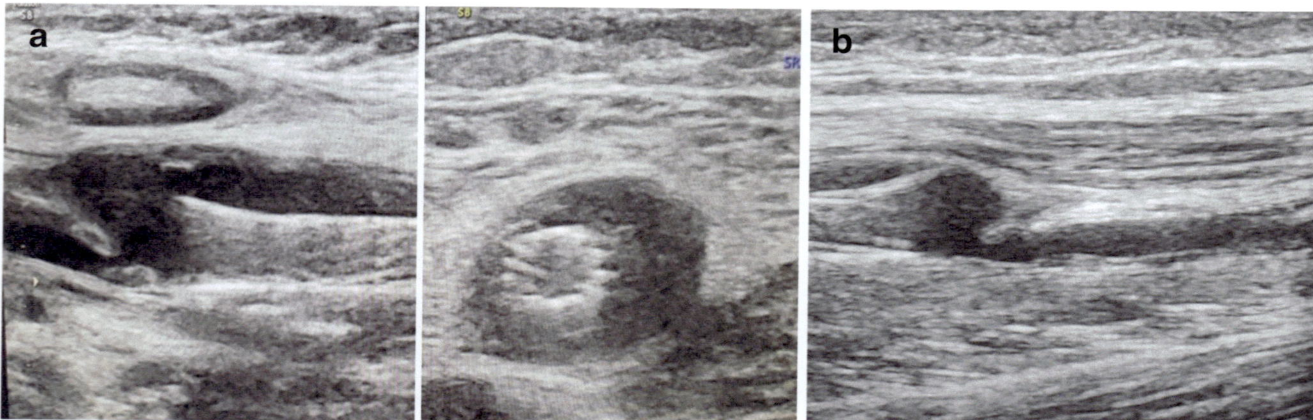

Fig. 17.1 (**a**) Ultrasound of the proximal right thigh (longitudinal) reveals high grade stenosis secondary to visible oblique flap in the proximal SFA and fusiform aneurysmal segment distal to it with a metal stent within the posterior aspect of the aneurysm segment. The transverse projection on the right reveals the stent lying along the right postero-lateral aspect of the aneurysmal femoral segment. (**b**) Ultrasound of the distal right thigh (longitudinal) reveals distal extent of the aneurysm further distal to the terminal stent ending with another focal stenosis secondary to a visible flap

G. D. Gangwani (✉)
Department of Interventional Radiology, Bhaktivedanta Hospital and Research Institute, Thane, Maharashtra, India

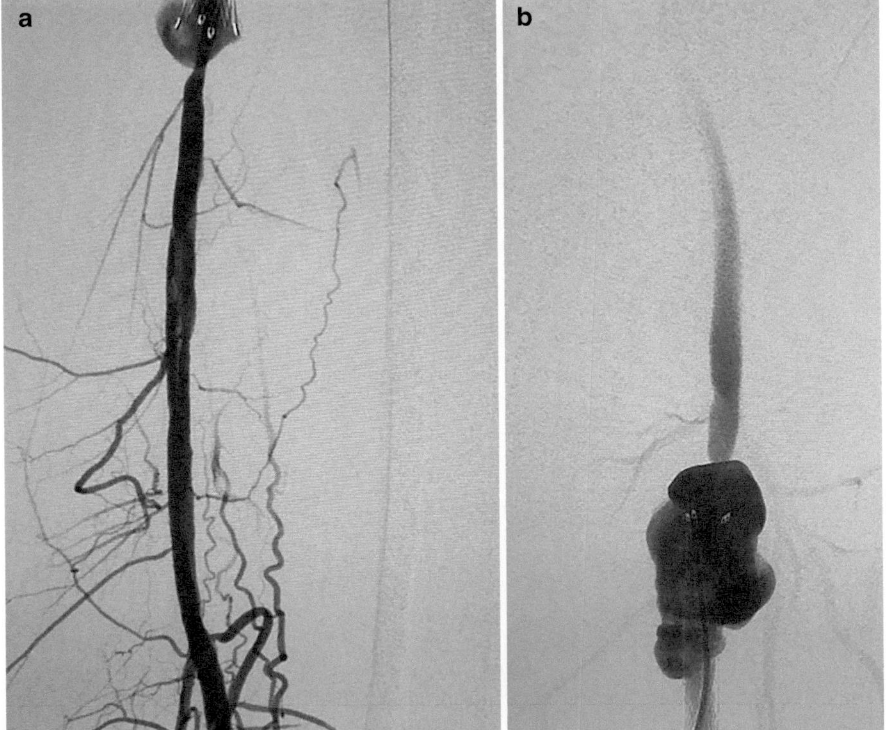

Fig. 17.2 (**a**) Retrograde popliteal digital subtraction angiogram (DSA) revealed the terminal extent of the fusiform aneurysm segment distal to the terminal stent struts. (**b**) Retrograde superficial femoral angiogram revealed proximal extent of the fusiform aneurysmal segment cranial to the proximal stent struts

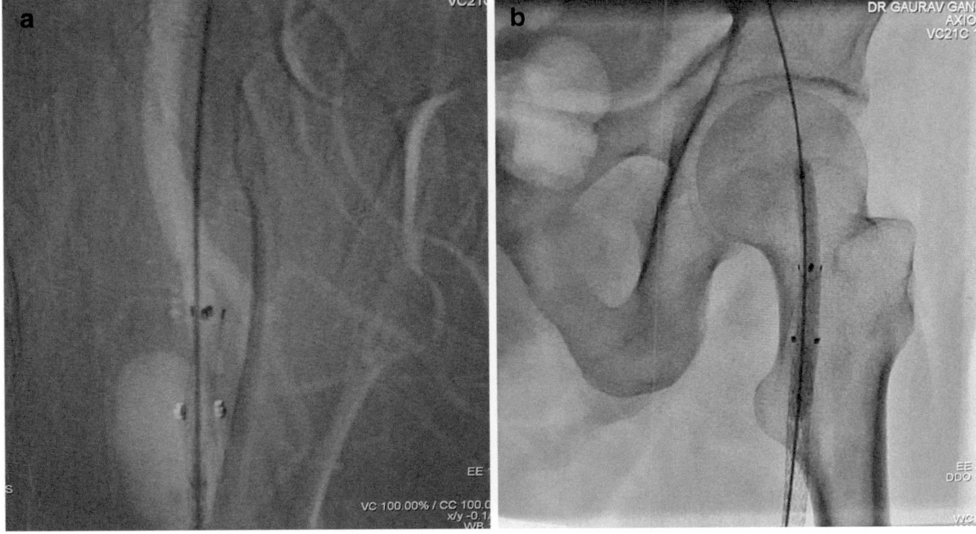

Fig. 17.3 (**a**) Road map image of right groin in lateral projection reveals proximal stent graft deployment with proximal extent distal to CFA bifurcation preventing jailing of profunda but proximal to the entry zone/flap of the aneurysm. (**b**) AP fluoroscopic projection of right hip with balloon dilatation within the proximal stent graft for sealing the entry zone

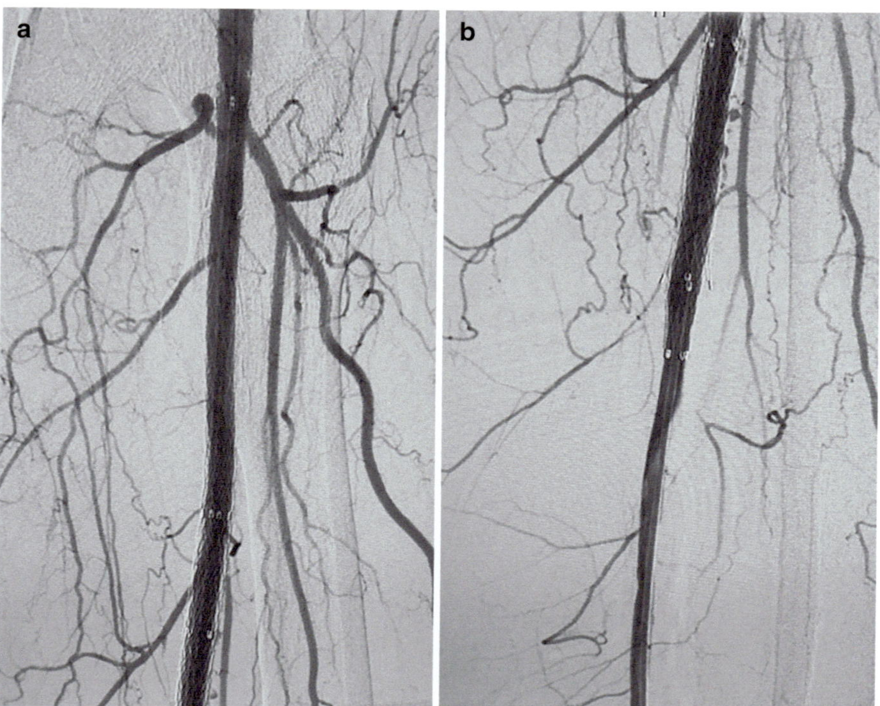

Fig. 17.4 (**a**) Right common femoral angiogram (DSA) suggestive of good antegrade flow across superficial femoral artery and complete occlusion or non-opacification of the aneurysm. (**b**) Right common femoral angiogram (DSA) with projection at level of distal SFA suggestive of good antegrade flow across distal superficial femoral artery and stent graft and complete occlusion or non-opacification of the aneurysm

"Musashi" Snuffbox Access for Simultaneous Arterial and Venous Access

Uei Pua

A 64-year-old with history of colo-rectal cancer was referred for microwave ablation of a solitary metastasis to the right adrenal gland. As the mass was partially encasing the inferior vena cava (IVC) (Fig. 18.1) and to allow for complete ablation without inadvertent IVC perforation, an imaging catheter was placed in the IVC (Fig. 18.2) to allow for contrast opacification during probe placement under CT fluoroscopy. Together with a need for intra-arterial blood pressure monitoring as a standard for adrenal ablation, decision was made for dual arterial and venous access over the anatomical snuffbox, an access we termed "Musashi Access."

Under US guidance, a vena comitans of the distal radial artery was first accessed within the anatomic snuffbox of the

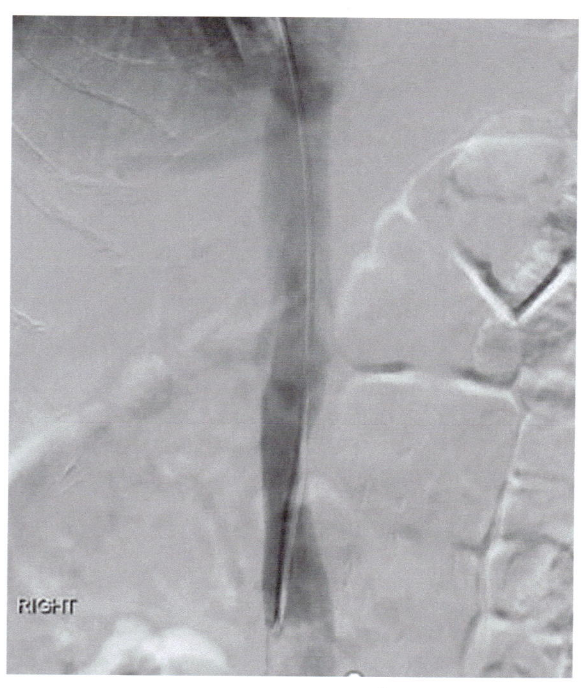

Fig. 18.2 Fluoroscopic image of the catheter position caudal to the region of ablation to allow good opacification of the IVC

left hand, using a trans-radial sheath set (5F Glidesheath Slender, Terumo, Tokyo, Japan), this was followed insertion of a 5F, 125 cm long catheter (Ultimate 1, Merit Medical, UT) with the tip positioned over L3 vertebral body (Figs. 18.3 and 18.4). A second sheath set was then used to access and place an arterial sheath in the distal radial artery using standard technique (Figs. 18.3 and 18.4). This was used for intra-arterial blood pressure monitoring. Two microwave ablation probes (PR 15; NeuWave Medical, Madison Wisconsin, USA) was positioned in a criss-cross fashion straddling the IVC under CT fluoroscopic guidance with intermittent IVC opacification (Fig. 18.5) by injection contrast through the diagnostic catheter. Complete ablation was achieved (Fig. 18.6) and the patient was discharged well.

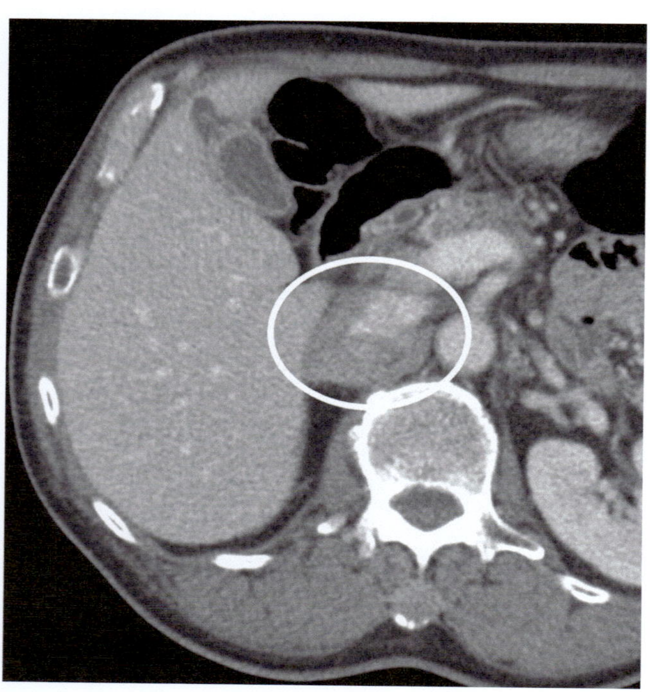

Fig. 18.1 CT image of the right adrenal metastasis partially encasing the IVC (circle)

U. Pua (✉)
Department of Diagnostic Radiology, Tan Tock Seng Hospital, Singapore, Singapore

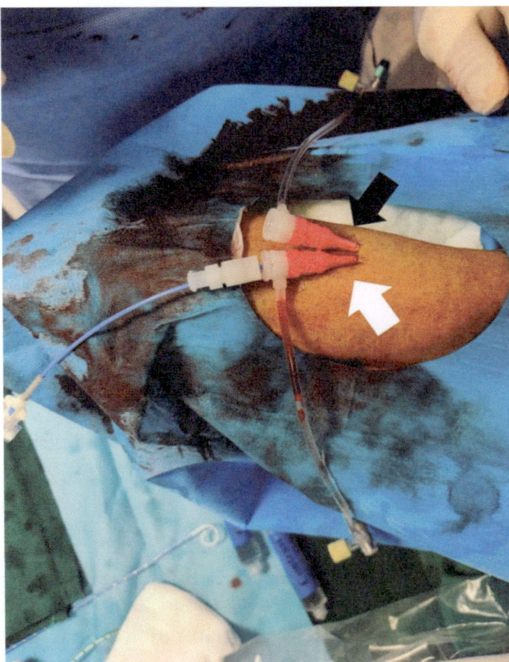

Fig. 18.3 Intra-operative picture of the left anatomical snuffbox with two radial sheaths in situ, in the distal radial artery (black arrow) and a vena comitans (white arrow) with a diagnostic catheter in situ

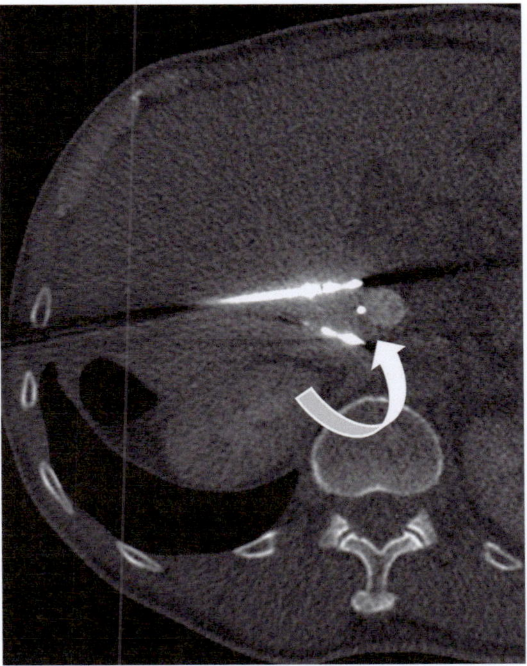

Fig. 18.5 Intra-operative CT image showing opacification of the IVC by injection of 10 cc of diluted contrast through the diagnostic venous catheter (curved arrow). Criss-cross placement of the microwave probes allowed for complete ablation of the tumor

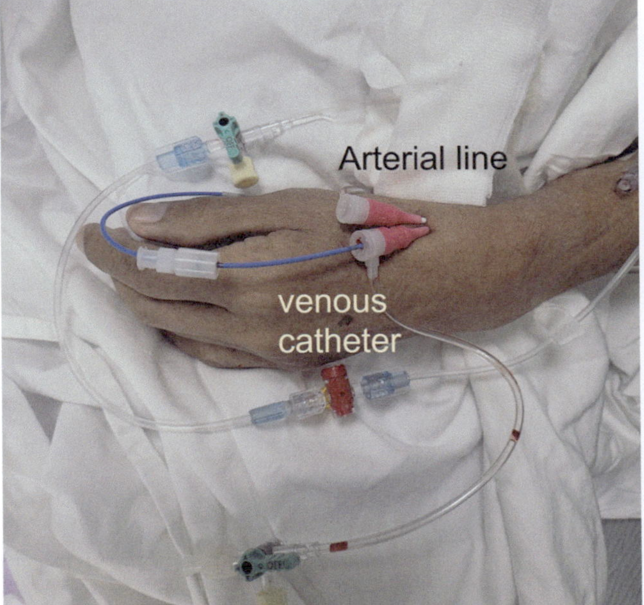

Fig. 18.4 Clinical photo of the dual access over the anatomical snuffbox. The access was closed using standard radial compression band

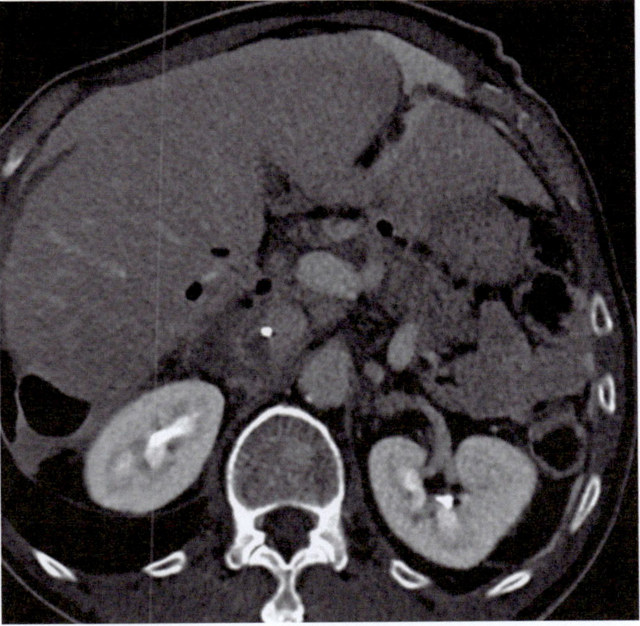

Fig. 18.6 Completion CT showing non-enhancement of the tumor consistent with complete ablation

This access is nicknamed after Miyamoto Musashi, who was a well-known samurai famous for his technique of using two swords to fight simultaneously.

Modified SAFARI Technique: Using a Re-entry Device and a Target Balloon to Connect Antegrade and Retrograde Subintimal Lumina

Athanasios Diamantopoulos and Romman Nourzaei

An 82-year-old man with chronic limb-threatening ischemia (CLTI), and ulcers, was referred for endovascular revascularization of his occluded popliteal artery following occlusion of a superficial femoral artery to proximal anterior tibial artery (ATA) bypass. His comorbidities included hypertension and dyslipidemia.

Using a 7Fr antegrade access, digital subtraction angiography (DSA) showed occlusion of the P2/P3 segments of the popliteal artery and proximal ATA with reconstitution at the distal anastomosis of the occluded bypass (Fig. 19.1a, b). Multiple intraluminal and subintimal attempts to cross the native artery through both antegrade and retrograde ATA approaches were unsuccessful despite the use of an antegrade re-entry device, resulting in two unconnected lumina (Fig. 19.2a). These were then bridged using a modified SAFARI technique. A 4 mm diameter × 40 mm long angioplasty balloon (Cook Medical, In, USA) was advanced retrograde from the ATA access whilst a re-entry "outback" catheter (CORDIS, Ca, USA) was advanced antegrade to the P1 segment. The balloon was inflated and the re-entry device was used to puncture it, thus connecting the subintimal planes (Fig. 19.2b). A 0.014″ STABILIZER ™ Plus Guidewire (Cordis, Ca, USA) was looped into the ruptured balloon and advanced out of the distal access (Fig. 19.2c). Thereafter, the guidewire was manipulated into the distal ATA. The occlusion was treated with antegrade angioplasty and two 5.5 mm diameter × 150 mm long overlapping SUPERA stents (ABBOTT, Il, USA) (Fig. 19.3a). Final DSA showed excellent flow with increased perfusion to the foot (Fig. 19.3b). Dual antiplatelet therapy (Aspirin 75 mg/d and Clopidogrel 75 mg/d) was begun. At 6-week follow-up the ulcers had become dry and demonstrated good healing.

A. Diamantopoulos (✉)
Department of Interventional Radiology, Guy's and St. Thomas'
NHS Foundation Trust, London, UK

School of Biomedical Engineering and Imaging Sciences, Faculty of Life Sciences and Medicine, Kings College London, London, UK
e-mail: athanasios.diamantopoulos@nhs.net;
athanasios.diamantopoulos@gstt.nhs.uk

R. Nourzaei
Department of Interventional Radiology, Guy's and St. Thomas'
NHS Foundation Trust, London, UK
e-mail: Romman.Nourzair@gstt.nhs.uk

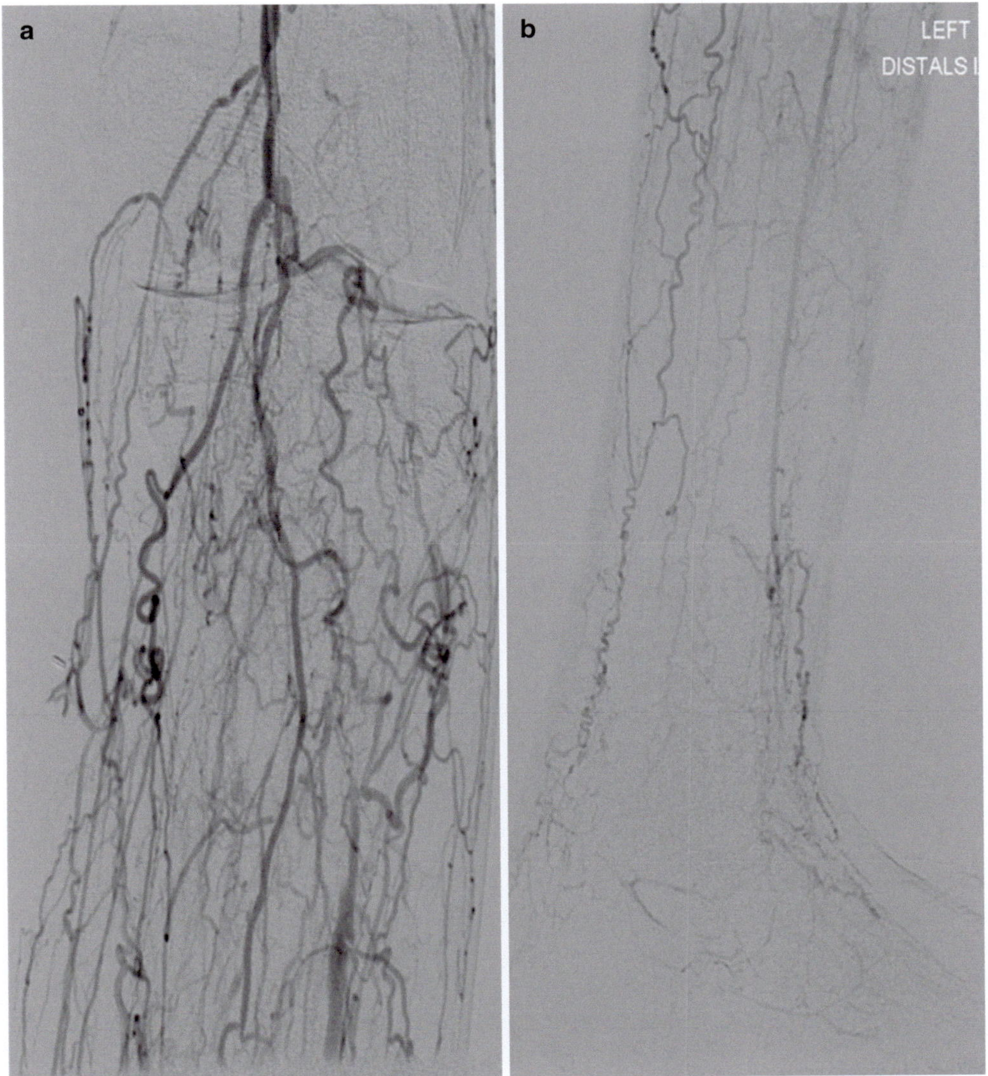

Fig. 19.1 Digital subtraction angiogram confirming (**a**), occlusion of the P2/P3 segments of the popliteal and proximal ATA (**b**). The mid ATA was patent with occlusion in its distal segment

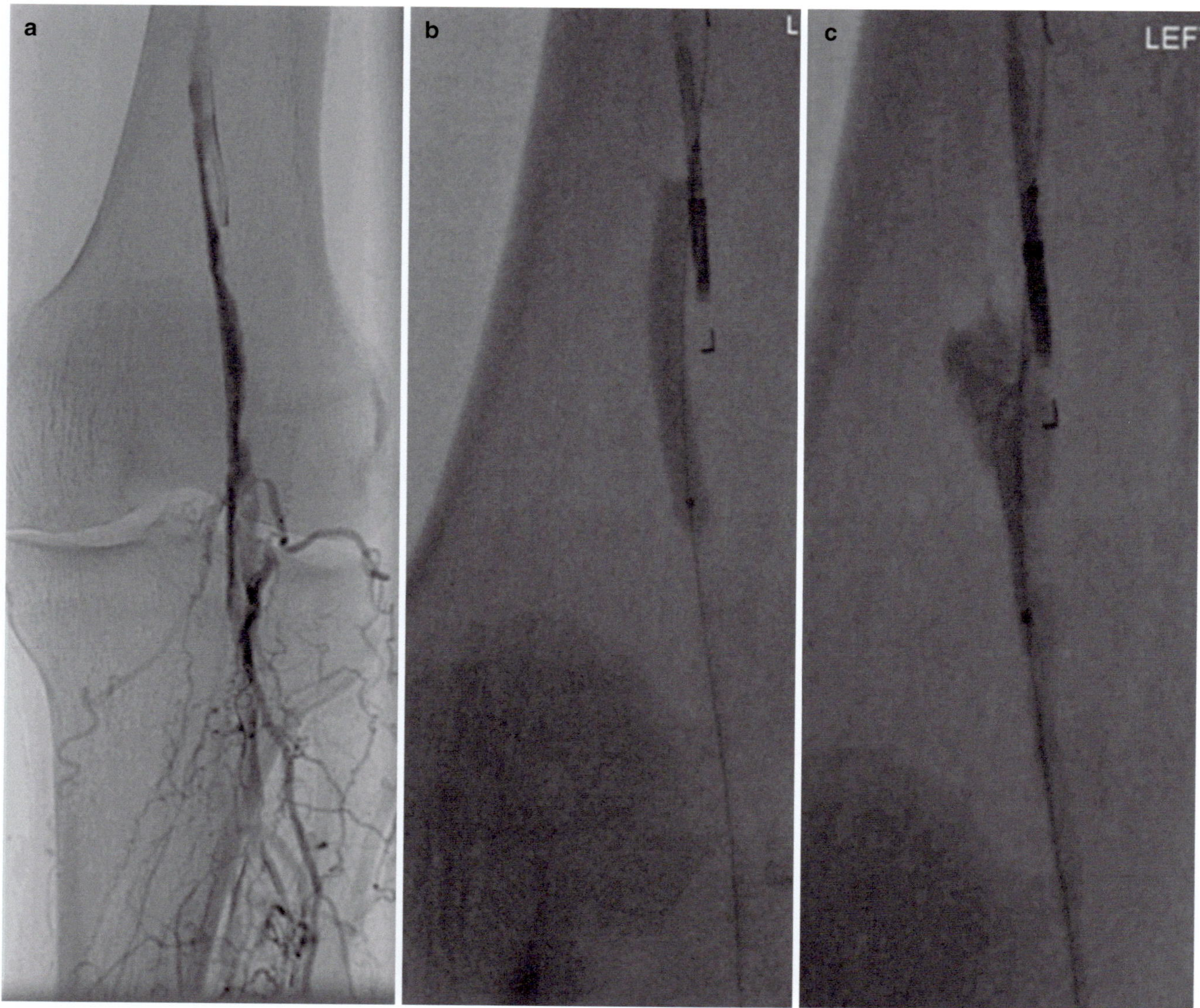

Fig. 19.2 Two nonconnected subintimal lumens following unsuccessful re-entry from both accesses (**a**). Re-entry catheter in the antegrade subintimal space at the level of P1 and inflated balloon in the retrograde subintimal space (**b**). Ruptured balloon with wire looped in it achieving connection of the subintimal lumens planes (**c**)

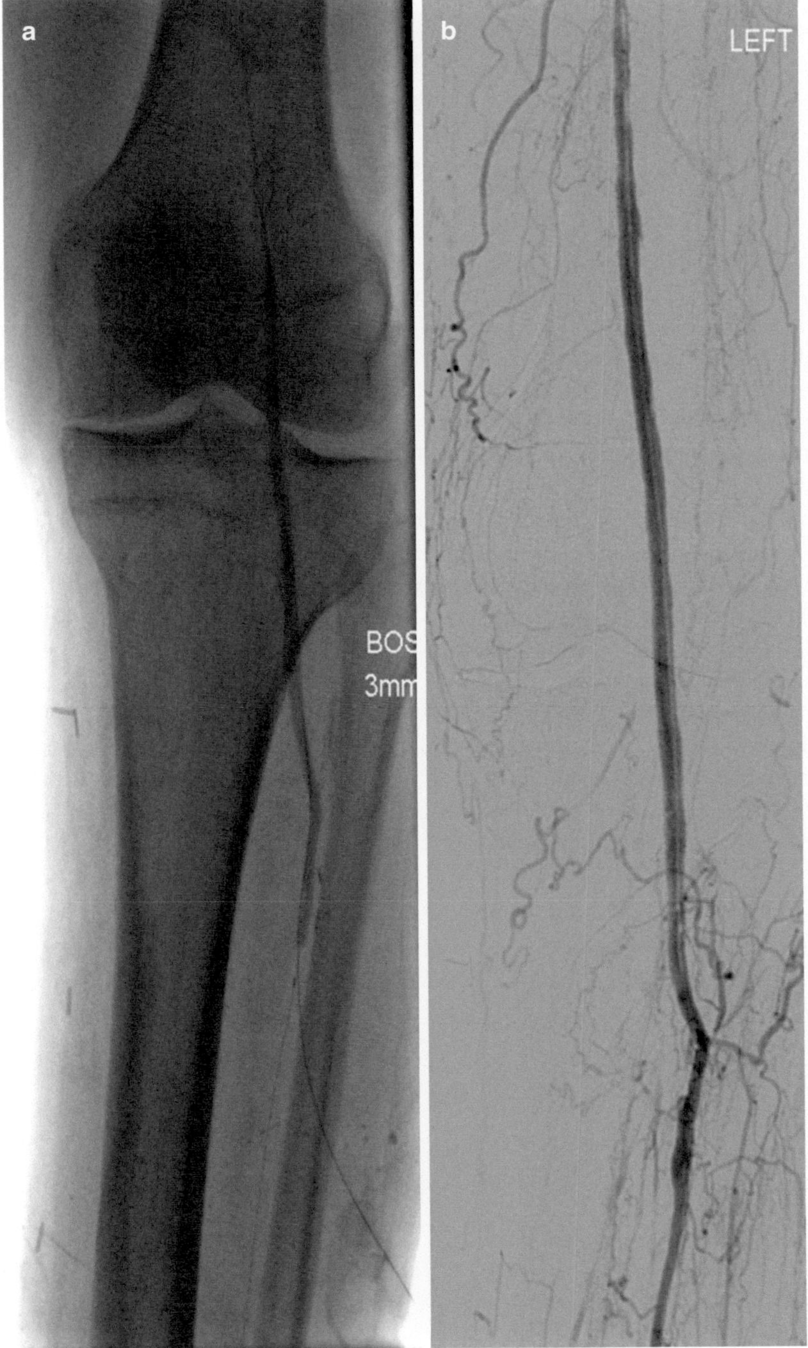

Fig. 19.3 The occlusion was then stented following Balloon angioplasty (**a**). Final DSA showed excellent flow through the previous occluded segment (**b**)

Carotid Retrograde Rescue through the Anterior Communicating Artery

Carlos Eduardo Baccin and Rafael Trindade Tatit

A 49-year-old man with hypertension presented with amaurosis fugax in the left eye and was diagnosed with occlusion of the left internal carotid artery (ICA) due to an arterial dissection. Dual antiplatelet therapy was started, leading to recanalization of the vessel and development of a cervical pseudoaneurysm diagnosed by MR angiography (10 mm diameter and 25 mm extension). Therefore, an interventional procedure was indicated.

The procedure was performed using a right transfemoral artery approach, under general anesthesia. A 6Fr Shuttle sheath was placed in the left ICA and a Derivo (flow diverter) stent (6.0 mm × 50 mm) delivered covering the pseudoaneurysm (Fig. 20.1a, b) [1, 2]. However, the proximal end spontaneously occluded (the so-called fish mouth phenomenon), requiring the infusion of intravenous abciximab to restore the flow though the left internal carotid artery. A left femoral access was required to navigate a shuttle sheath and a distal access catheter in the right ICA and a microcatheter with a 0.14 microguidewire through the anterior communicating artery (Fig. 20.1c), obtaining retrograde access to open the proximal stent end that had migrated into the pseudoaneurysm. Then, in an anterograde manner, a microcatheter and microguidewire were advanced into the stent lumen to deliver a new Derivo stent (6.0 mm × 40 mm) inside the existing one, extending to the proximal ICA. Finally, a Solitaire stent (6 mm × 20 mm) was also implanted to ensure the opening of the Derivo stent in the proximal ICA (Fig. 20.1d).

A few hours after the procedure, the patient developed a headache and reduced level of consciousness due to subarachnoid hemorrhage diagnosed by computed tomography (Fig. 20.2). Platelet transfusion was performed with recovery of the neurological status a few days later whilst maintaining dual antiplatelet therapy. The patient recovered well, without neurological deficits, and 6-month follow-up angiography showed exclusion of the pseudoaneurysm with patency of the adjacent ICA, with remodeling and recovery of its caliber (Fig. 20.3).

C. E. Baccin (✉)
Department of Interventional Neuroradiology, Hospital Israelita
Albert Einstein, São Paulo, São Paulo, Brazil

R. T. Tatit
Department of Medicine, Faculdade Israelita de Ciências da Saúde
Albert Einstein, São Paulo, São Paulo, Brazil

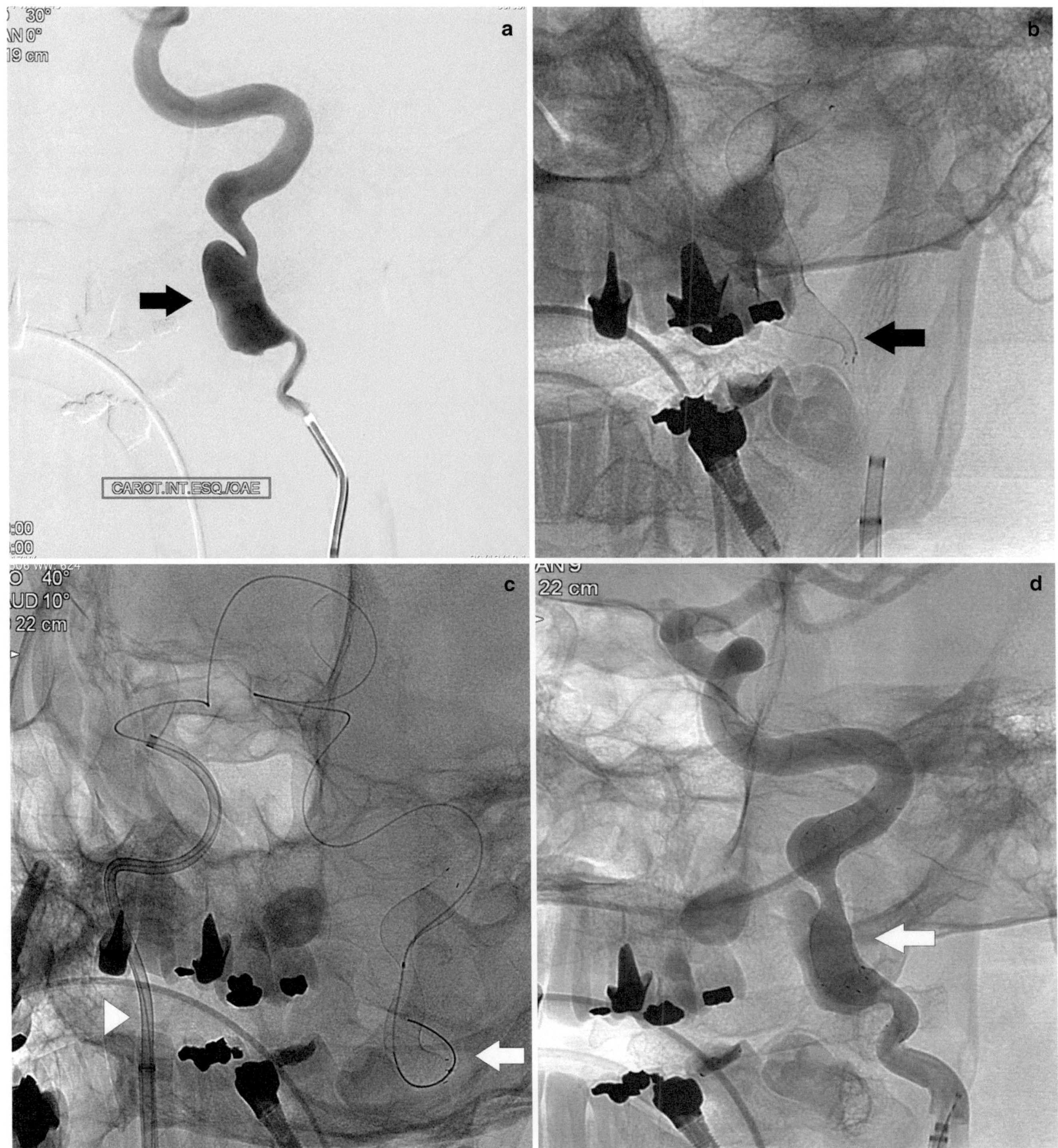

Fig. 20.1 (**a**, **b**) Digital subtraction angiography showing a 6Fr shuttle in the left ICA and a Derivo stent placed covering the pseudoaneurysm with its proximal end narrowed (arrow). (**c**) Digital subtraction angiography showing the left carotid retrograde rescue through the right ICA (arrowhead) and anterior communicating artery opening the proximal stent extremity that migrated into the pseudoaneurysm (arrow). (**d**) Digital subtraction angiography showing final result after delivery of multiple stents and coverage of the pseudoaneurysm neck (arrow)

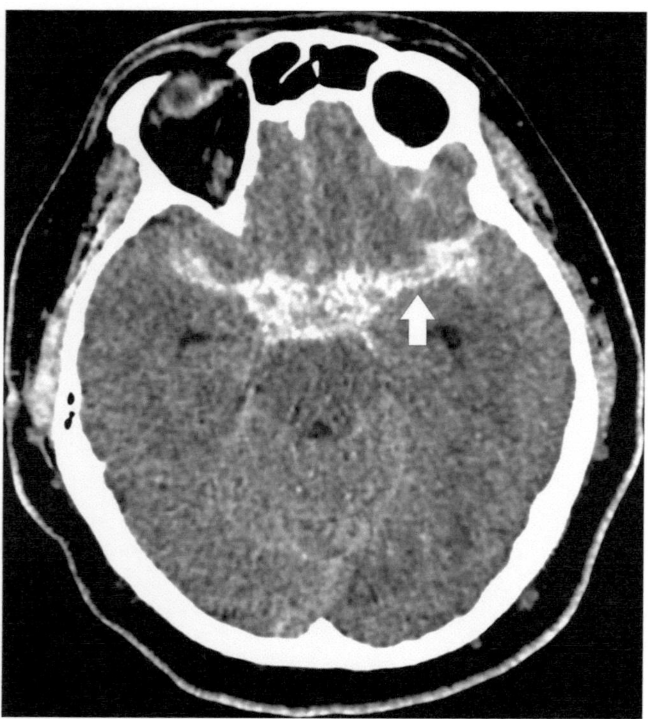

Fig. 20.2 Computed tomography imaging post-procedure demonstrating extensive subarachnoid hemorrhage (arrow)

Bibliography

1. Akgul E, Onan HB, Akpinar S, Balli HT, Aksungur EH. The DERIVO embolization device in the treatment of intracranial aneurysms: short- and midterm results. World Neurosurg. 2016;95:229–40. https://doi.org/10.1016/j.wneu.2016.07.101.
2. Martínez-Galdámez M, Rodríguez C, Hermosín A, et al. Internal carotid artery reconstruction with a "mega flow diverter": first experience with the 6×50 mm DERIVO embolization device. Neurointervention. 2018;13(2):133–7. https://doi.org/10.5469/neuroint.2018.00934.

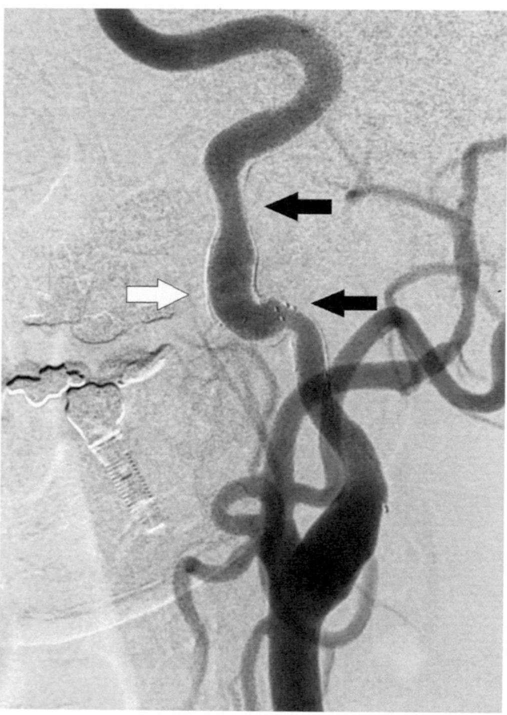

Fig. 20.3 Digital subtraction angiography 6-month follow-up showing exclusion of the pseudoaneurysm (white arrow), remodeling and recovery of the ICA's caliber (black arrows)

Combined Endovascular and "Minimally Invasive" Removal of Traumatic Nail Gun Injury to the Skull and Face

Zachary T. Berman, David R. Santiago-Dieppa, Jillian Plonsker, and Scott Olson

A 29-year-old male was assaulted with a pneumatic nail gun, implanting four intracranial and one extracranial nail into his skull (Fig. 21.1). He was intubated prior to arrival for decline in mental status, therefore no baseline neurologic exam was obtained.

After a non-contrast computed tomography scan was obtained, a multidisciplinary decision was made to attempt extraction of the nails in the angiography suite to allow for immediate vessel embolization in the event of hemorrhage. Initial digital subtraction and rotational cone beam angiograms were obtained demonstrating injury to the left internal maxillary artery (Fig. 21.2a), but no obvious injury to the intracranial anterior circulation arteries (Fig. 21.3a, b). The extracranial nail was removed and brisk hemorrhage from the nail tract was encountered clinically as well as on angiography (Fig. 21.2b). Embolization was performed at the level of the injury with pushable microcoils through the prepositioned microcatheter which resolved the hemorrhage (Fig. 21.2c).

All intracranial nails were removed by making a small incision over the nail head and extracted using vise grip pliers (Fig. 21.3c). The nail tracts were irrigated with antibiotic saline and injected with hemostatic agents. No hemorrhage was encountered from the intracranial nail extraction sites. Repeat angiography confirmed that there was no intracranial extravasation as well (Fig. 21.3d). The scalp incisions were closed in the standard fashion.

Fig. 21.1 Anteroposterior skull radiograph demonstrating the four intracranial (arrows) and one extracranial nails (curved arrow)

The patient did well and was ambulatory upon discharge 7 days later with only minimal (4 out of 5) weakness in his right upper and lower extremities. His sensation was grossly intact. He was subsequently lost to follow-up.

Z. T. Berman (✉)
Department of Radiology, University of California, San Diego, La Jolla, CA, USA
e-mail: ZBerman@health.ucsd.edu

D. R. Santiago-Dieppa · J. Plonsker
Department of Neurosurgery, University of California, San Diego, La Jolla, CA, USA
e-mail: drsantiagodieppa@health.ucsd.edu;
jhplonsker@health.ucsd.edu

S. Olson
Department of Neurosurgery and Radiology, University of California, San Diego, La Jolla, CA, USA
e-mail: seolson@health.ucsd.edu

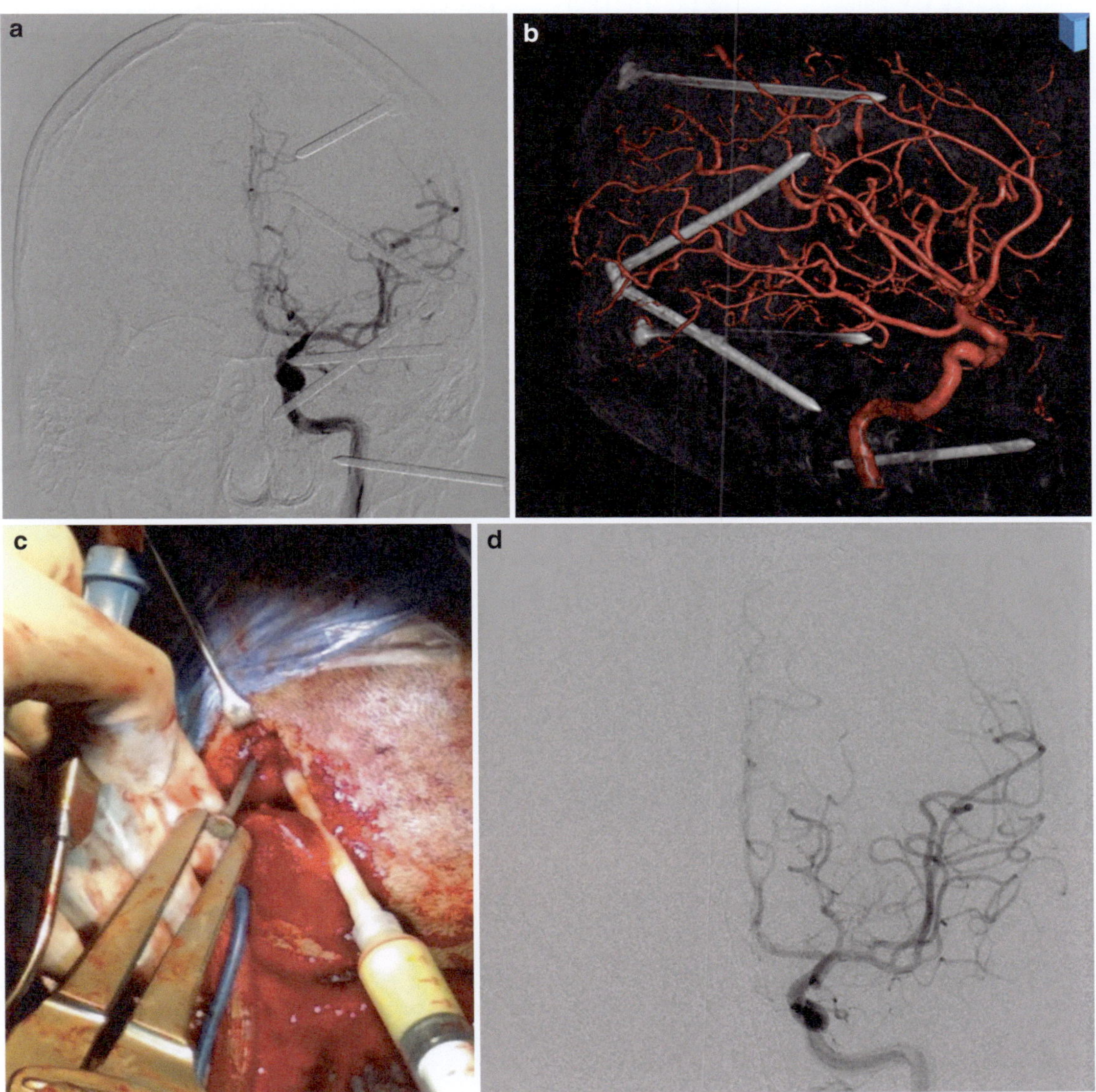

Fig. 21.2 (**a**) Digital subtraction angiogram (DSA) of the left internal maxillary artery demonstrates the extracranial nail traversing the expected path of the distal branches (arrow) (**b**) extravasation through the nail tract after removal (curved arrow) (**c**) post embolization DSA confirms resolution of the extravasation

Fig. 21.3 (**a**) DSA and (**b**) rotational cone beam angiography of the left anterior circulation demonstrates a normal appearance of the anterior and middle cerebral artery branches without extravasation prior to nail removal. (**c**) Nail removal within the interventional suite (**d**) DSA after nail removal shows no extravasation nor vessel occlusion

Common Carotid Artery Pseudoaneurysm

22

Thomas Barge and Raman Uberoi

A 73-year-old female presented with acute-on-chronic renal failure, pulmonary edema, and hyperkalemia. Past medical history included ischemic heart disease, and transient ischemic attacks, for which she had undergone prior right internal carotid stent placement. She was admitted for acute hemodialysis.

A right internal jugular vein (IJV) 14.5 French non-tunneled dual lumen dialysis catheter was inserted. Ultrasound was used to mark the site of insertion, but not used "real-time" during IJV puncture (Fig. 22.1a). The catheter was used uneventfully. Note the subtle leftward deviation of the trachea, most apparent when compared with a chest radiograph obtained 5 months earlier (Fig. 22.1b).

Due to ongoing dyspnea despite fluid removal during hemodialysis, a contrast-enhanced venous phase chest CT scan was obtained 3 days following insertion of the dialysis catheter. This demonstrated a 55 × 38 × 60 mm superior mediastinal mass abutting the right common carotid artery (CCA) and causing leftward displacement of the trachea (Fig. 22.2). The dialysis line was appropriately sited within the right IJV.

A CT angiogram performed shortly after the initial CT chest did not definitively demonstrate the origin of the mass and therefore a duplex ultrasound was performed. This demonstrated a partly thrombosed pseudoaneurysm arising from the right CCA, with a short 2 mm long neck, 5 mm in diameter (Fig. 22.3). A small CCA to IJV arteriovenous fistula was present (Fig. 22.3). This most likely arose following a through-and-through RIJ puncture during the insertion of the dialysis catheter.

Due to the interval partial thrombosis of the sac between the initial CT and duplex US, which were performed 1 day apart, the pseudoaneurysm was initially managed conservatively. Direct sac thrombin injection was considered high risk due to the short neck and risk of distal thrombosis or embolization into the right CCA. Serial sonography over a 3-month period showed no interval sac size reduction, and a persistent patent central component. We decided to stent the right CCA to cover both the pseudoaneurysm neck and arteriovenous fistula.

Using a right common femoral approach, a single Proglide closure device (Abbott Laboratories, Chicago, USA) was

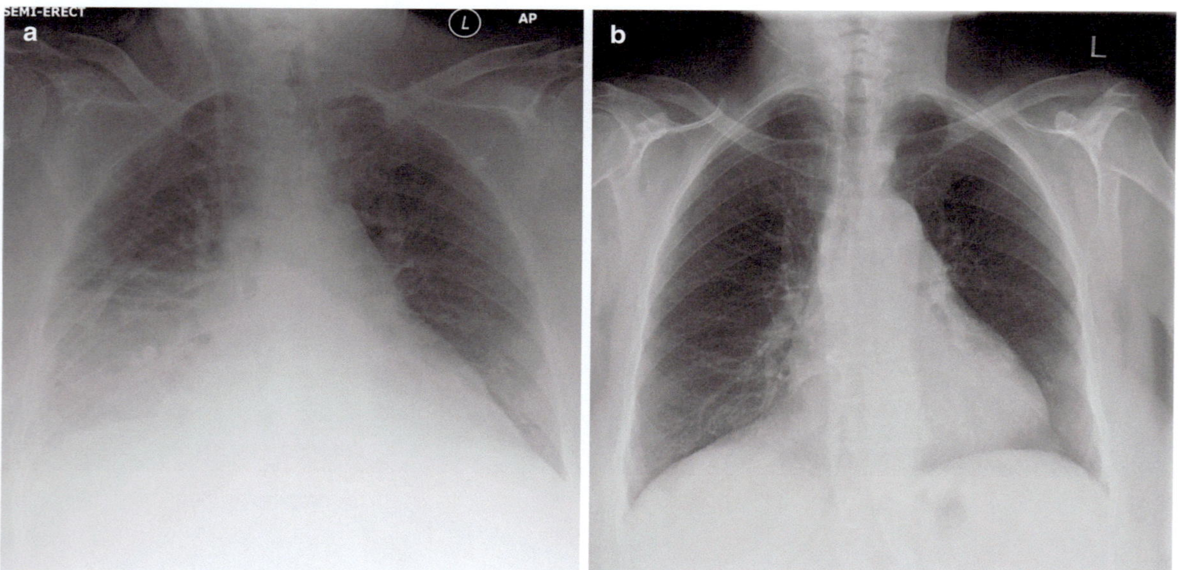

Fig. 22.1 (**a**) Chest radiograph (CXR) following insertion of the right internal jugular non-tunneled hemodialysis catheter. Note the leftward deviation of the trachea. (**b**) Comparison CXR from 5 months earlier demonstrates the central position of the trachea

T. Barge · R. Uberoi (✉)
Department of Radiology, John Radcliffe Hospital,
Oxford, Oxon, UK
e-mail: Tom.Barge@doctors.org.uk; raman.uberoi@ouh.nhs.uk

Z. J. Haskal (ed.), *Extreme IR*, https://doi.org/10.1007/978-3-031-24251-9_22

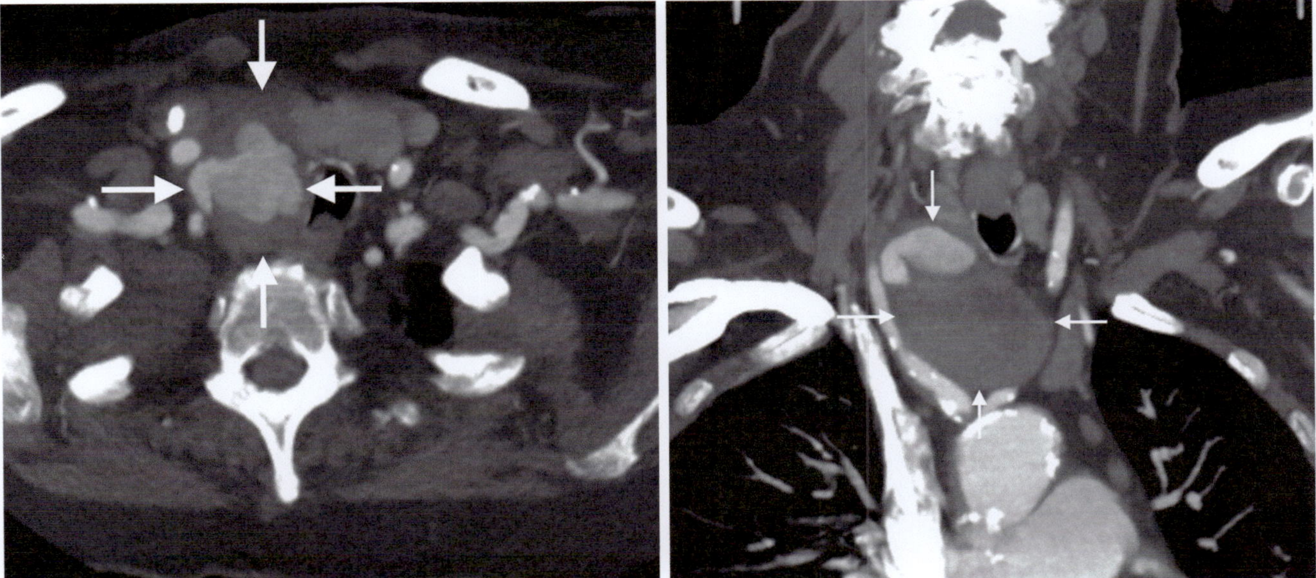

Fig. 22.2 Axial and coronal maximum intensity projection CT image demonstrates a portion of the enhancing right superior mediastinal mass (arrowed) and the presence of the RIJ dialysis catheter

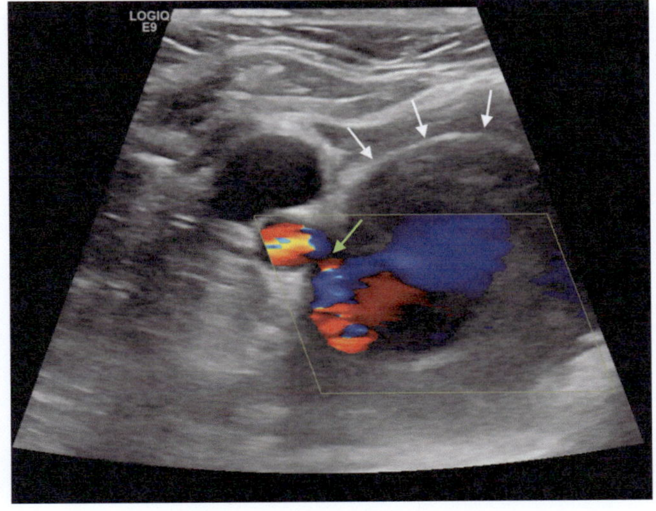

Fig. 22.3 Duplex sonography shows the short neck of the right CCA pseudoaneurysm (Green arrow) and IJV arteriovenous fistula. White arrows delineate the anterior border of the partly thrombosed pseudoaneurysm. The jugular vein is seen at the upper left (without color)

pre-deployed and a 6 French sheath inserted. A 5F Berenstein catheter was navigated to the right common carotid artery. Digital subtraction angiography demonstrated filling of the pseudoaneurysm from the right CCA, and a persistently patent sac (Fig. 22.4). 5000 units of heparin were administered and the sheath was exchanged for a 10 French 45 cm Flexor sheath (Cook Medical, Bloomington, USA); its tip was placed in the proximal right common carotid artery. A 9 × 50 mm Viabahn covered stent (Gore Medical, Flagstaff, USA) was deployed in the common carotid, with cessation of filling of the pseudoaneurysm (Fig. 22.5). Hemostasis was achieved with the pre-deployed Proglide, augmented by a 6 French Angioseal (Terumo Corporation, Tokyo, Japan).

She was prescribed a 6-month course of dual antiplatelet therapy with aspirin and clopidogrel, followed by lifelong clopidogrel. She remains dialysis dependent via a tunneled long-term left IJV dialysis catheter. A follow-up CT performed 5 months following stent placement confirms continued thrombosis of the pseudoaneurysm and patency of the stent (Fig. 22.6).

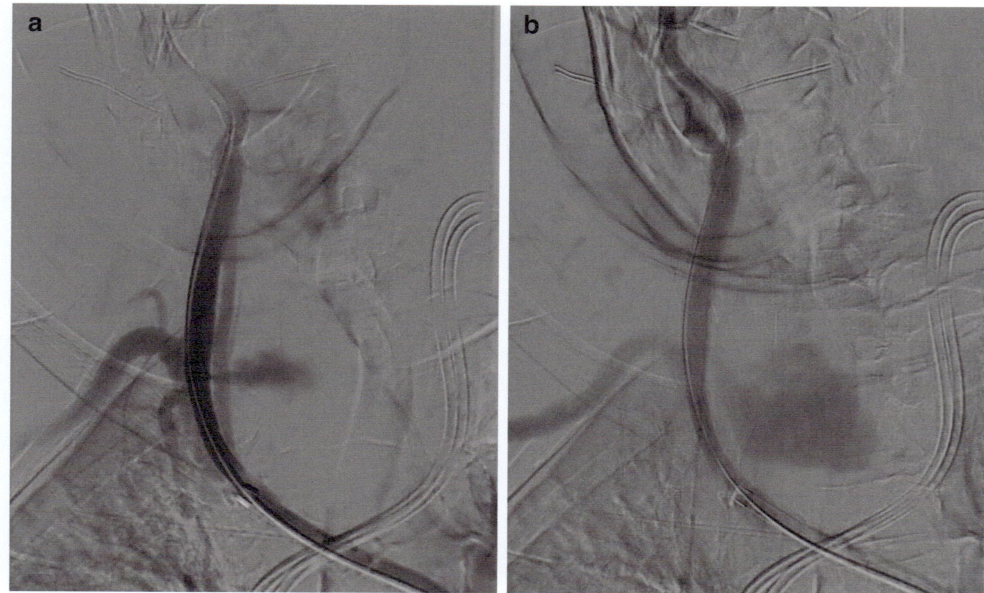

Fig. 22.4 (**a**) Digital subtraction angiogram (DSA) demonstrates a contrast jet from the right CCA into the pseudoaneurysm. Note the presence of an existing right ICA stent. (**b**) Slightly delayed DSA image demonstrating filling of the right CCA pseudoaneurysm sac

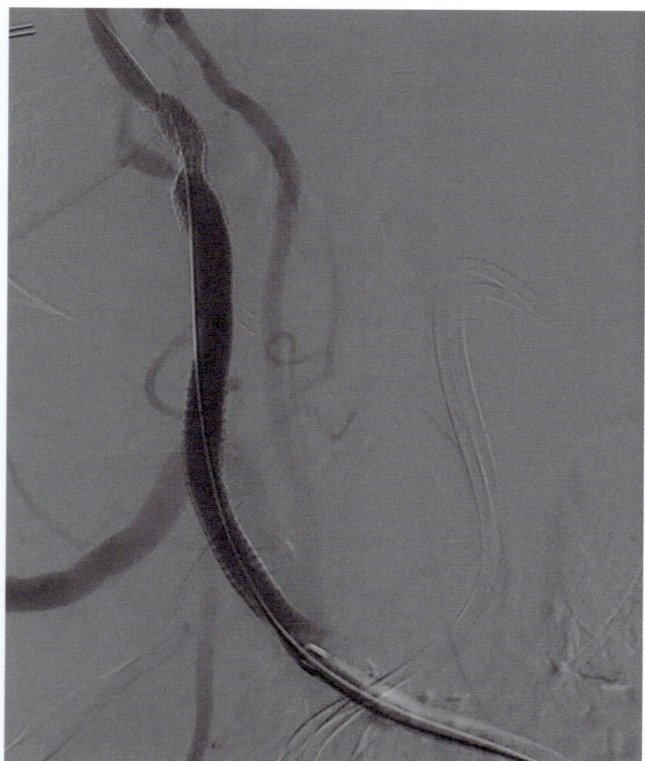

Fig. 22.5 Completion DSA shows the final position of the Gore Viabahn covered stent, covering the pseudoaneurysm neck and arteriovenous fistula

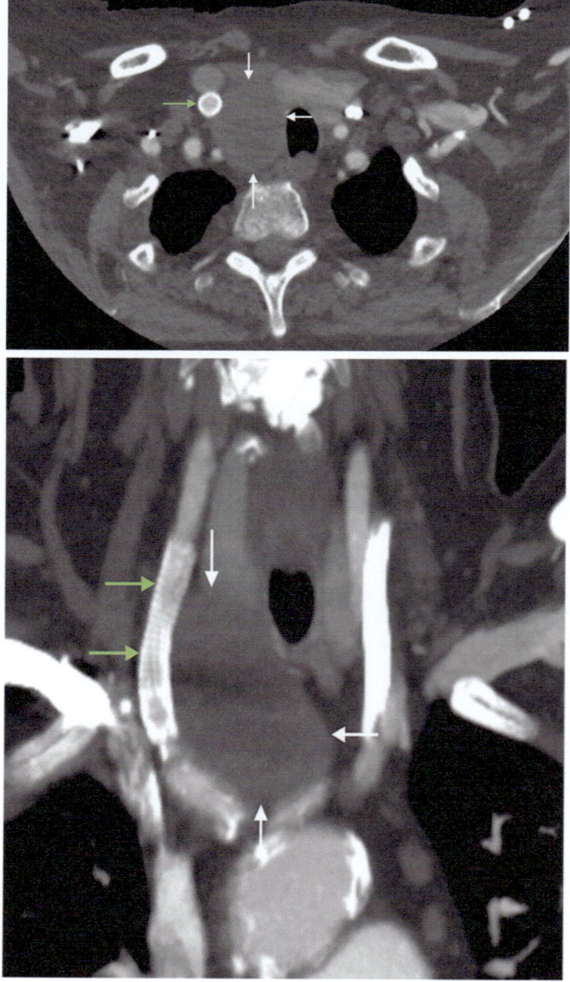

Fig. 22.6 Axial and coronal images from the 5-month follow-up CT image demonstrates the common carotid stent (Green arrows) and the thrombosed pseudoaneurysm

Ultrasonic Thrombectomy and Stent Placement for Life-Threatening SVC Syndrome in an Infant: Acute and Long-Term Outcomes

Ziv J Haskal

A 7-month-old infant girl with a protein losing enteropathy underwent surgical placement of a left subclavian tunneled catheter for total parenteral nutrition infusion at 2 months. Within 3 months hence, she developed progressive severe head, facial, upper extremity, periorbital, and lid edema (Fig. 23.1).

The catheter had withdrawn to abut the SVC (Fig. 23.2); sonography revealed the right and left internal jugular (IJ), and subclavian veins as thrombosed. By venography, the left and innominate vein and superior vein cava (SVC) were also occluded; these were recanalized with 3–6 mm angioplasty balloons (to expand the fibrin sheath), followed by ultrasonic thrombectomy device (OmniWave, OmniSonics Medical Technologies) (Fig. 23.3a) and repeat prolonged PTA (Fig. 23.3b) tPA was contraindicated due to coincidental gastrointestinal bleeding.

Despite anticoagulation, her swelling progressed over the next 2 days. All veins had re-thrombosed; despite repeat prolonged dilation, patency was not maintainable, thus 6 mm diameter by 60 mm long nitinol stent (SMART, Cordis) was placed, however thrombus remained as well as retrograde left IJ vein flow (Fig. 23.4). The stent was extended into the left IJ vein and brisk antegrade flow resulted (Fig. 23.5).

Facial swelling rapidly diminished, disappearing at 3 days. A 5Fr tunneled infusion catheter was placed through the IJ stent. For TPN. As an infant, she maintained a high percentile head circumference measurement (Fig. 23.6) and underwent one venogram several years later for transient symptoms. At 6- and 13-year follow-up (Fig. 23.7), she is healthy. An incidental chest radiograph showed separation and discontinuity of all the stent. Despite this, she remains free of any related symptoms or visible collateral veins (Fig. 23.8).

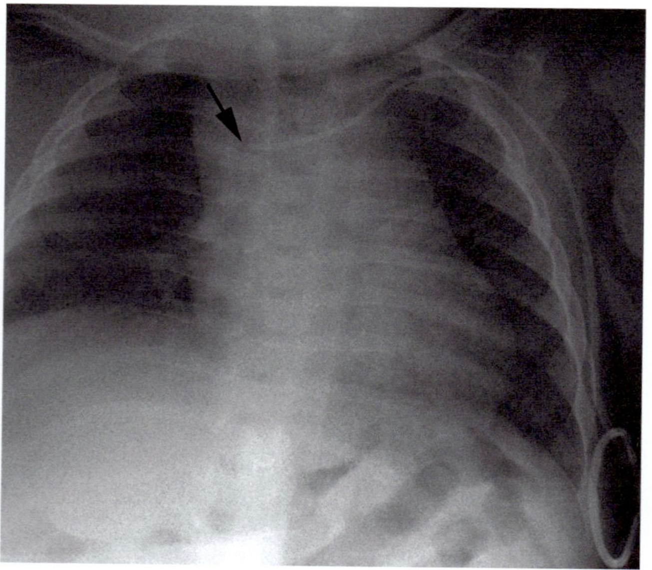

Fig. 23.1 Chest radiograph demonstrates the position of the left tunneled subclavian catheter. Its tip lay at the junction of the left innominate vein and SVC (arrow)

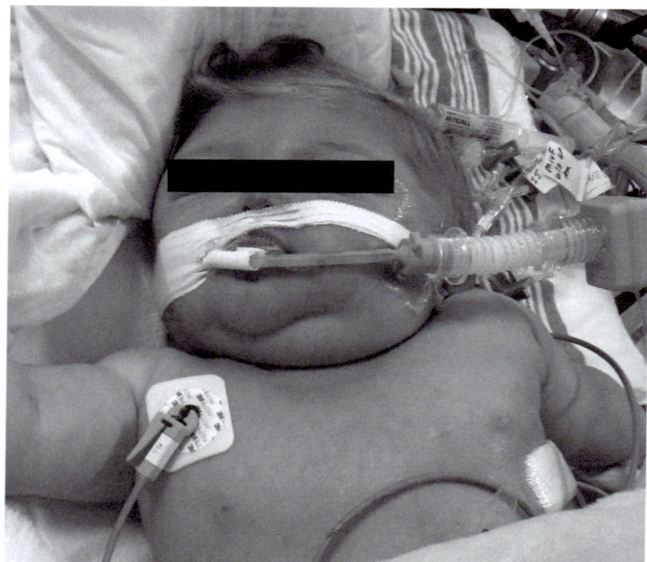

Fig. 23.2 Photograph of the infant at the peak of her superior vena cava (SVC) syndrome and upper extremity edema. Severe periorbital and facial swelling is present

Z. J Haskal (✉)
Department of Radiology and Medical Imaging, Interventional Division, University of Virginia, Charlottesville, VA, USA

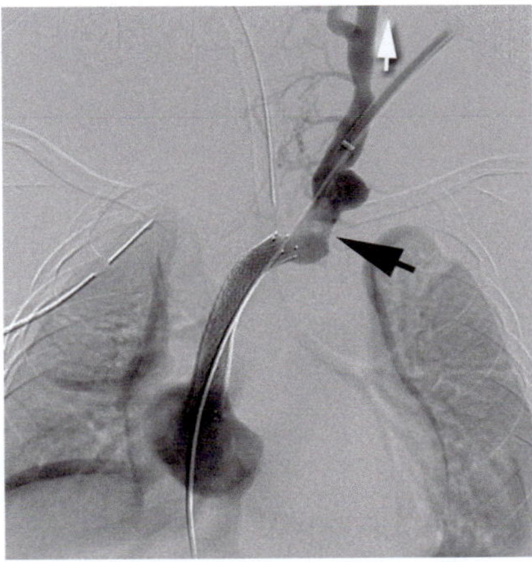

Fig. 23.3 (**a**) Left internal jugular venography demonstrates thrombus within the left internal, innominate and super vena cava, and a stenosis at the junction of the left internal jugular and innominate veins is seen (arrowhead). The OmniSonics catheter is positioned across the thrombus. (**b**) The left IJV stenosis has improved after angioplasty. Despite repeated dilation of the innominate vein and SVC, and boluses of heparin, complete recoil of the innominate/ SVC stenosis occurred, followed rethrombosis of the affected veins

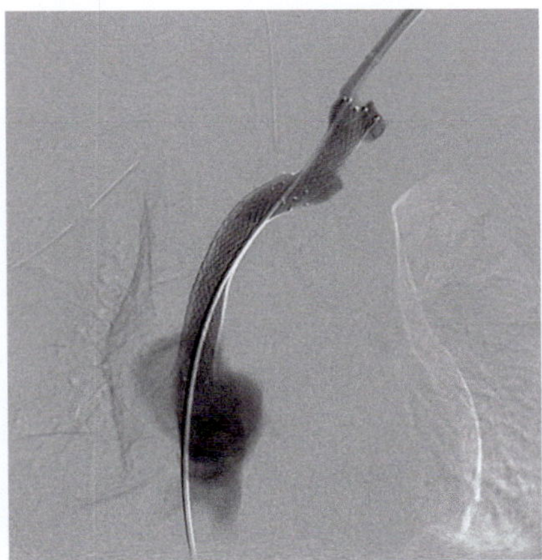

Fig. 23.4 After first stent placement into the innominate-SVC segment, there is prograde SVC flow, however clot reformed at the jugular stenosis (black arrow). Retrograde flow in the jugular is seen (white arrow)

Fig. 23.5 Brisk prograde decompressive flow is seen in this left internal jugular venogram, performed after placement of the coaxial second stent (extended across the jugular stenosis)

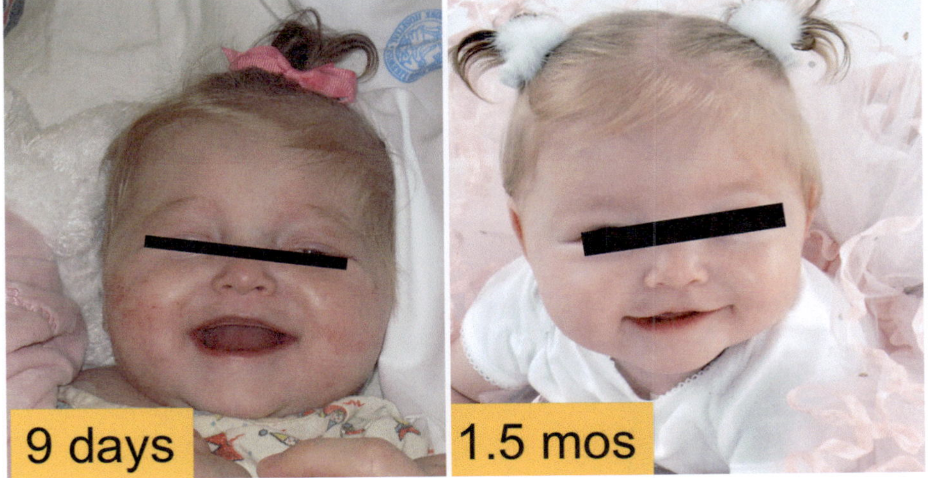

Fig. 23.6 At 9-day and 1.5-month follow-up, she was free of SVC syndrome symptoms

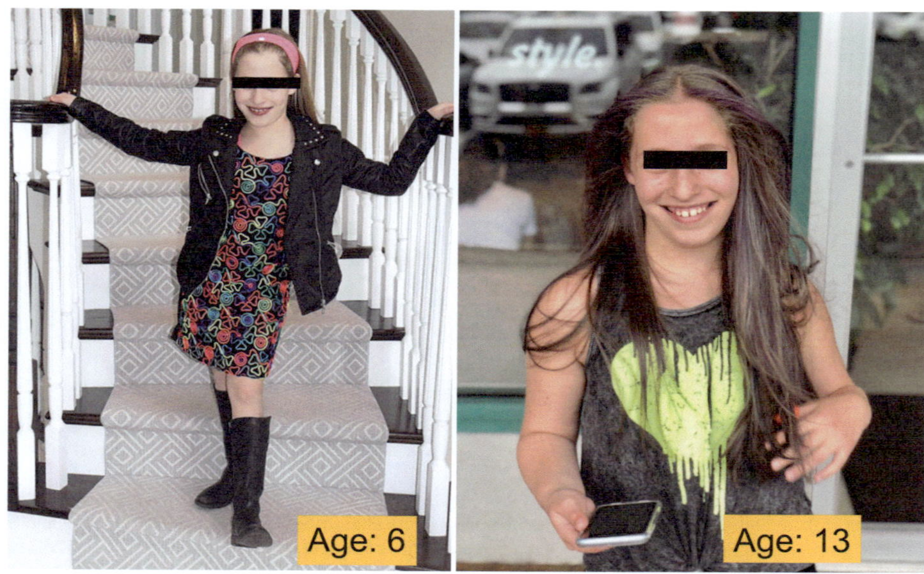

Fig. 23.7 At 6 and 13 years of age, she has had no symptom recurrence nor attributable symptoms

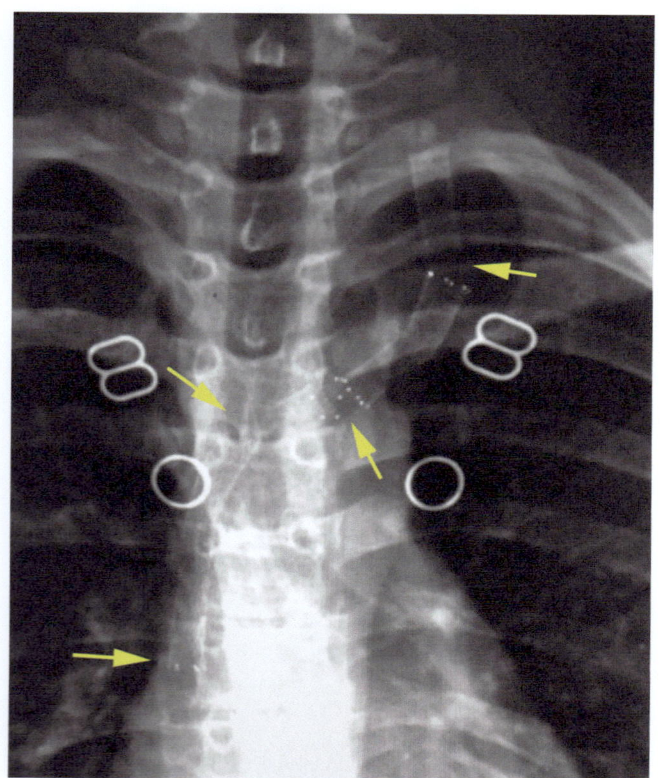

Fig. 23.8 A recent incidental chest radiograph shows complete disassociation of the stents, with gaps (arrows) between the stents, as the patient has grown to young adulthood. She remains free of symptoms

Bibliography

1. Gerling S, Klinge J, Singer H, Hofbeck M. Successful treatment of superior vena cava thrombosis in a neonate. Eur J Pediatr. 2002;161:466–7.
2. Hausler M, Hubner D, Hornchen H, Muhler EG, Merz U. Successful thrombolysis of inferior vena cava thrombolysis in a preterm neonate. Clin Pediatr (Phila). 2001;40:105–8.
3. Salonvaara M, Riikonen P, Kekomaki R, Heinonen K. Clinically symptomatic central venous catheter-related deep venous thrombosis in newborns. Acta Paediatr. 1999;88:642–6.
4. Tzifa A, Marshall AC, McElhinney DB, Lock JE, Geggel RL. Endovascular treatment for superior vena cava occlusion or obstruction in a pediatric and young adult population: a 22-year experience. J Am Coll Cardiol. 2007;49:1003–9.

Sharp Recanalization of Chronic Total Venous Occlusions of the Superior Vena Cava at the Cavoatrial Junction

Mohammad Arabi

An 18-year-old female with systemic lupus required chronic medication infusions through a subcutaneous implantable port for 5 years. She presented with a dysfunctional catheter due to chronic superior vena cava (SVC) occlusion. Central venography showed occlusion of the infra-azygos SVC to cavoatrial junction (Fig. 24.1a). Initial attempts to cross the occlusion were unsuccessful. After placing a loop snare within the right atrium as a target, sharp recanalization of the occluded SVC was performed using a gently curved 22 g Chiba needle inserted via a 5 Fr braided sheath in the jugular vein access (Fig. 24.1b). Using the resultant through-and-through wire, a transjugular 5 mm balloon and 10 mm diameter transfemoral balloon expandable stent graft (Lifestream, Bard, USA) were introduced. This allowed for immediate stent deployment after initial angioplasty to minimize the risk of potential SVC rupture and pericardial tamponade ("balloon-stent chain" technique) (Fig. 24.1c, d). The stent was post-dilated to 12 mm, and final venography showed restored direct flow into the right atrium. (Fig. 24.1e) The tip of the port-A-cath was repositioned into the SVC after stent placement. The SVC stent required few angioplasty procedures to maintain patency, and the catheter remains functional five years after the index procedure.

M. Arabi (✉)
Medical Imaging Department, King Abdulaziz Medical City,
Ministry of National Guard Health Affairs, Riyadh, Saudi Arabia

Z. J. Haskal (ed.), *Extreme IR*, https://doi.org/10.1007/978-3-031-24251-9_24

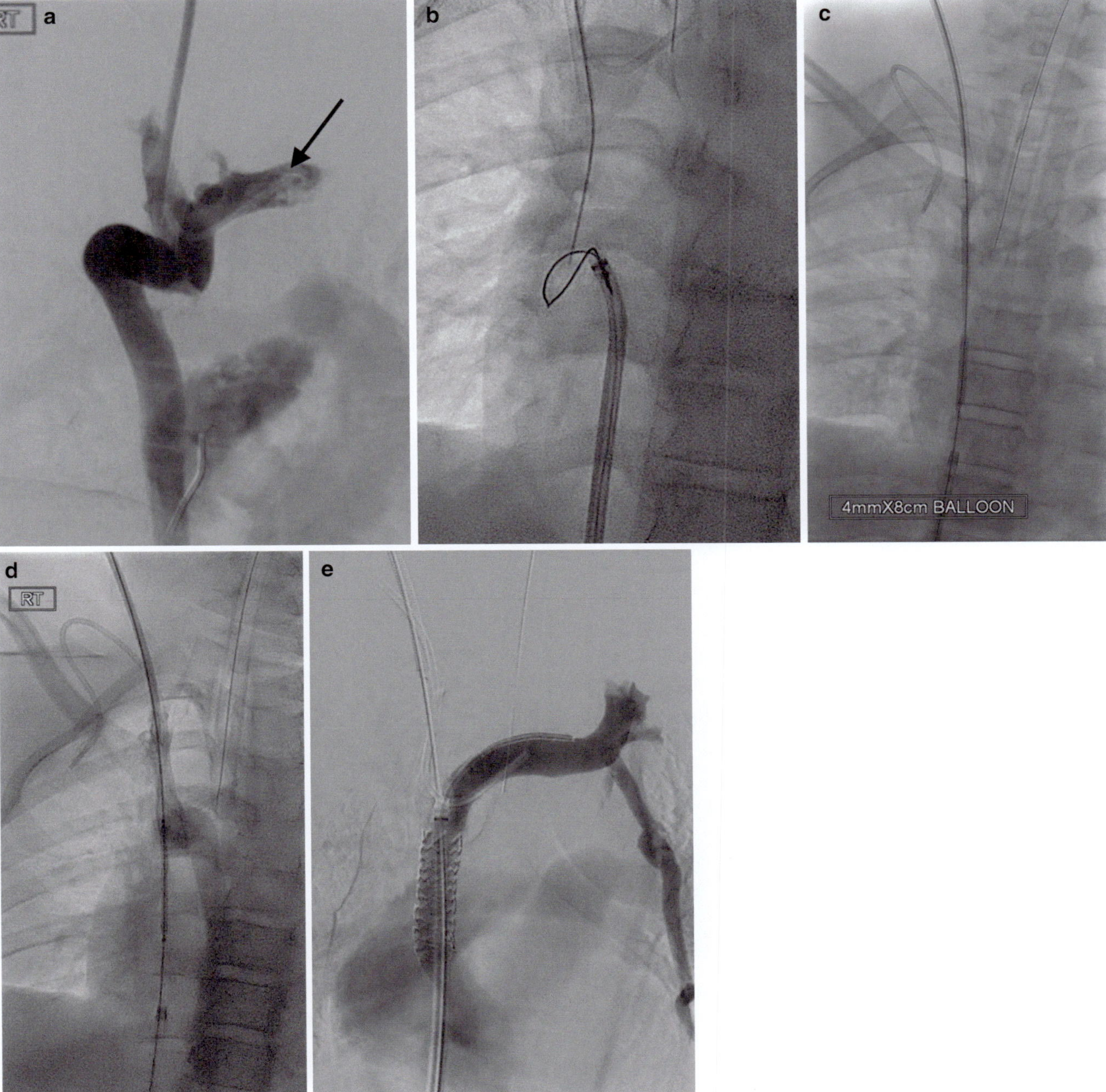

Fig. 24.1 (a) Simultaneous central venography from the jugular and femoral accesses showed long segment of infra-azygos SVC occlusion involving the cavoatrial junction. The tip of the port-A-cath (arrow) was positioned in the left brachiocephalic vein prior to the attempted recanalization. (b) Single shot shows the Chiba needle targeting the snare in the right atrium. (c) Predilatation of the trans mediastinal tract using a 5 mm balloon introduced over the floss wire. (d) Demonstrates the balloon mounted stent graft positioned across the recanalized SVC segment over the same floss wire immediately after removal of the predilatation balloon. (e) Completion venography shows patent stent with no extravasation. The tip of the port-A-cath was repositioned into the SVC after the stent placement (not shown)

Balloon Targeted Sharp Recanalization and Neo-SVC Reconstruction Via Transhepatic Access

Kyle Pate and Saher Sabri

A 37-year-old male with end-stage renal disease presented with prior failed attempted thrombectomy of a right-sided Hero graft (Merit Medical, South Jordan, UT). CT venography demonstrated chronic occlusion of the superior vena cava (SVC), brachiocephalic, external iliac, and common femoral veins with extensive calcifications (Fig. 25.1a, b).

A staged recanalization and SVC reconstruction and recreation of the Hero graft was planned. Initial attempts to recanalize the SVC via an antegrade approach from the right neck were unsuccessful (Fig. 25.2). Due to calcified long segment iliac vein occlusions, a trans-hepatic access was obtained.

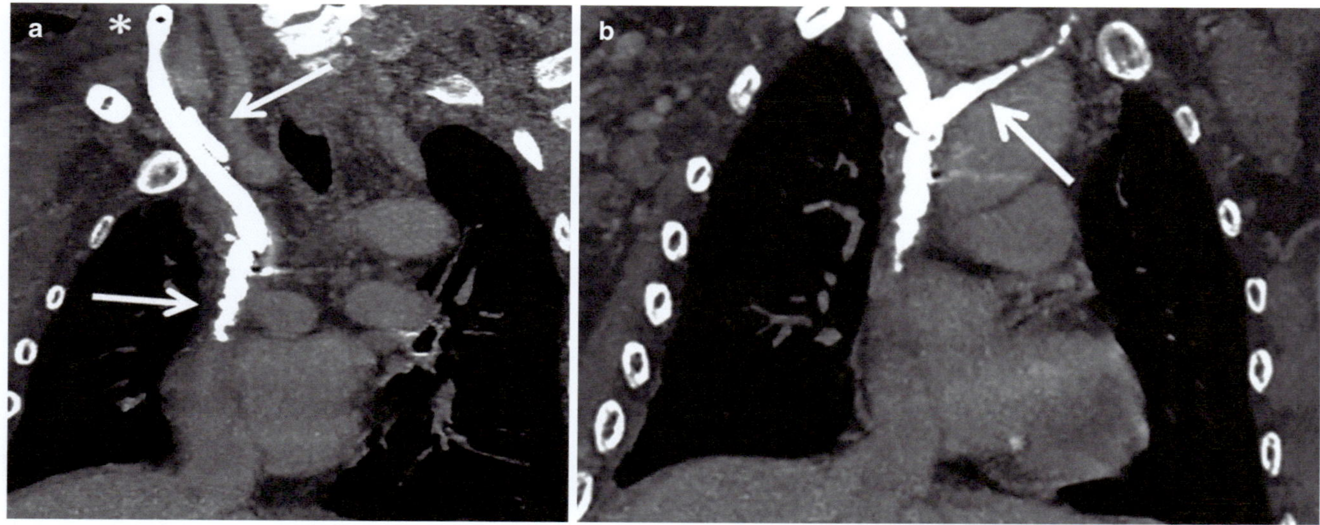

Fig. 25.1 (**a**) Coronal oblique MIP reformat showing chronic occlusion of the SVC and right brachiocephalic vein with calcifications (arrows). Air within the occluded Hero graft (*) is related to a recent thrombectomy attempt. (**b**) Coronal MIP reformat showing chronic occlusion of the left brachiocephalic vein with calcifications (arrow)

K. Pate · S. Sabri (✉)
Department of Interventional Radiology, MedStar Georgetown University Hospital, Washington, DC, USA
e-mail: saher.s.sabri@medstar.net

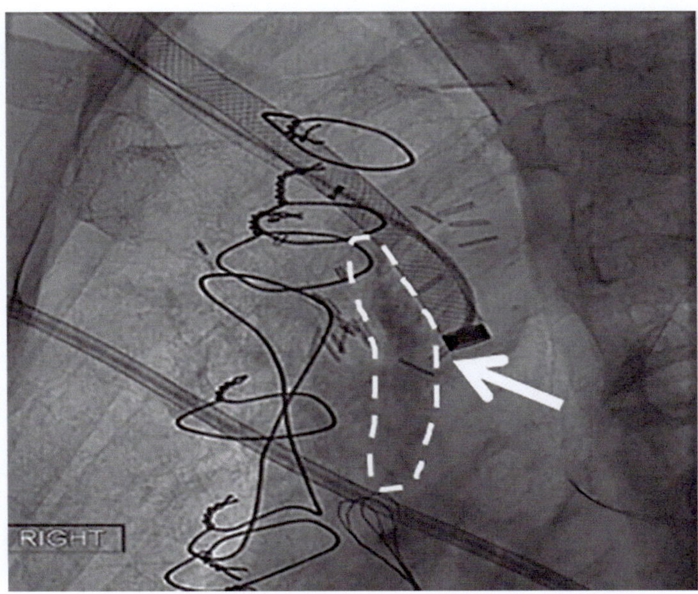

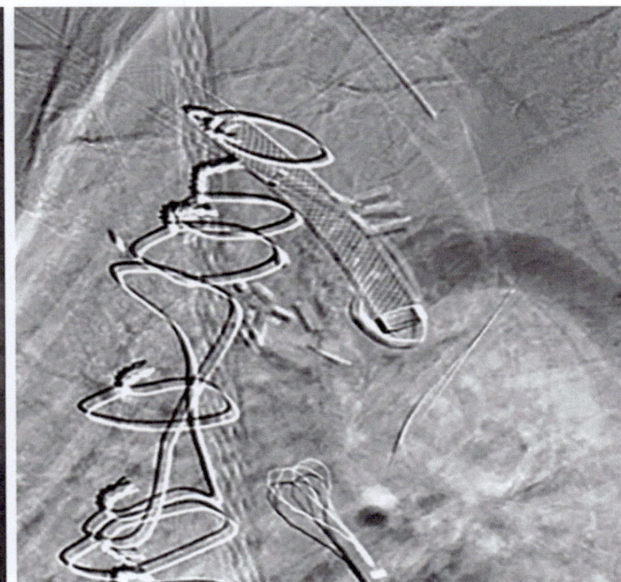

Fig. 25.2 (Left) Single intraprocedural exposure shows the catheter tip from the right neck access adjacent to the tip of the Hero graft. Calcifications represent the chronic SVC occlusion (dashed line).

(Right) DSA from the right neck shows filling of an enlarged azygous vein, no communication with the right atrium

A 10 French sheath (Cook Medical, Bloomingdale, IN) was placed in the right atrium and a 21-gauge Chiba needle was advanced co-axially through a Colapinto needle (Cook Medical, Bloomingdale, IN) toward the SVC. Using the SVC calcifications as a guide, the Chiba needle was advanced alongside the occluded proximal SVC (Fig. 25.3). A stiff 0.018-inch wire was advanced in the mediastinum, and a 4 mm angioplasty balloon was advanced over the wire and inflated as a target for sharp recanalization. From the right supraclavicular region, a micropuncture needle was advanced percutaneously and used to puncture the balloon (Fig. 25.4). Once through-and-through wire access was achieved, positioning was confirmed on cone beam CT. Venoplasty was used to create a neo-SVC followed by placement of a balloon expandable covered stent (Viabahn VBX, Gore Medical, Flagstaff, AZ) which was dilated to 10 mm. Finally, a tunneled transhepatic dialysis catheter was left in place. The patient underwent partial explantation of the Hero graft. One month later, after stent graft incorporation, the patient underwent successful placement of a new Hero graft (Fig. 25.5). The transhepatic catheter was later removed and the tract embolized using metallic coils. The patient's Hero graft was functioning 9 months post SVC reconstruction.

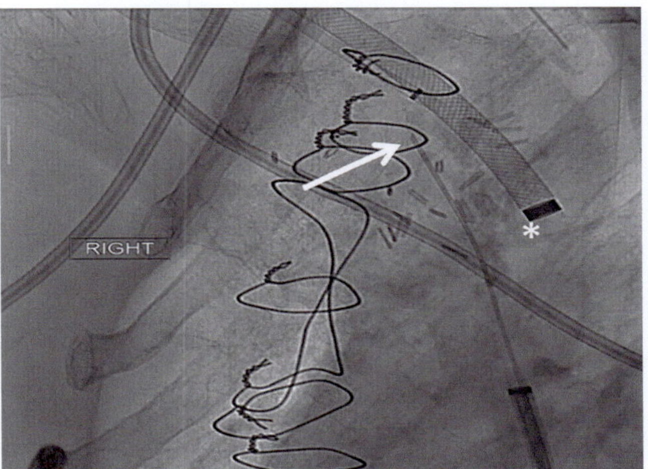

Fig. 25.3 Intraprocedural exposure showing a Chiba needle advanced coaxially from the transhepatic access. The tip of the needle (arrow) is alongside the occluded proximal SVC as marked by the adjacent calcifications (*) and Hero graft more medially

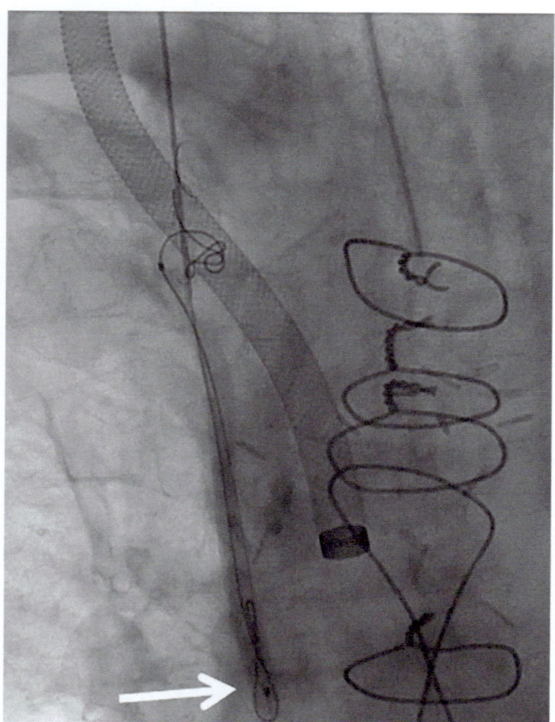

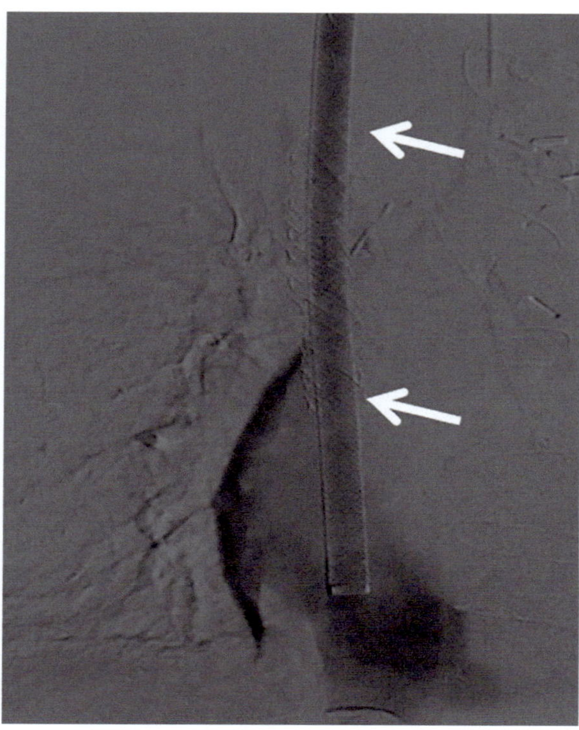

Fig. 25.4 Single cine image captured during puncture of the angioplasty balloon located in the neo-SVC. The wire is being advanced through the micropuncture needle and can be seen coiling in the caudal portion of the balloon (arrow)

Fig. 25.5 DSA following contrast injection through the Hero graft. The Hero graft traverses the covered stent (arrows) in the neo-SVC. Contrast flows freely into the right atrium

Extra-Anatomical Venous Bypass Through a Malignant Tumor for Palliation of Massive Arm Edema

Yasuaki Arai and Miyuki Sone

A man in his early 40s presented with severe edema of his right upper extremity caused by a malignant peripheral nerve sheath tumor of the brachial plexus and nodal metastases (Figs. 26.1 and 26.2). He had undergone surgical resection, chemotherapy and radiation, however the tumor recurred and metastasized to his lungs and bone. Amputation of his right arm was scheduled in consideration of his paralyzed, swollen, and heavy arm and considerable deterioration of his quality of life.

Right arm venography of the right arm showed occlusion of the right brachial vein and numerous collateral vessels (Fig. 26.3). Endovascular recanalization failed because the occlusion could not be traversed.

Using a right internal jugular vein, the stiff end of an 0.035 inch guidewire was advanced into the tumor, followed by balloon dilatation (Fig. 26.4) and placement of a bare metallic stent (8 mm diameter × 4 cm long) to create a "space" inside of the tumor.

A combination of sharp and blunt tunneling with a needle and a guidewire was performed to establish an extra-anatomical route from the antecubital vein toward the inner lumen of the stent that had been placed as a target. A 0.035 in. guidewire was pulled through from the right brachial vein into the right internal jugular vein using a loop snare (Fig. 26.5). The intratumoral tunnel was dilated with a 6-mm balloon catheter, and two VIABAHN stent grafts (6 mm × 10 cm) were deployed (Fig. 26.6). Final venography demonstrated brisk unimpeded venous return to the right atrium (Fig. 26.7). His right arm edema significantly improved over 2 weeks (Fig. 26.8). The amputation surgery was cancelled.

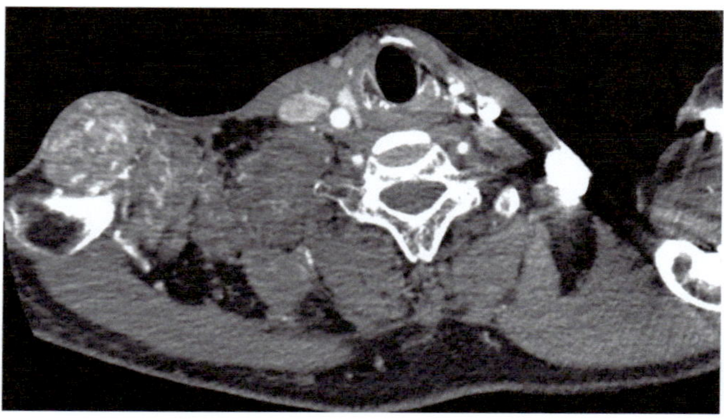

Fig. 26.2 Contrast-enhanced CT shows a huge tumor in the right shoulder region

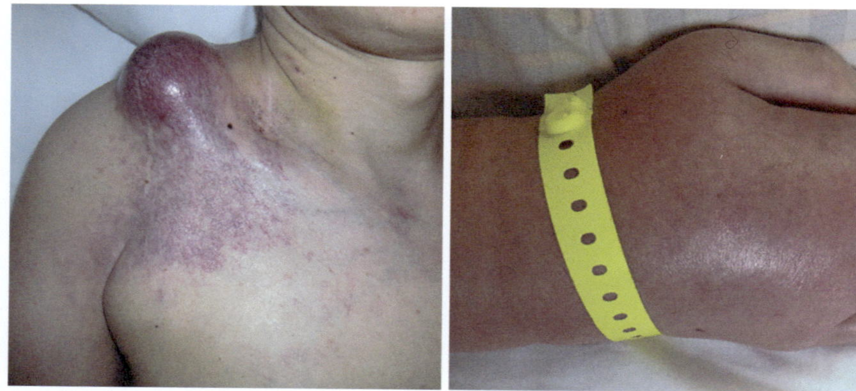

Fig. 26.1 Severe right upper extremity edema caused by a huge tumor in shoulder region

Y. Arai (✉) · M. Sone
Department of Diagnostic Radiology, National Cancer Center,
Tokyo, Japan
e-mail: arai-y3111@mvh.biglobe.ne.jp

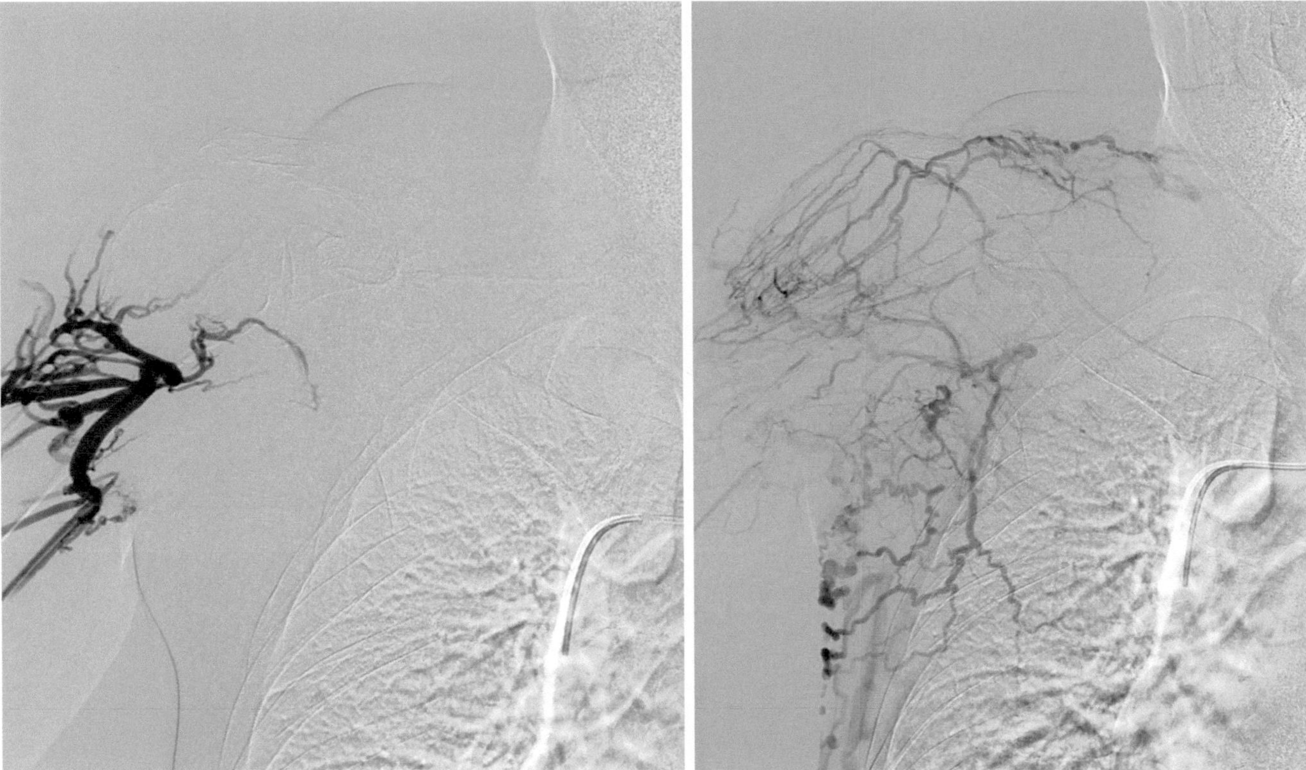

Fig. 26.3 The right arm venography showed the occlusion of the right brachial vein and numerous collateral veins

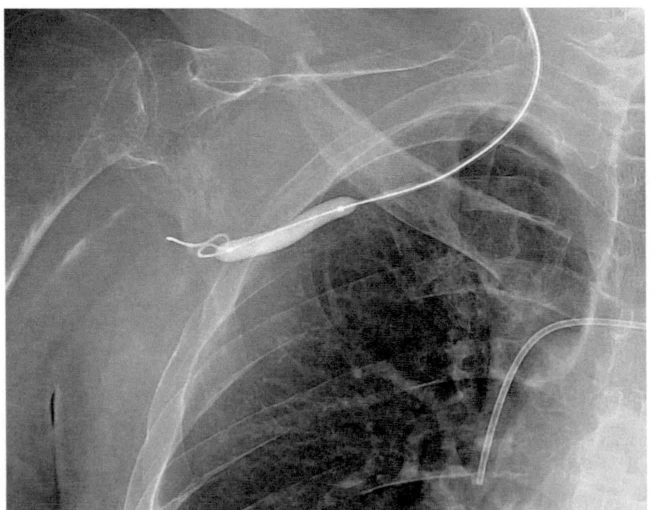

Fig. 26.4 The space was made with the inflation of balloon catheter inserted via the left internal jugular vein

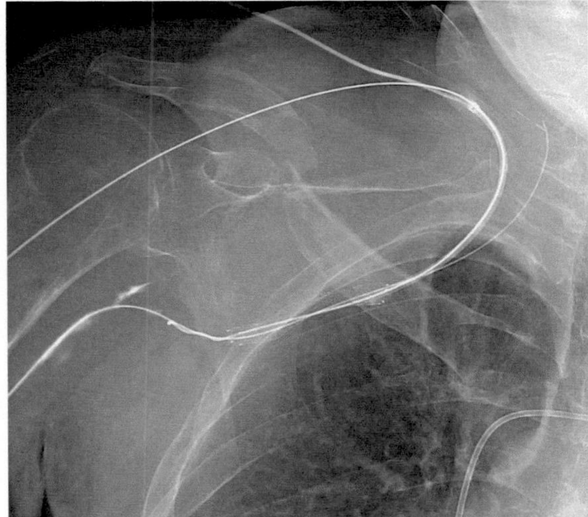

Fig. 26.5 Using the stent as a target, a 0.035 inch guidewire was pulled through from the right brachial vein to the right internal jugular vein using a loop snare

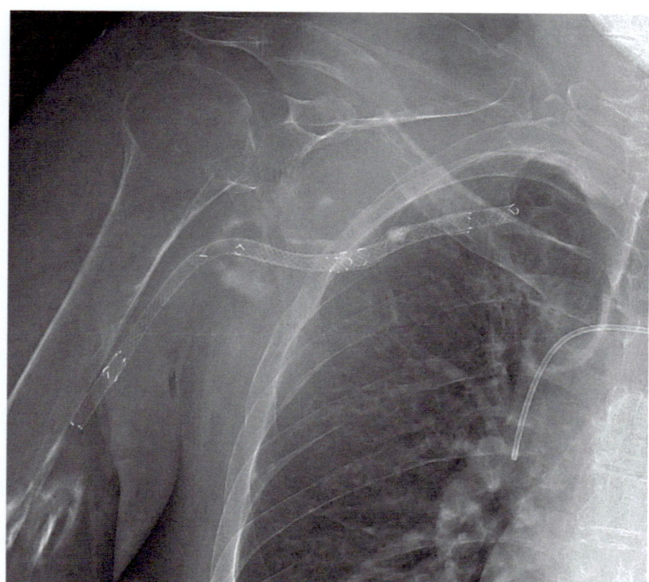

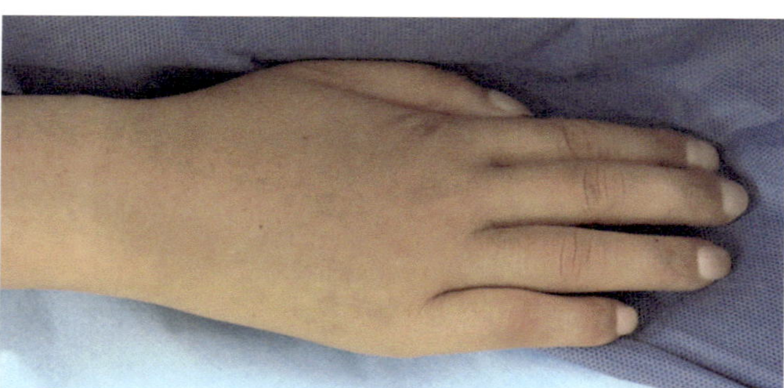

Fig. 26.8 The edema of the right upper limb was significantly improved 2 weeks later

Fig. 26.6 Two VIABAHN stent grafts were placed communicating between the right brachial vein and the right jugular vein

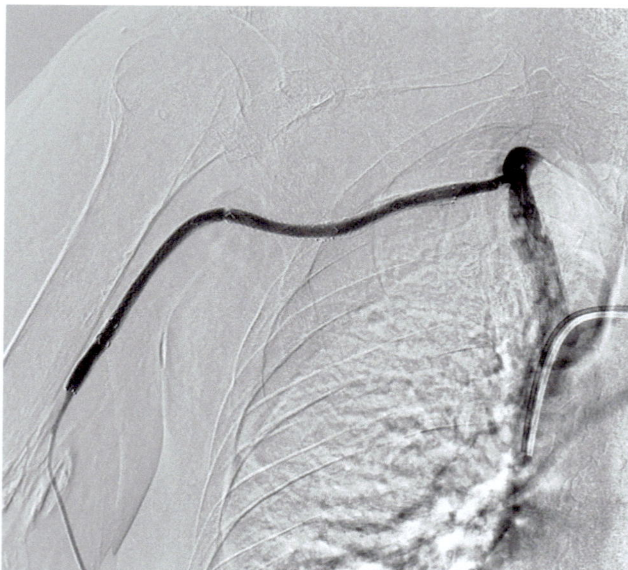

Fig. 26.7 The venography via the right brachial vein showed the smooth venous return to the right atrium

Michael Markovitz and Glenn Hoots

A 68-year-old male with Factor V Leiden had a permanent VenaTech inferior vena cava (IVC) filter (B. Braun, Melsungen, Germany) placed for recurrent thrombosis despite anticoagulation [1]. Incidental imaging 4 years later showed a tilted filter with struts extending posteriorly beyond the IVC (Fig. 27.1). Despite being aware that the filter was technically permanent, the patient insisted on attempted filter retrieval.

Jugular-directed forceps were used to bring the filter legs together, allowing them to be snared from a femoral approach. Whilst distracting the filter, the 18 Fr sheath kinked and mangled it (Fig. 27.2). The main filter body was retrieved from above and retained caval struts individually removed with forceps. A fragment embolized to the proximal pulmonary artery was snared and removed. Additional fragments had embolized to the left lung and right heart; the risk

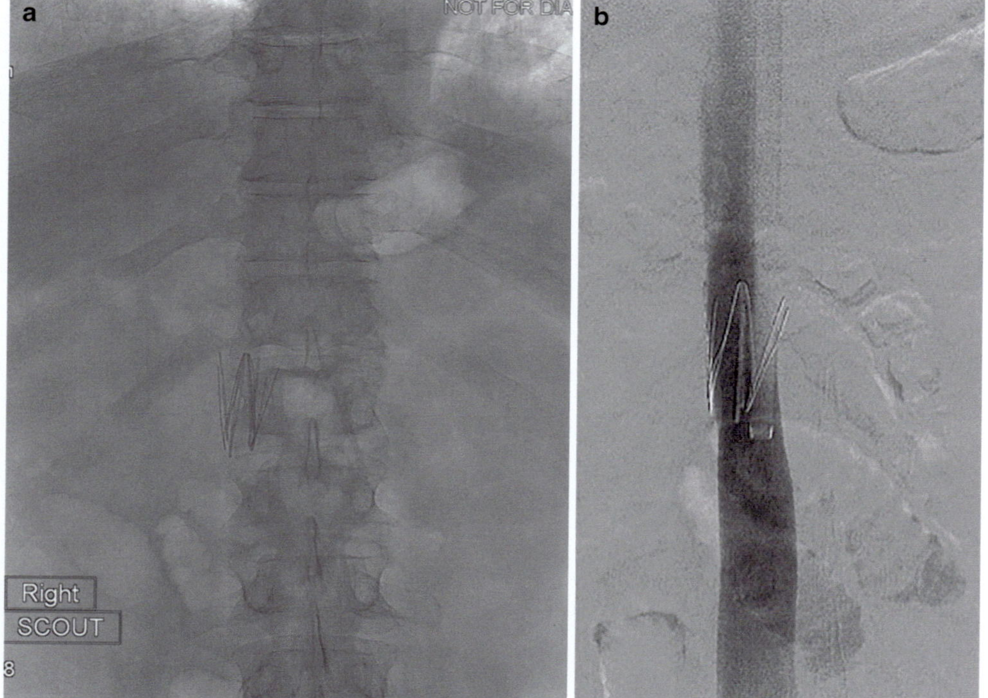

Fig. 27.1 (**a**) AP and bilateral oblique (not shown) scout images demonstrate a permanent VenaTech IVC filter tilted anteriorly. (**b**) Digital subtracted inferior venacavogram shows the posteromedial struts outside the IVC lumen

M. Markovitz (✉)
Department of Radiology, University of South Florida,
Tampa, FL, USA
e-mail: michaelmarkovitz@usf.edu

G. Hoots
Department of Radiology, Tampa General Hospital, Florida
Interventional Specialists, University of South Florida,
Tampa, FL, USA

Z. J. Haskal (ed.), *Extreme IR*, https://doi.org/10.1007/978-3-031-24251-9_27

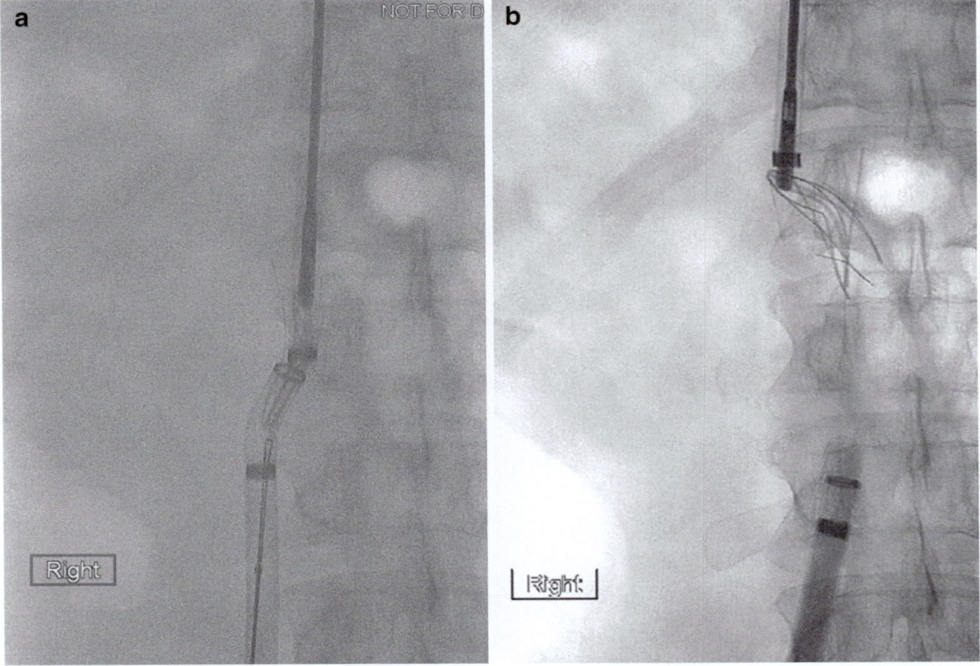

Fig. 27.2 (**a**) AP fluoroscopic image demonstrates kinking of the right femoral vein sheath within the IVC (**b**) with mangling of the filter upon sheath retraction

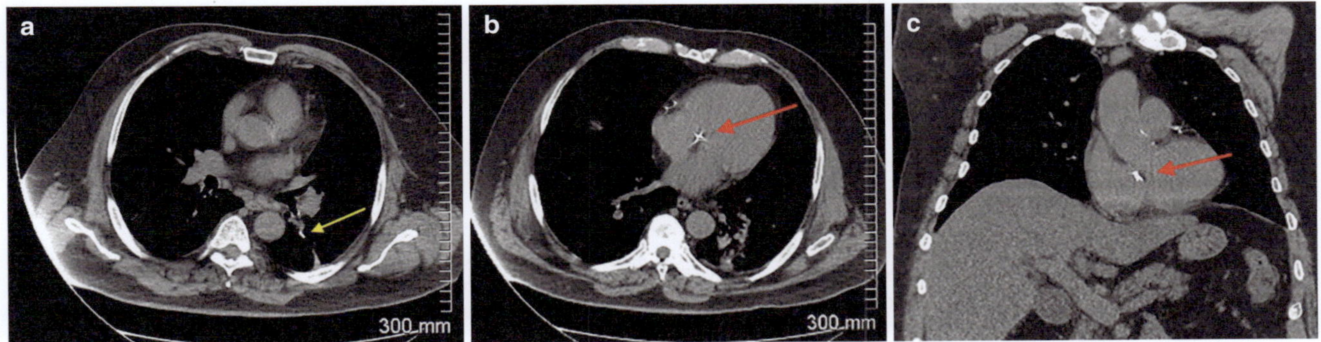

Fig. 27.3 (**a**) Axial computed tomography (CT) shows a metallic density in a peripheral branch of the left lower lobe superior segmental artery (yellow arrow) consistent with fractured filter fragment. (**b**) Axial and (**c**) coronal CT demonstrate additional metallic density along the medial tricuspid valve (red arrows)

of retrieving these was deemed excessive. Final venography affirmed an intact IVC. CT demonstrated filter fragments in a peripheral branch of the left lower lobe superior segmental artery (7 mm) and the tricuspid valve (3 mm) (Fig. 27.3). At 2-month follow-up, he was asymptomatic. To avoid CT radiation, chest radiography was performed: known filter fragments were not seen (Fig. 27.4). Further imaging was deferred as the small fragments were considered unlikely to cause a complication or migrate.

Removal of nearly every permanent filter has been reported, intact or in piecemeal fashion [2, 3]. Fluoroscopy and fused intracardiac echocardiography to remove intracardiac struts has been described [4]. This case emphasizes the challenges and unique risks of such permanent filters, especially ones where multiple struts make long segments of wall contact, such as the VenaTech and TrapEase filters.

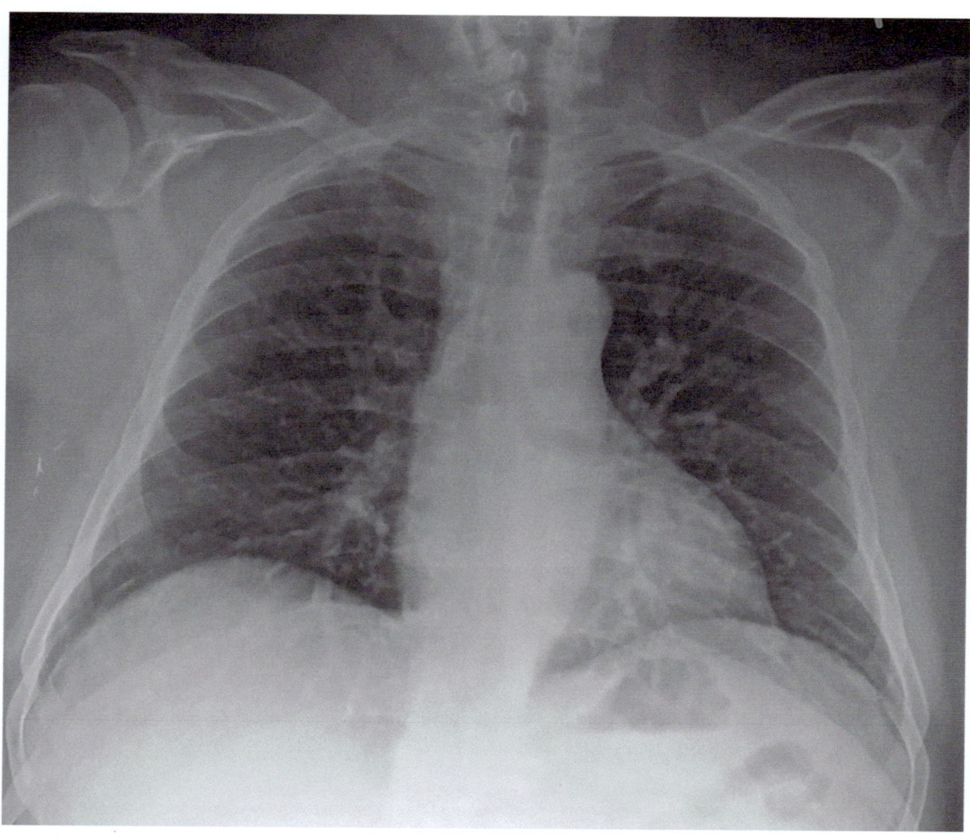

Fig. 27.4 Chest radiograph obtained 2 months after filter retrieval demonstrating no acute findings. Known left lung and right heart filter fragments are not visualized

Bibliography

1. Millward S, Peterson R, Moher D, Lewandowski B, Burbridge B, Aquino J, Formoso A. LGM (vena tech) vena Caval filter: experience at a single institution. J Vasc Interv Radiol. 1994;5:351–6.
2. Kuo WT, Deso SE, Robertson SW. Vena tech LGM filter retrieval 16 years after implantation: piecemeal removal by intentional mechanical fracture. J Vasc Interv Radiol. 2013;24:1731–7.
3. Ahmed O, Hadied MO, Madassery S. Retrieval of a permanent VenaTech LGM filter 18 years after implantation using a novel removal method. J Vasc Surg Venous Lymphat Disord. 2018;6:526–9.
4. Hannawa KK, Good ED, Haft JW, Williams DM. Percutaneous extraction of Embolized Intracardiac inferior vena cava filter struts using fused Intracardiac ultrasound and Electroanatomic mapping. J Vasc Interv Radiol. 2015;26:1368–74.

Zachary Haber and Mona Ranade

A rare complication of inferior vena cava (IVC) filters is upper gastrointestinal bleeding (UGIB) secondary to caval-duodenal fistula. Here, we present the same complication managed by a minimally invasive percutaneous approach.

A 61-year-old male with complex surgical history for retroperitoneal liposarcoma, presented to the ED for UGIB secondary to duodenal perforation by his indwelling IVC filter strut. Chronic filter-related iliocaval thrombosis was noted on imaging (Fig. 28.1). Vascular access was obtained, venogram was performed (Fig. 28.2). Complex IVC filter removal and through access from IJ to bilateral femoral vein was obtained with a gooseneck snare and serial balloon venoplasty was performed. Venography demonstrated active extravasation around filter strut into duodenum (Fig. 28.3a). To ensure re-entry, two kissing Vici stents (Boston Scientific, Marlborough, MA) were placed (Fig. 28.3b). Using endobronchial forceps, advanced through a 16 French sheath, the IVC filter was removed. The caval-duodenal fistula was then cannulated with a Progreat Omega microcatheter (Terumo, Tokyo, Japan) and embolization was performed with a 1:1 n-Butyl cyanoacrylate and Lipiodol (Guerbet, Villepinte, France) mixture (Fig. 28.4). Venography with glue cast (arrow) and coronal CT images confirmed resolution of the caval-duodenal fistula (Fig. 28.5). On post-procedure day 2, the patient resumed a normal diet and had no further episodes of UGIB.

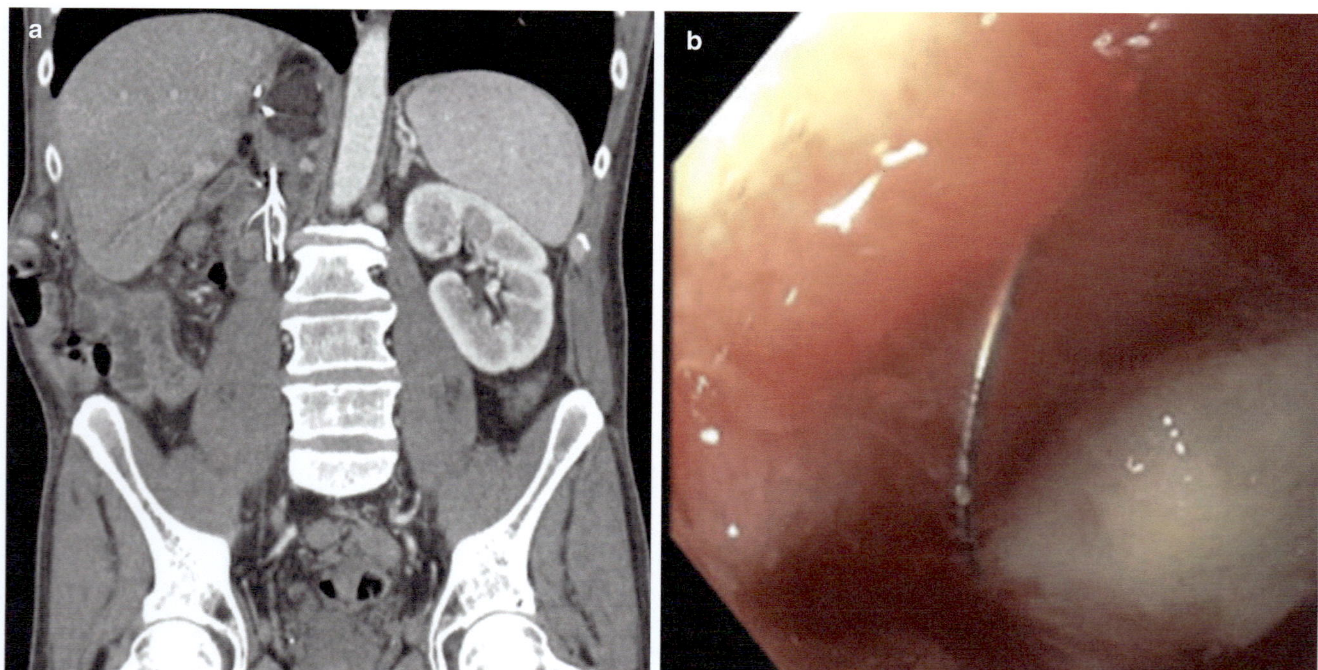

Fig. 28.1 (**a**) Coronal CT demonstrates IVC filter with strut within duodenum. (**b**) Endoscopy photograph confirms perforated filter strut

Z. Haber · M. Ranade (✉)
Department of Interventional Radiology, University of California, Los Angeles, CA, USA
e-mail: zhaber@mednet.ucla.edu; mranade@mednet.ucla.edu

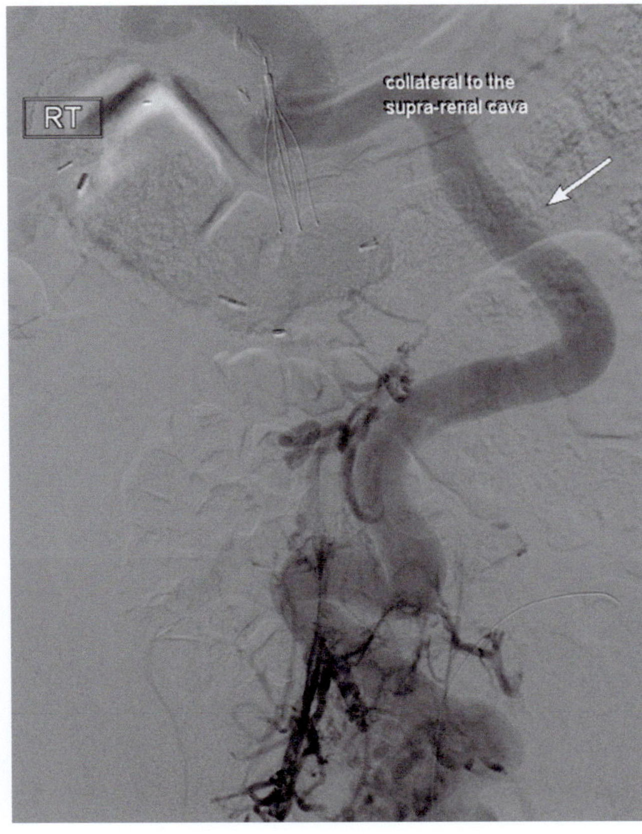

Fig. 28.2 Venogram demonstrates iliocaval thrombosis

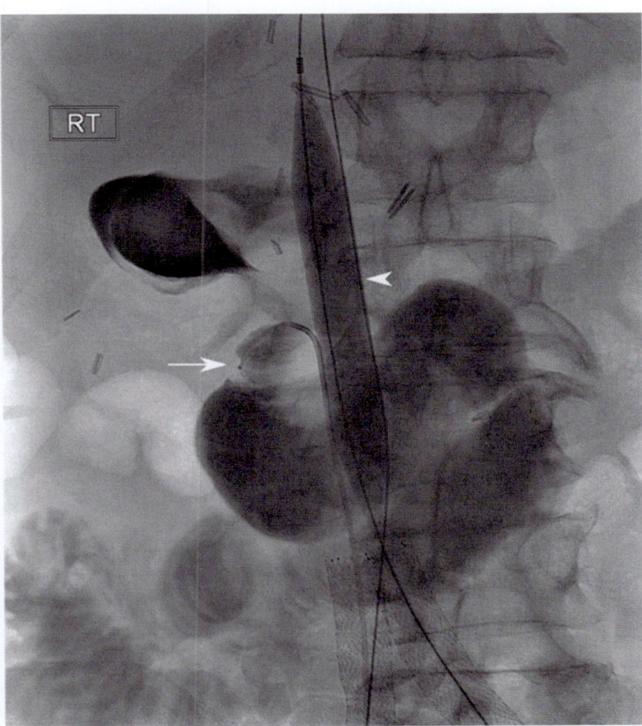

Fig. 28.4 Spot fluoroscopic image with microcatheter within caval-duodenal fistula (arrow) and inflated balloon within IVC to protect from non-target embolization (arrowhead)

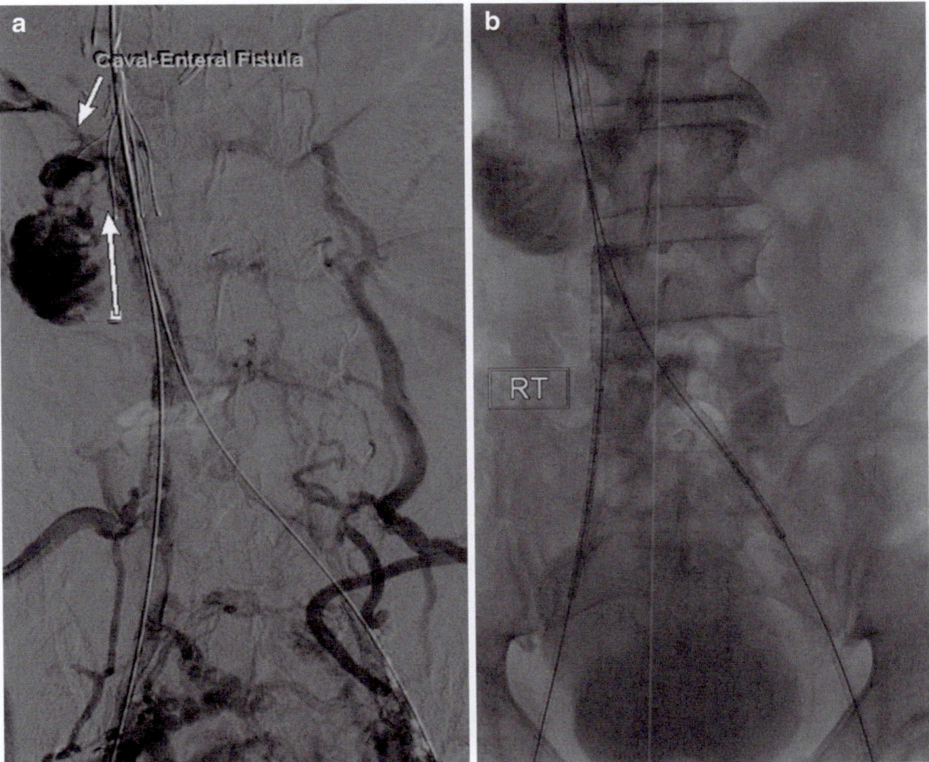

Fig. 28.3 (**a**) Venogram demonstrates active extravasation around filter strut into duodenum. (**b**) Spot fluoroscopic image shows placement of two 14 × 90 mm stents within the iliocaval system

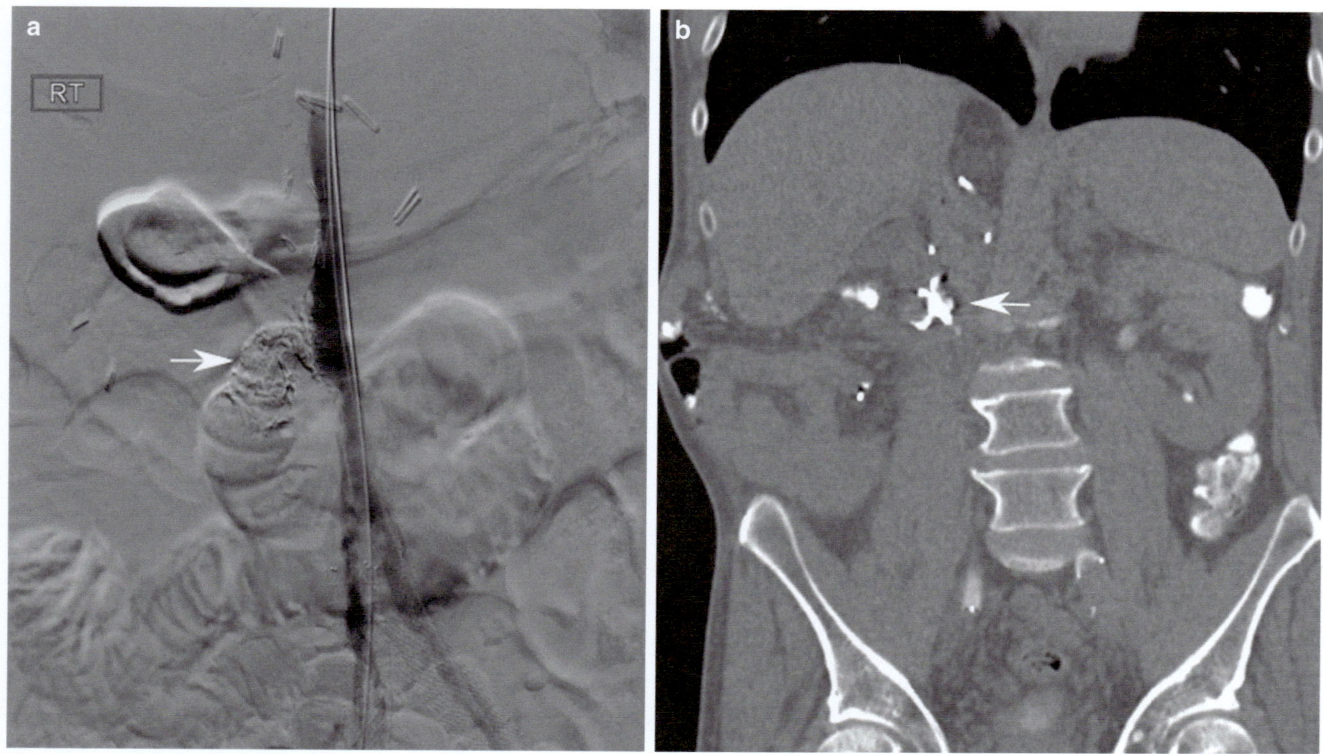

Fig. 28.5 (**a**) Venogram with glue cast (arrow) with resolution of caval-duodenal fistula. (**b**) Coronal CT correlate with glue cast seen (arrow)

Stent-Excluded IVC Filter Causing Severe Abdominal Pain: The Porthole Retrieval Technique

Raghuram Posham, Robert Lookstein, and Aaron Fischman

A 43-year-old female developed sudden severe abdominal pain and intractable vomiting. She had a history of DVT, PE, and symptomatic IVC-filter associated iliocaval thrombosis requiring prior multiple interventions. She ultimately underwent complete iliocaval reconstruction with stent-exclusion of the filter. On arrival, a CT scan showed one strut of the filter eroding into the duodenum (Fig. 29.1).

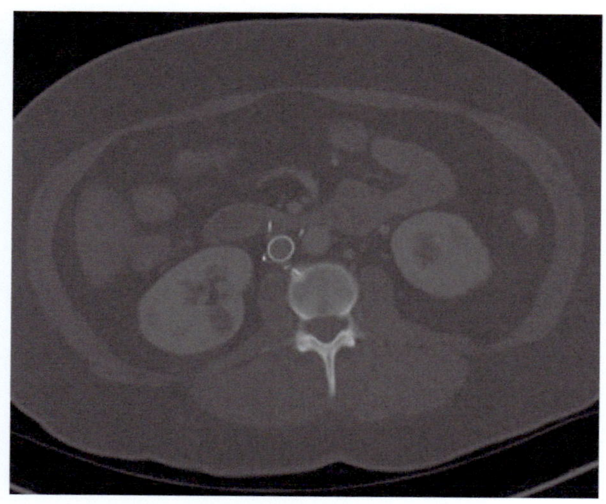

Fig. 29.1 Contrast-enhanced computed tomography axial image at the inferior aspect of the inferior vena cava (IVC) filter (Günther Tulip, Cook Medical Inc., Bloomington, IN) shows penetration of the anterior strut into the duodenum

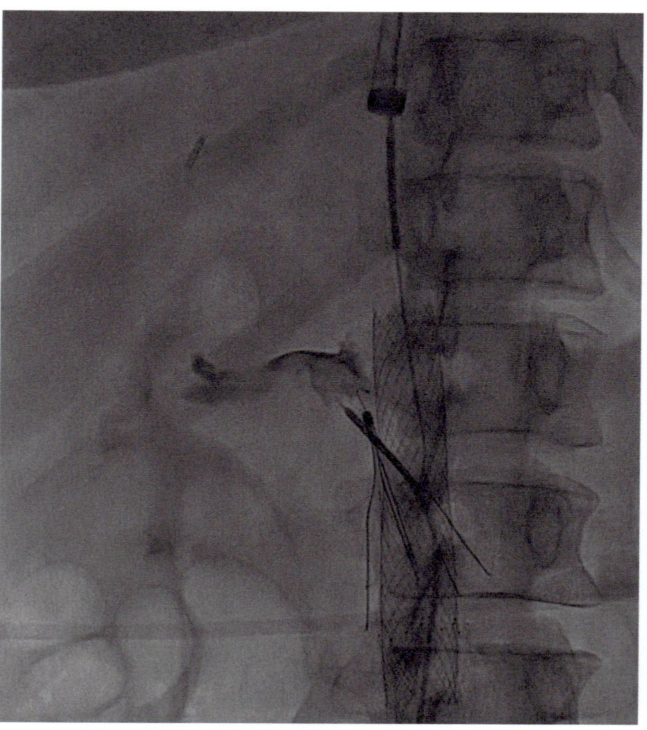

Fig. 29.2 The right renal vein is catheterized using a 5-F × 65 cm, Multipurpose A glide catheter, and 150 cm, 0.038 in Angle Gllidewire (Terumo, Somerset, NJ) through the interstices of the Wallstent (Boston Scientific, Watertown, MA). The hook of the filter is seen near the origin of the renal vein

Attempts to dissect along the right side of the stent were unsuccessful as the stent was completely endothelialized. The right renal vein was successfully catheterized through the stent interstices (Fig. 29.2), showing the filter neck within the proximal renal vein. A wire was successfully directed back into the stent for through-and-through access (Fig. 29.3a). Sequential venoplasty was performed through the interstices to create a "port-hole" in the stent next to the filter neck (Fig. 29.3b).

An 18-Fr sheath was advanced from the internal jugular vein through the defect using the "swallow-the-balloon" technique (Fig. 29.4), allowing endoscopic forceps to engage the filter neck and pull it into the sheath (Fig. 29.5). A bal-

R. Posham (✉) · R. Lookstein · A. Fischman
Department of Interventional Radiology, Mount Sinai Hospital, New York, NY, USA
e-mail: Raghuram.posham@mountsinai.org;
Robert.lookstein@mountsinai.org;
aaron.fischman@mountsinai.org

Z. J. Haskal (ed.), *Extreme IR*, https://doi.org/10.1007/978-3-031-24251-9_29

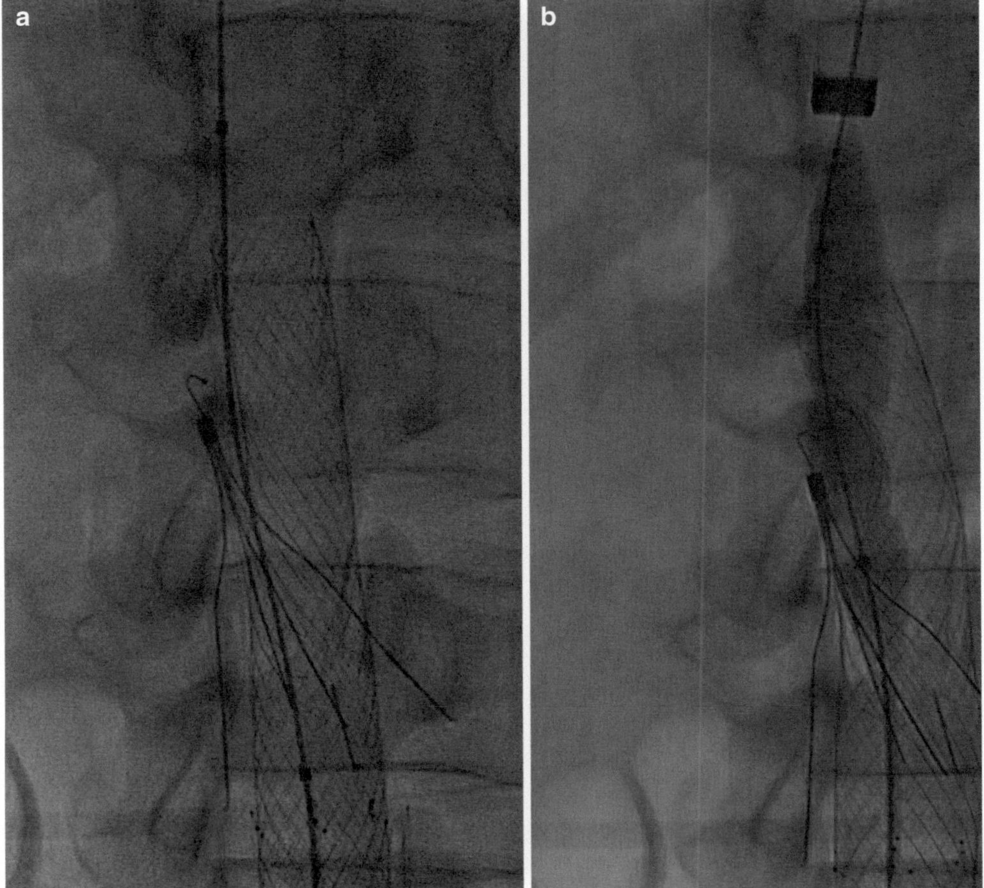

Fig. 29.3 (**a**) The wire is passed back into the stent lumen and snared from above (6Fr × 120 cm, 20 mm loop diameter gooseneck snare, Medtronic, Minneapolis, MN) for through-and-through access through stent interstices. (**b**) Sequential venoplasty was performed through the interstices using 4 mm–12 mm × 60 mm balloon (Charger, Boston Scientific, Watertown, MA) to create a "port-hole" fenestration in the wall stent in direct apposition to the filter neck

loon was simultaneously inflated over a safety wire in the stent to free the filter legs from the surrounding soft tissue, prevent stent crumpling as the filter was pulled into the sheath, and provide hemostasis in case of IVC rupture (Fig. 29.6).

Following retrieval, a cone-beam CT was performed demonstrating a patent stent with adequate opposition to the IVC lumen. The patient tolerated the procedure well and was discharged 2 days later with complete resolution of abdominal pain. She remained asymptomatic at 3-month follow-up (Fig. 29.7).

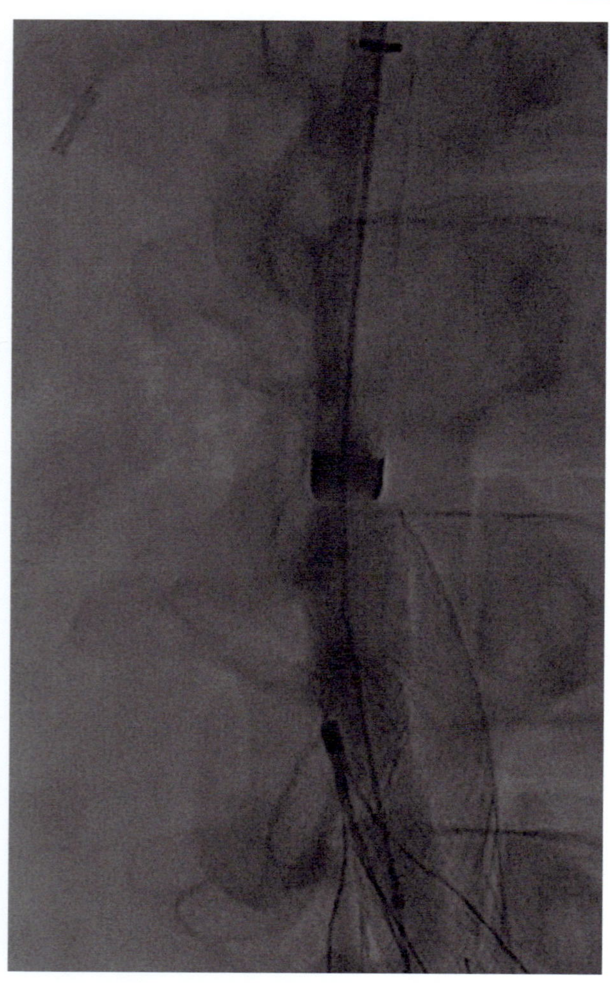

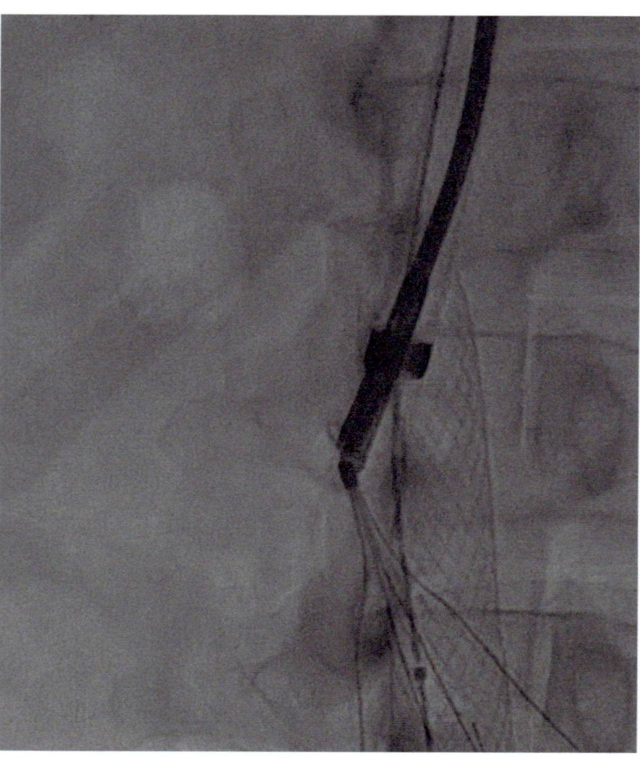

Fig. 29.5 Crocodile Jaw Grasping Forceps (model 4162; LYMOL Medical Corp, Woburn, Massachusetts) are advanced through the sheath to directly grasp the filter neck

Fig. 29.4 An 18Fr sheath (18Fr × 40 cm Check-Flo Performer Introducer, Cook Medical Inc., Bloomington, IN) is advanced through the "port-hole" fenestration using the swallow-the-balloon technique, i.e., pushing the sheath over a gradually deflating balloon to minimize step-off

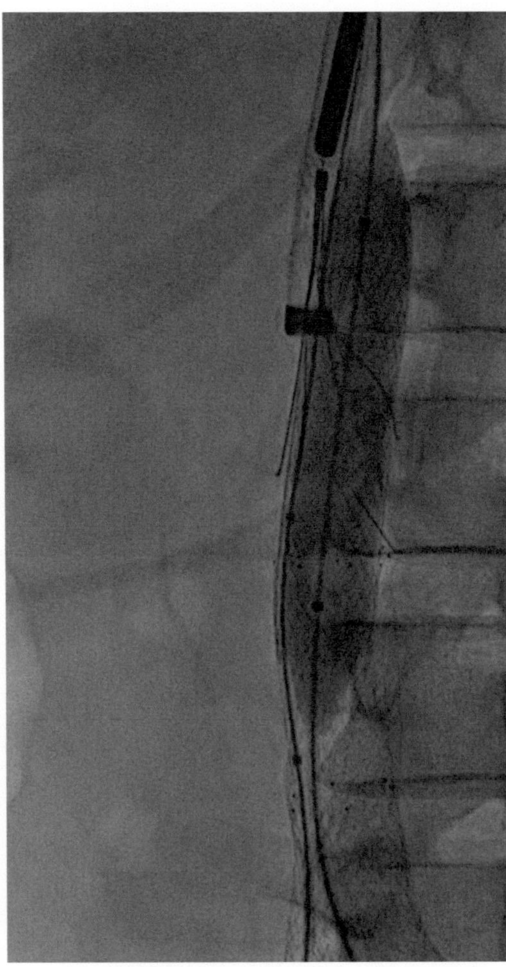

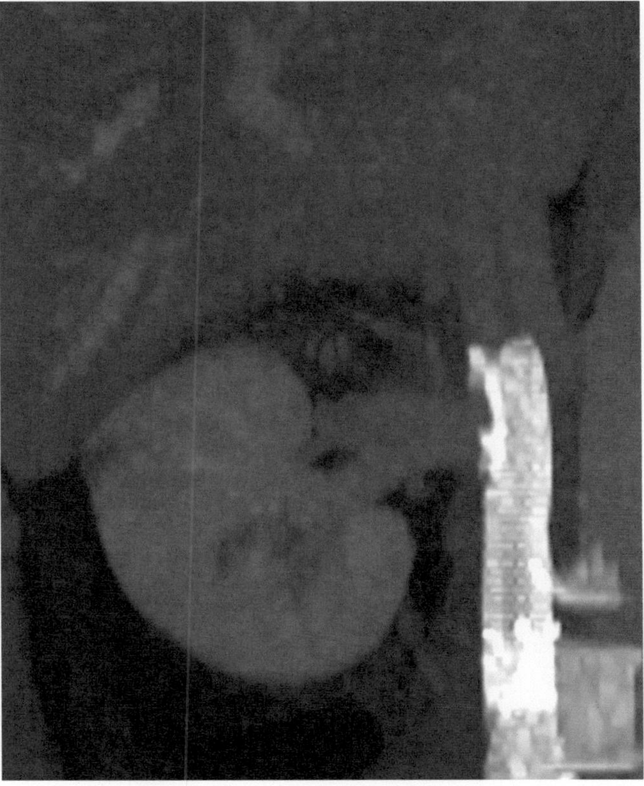

Fig. 29.7 Computed Tomography Maximum Intensity Projection (CT-MIP) images obtained at 3 months post procedure shows the "porthole" at the level of the right renal rein, and the remainder of the stent in good apposition to the IVC wall. There is no evidence of thrombosis, hematoma, or other abnormality

Fig. 29.6 From a left CFV access, a 14 mm × 6 cm Balloon (XXL Balloon, Boston Scientific, Watertown, MA) was simultaneously inflated over a safety wire in the IVC stent lumen to assist in freeing the filter legs from the surrounding soft tissue, prevent crumpling of the stent as the filter was pulled into the sheath, and provide temporary hemostasis in case of IVC rupture

AngioVac Thrombectomy of Two-Month-Old Iliocaval Thrombosis in a 15-Year-Old Resulting from Gunshot Wound and Surgical Caval Ligation

Ziv J Haskal

A 15-year-old male received an accidental gunshot to the abdomen resulting in pulseless electrical activity arrest, open thoracotomy, hemorrhagic shock and injuries to gastrointestinal, liver, and pancreatic injuries. A bleeding inferior vena cava (IVC) injury was primarily repaired. With ongoing resuscitation and emergent transfer, he underwent reoperations, washout of abscesses, and bullet removal (Fig. 30.1). CT imaging demonstrated infrarenal thrombus in the IVC extending into the common iliac veins (Fig. 30.2). He was discharged after 1 month and was readmitted 3 weeks later for thrombectomy.

Whilst under general anesthesia, femoral and jugular venography demonstrated the ilio-midcaval thrombosis(Fig. 30.3). Probing the surgical site of occlusion led to opacifying abdominal lymphatic trunks that filled the thoracic duct without leak (Fig. 30.4). The hard occlusion, at the surgical clips was traversed with sharp recanalization from the jugular to femoral axis. This was dilated with serial balloons to 14 mm without extravasation, after which the AngioVac circuit was assembled and the jugular cannula activated in the upper IVC.

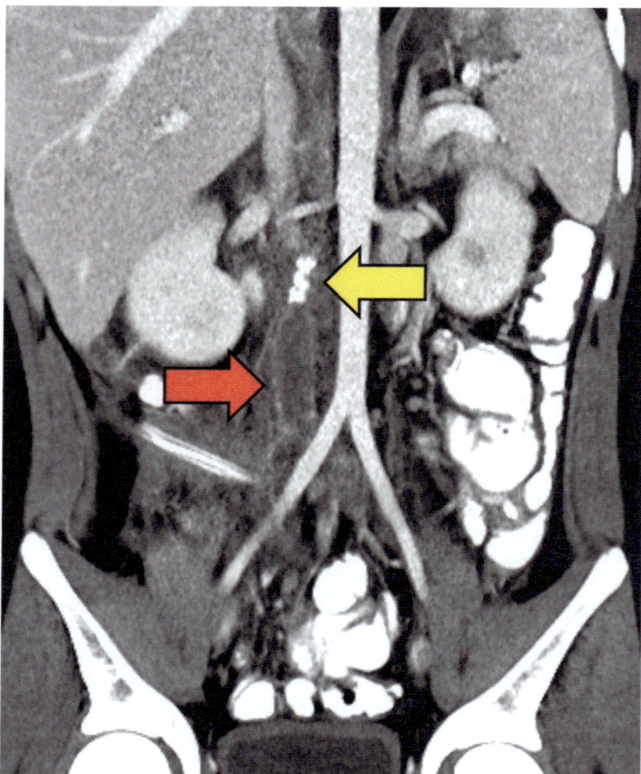

Fig. 30.2 Coronal CT at week 3 demonstrates the lower caval thrombosis (red arrow), and the surgical clips at its ligation (yellow arrow); cephalad of this, the IVC is patent

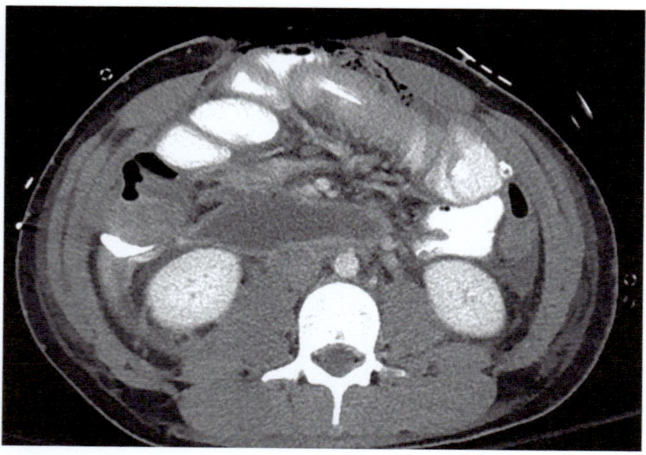

Fig. 30.1 CT image after third operation demonstrates open abdomen, mid abdominal abscess (multiple others were present, not shown), lack of caval opacification

Transfemoral occlusion and angioplasty balloons and Arrow PTD were used to macerate and push thrombus toward the suction cannula (Figs. 30.5 and 30.6). Four collection baskets were filled with extracted hard rubbery thrombus. Stents were deferred given his age and expected growth. After final 16 mm IVC dilation, prograde flow was present in the iliac and femoral veins, with residual adherent clot in the left iliac vein at end (Fig. 30.7). Enoxaparin anticoagulation was initiated and he was discharged after 1 day. His leg swelling resolved at follow-up. At 5 years, he has no leg swelling and no venous claudication.

Z. J Haskal (✉)

Department of Radiology and Medical Imaging, Interventional Division, University of Virginia, Charlottesville, VA, USA

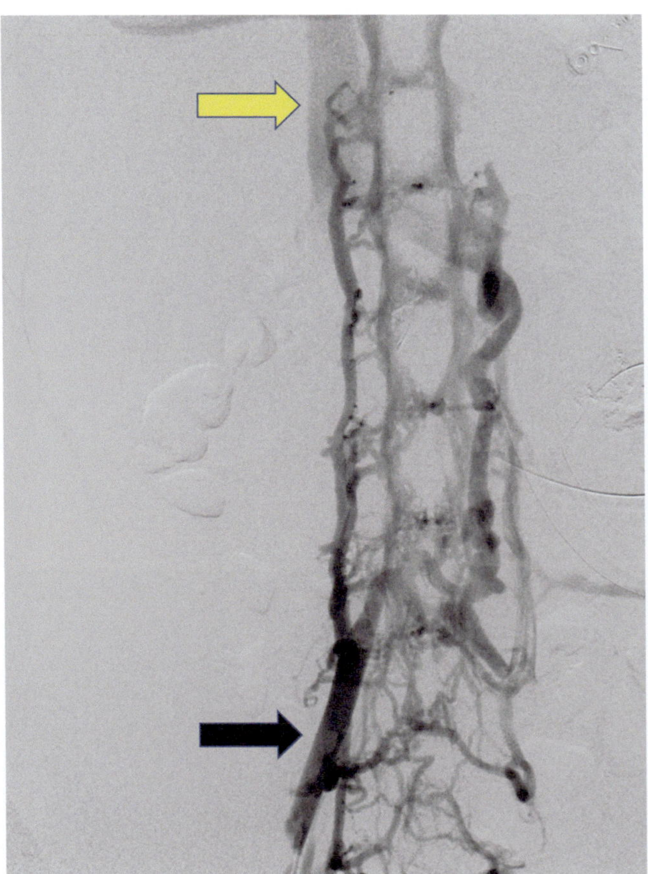

Fig. 30.3 Initial transfemoral venogram demonstrates partial patency of the right iliac vein (black arrow), complete caval thrombosis and extensive paravertebral collaterals, and reconstitution of the patent upper IVC (yellow arrow)

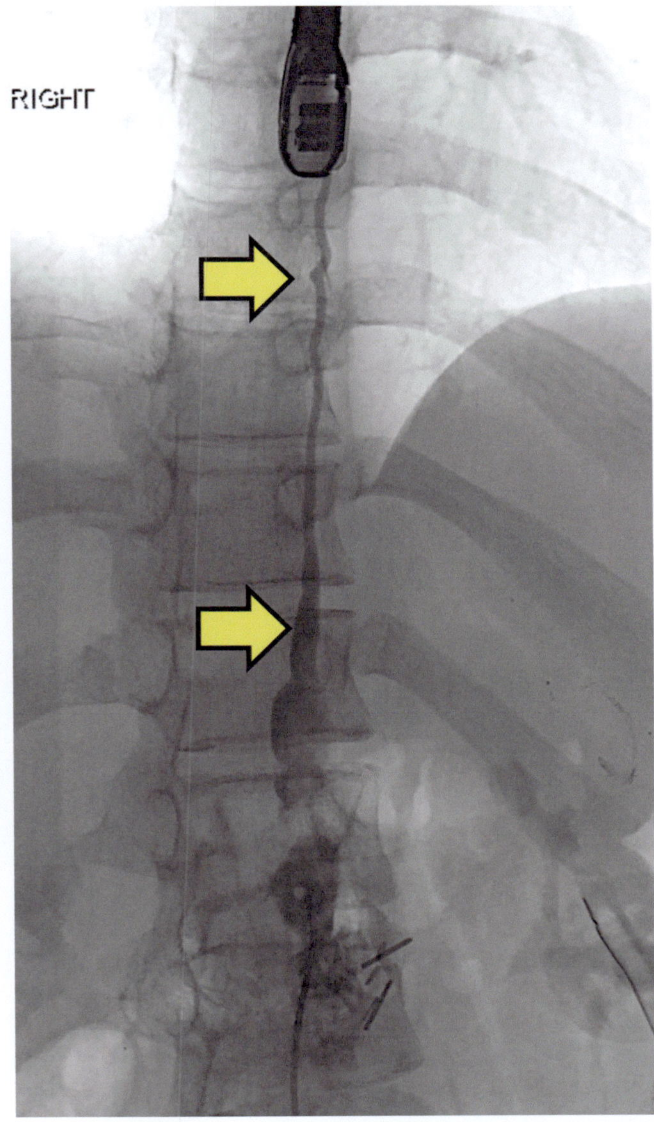

Fig. 30.4 Contrast injection during attempts to traverse the surgical occlusion fills an abdominal lymphatic trunk in continuity with the thoracic duct

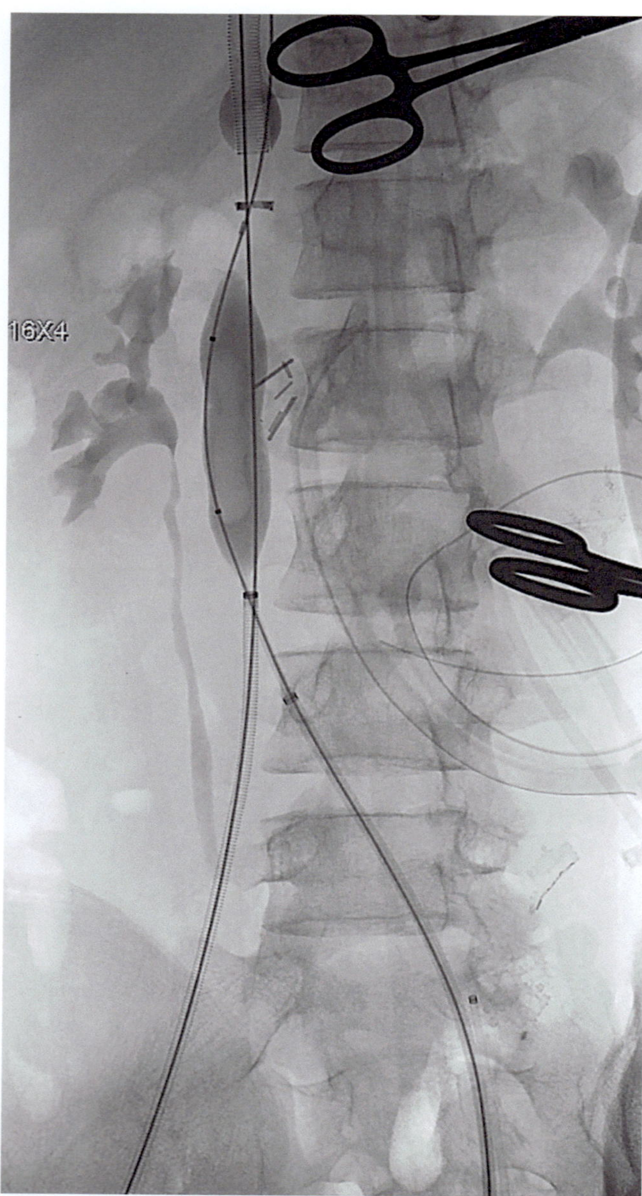

Fig. 30.5 Through and through jugular to right femoral wire access has been established. A left transfemoral 16 mm balloon has been inflated centered at the level of the surgical clips (prior occlusion). The inflated AngioVac cannula is seen at the top. A small caliber left femoral arterial sheath is also present

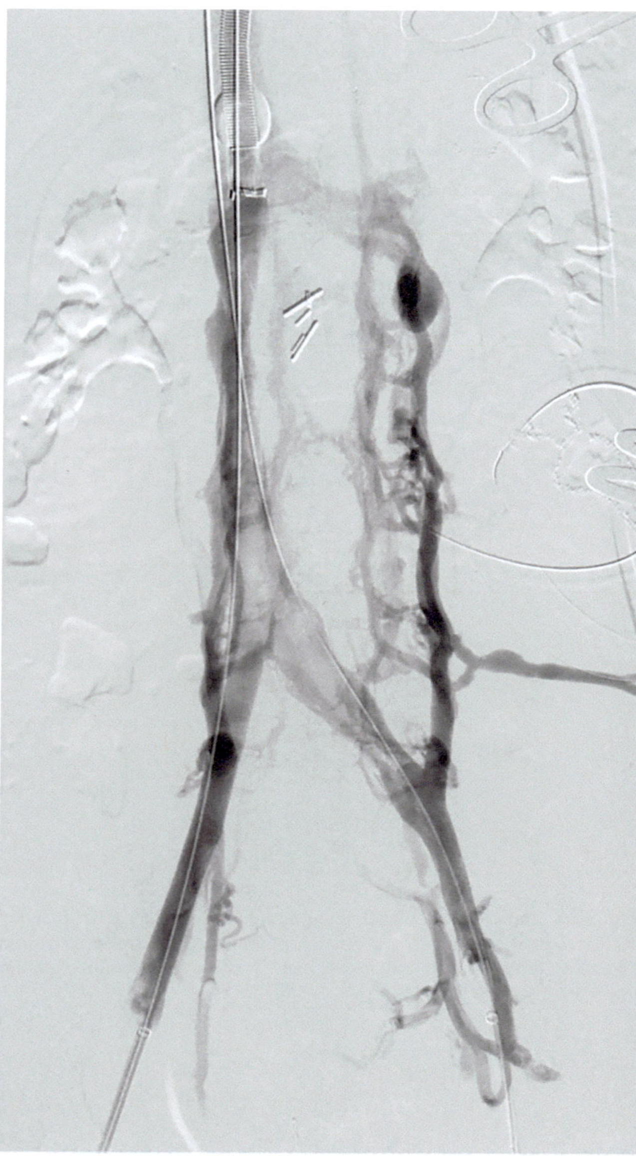

Fig. 30.6 Inferior vena cava gram after partial thrombectomy and 14 mm midcaval angioplasty. The AngioVac catheter is faintly seen at the top

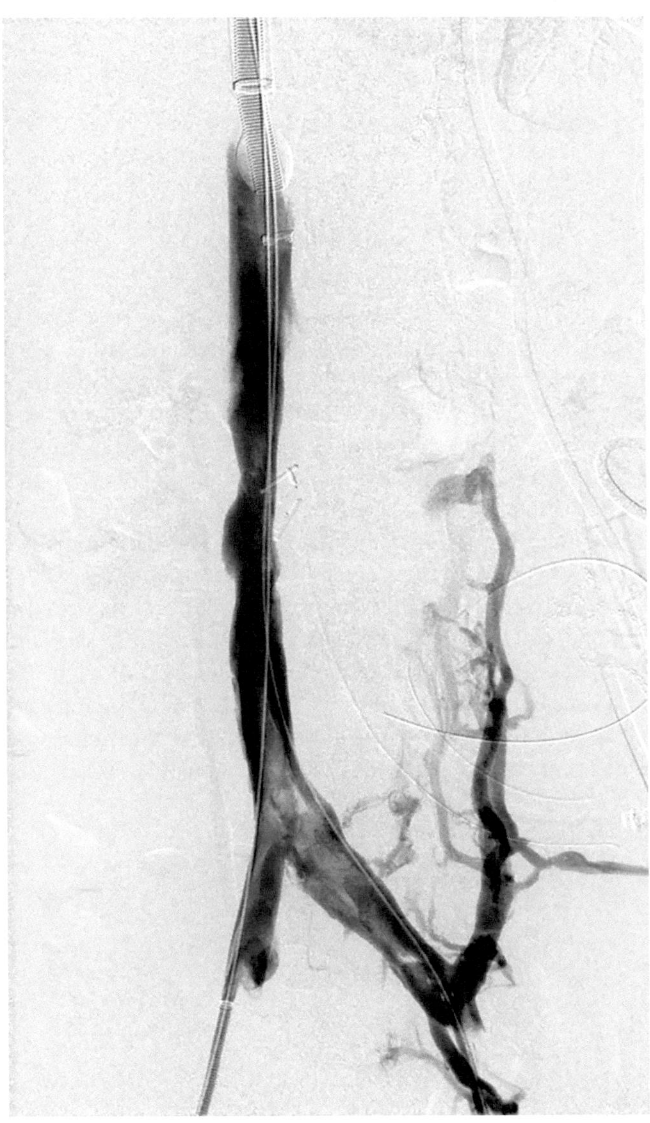

Fig. 30.7 IVC venogram demonstrates restoration of caval patency. Some caudal partial thrombus remains

Single-Session Total IVC and Iliofemoral Endovascular Construction for Caval Agenesis

Mina S. Makary

A 30-year-old male with congenital IVC atresia and chronic bilateral iliofemoropopliteal thrombotic occlusions presented with progressive worsening of debilitating lower extremity edema. Abdomen and pelvis CT redemonstrated absence of the IVC and new subacute-on- chronic bilateral iliofemoral thromboses and numerous retroperitoneal and body wall venous collaterals. Duplex ultrasound evaluation demonstrated similar findings in both femoral and popliteal veins.

Bilateral popliteal and right internal jugular vein approaches confirmed prior findings, including a small suprahepatic IVC remnant (Fig. 31.1). Blunt recanalization of both popliteal, femoral, and iliac veins was performed using directional catheters and guidewires. IVC construction was performed using antero- and retro-grade blunt and sharp techniques, including the Rösch-Uchida transjugular liver access targeting an inflated balloon with fluoroscopic and cone-beam CT triangulation (Fig. 31.2). IVUS was used to confirm passage of guidewire through bilateral lower extremities and the neo-IVC. The 24F Inari FlowTriever was used to aspirate clot, followed by venoplasty. Twenty mm diameter Abre (Medtronic) venous stents were deployed within neo-cava and kissing 16 mm stents for the iliac and central femoral veins followed by balloon dilation (Figs. 31.3 and 31.4). Dual antiplatelet and anticoagulant was initiated. He had near-complete resolution of lower extremity symptoms at 2-week follow-up. At 6 months, he was functional and able to return to work, having been previously disabled.

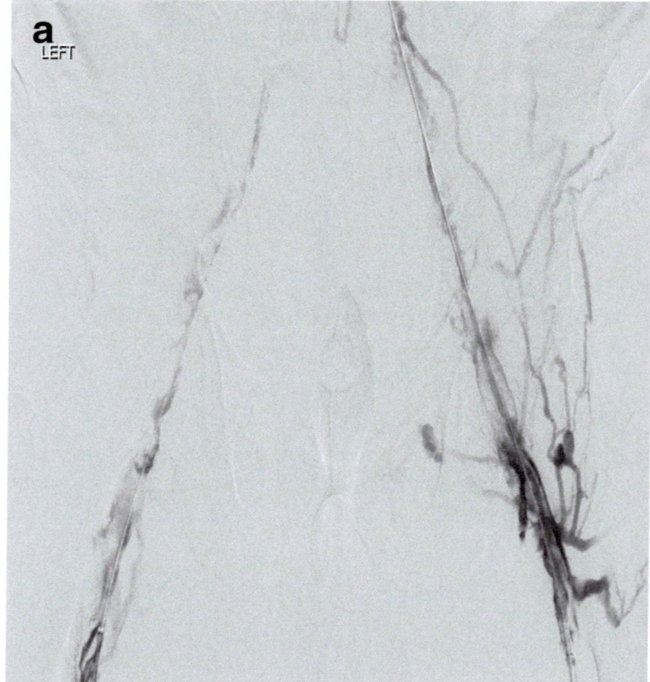

Fig. 31.1 Conventional diagnostic venography demonstrated (**a**) occlusion of the bilateral iliofemoral veins and development of venous collaterals, (**b**) absence of IVC with drainage through the para-lumbar venous plexus, and (**c**) presence of a small suprahepatic venous remnant which was used in subsequent venous construction

M. S. Makary (✉)
Division of Vascular and Interventional Radiology, Department of Radiology, The Ohio State University Wexner Medical Center, Columbus, OH, USA
e-mail: mina.makary@osumc.edu

Fig. 31.1   (continued)

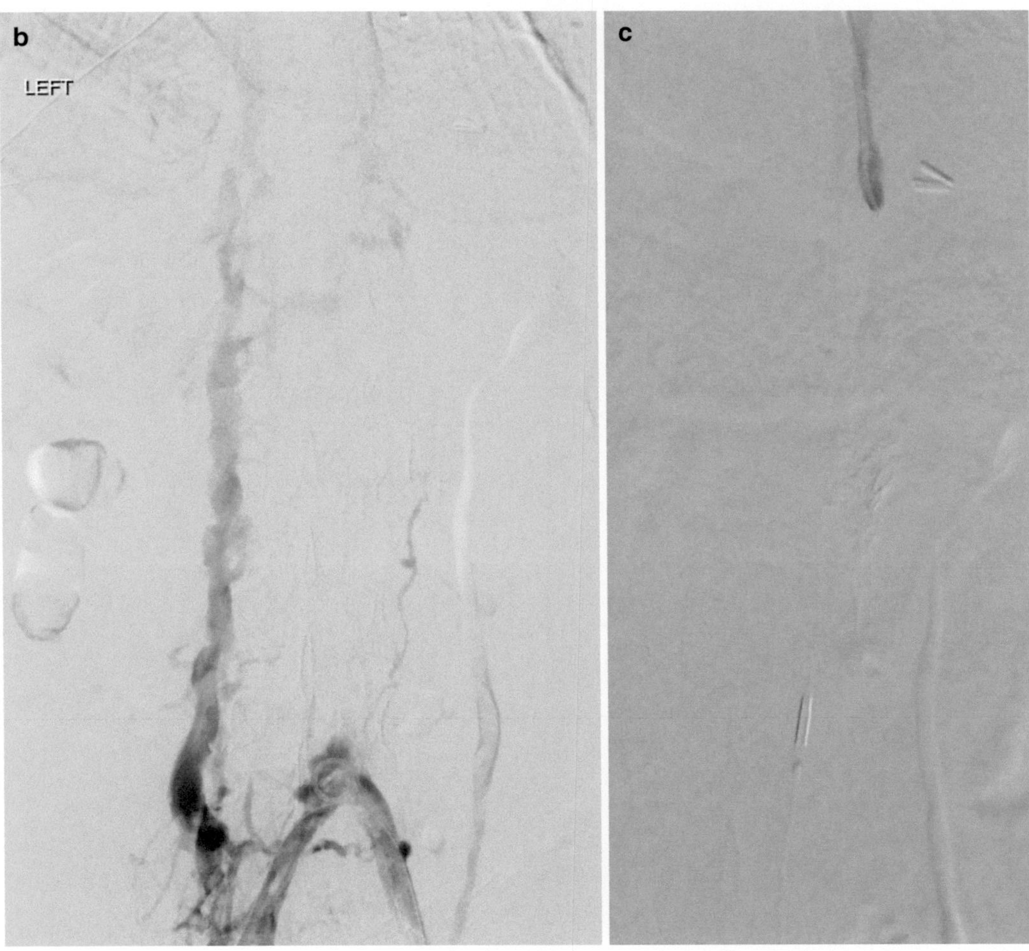

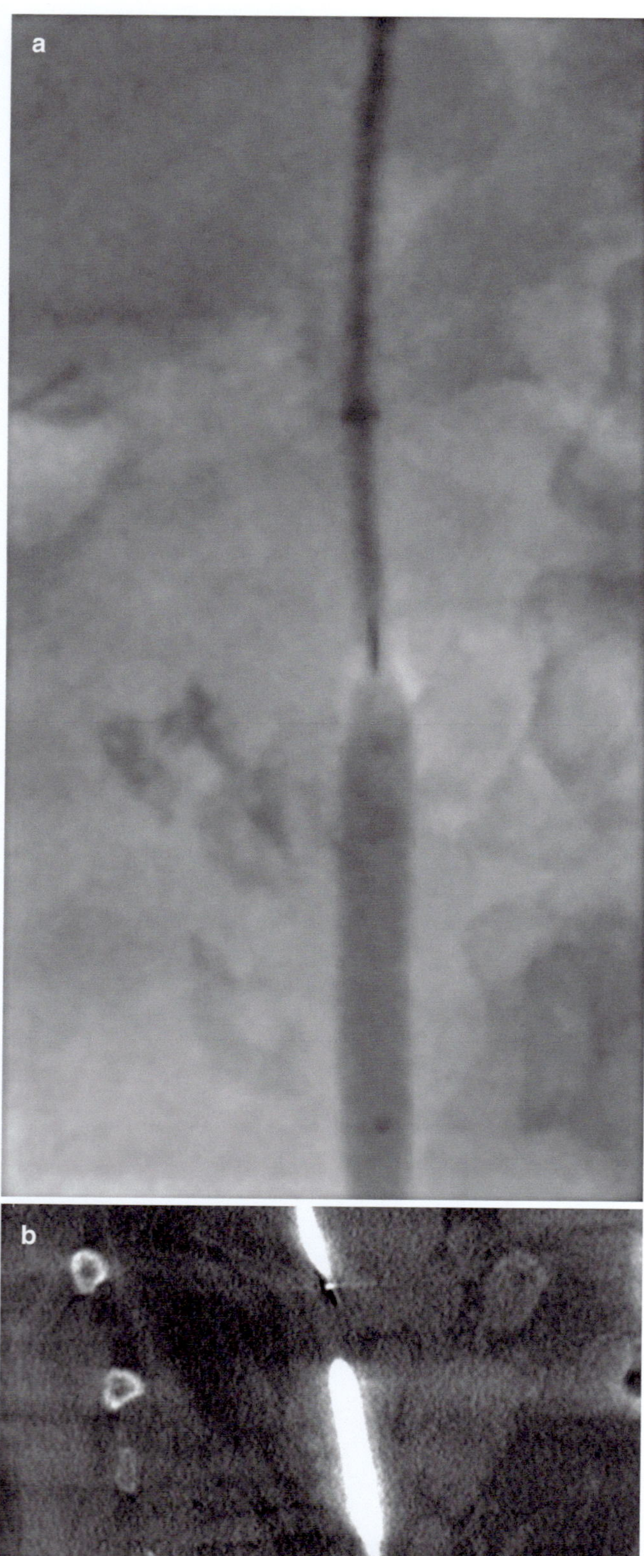

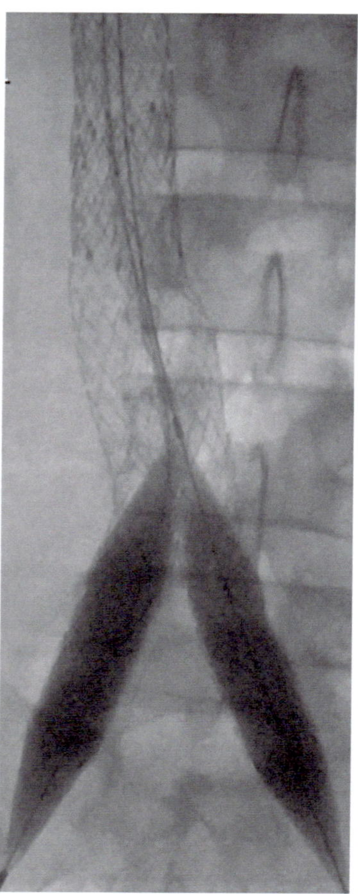

Fig. 31.3 Caval construction with overlapping 20 mm venous stents, followed by kissing 16 mm stents for the iliac and central femoral veins with corresponding venoplasty

Fig. 31.2 Caval construction with sharp techniques utilizing a Rösch-Uchida transjugular liver access needle in a suprahepatic venous remnant targeting an inflated balloon placed in the lower retroperitoneum via the popliteal access, with (**a**) fluoroscopic and (**b**) cone-beam CT triangulation

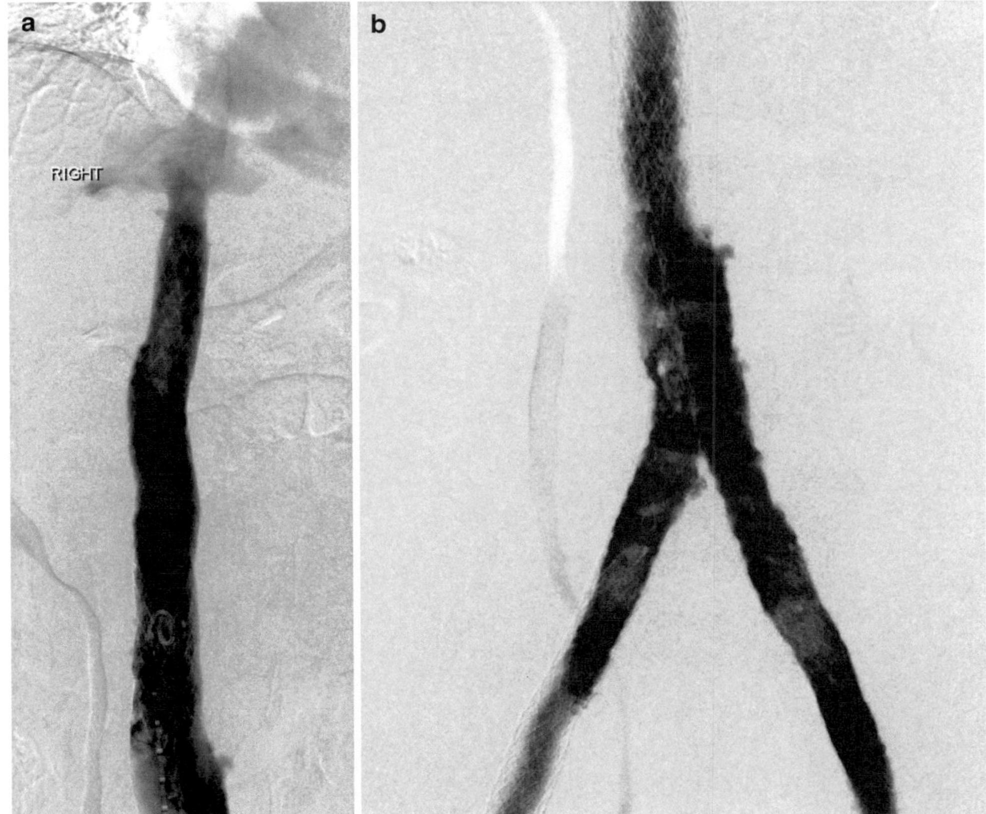

Fig. 31.4 Completion venography demonstrating a patent (**a**) neo-IVC and (**b**) iliofemoral veins, with contrast flow to the right atrium

Sebouh Gueyikian

A 38-year-old female with recurrent left leg DVT since age of 20 had failed stenting of a May-Thurner lesion. Prior surgical inferior vena cava (IVC) and bi-iliac vein reconstruction was aborted mid-procedure after resection of the IVC bifurcation and a portion of venous stent. Sixteen years later, she presented with bilateral leg swelling and pelvic pressure.

Computed tomography showed chronically occluded common iliac veins and hypertrophied bilateral gonadal veins draining into the patent infrarenal IVC. Under general anesthesia, right jugular and bilateral common femoral venous accesses were established (Figs. 32.1 and 32.2). The PowerWire RF (Baylis Medical) was advanced under fluoroscopy and cone-beam CT guidance from the cephalic aspect of the right common iliac vein (CIV) to the IVC across a 9 cm retroperitoneal gap. A 4 mm by 6 cm Conquest balloon (Bard) was deployed as a target along this path.

The left CIV stent was crossed using the PowerWire RF. A right common iliac arterial injury (Fig. 32.3) was repaired with a 7 mm by 5 cm Viabahn (Gore) stent-graft. Bilateral CIV to IVC access was achieved and angioplastied with two 14mm Atlas (Bard) balloons. Two 14 mm by 12 cm Vici stents (Boston Scientific) were deployed. Immediately thereafter, she became tachycardic and hypotensive. Venography showed active extravasation along the right IVC (Fig. 32.4). Two 13 mm by 10 cm Viabahn stent-grafts (Gore) were deployed to span this area. Venography showed persistent extravasation (Fig. 32.5). Prolonged bilateral balloon tamponade was unsuccessful. Massive transfusion protocol was initiated. Ongoing bleeding was suspected from the right gonadal vein into the portion of IVC adjacent to entry sites of the stents. Thirteen millimeter by 10 cm Viabahn (Gore) stent-grafts were deployed caudally and bilaterally and the right internal iliac vein was covered by stent-graft (Fig. 32.6). Her hemodynamics immediately improved and she became normotensive. Completion cone-beam CT showed a large retroperitoneal hematoma (Fig. 32.7). She was observed in an ICU and discharged within 48 h. At 1-year follow-up, she maintains resolution of all symptoms.

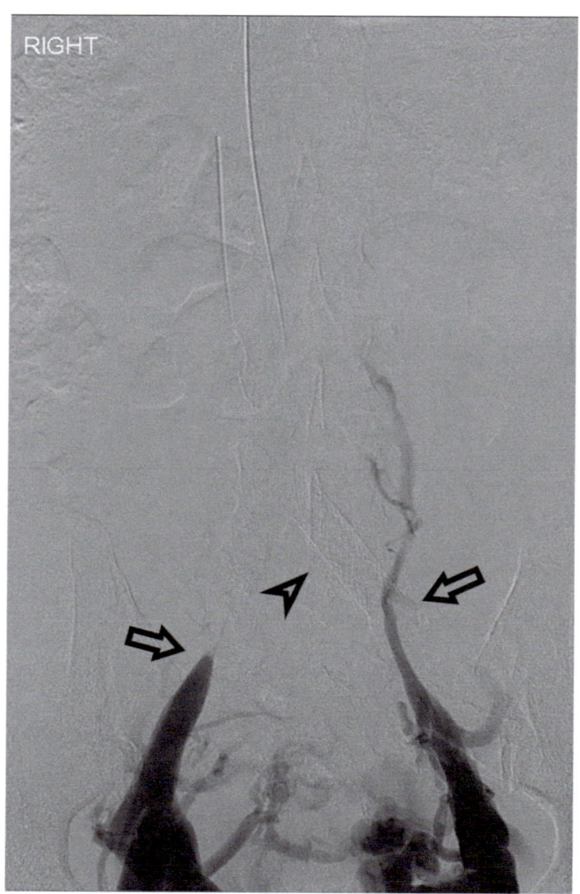

Fig. 32.1 Digital subtraction angiogram (DSA) of early pelvic venogram from bilateral common femoral venous access shows occlusion of the bilateral common iliac veins (Arrows). Partially resected left common iliac vein stent is chronically occluded (Arrowhead)

S. Gueyikian (✉)
Department of Interventional Radiology, Northshore University
Healthcare System, Evanston, IL, USA

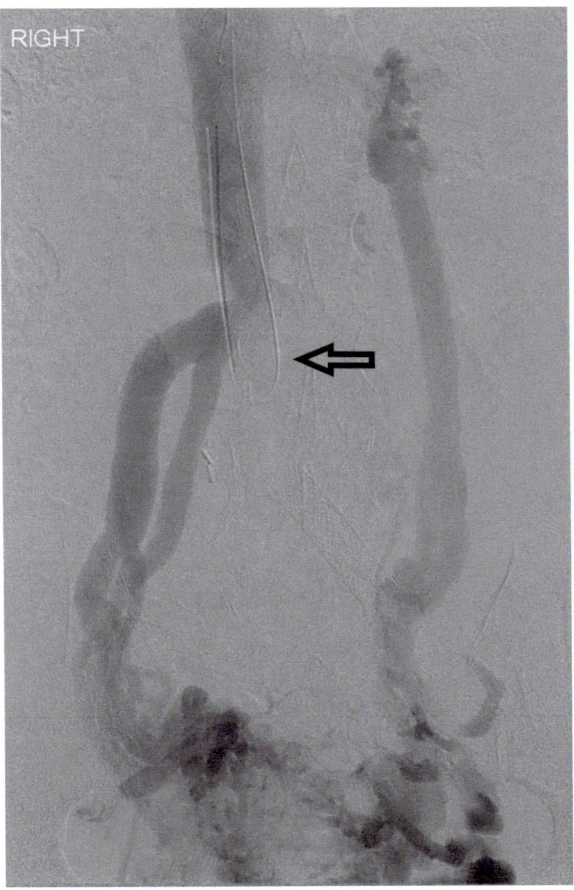

Fig. 32.2 DSA of delayed pelvic venogram shows pelvic venous drainage to the enlarged bilateral gonadal veins. The right duplicated gonadal vein drains into the infrarenal IVC. The left gonadal vein drains into the left renal vein. A 0.035 Benson wire (Cook) (Arrow) was coiled in the most inferior aspect of the IVC as target

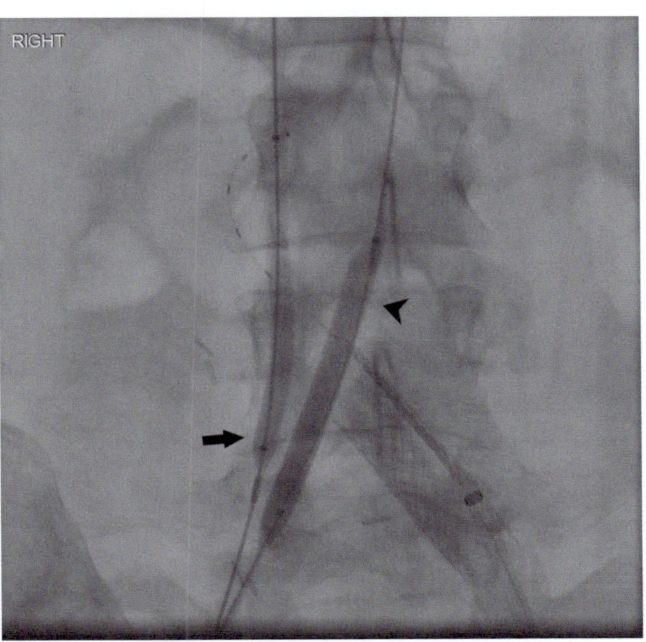

Fig. 32.3 Angled catheter and sheath were advanced through the left CIV stent using the PowerWire RF (Baylis). A 4 mm by 6 cm Conquest balloon (Bard) was used as a target (Arrow) in the newly formed retroperitoneal pathway to IVC. A 7 mm by 10 mm Mustang Balloon (Bard) was placed in the right common iliac artery (Arrowhead) to tamponade recent arterial perforation and act as a marker to avoid. This was ultimately treated with a stent-graft placement. A new path on the left, inferior to the occluded stent was ultimately created

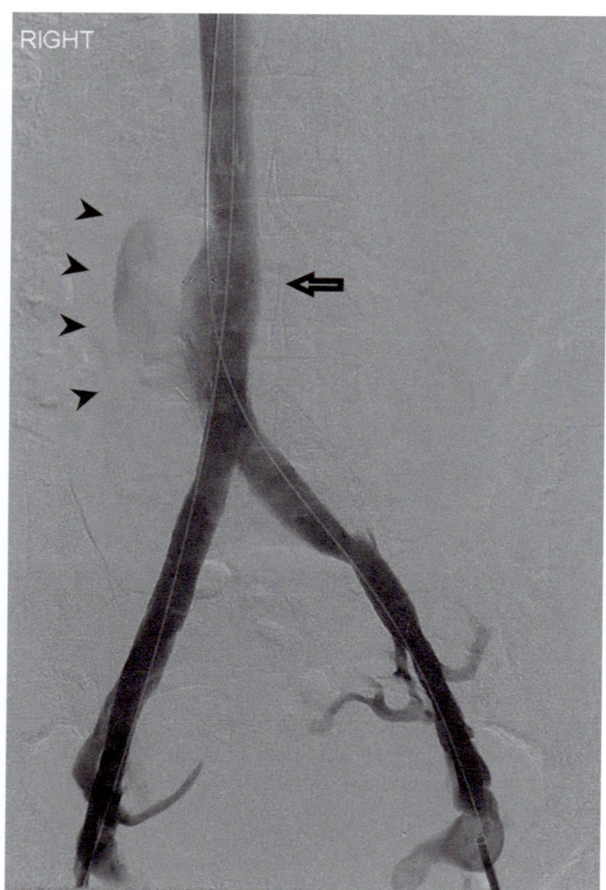

Fig. 32.4 DSA demonstrates bilateral newly constructed common iliac venous system and IVC as well as large right-sided active extravasation (Arrowheads). The superior end of the stent complex (Arrow) appears to end at the mid level of the extravasation

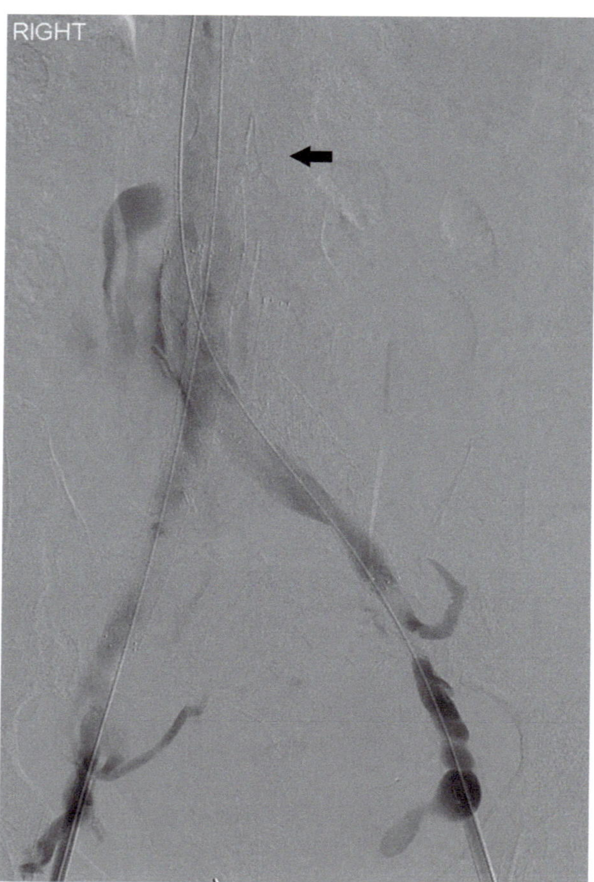

Fig. 32.5 DSA persistent filling of extravasation despite deployment of covered stents placed from the level of CIV to above the extravasation. The superior end of the covered stents (Arrow) is above the area of extravasation. Patient continued to actively bleed and be hypotensive due to filling of Inferior IVC from the right gonadal vein

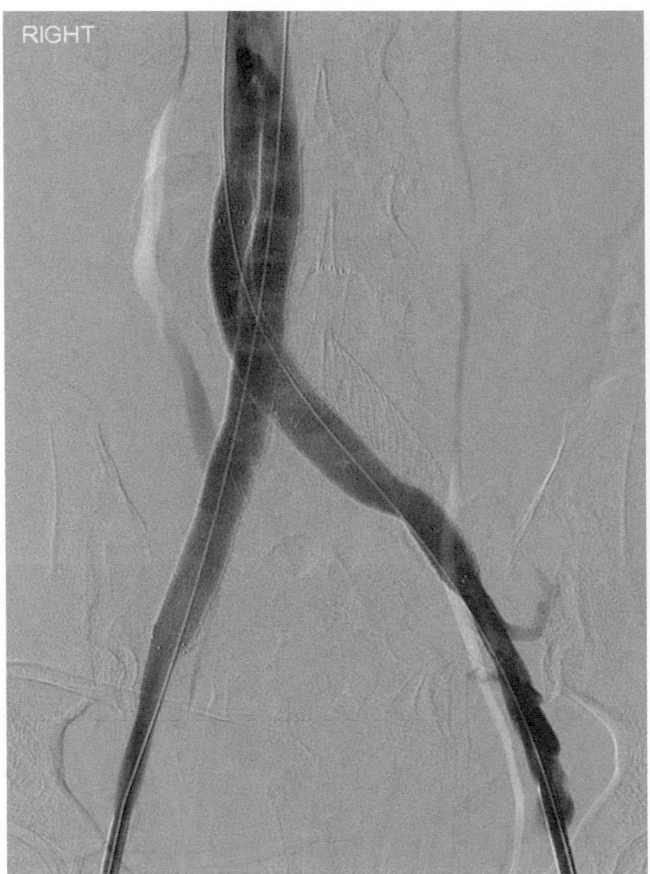

Fig. 32.6 DSA shows patent bilateral external iliac veins and common iliac veins. There is no longer any filling of the right internal iliac vein nor the area of extravasation. The patient's hemodynamics immediately responded to covering the inflow of the right gonadal vein

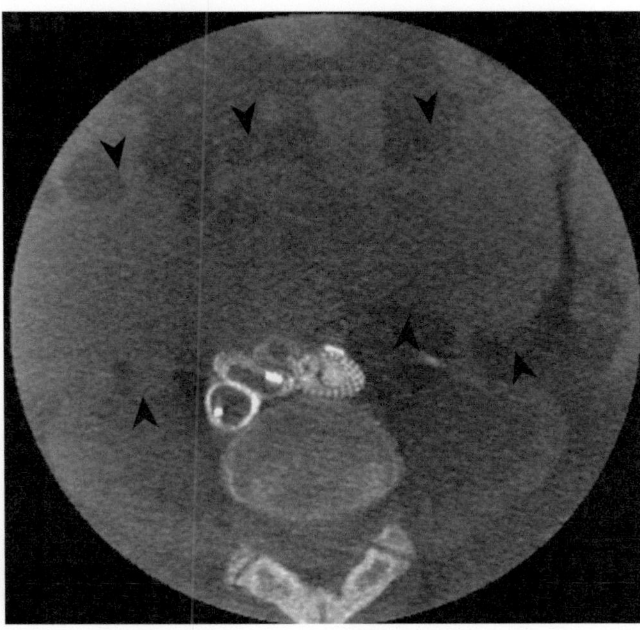

Fig. 32.7 Axial cone-beam reconstruction image. This demonstrates the newly formed stent complex posteriorly and large retroperitoneal hematoma (Arrowheads)

Part IV

Portal Hypertension

TIPS Surprise and Massive Extravasation: Never Underestimate a "Small" Splenic Aneurysm

Elias Brountzos

A 60-year-old man with portal hypertension presented with severe bleeding from ileal loop varices. He had a history of bladder cancer treated by cystectomy and ileal loop. Multidisciplinary review led to therapeutic transjugular intrahepatic portosystemic shunt [TIPS] creation. Pre-interventional CT depicted a small splenic aneurysm at the porto-splenic junction (Fig. 33.1).

The TIPS procedure was performed under general anesthesia. The portal vein was catheterized via the middle hepatic vein using a Rosch Uchida TIPS set (Cook Bloomington, In). Figure 33.2 depicts the ileal loop varices. Using our standard technique, a super stiff guidewire was inserted, which took an abnormal course into the abdomen (Fig. 33.3).

Contrast venography depicted massive extravasation of the contrast medium in the peritoneal cavity (Fig. 33.4). The patient became hemodynamically unstable, requiring rapid blood transfusion, and resuscitation with vasoconstrictive agents (pressors).

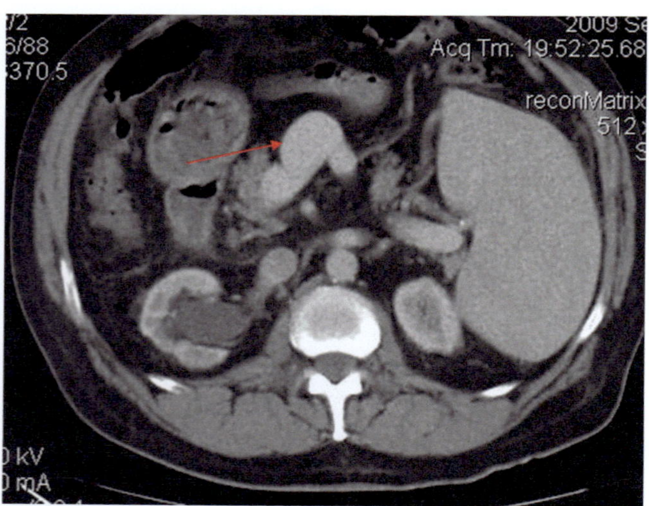

Fig. 33.1 Axial contrast-enhanced pre-TIPS CT scan of the abdomen demonstrates aneurysmal enlargement of the central, juxta-portal splenic vein (red arrow)

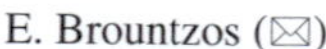

E. Brountzos (✉)

2nd Department of Radiology, Medical School National and Kapodistrian University of Athens, General University Hospital Attikon, Haidari, Greece

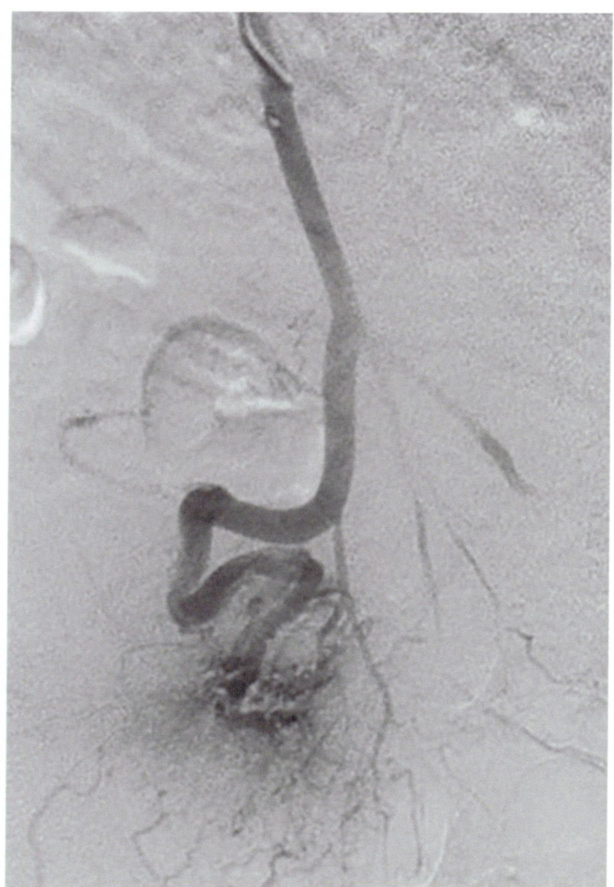

Fig. 33.2 Selective digital subtraction mesenteric venography during TIPS creation demonstrates retrograde filling of ileal varices

A 18 mm diameter × 40 mm long angioplasty balloon was inflated for 4 min to control the hemorrhage. Thereafter, a 10 mm diameter × 60 mm long TIPS endograft (Viatorr, W. L. Gore & Associates, Inc) was used to complete the TIPS and decrease splenoportal vein pressures.

Despite this, repeat angiography showed continued hemorrhage. A 20 mm diameter × 40-mm long balloon was tried for translesional hemostasis; however, the extravasation became even greater (Fig. 33.5). Thus a cuff 26 mm diameter × 30-mm long aortic endograft cuff (W. L. Gore & Associates, Inc.) (arrow) was deployed across the splenic aneurysm without success (Fig. 33.6).

Z. J. Haskal (ed.), *Extreme IR*, https://doi.org/10.1007/978-3-031-24251-9_33

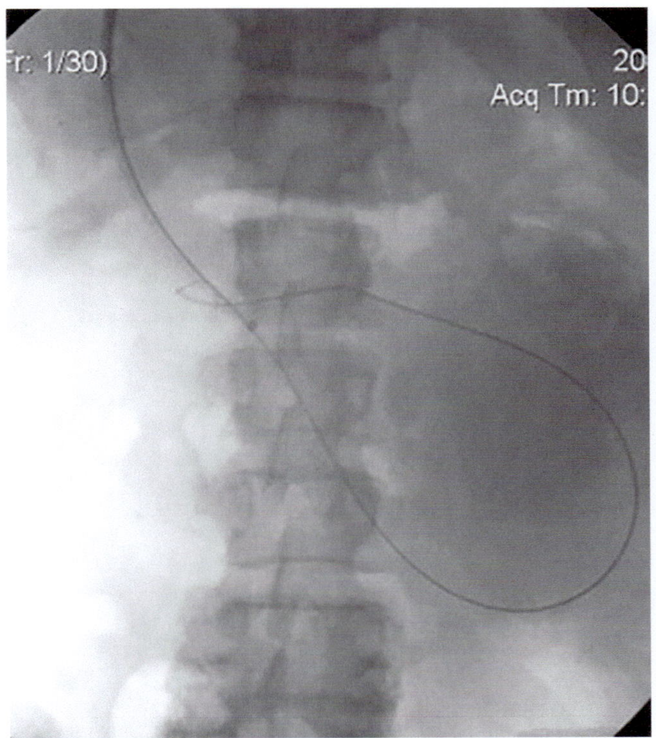

Fig. 33.3 Spot radiograph during TIPS creation. A sheath is present in the portal vein. The stiff guidewire exits the sheath and makes a broad loop within the abdomen, not corresponding to an intraluminal structure

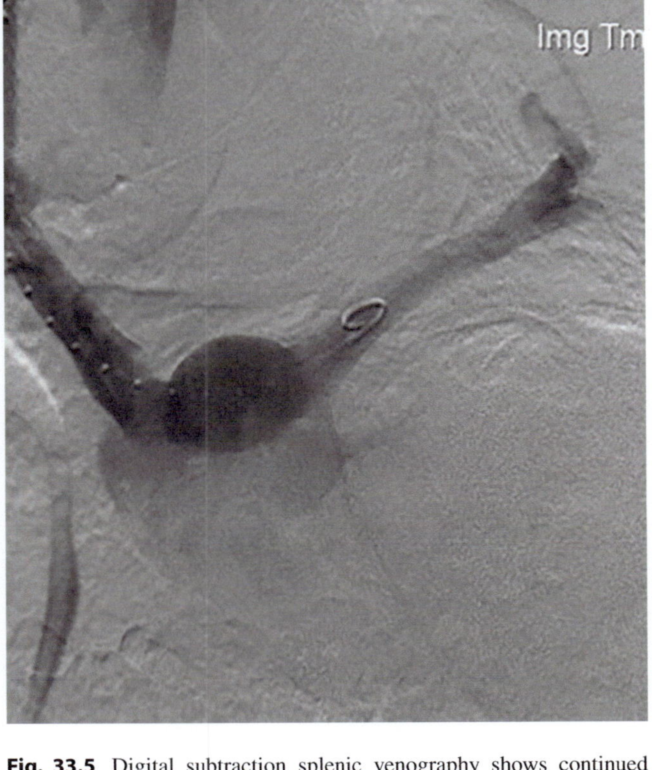

Fig. 33.5 Digital subtraction splenic venography shows continued contrast extravasation despite several minutes of splenic vein tamponade with a 2 cm diameter balloon

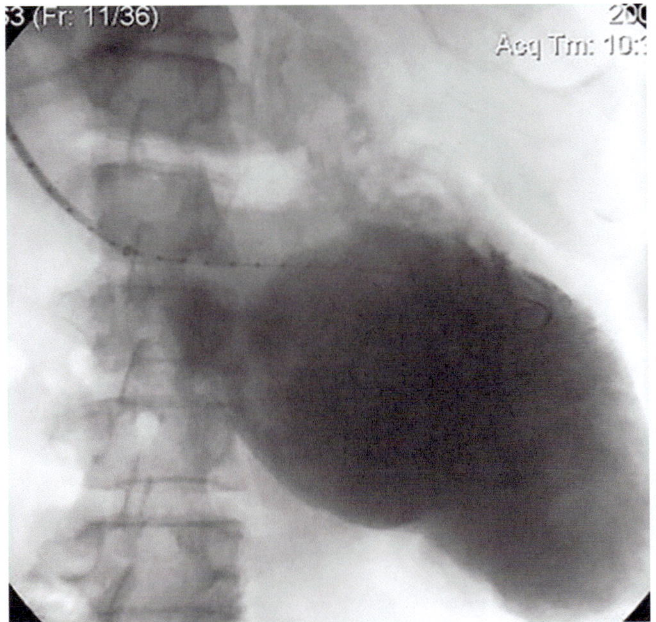

Fig. 33.4 Spot radiograph shortly thereafter demonstrates massive-free extravasation of contrast into the peritoneal cavity

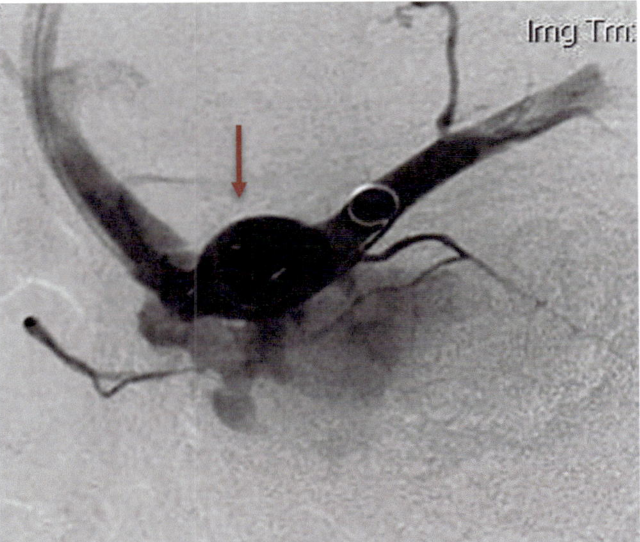

Fig. 33.6 Repeat splenic venography after placement of a central splenic vein 2.6 cm aortic cuff endograft demonstrates continues extravasation

Finally, a bare 12 mm diameter × 60-mm long metal stent was deployed into the SMV to protect its patency Fig. 33.7, arrow) and an additional aortic cuff 28 mm diameter × 30-mm long was placed peripheral to the previous one (arrow), after which stopped the hemorrhage. (Fig. 33.8). The patient recovered and was discharged after 5 days.

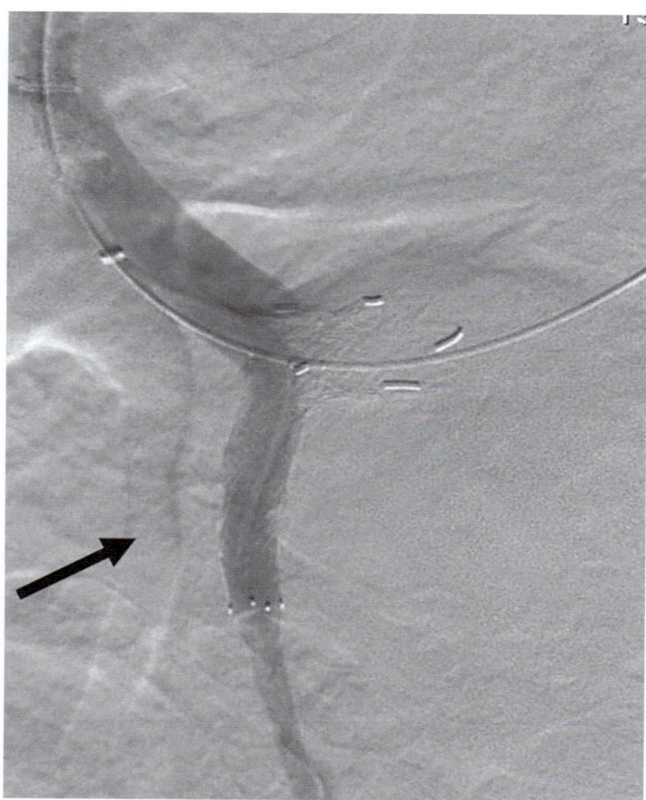

Fig. 33.7 Mesenteric venography after placement of an uncovered metal stent within the central superior mesenteric vein demonstrates its patency. The stent was placed to prevent jailing of the SMV

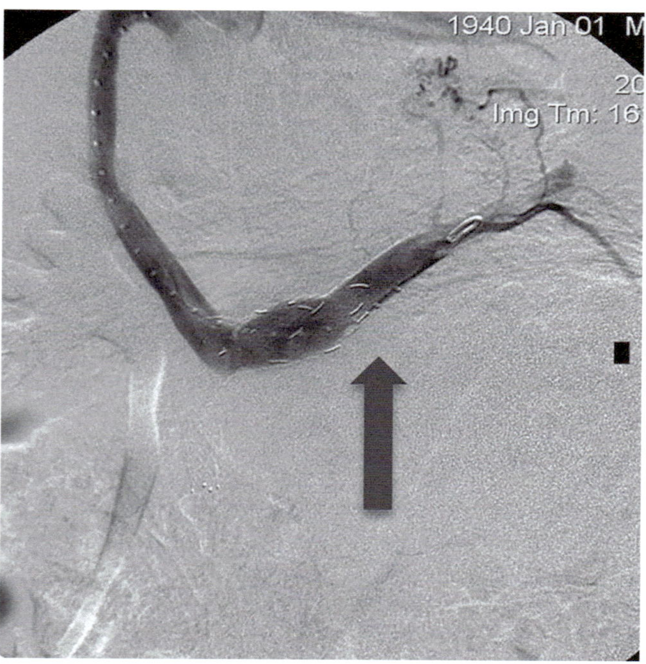

Fig. 33.8 Final splenic venography after placement of an additional 2.8 cm coaxial aortic cuff into the splenic vein shows cessation of the extravasation, patency of the splenic and portal veins and the TIPS

The patient was followed up clinically and with Doppler Sonography at 1, 3, and every 6 months thereafter. At 36 months, he remained free of recurrent ileal loop bleeding, and imaging confirmed patency of the splenic, mesenteric, and portal veins and TIPS.

Portal Hypertension due to a Pancreatic Pseudocyst Fistula into the Portal Vein: Treatment with Extended TIPS

34

Christoph A. Binkert

A 44-year-old patient with chronic alcoholic pancreatitis presented with a pseudocyst invading the portal vein causing portal hypertension, extensive ascites, and gastrointestinal bleeding. The patient was in a cachectic condition and palliative services were involved. CT showed multiple pancreatic pseudocysts. One pseudocyst, proven so by aspiration of pancreatic enzymes, had invaded the portal vein (Fig. 34.1). Such pancreatic-portal vein fistulas are uncommon, but potentially life threatening [1–3].

After drainage of 3 L of ascites the inferior mesenteric vein (IMV) was accessed transabdominally using ultrasound guidance. An AccuStick Introducer System (Boston Scientific) was then advanced into the IMV and venography was performed (Fig. 34.2a). A guidewire was manipulated through the occluded vein into the pseudocyst. The pseudo-cyst was filled with contrast (Fig. 34.2b). The pseudocyst was then accessed with a Rösch-Uchida TIPS set (Cook Medical) using a TIPS approach and a wire was placed within the pseudocyst (Fig. 34.2c). A catheter was then advanced alongside the previous guidewire into the IMV. After confirming the connection to the IMV (Fig. 34.2d), the entire tract was ballooned with 8–10 mm. Three overlapping Fluency (BD Bard) stent-grafts were placed connecting the IMV with the IVC (Fig. 34.2e).

The patient recovered well after the procedure. Three months later, a stenosis at the central end of the TIPS was detected by sonography due to straightening and foreshortening of the most central stent graft. A bridging stent graft (Viatorr, Gore) was successfully placed (Fig. 34.3). At 21-month follow-up, CT confirms patency of the stents and no ascites (Fig. 34.4). The patient is clinically well.

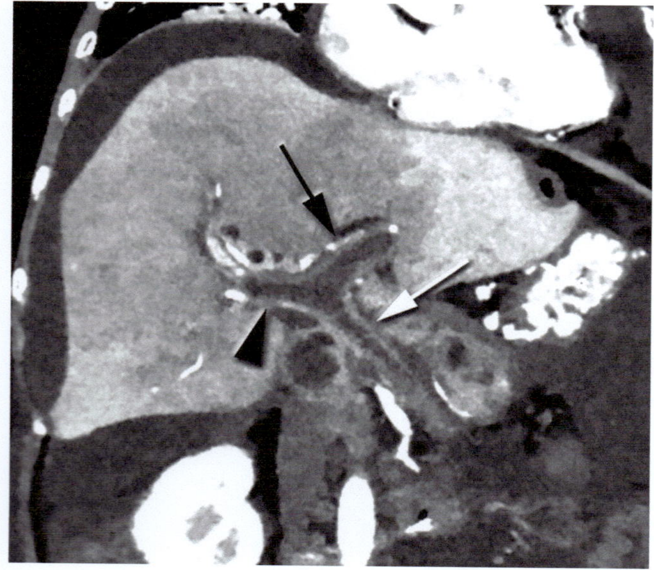

Fig. 34.1 CT shows hypodense cyst within the main portal vein (white arrow), left portal vein (black arrow), and right portal vein (black arrowhead)

C. A. Binkert (✉)
Institute of Radiology and Nuclear Medicine, Kantonsspital Winterthur, Winterthur, Switzerland
e-mail: Christoph.binkert@ksw.ch

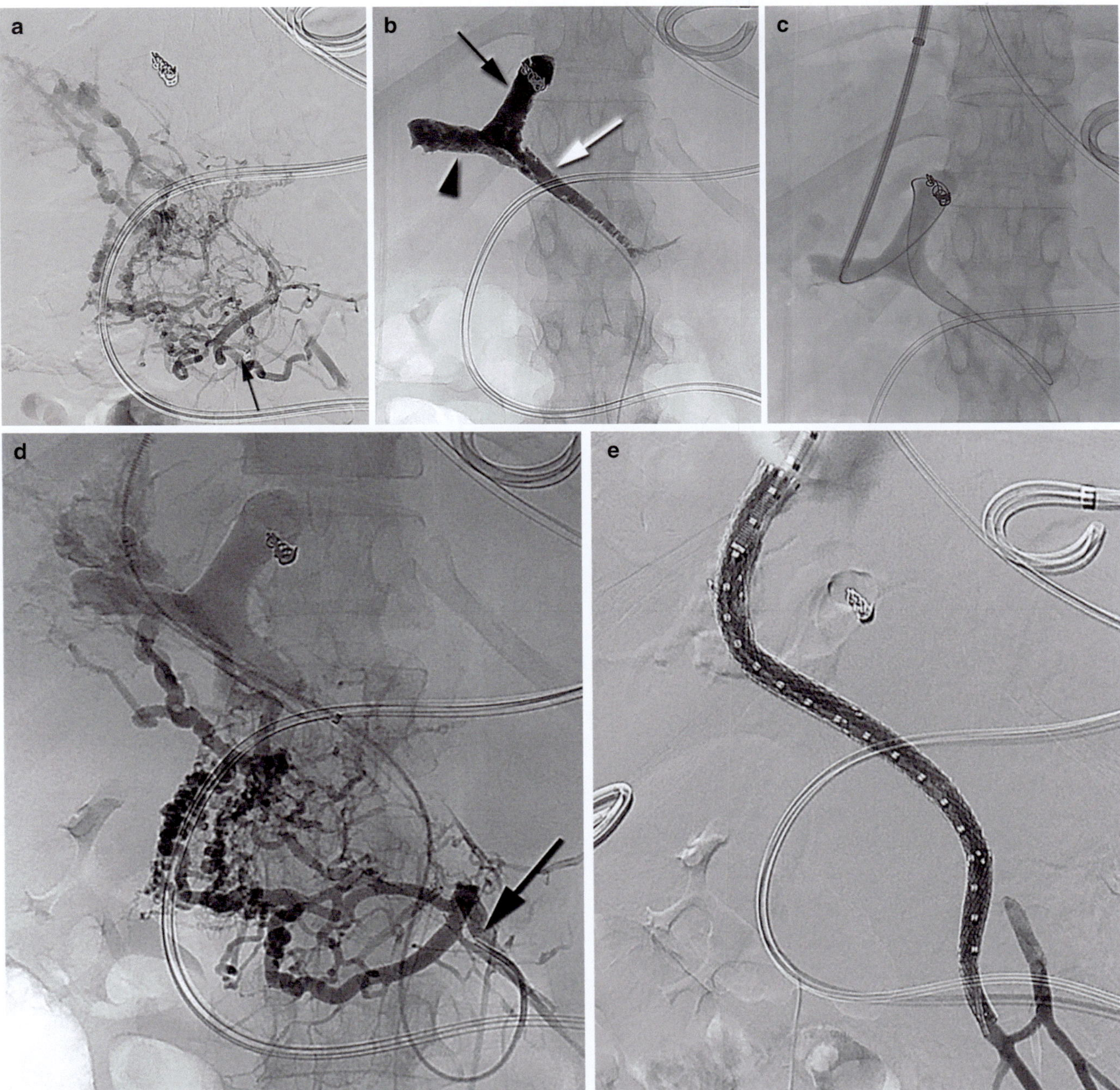

Fig. 34.2 (**a**) Digital subtraction angiography(DSA) through the IMV catheter (black arrow at catheter tip) shows multiple collateral vein and developing cavernous transformation of the portal vein. (**b**) Fluoroscopic imaging shows contrast injection into the pancreatic pseudocyst invading the main portal vein (white arrow), left portal vein (Black arrow), and right portal vein (black arrowhead). (**c**) The TIPS cannula is within the pseudocyst located in right portal vein with guidewire looped in the pseudocyst in the left portal vein, and tip in the main portal vein. Coils from embolization of the transhepatic liver access after pseudocyst puncture are visible. (**d**) Catheter has been advanced out of the pancreatic pseudocyst into the IMV with its tip in a side branch of the IMV (black arrow). (**e**) IMV DSA shows a widely patent stent-grafted connection between IMV and inferior vena cava without any collaterals

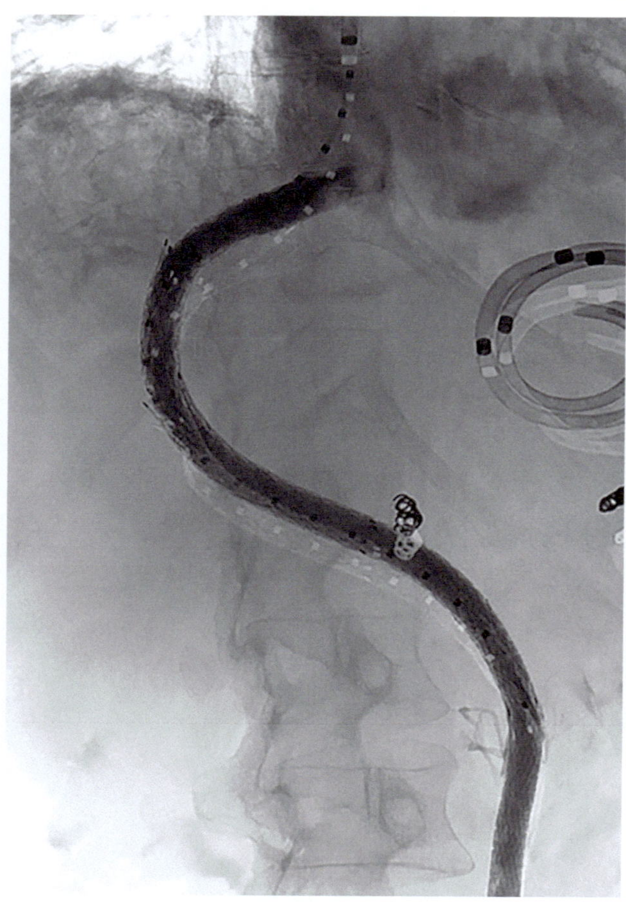

Fig. 34.3 Venography after stent grafts were extended to the inferior vena cava (after shortening of the prior stent grafts leading to a stenosis at the central end of the devices)

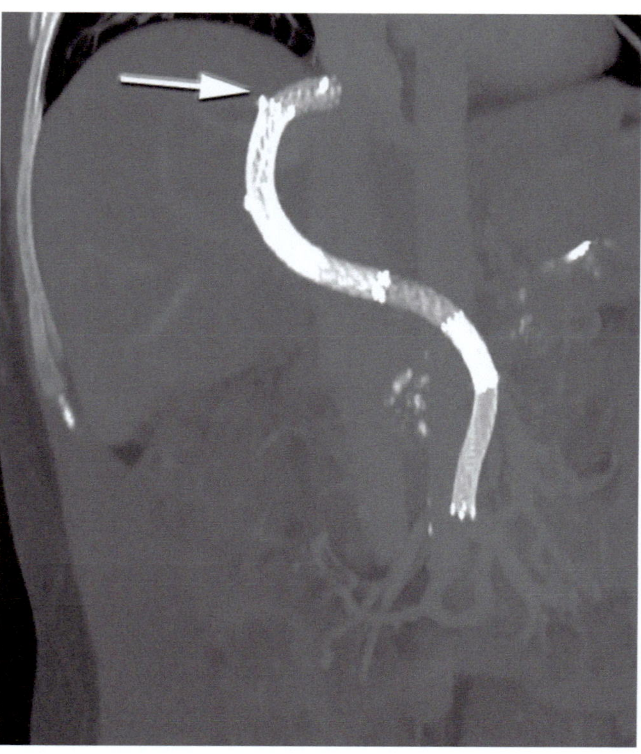

Fig. 34.4 Coronal maximum intensity projection (MIP) reconstruction of the CT shows the patent, extended TIPS from IMV to inferior vena cava. The initial, central end of the stent graft is marked with a white arrow. The secondary stent graft extension is seen between the white arrow and the inferior vena cava

Bibliography

1. Eccles J, et al. Pancreatic pseudocyst-portal vein fistula with refractory hepatic pseudocyst: two cases treated with EUS cyst-gastrostomy and review of the literature. Endosc Int Open. 2019;07:E83–6.
2. Raza SS, et al. Spontaneous pancreatic pseudocyst–portal vein fistula: a rare and potentially life-threatening complication of pancreatitis. Ann R Coll Surg Engl. 2013;95:e7–9.
3. Masuda S, et al. Pancreatic pseudocyst-portal vein fistula: a case treated with EUS-guided cyst-drainage and a review of the literature. Clin J Gastroenterol. 2020;13:597–606.

Direct Transhepatic Varico-Caval Shunt for the Treatment of Portal Varices

Panagiotis M. Kitrou, Konstantinos Katsanos, and Dimitrios Karnabatidis

A 34-year-old male was admitted for small bowel variceal bleeding requiring multiple blood transfusions. He had undergone an appendectomy at the age of 7 with an iatrogenic complication of portal vein thrombosis. A surgical splenorenal shunt had prevented hemorrhage for some time, but ultimately failed. Imaging showed large varices present at the level of porta hepatis adjacent to the inferior vena cava (Fig. 35.1); thus, a decision was made to create a porto-varico-caval shunt.

A snare was introduced from the right internal jugular to the inferior vena cava (IVC) (Fig. 35.2). Using imaging guidance, a transhepatic needle was advanced through the varicose vein and into the inferior vena cava (Fig. 35.3). A guidewire was introduced and the needle which was then exchanged for a sheath. The wire was snared within the IVC and exteriorized to provide a through-and-through wire (Fig. 35.4).

The shunt "connection" was dilated and then an ePTFE covered stent was deployed from the jugular approach and post-dilated (Figs. 35.5 and 35.6). Final venography showed direct decompressive flow (Fig. 35.7). The transhepatic tract was coil embolized. Computed tomographic imaging demonstrates the shunt course (Fig. 35.8). At a second setting, direct percutaneous foam sclerotherapy of the bowel varices using 4 mL of 2% Polidocanol mixed with 16 mL of air was performed under sonographic guidance. Three month endoscopy showed marked improvement in the appearance of the small bowel. He remained free of symptoms through 6 months of follow-up.

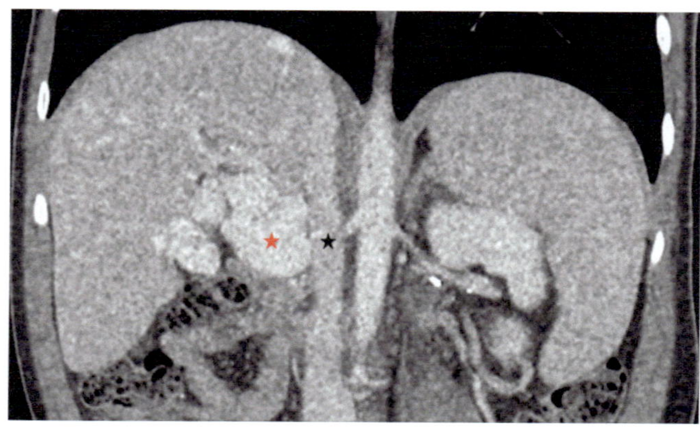

Fig. 35.1 CT imaging showing varicose veins at the porta hepatis (red star) next to the inferior vena cava (black star)

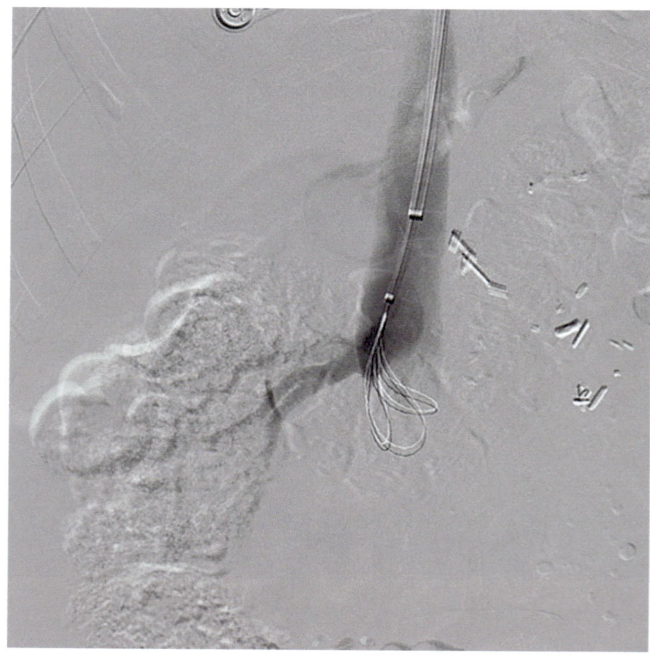

Fig. 35.2 Cavography shows the trilobed snare within the mid IVC

P. M. Kitrou (✉) · K. Katsanos · D. Karnabatidis
Department of Interventional Radiology, Patras University Hospital, Patras, Greece
e-mail: katsanos@upatras.gr; karnaby@upatras.gr

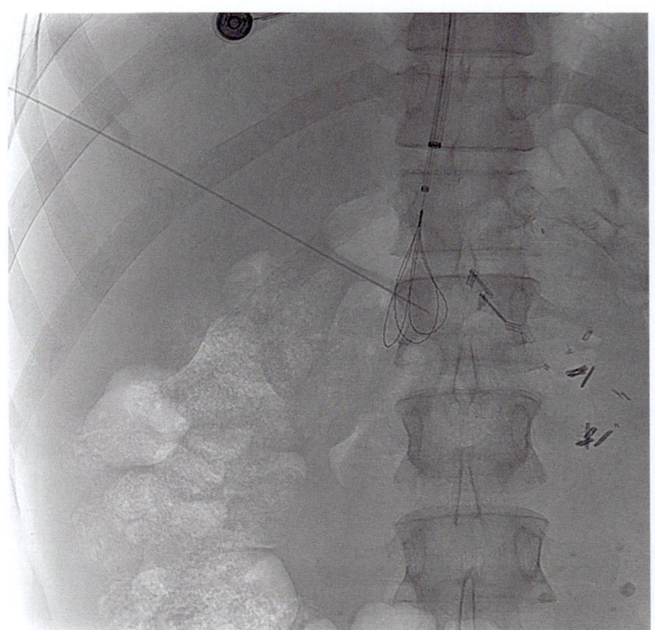

Fig. 35.3 Transhepatic needle insertion through the varicose vein and into the IVC, entering the snare target

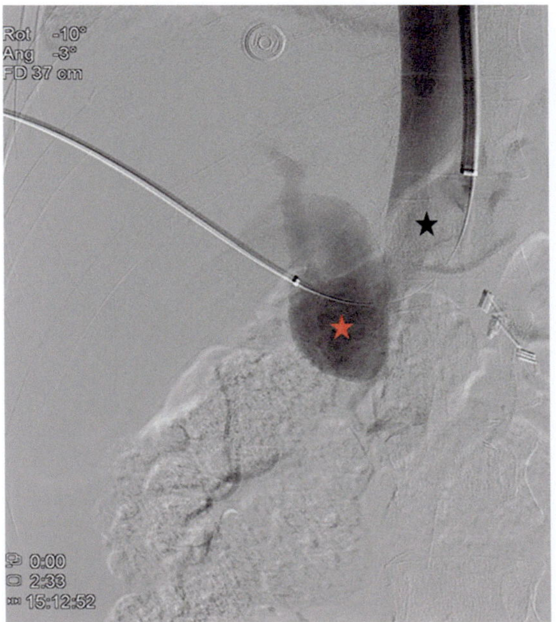

Fig. 35.4 Simultaneous venography using both jugular and transhepatic sheaths. (red star: varicose vein, black star: IVC)

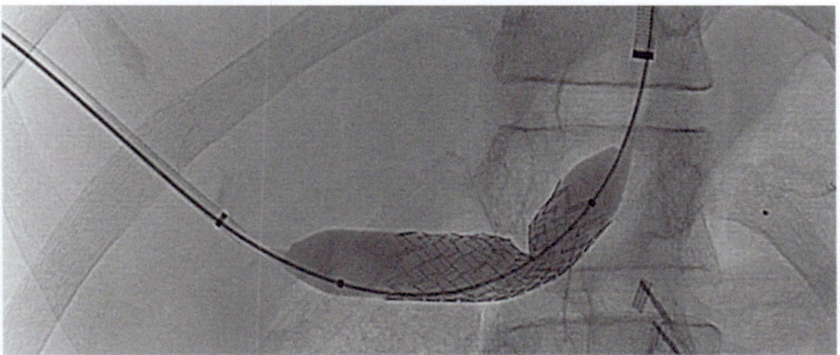

Fig. 35.5 Spot radiograph of during early stent dilation

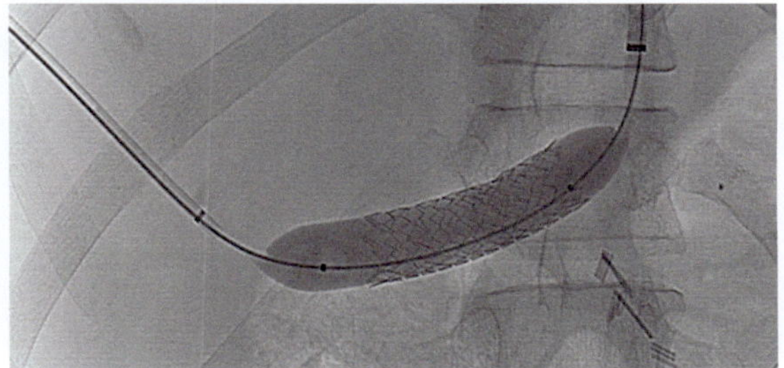

Fig. 35.6 Full expansion of the stent was achieved with further balloon inflation

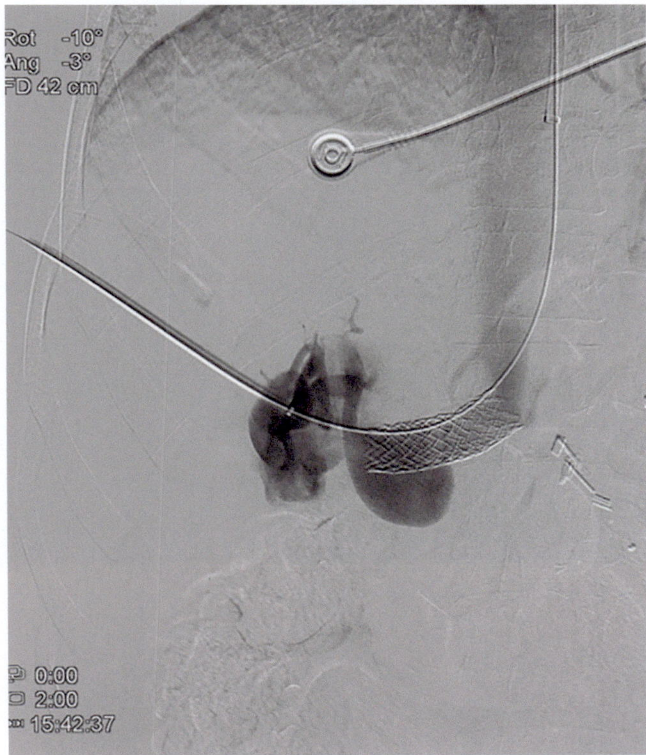

Fig. 35.7 Final venogram from the varicose sheath showing a direct flow to the IVC

Fig. 35.8 Coronal CT image shows the stent graft lined shunt (red star) and streak artifact from the liver tract embolization coils (black star)

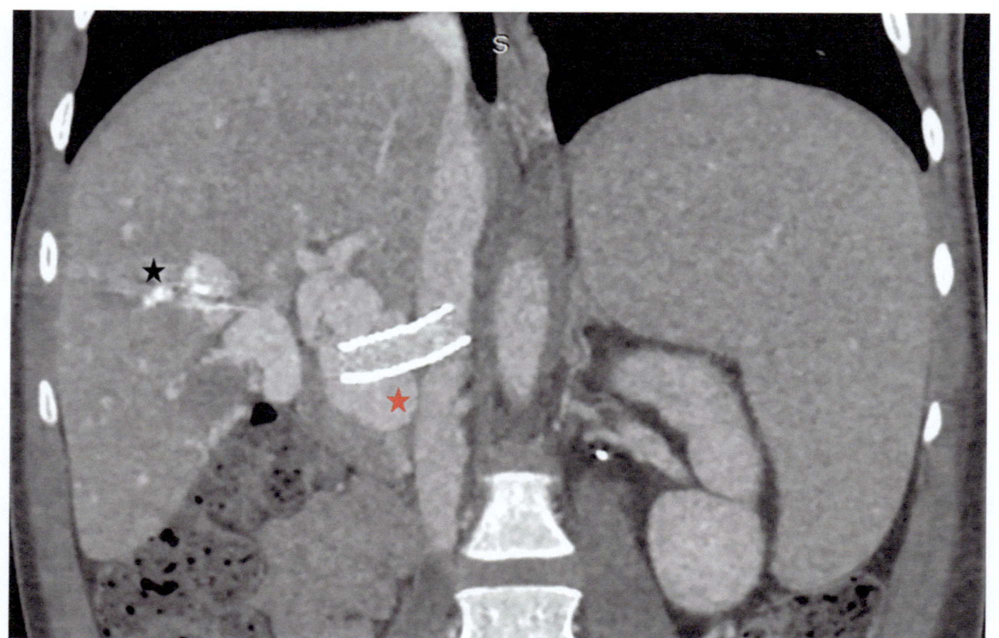

Emergent Stent Graft for Traumatic Laceration of the Right Portal Vein

Matthew Henry, John F. Angle, and Ziv J Haskal

A 36-year-old male presented with a stab wound in the right upper quadrant. In the operating room, a laceration was identified adjacent to the porta hepatitis. A Foley catheter was placed into the laceration within the liver to assist with hemostasis (Fig. 36.1). The patient was subsequently brought to the interventional radiology suite with the abdomen open. Angiography of the celiac and superior mesenteric arteries did not demonstrate extravasation.

The middle colic vein was catheterized under direct visualization. Portal venogram demonstrated proximal right portal vein active extravasation which was unsuitable for direct surgical repair (Fig. 36.2). Coil-embolization was not possible due to the proximity to the portal vein bifurcation. Therefore, a 20 mm–20 mm–55 mm covered stent (Endologix, Irvine, CA) was placed in the main portal vein extending into the left portal vein across the origin of the injured right portal vein (Fig. 36.3). Ensuing venogram demonstrated an endoleak with continued filling of the right portal vein origin (Fig. 36.3). A safety catheter had been left outside the endograft with the tip in the right portal vein. The right portal vein was coil embolized with Nester 0.035 coils (Cook Medical, Bloomington, IN) (Fig. 36.4). Afterward, the patient underwent a right hepatectomy due to inadequate perfusion.

One year later, the patient received a biliary drainage catheter due to a leaking biliary duct along the right hepatectomy margin (Fig. 36.5). At 4 years follow-up, he presented with several weeks of increasing continuous mid abdominal pain and occlusion of the main, left portal veins, and stent graft (Fig. 36.6). A transjugular approach was used to enter the occluded portal vein, drill through the hard organized thrombus, perform balloon maceration, and thrombectomy (Fig. 36.7). The main portal vein and stent graft were lined with a 14 × 60 mm Wallstent and an 8 mm diameter Viatorr-lined TIPS was created to enhance further clot lysis (Fig. 36.8). His pain was markedly reduced within 1 day. Whilst portal stent placement is routine for stenoses or occlusions, the acute use of a large caliber endograft for acute portal vein hemorrhage control is rare.

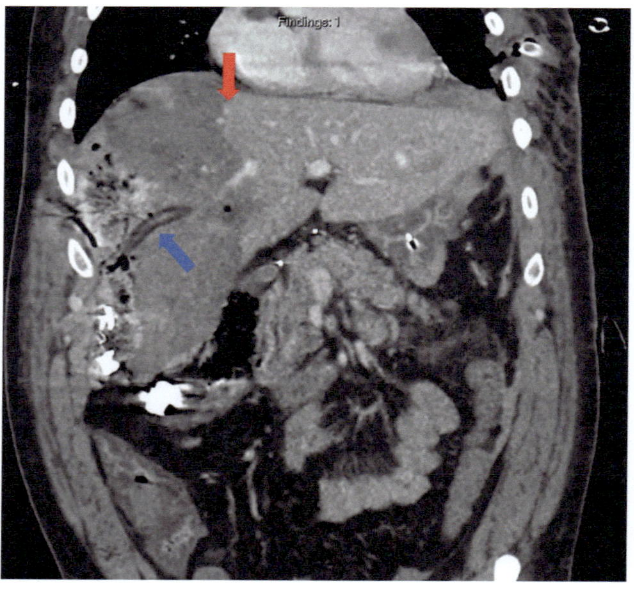

Fig. 36.1 CT scan following the initial operation showing the Foley catheter (blue arrow) and a perfusion demarcation line (red arrow)

M. Henry
Medical College of Wisconsin, Milwaukee, WI, USA

J. F. Angle (✉)
Department of Radiology and Medical Imaging, UVA Health, Charlottesville, VA, USA
e-mail: JFA3H@VIRGINIA.EDU

Z. J Haskal
Department of Radiology and Medical Imaging, Interventional Division, University of Virginia, Charlottesville, VA, USA

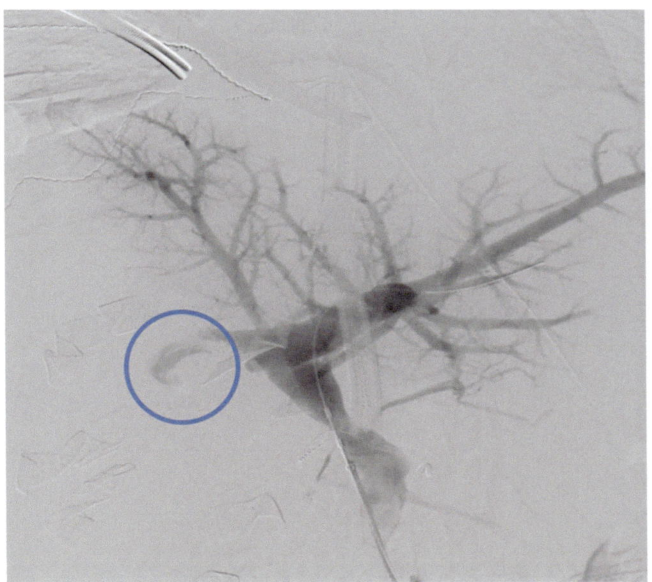

Fig. 36.2 Portal venogram demonstrating extravasation from the right portal vein (blue circle)

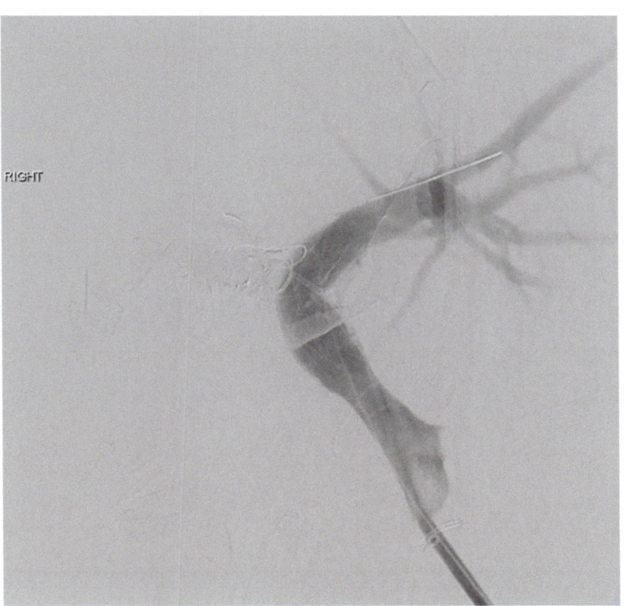

Fig. 36.4 Venogram showing resolution of the endoleak following coil deployment

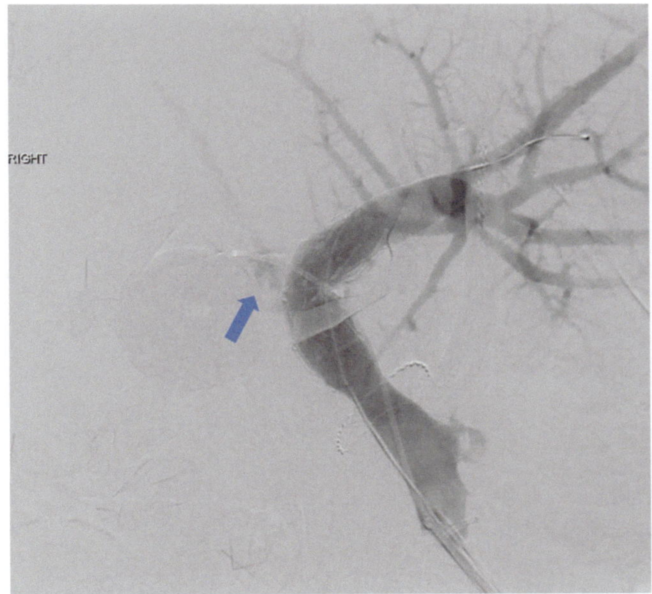

Fig. 36.3 Following stenting of the main portal vein into the left portal vein, an endoleak is appreciated (blue arrow)

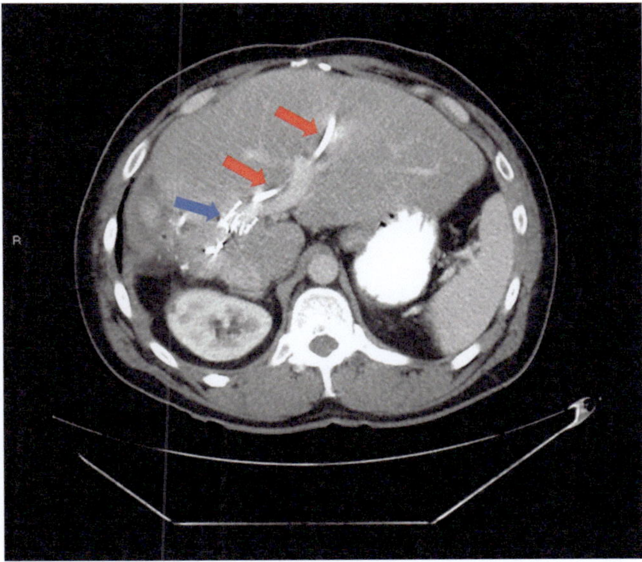

Fig. 36.5 CT scan 1 year later demonstrating the portal vein stent (blue arrow) and the biliary catheter (red arrows)

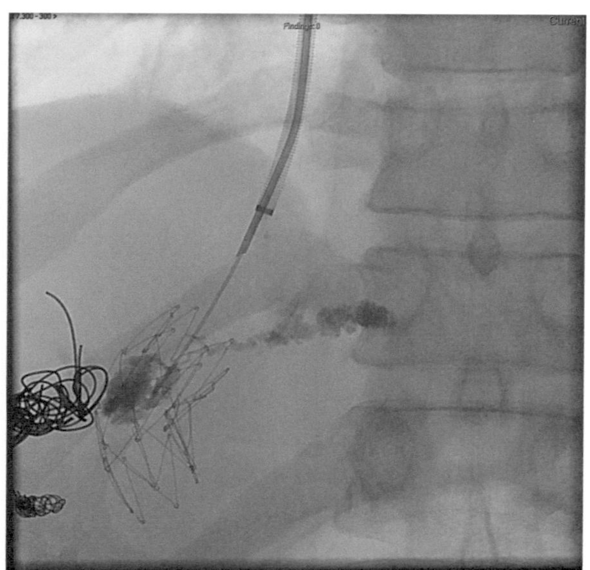

Fig. 36.6 TIPS and portal vein thrombectomy 4 years later. A coaxial 21 g needle is used to enter and opacify the densely occluded left portal vein

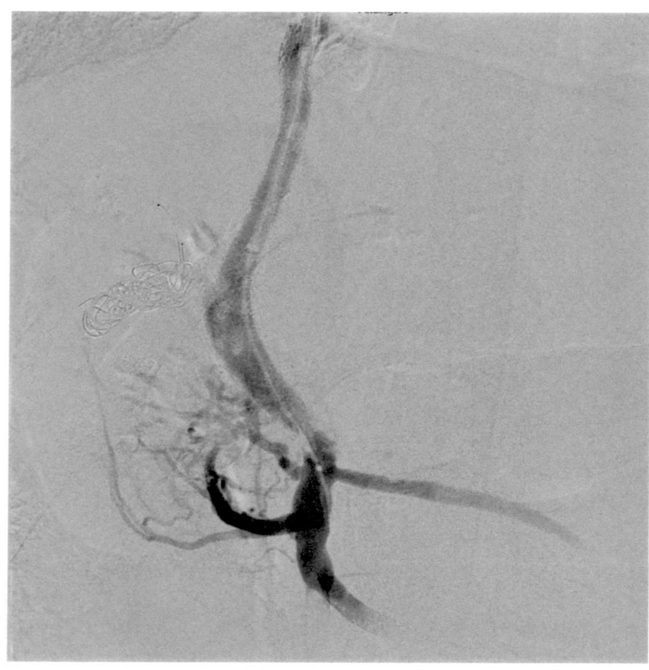

Fig. 36.8 Final venography after mechanical thrombectomy of the main portal vein, stent placement, and creation of an 8 mm TIPS between a 5 mm middle hepatic vein and left portal vein. Final porto-systemic gradient was 3 mmHg

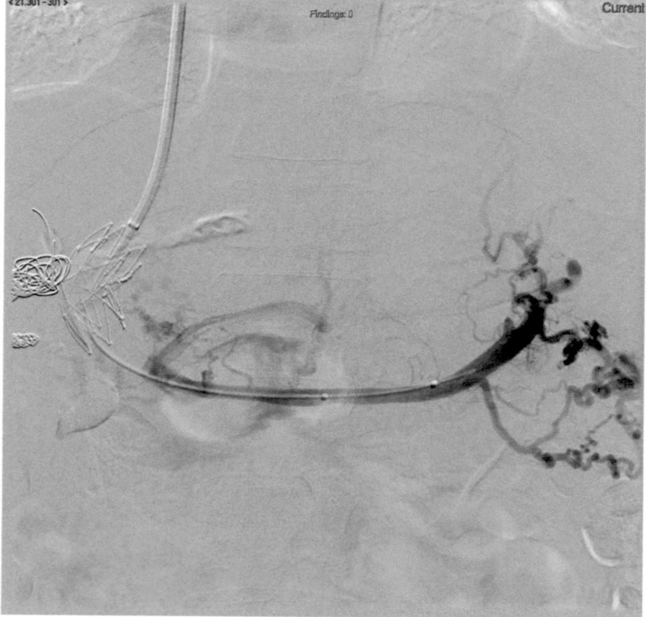

Fig. 36.7 Initial splenic venography demonstrates occlusion of the main portal vein and stent graft. Initial splenic pressure was 27 mmHg, and spleno-atrial gradient was 17 mmHg

Angio-CT Guided Sharp Recanalization of Superior Mesenteric Venous Occlusion for Treatment of Bleeding Jejunal Varices

Ethan Ungchusri, Elliot Berger, Jeffery Leef, and Osman Ahmed

A 51-year-old man with history of ulcerative colitis, proctocolectomy, and ileostomy, MELD score of 16, presented with large volume bloody ileostomy output and hypotension. Endoscopic control of bleeding jejunal varices was unsuccessful.

In the preceding 6 months, the patient had three similar presentations of GI bleeding with two unsuccessful attempts at variceal embolization. Initially, a transhepatic-portal venogram demonstrated a chronic, "flush" occlusion of the superior mesenteric vein (SMV) preventing access to the jejunal varices (Fig. 37.1). Subsequent attempt at embolization through direct mesenteric venous collaterals was precluded by lack of stomal varices and overlying bowel gas which prevented ultrasound-guided direct puncture of the SMV.

On the third attempt, using Angio-CT, the SMV was cannulated in retrograde fashion (Fig. 37.2). Through this access, the dilated jejunal varices were selected with a microcatheter (Fig. 37.3) and embolized with gelatin foam and microcoils (Fig. 37.4). Under a combination of CT and fluoroscopic guidance, a microsnare was then deployed through the SMV and targeted with a Rosch-Uchida needle advanced through a transjugular portal venous access (Fig. 37.5). The pressure gradient across this occlusion was 17 mmHg. After achieving through-and-through access (Fig. 37.6), self-expanding Zilver® stents (Cook Medical) were deployed to recanalize the occluded SMV segment followed by creation of a portosystemic shunt (Fig. 37.7). Upon completion, the gradient was reduced to 6 mmHg. The patient's stomal bleeding immediately resolved however his hospital course was complicated by acute kidney injury, secondary to hypotension, resulting in end-stage renal disease. Follow-up examination at 7, 13, and 16 months affirmed shunt patency and no further clinical episodes of gastrointestinal bleeding. At the 16-month follow-up, the patient's MELD score had increased to 21.

E. Ungchusri (✉)
Department of Radiology, University of Chicago Medical Center, Chicago, IL, USA
e-mail: ethan.ungchusri@uchospitals.edu

E. Berger
College of Osteopathic Medicine, Des Moines University, Des Moines, IA, USA
e-mail: elliot.berger@dmu.edu

J. Leef · O. Ahmed
Department of Vascular and Interventional Radiology, University of Chicago Medical Center, Chicago, IL, USA
e-mail: jleef@radiology.bsd.uchicago.edu;
oahmed@radiology.bsd.uchicago.edu

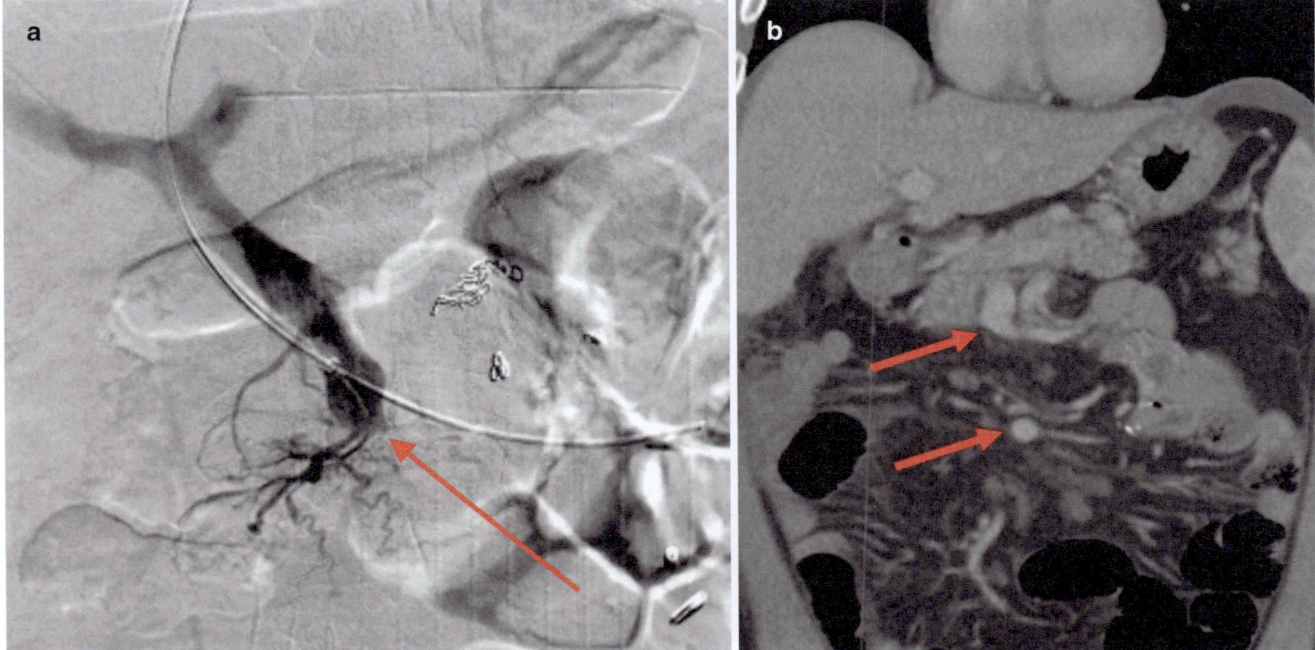

Fig. 37.1 (**a**) Transhepatic portal venogram demonstrating chronic occlusion of superior mesenteric vein (straight arrow). (**b**) Corresponding pre-procedure CT delineates length and chronic appearance of SMV occlusion (red arrows)

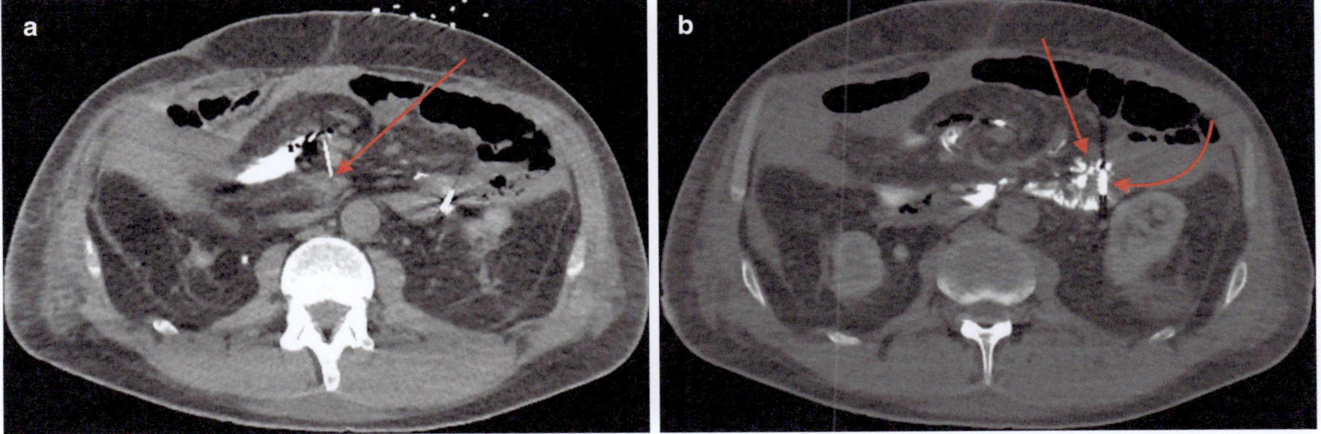

Fig. 37.2 (**a**) Angio-CT guided percutaneous microcatheter (straight arrow) access of the superior mesenteric vein. (**b**) CT angiogram through percutaneous access of superior mesenteric vein demonstrating jejunal varices (straight arrow) and endoscopic clip (curved arrow)

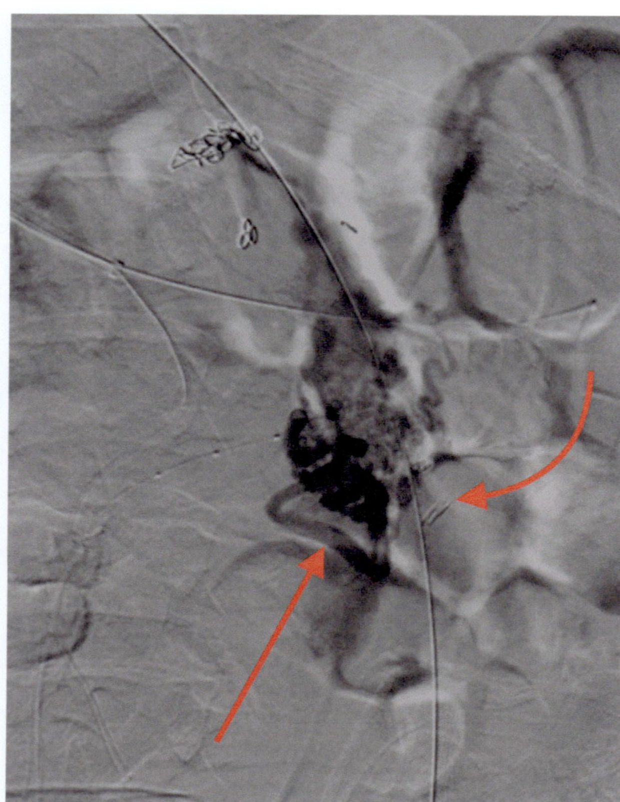

Fig. 37.3 Angiogram through microcatheter demonstrating jejunal varices (straight arrow) and endoscopic clip (curved arrow)

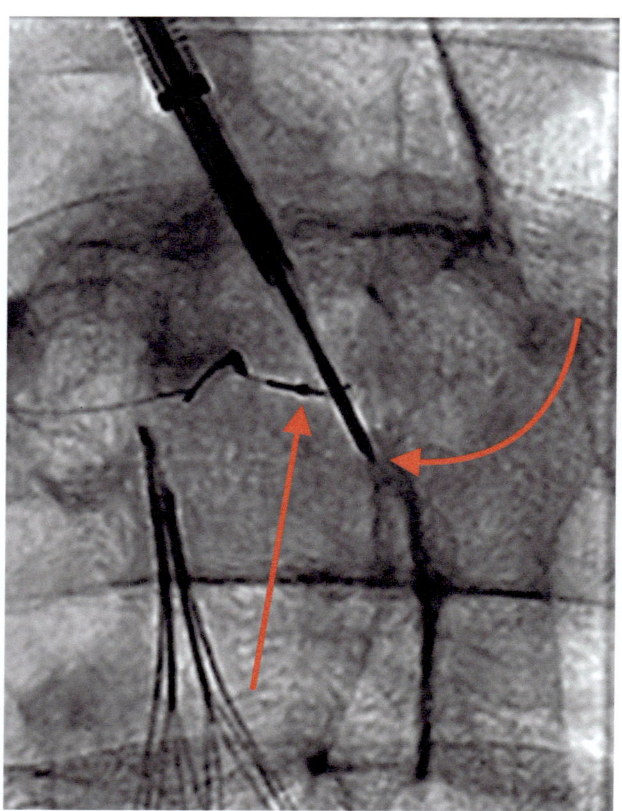

Fig. 37.5 Microsnare (straight arrow) from direct SMV access targeted with Rosch-Uchida needle (curved arrow) from transhepatic portal venous access

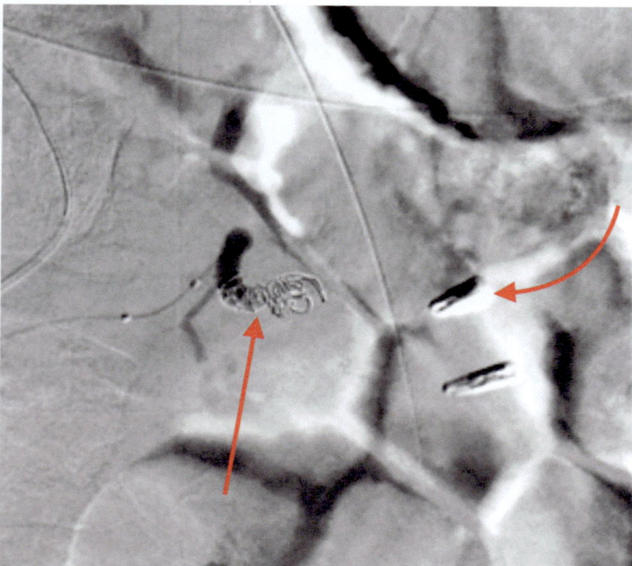

Fig. 37.4 Angiogram after coil (straight arrow) embolization of jejunal varices in the region of endoscopically visualized bleeding marked with endoscopic clips (curved arrow)

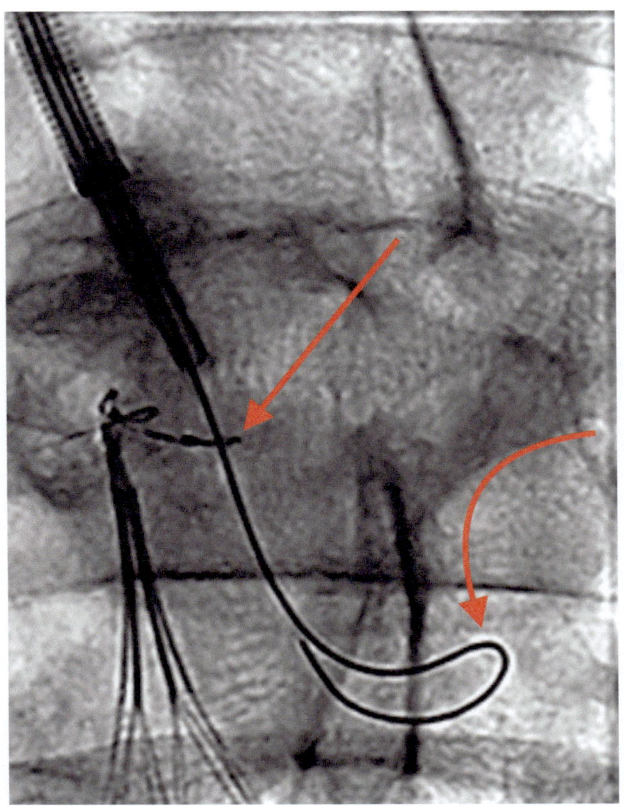

Fig. 37.6 Microsnare (straight arrow) used to capture microwire (curved arrow) to achieve through-and-through access

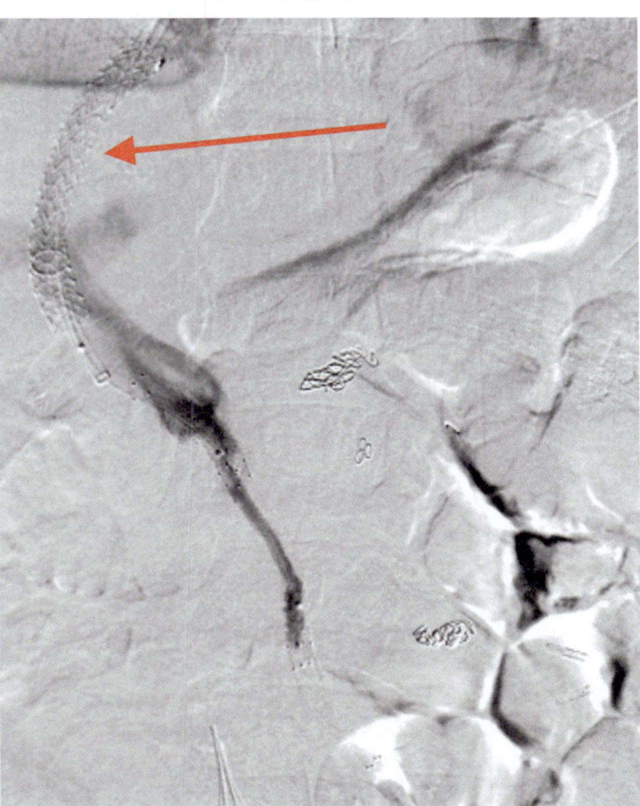

Fig. 37.7 Completion mesenteric venogram demonstrating recanalized SMV and brisk flow through intrahepatic portosystemic shunt (straight arrow)

Double-Barrel Flow Reducing Stents for Hypoplastic Portal System Development in a Congenital Portosystemic Shunt [CPSS]

Eli Atar, Aenov Cohen, and Elchanan Bruckheimer

Congenital portosystemic shunts (CPSS) divert portal venous flow into the systemic circulation causing hyperammonemia and diminished fetal portal flow resulting in portal hypoplasia which may only be identifiable by balloon occlusion of the shunt [1, 2]. Acute shunt closure in patients with portal hypoplasia can cause excessive portal hypertension. A staged transcatheter shunt reduction is recommended [2] to increase portal flow with consequent vessel growth in lieu of surgical shunt reduction or liver transplantation [2–4].

A 10-month-old boy was referred for angiographic assessment of a CPSS. Digital subtraction angiography (DSA) of the superior mesenteric artery (SMA) demonstrated the mesenteric venous system bypassing the liver through the large CPSS; there was no visible portal system (Fig. 38.1). A 7 mm balloon was used to temporarily occlude the shunt while contrast was injected, demonstrating severely hypoplastic intrahepatic portal branches (Fig. 38.2). The portal pressure rose to 40 mmHg during balloon inflation. Staged closure using a "bow-tie" covered stent [2] was not possible due to the patient's size and shunt course. Continued flow around placed plugs or coils, for partial closure, can prove unreliable or unsafe. We decided to divide the single 7 mm lumen of the shunt by implanting two parallel 4 mm coronary stents to increase venous resistance, and, if insufficient, occlude one stent while the other stent would act as a "vent." Using internal jugular and femoral venous accesses, 0.014" guide wires were placed across the shunt and two coronary bare metal stents were deployed in parallel (Fig. 38.3). SMA

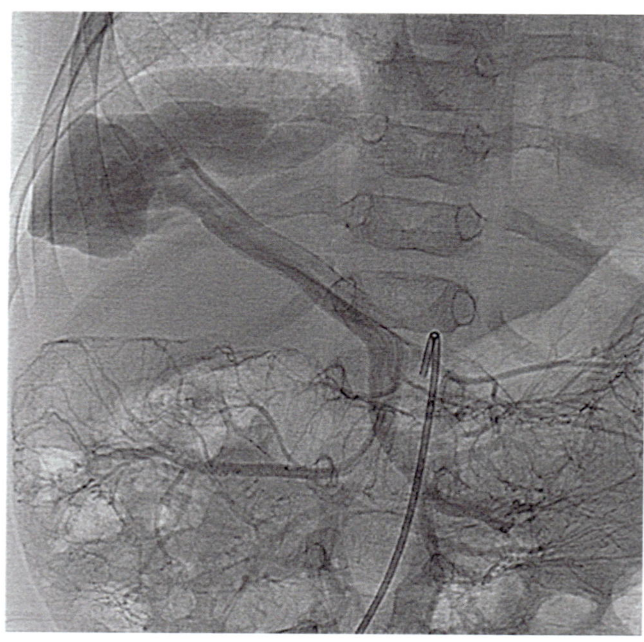

Fig. 38.1 Portal phase of contrast Injection in the SMA demonstrating the shunt with absence of intrahepatic portal vessels; a large varix and multiple draining veins is present

angiography 4 months later demonstrated a developing portal system (Fig. 38.4) and a year later demonstrated spontaneous occlusion of both stents and a normal intrahepatic portal system (Fig. 38.5). This approach has been applied, with or without plugs, in a series of CPSS patients.

E. Atar (✉)
Department of Radiology, Rabin Medical Center,
Petah Tikva, Israel

A. Cohen
Department of Radiology, Rabin Medical Center and Schneider
Children's Medical Center, Petah Tikva, Israel

E. Bruckheimer
Department of Pediatric Cardiology, Schneider Children's Medical
Center, Petah Tikva, Israel
e-mail: elchananb@bezeqint.net

© The Author(s), under exclusive license to Springer-Nature Switzerland AG 2023
Z. J. Haskal (ed.), *Extreme IR*, https://doi.org/10.1007/978-3-031-24251-9_38

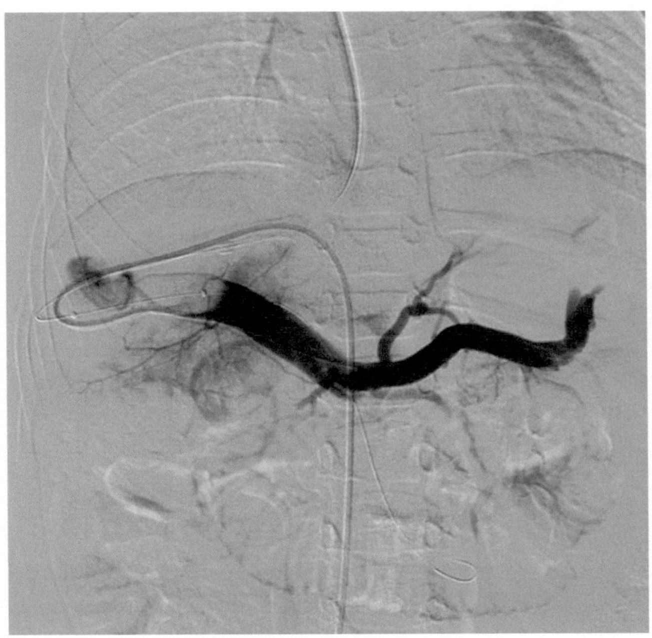

Fig. 38.2 Angiography during balloon occlusion placed proximal to the varix demonstrates the patent main portal vein and splenic vein with extremely hypoplastic intrahepatic portal branches

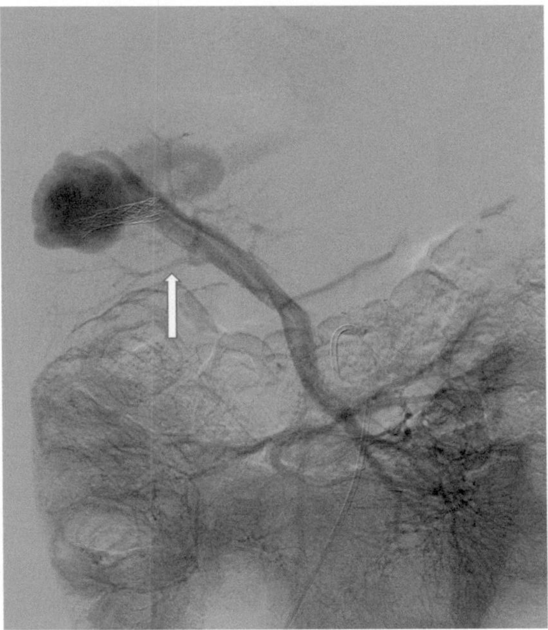

Fig. 38.4 SMA angiography performed 3 months after stent deployment—the stents are still patent; however, there is significantly reduced flow through the shunt. The portal system branches are now evident **without** balloon occlusion (arrow)

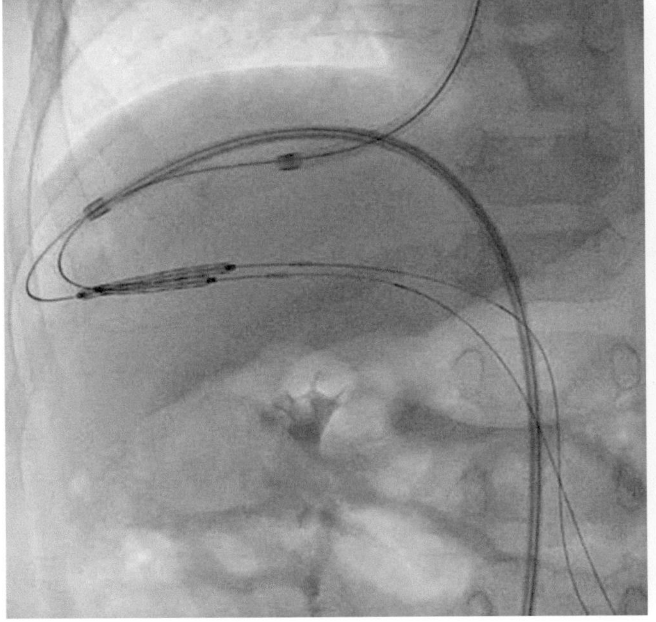

Fig. 38.3 Two parallel coronary stents are positioned within the shunt prior to deployment. The stents were inserted via the right femoral and jugular veins

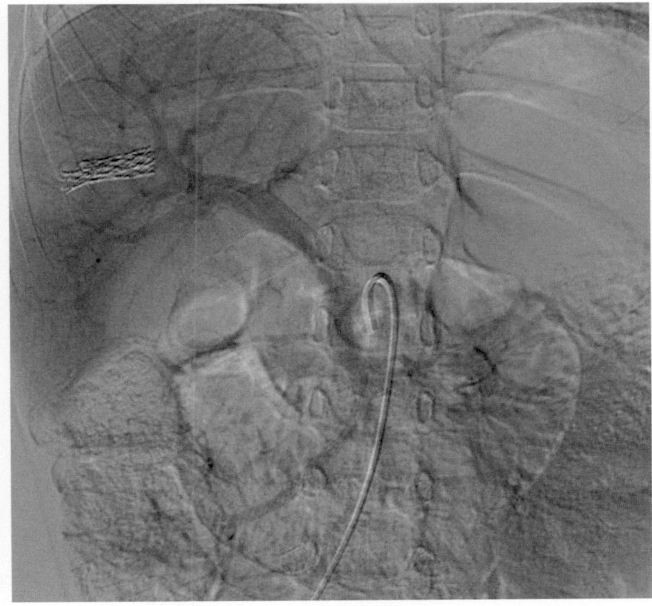

Fig. 38.5 SMA angiography performed 10 months later demonstrates normal intrahepatic portal veins. The stents are occluded and there is no flow into the shunt

Bibliography

1. Witters P, Maleux G, George C, et al. Congenital veno-venous malformations of the liver: widely variable clinical presentations. J Gastroenterol Hepatol. 2008;23:e390–4.
2. Bruckheimer E, Dagan T, Atar E, Schwartz M, Kachko L, Superina R, Amir G, Shapiro R, Birk E. Cardiovasc Interv Radiol. 2013;36(6):1580–5.
3. Tercier S, Delarue A, Rouault F, Roman C, Bréaud J, Petit P. Congenital portocaval fistula associated with hepatopulmonary syndrome: ligation vs liver transplantation. J Pediatr Surg. 2006;41:e1–3.
4. Lautz TB, Tantemsapya N, Rowell E, Superina RA. Management and classification of type II congenital portosystemic shunts. J Pediatr Surg. 2011;46:308–14.

Embolization of a Large Inadvertent Iatrogenic Arterioportal Shunt

39

George R. Wong, Clayton W. Commander, and Maureen P. Kohi

A 10-year-old female with portal hypertension secondary to extrahepatic portal vein occlusion presented with variceal hemorrhage. A meso-portal bypass (Rex shunt) was created whereby an interposed venous conduit was used to anastomose the superior mesenteric vein to the left portal vein restoring antegrade flow to the liver. Postoperatively, the patient complained of postprandial abdominal pain. Sonography revealed a focally elevated velocity within the shunt (285 cm/s). Transhepatic portography was performed with angioplasty of an in-shunt stenosis.

Her pain persisted and repeat shunt sonography demonstrated a markedly elevated velocity (786 cm/s). Portogram again showed stenosis; therefore, a stent was placed with improvement of the pressure gradient (Fig. 39.1). Her abdominal pain persisted, and a CT was obtained showing simultaneous opacification of the intrahepatic portal veins and abdominal aorta (Fig. 39.2), indicating the shunt now connected the superior mesenteric artery to the left portal vein (Fig. 39.3).

Shunt embolization was undertaken. By transhepatic portal venography, the shunt was 16.5 mm in diameter, exceeding vascular plugs considered large enough for safe embolization. Therefore, an Optease IVC filter was positioned within the shunt (Fig. 39.4) serving as a scaffold for detachable coils which were deployed within the filter with occlusion of the shunt (Fig. 39.5). Gastroenterologists band-ligated her esophageal varices. The patient's abdominal pain subsequently resolved.

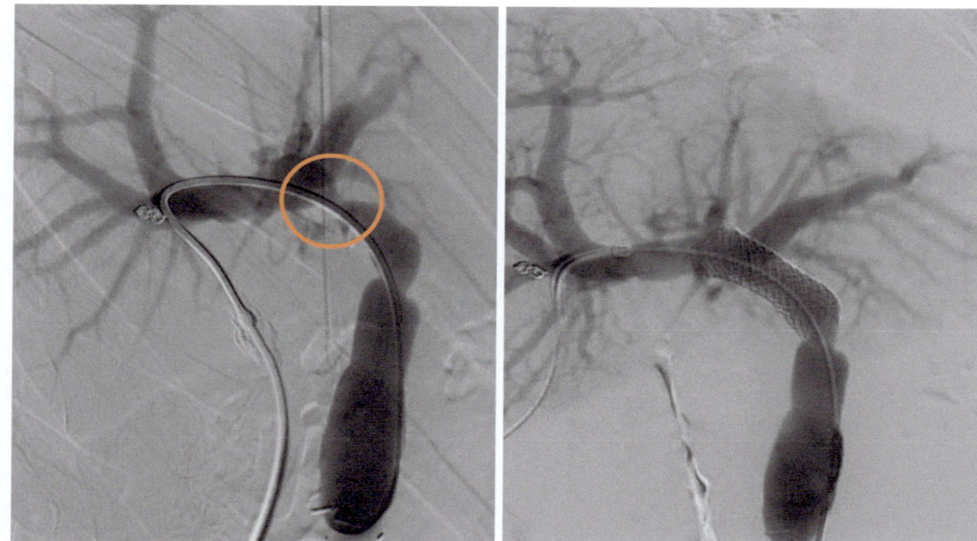

Fig. 39.1 In the left, there is a focal stenosis of the downstream aspect of the Rex shunt. In the right, a 14 × 20 mm Wallstent was placed, and angioplasty performed with a 10 mm × 6 cm balloon. Gradient decreased from 29 mmHg to 4 mmHg

The authors have no relevant financial disclosures.

G. R. Wong (✉) · C. W. Commander · M. P. Kohi
Department of Radiology, University of North Carolina School of Medicine, Chapel Hill, NC, USA
e-mail: george.wong@unchealth.unc.edu

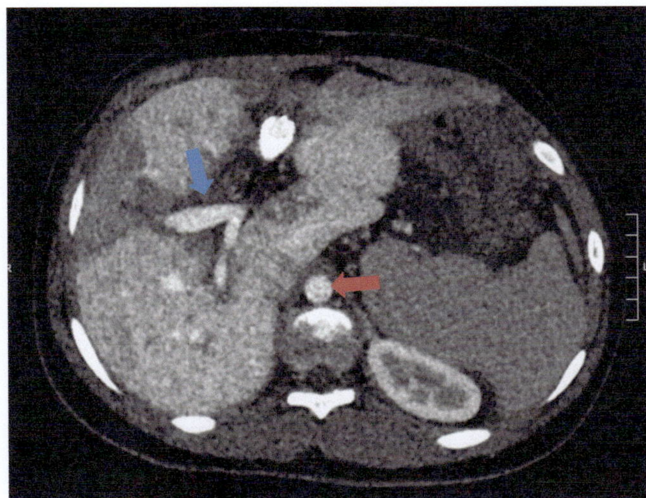

Fig. 39.2 Contrast-enhanced CT with simultaneous opacification of the intrahepatic portal veins (blue arrow) and abdominal aorta (red arrow)

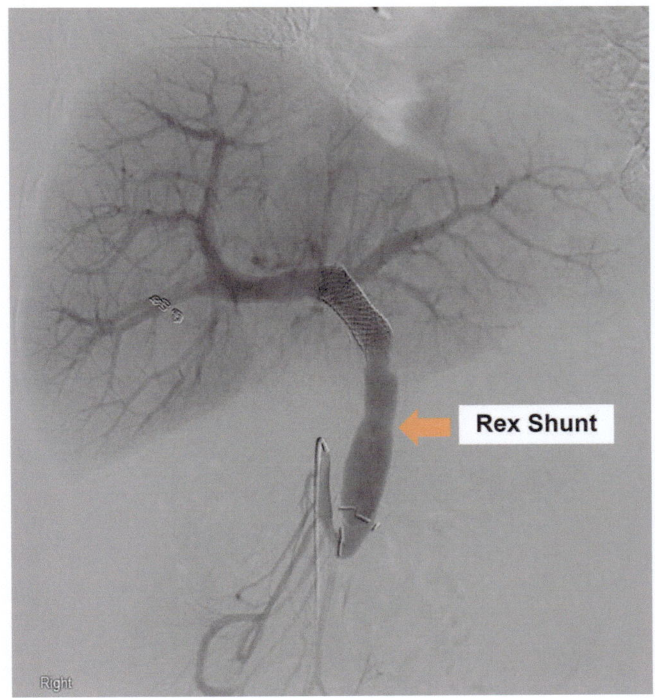

Fig. 39.3 DSA from the superior mesenteric artery shows opacification of the Rex shunt

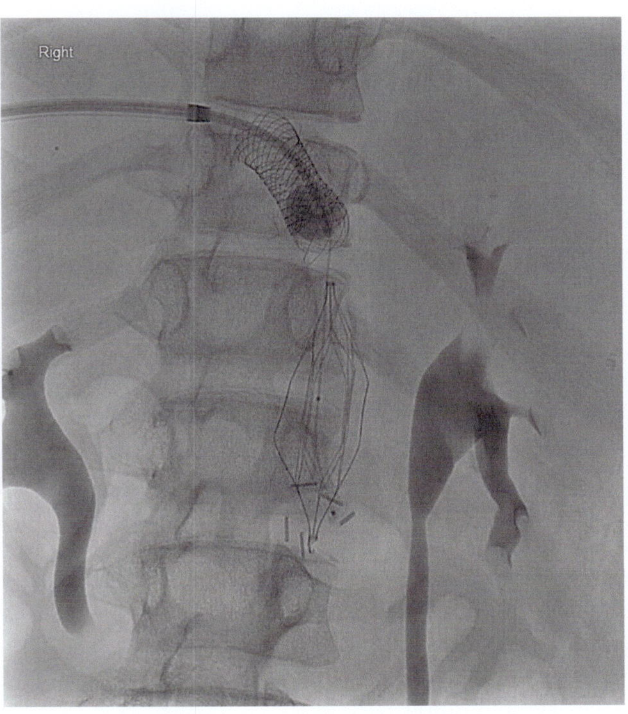

Fig. 39.4 An Optease (Cordis Corporation, Miami Lakes, FL) IVC filter was deployed in the upstream aspect of the shunt

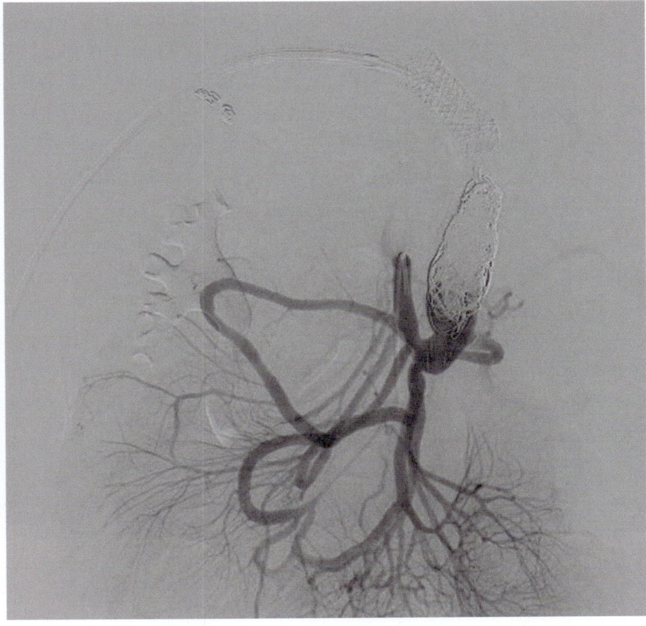

Fig. 39.5 Post-embolization SMA angiogram shows occlusion of the arterioportal shunt

Pancreatitis-Related Portal Vein Aneurysm Treated with Stent-Assisted Coil Embolization

R. Torrance Andrews, Abdul Rehman Mustafa, and Kaj H. Johansen

A 36-year-old woman with a recent history of pancreatitis treated with a pancreatic duct stent had persistent right upper abdominal pain and focal tenderness, despite resolution of her pancreatitis and passage of her stent. Imaging revealed a 2.9 cm portal vein aneurysm (Fig. 40.1). The aneurysm arose off the terminus of the portal vein, at the origin of the three portal vein branches (Fig. 40.2). She did not have cirrhosis on imaging, and her liver function was normal; the uninvolved portal vein measured 10 mm in diameter. The portal vein aneurysm was managed with percutaneous stent-assisted embolization.

The main portal vein was catheterized from a left transjugular and aneurysm from right transhepatic approach. A 14 mm diameter × 60 mm long bare-metal stent (Protégé; Medtronic, Dublin, Ireland) was deployed within the terminal portal vein, "trapping" the transhepatic catheter within the aneurysm sac (Fig. 40.3). The latter catheter was used to fill aneurysm sac with 10 and 12 mm diameter pushable metallic and fibered coils (10- and 12-mm Nester coils; Cook Medical, Bloomington, IN) (Fig. 40.4). After embolization, both catheters were withdrawn without tract embolization.

Postoperatively, her right upper quadrant pain resolved. The patient had normal post-procedure liver function studies and was discharged home 2 days later. The patient remained asymptomatic since intervention. CT follow-up at 5 years demonstrated patency of the portal vein and absence of progression of the aneurysm (Fig. 40.5). Artifact from the coils prevented full assessment of potential recanalization within the aneurysm.

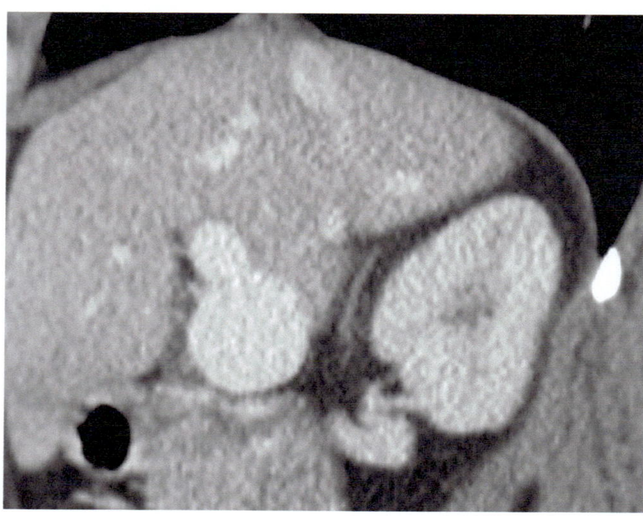

Fig. 40.1 Sagittal CT with venous contrast during the portal phase showing a saccular aneurysm at the portal bifurcation

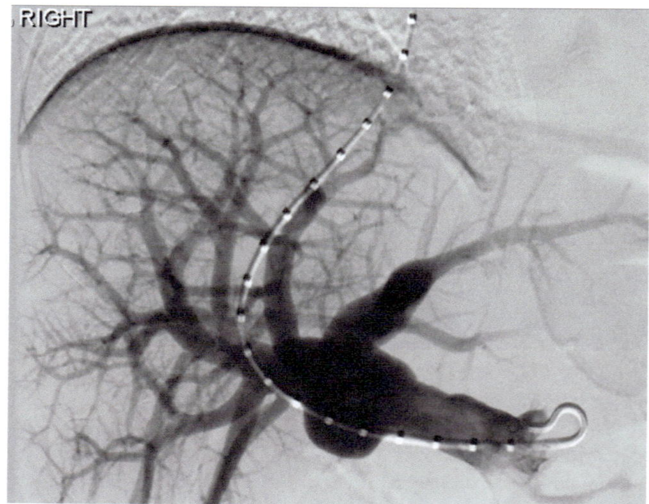

Fig. 40.2 Digital subtraction portogram demonstrating the relationship of three main portal branches to the aneurysm; all three arise within the aneurysmal segment, such that placing a covered stent into any one branch would exclude the other two

R. T. Andrews · K. H. Johansen
Department of Interventional Radiology, Swedish Medical Center, First Hill Campus, Seattle, WA, USA
e-mail: randrews@radiax.com; Kaj.Johansen@swedish.org

A. R. Mustafa (✉)
College of Medicine, Alfaisal University, Riyadh, Saudi Arabia

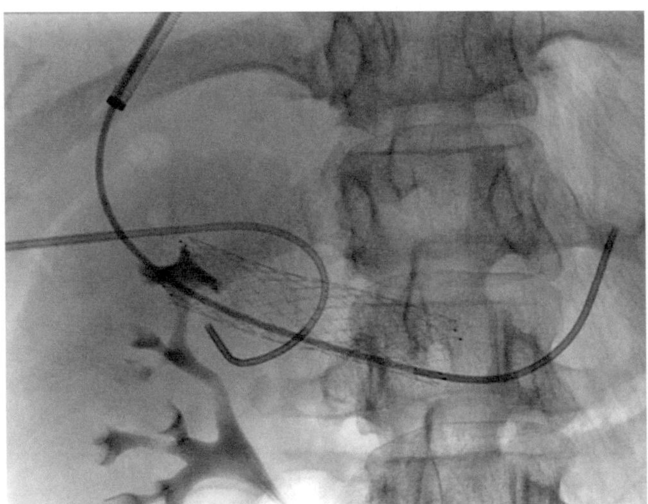

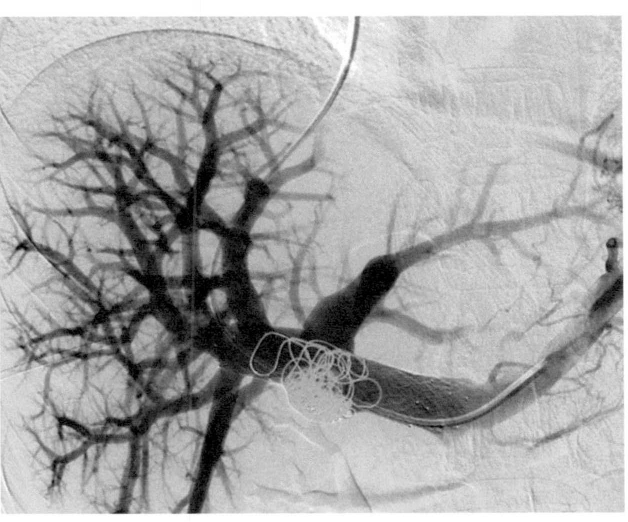

Fig. 40.3 A catheter for coil delivery has been introduced by direct portal puncture and is looped within the aneurysm. A bare stent, placed using a transjugular approach, extends from the main portal vein into the right posterior portal branch and excludes the embolization catheter from the flow channel

Fig. 40.4 Digital subtraction portogram following stent-assisted coil embolization demonstrates exclusion of the aneurysm with preservation of flow in all three portal branches arising from the treated segment

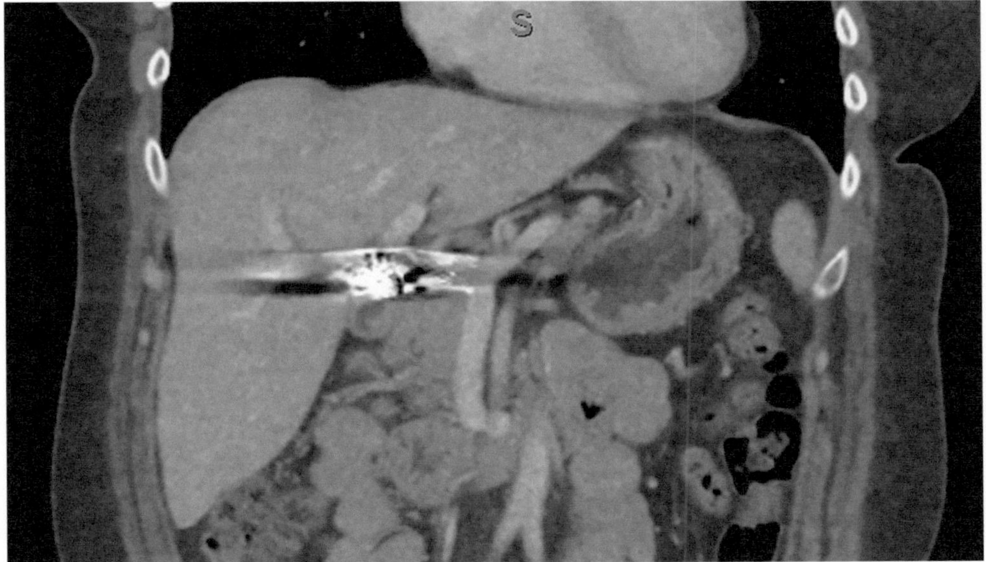

Fig. 40.5 Five-year coronal contrast-enhanced CT image demonstrated normal flow in the portal vein and metallic artifact obscuring the aneurysm (the size of which was stable)

Percutaneous Porto-Mesenteric Venous Endoconduit Creation to Restore Portal Venous Flow

Roberto Galuppo, Merve Ozen, Chadi Diab, and Malay B. Shah

A 64-year-old male who underwent orthotopic liver transplant for alcoholic cirrhosis complicated by portal vein (PV) thrombosis and allograft rejection requiring re-transplantation with portocaval hemitransposition. The donor PV was anastomosed to the recipient IVC with constriction of the suprahepatic IVC to divert venous flow into the liver. Seven years later, the recipient developed refractory life-limiting hepatic encephalopathy despite adequate liver function. Review of the cross-sectional imaging showed the PV in proximity from the native splenorenal shunt (SRS) with intervening liver parenchyma (Fig. 41.1). Diagnostic arteriography and venography with intravascular ultrasound evaluation of the PV and SRS (Figs. 41.2 and 41.3) was performed to assess for feasibility of creating an endovenous conduit in between these structures. Delayed arteriograms revealed small intrahepatic portal venous branches with hepatofugal flow towards the IVC. The splenomesenteric (SM) venous outflow was directed into systemic circulation via the SRS. A staged procedure consisting of an initial creation of endovenous conduit between the PV and the SRS, followed by embolization of the SRS was agreed upon during a multidisciplinary conference.

Percutaneous transhepatic access to the portocaval shunt (PCS) was obtained. The intravascular ultrasound catheter was utilized to guide a Rösch-Uchida needle into the SRS through the intervening liver parenchyma (Figs. 41.4, 41.5, and 41.6). A stent graft was deployed from the SM conflu-

The authors have no relevant financial disclosures.

R. Galuppo (✉) · M. Ozen · C. Diab
Department of Radiology, University of Kentucky, College of Medicine, Lexington, KY, USA
e-mail: rga228@uky.edu; moz226@uky.edu; Chadi.Diab@uky.edu

M. B. Shah
Department of Surgery, University of Kentucky, College of Medicine, Lexington, KY, USA
e-mail: malay.shah@uky.edu

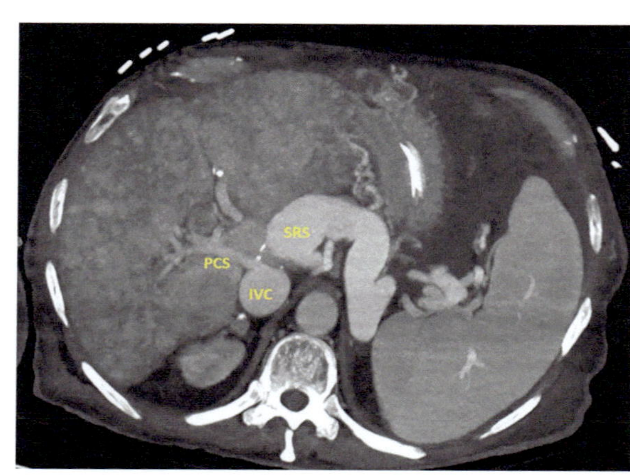

Fig. 41.1 Axial maximum intensity projection reformat of contrast-enhanced computed tomography shows the portocaval transposition (PCS) and splenorenal shunt (SRS) with small portion of intervening liver (*)

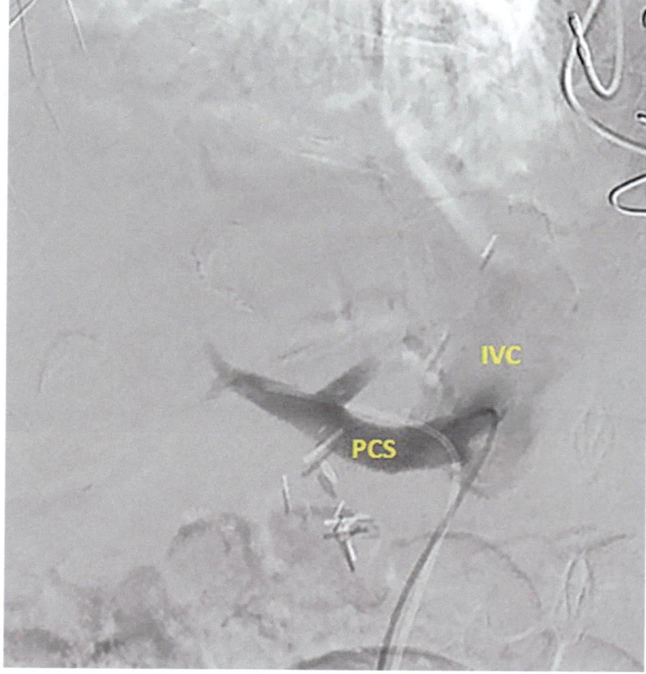

Fig. 41.2 Digital subtraction angiogram (DSA) of the portocaval shunt (PCS) with relatively small intrahepatic portal branches and hepatofugal flow into the IVC

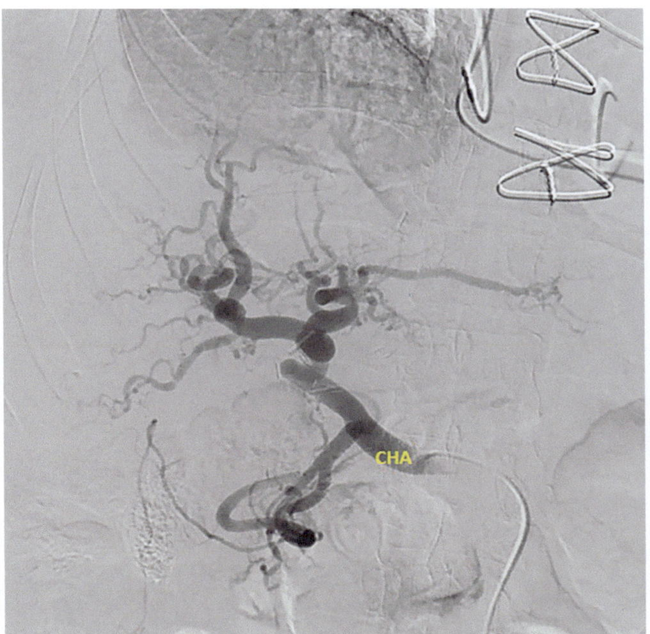

Fig. 41.3 Common hepatic artery DSA shows hypertrophied hepatic arteries

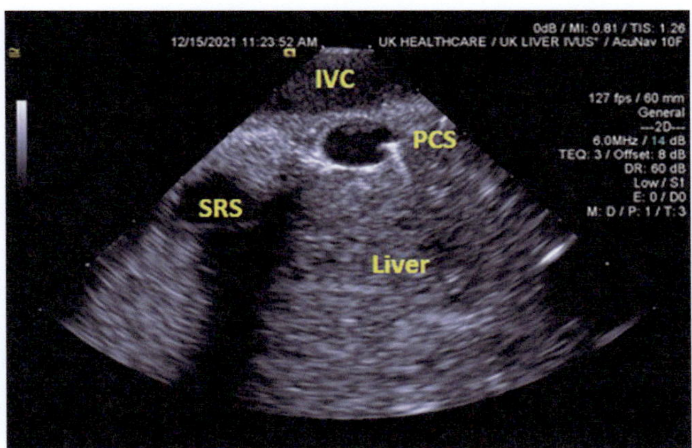

Fig. 41.4 Intravascular ultrasound images from ACUSON AcuNav intracardiac echocardiography catheter (ICE) (Siemens, PA, USA) within the IVC introduced via left femoral approach shows relation of the IVC, PCS with guidewire, SRS, and the liver

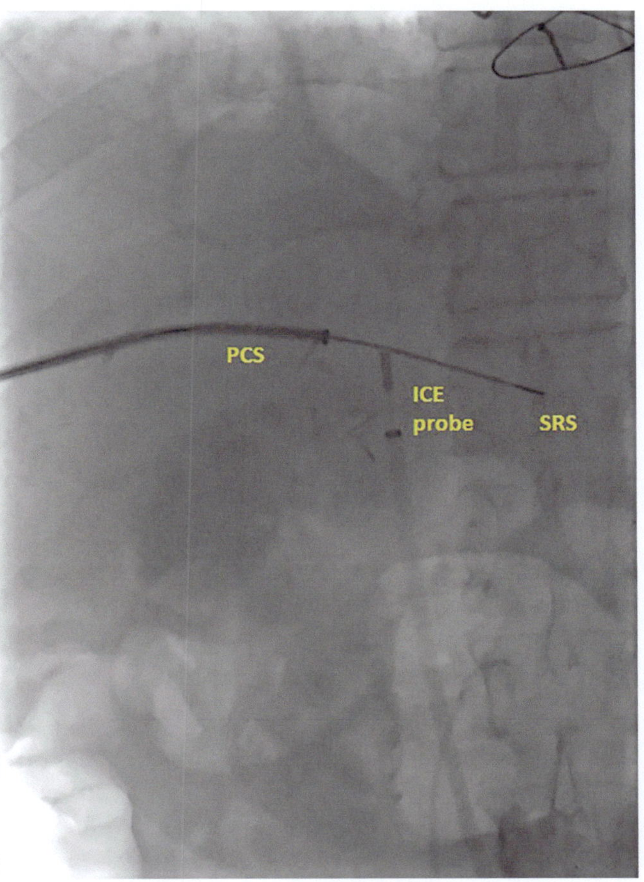

Fig. 41.5 Fluoroscopy digital image show ICE probe within the IVC, introduced via left femoral approach, providing guidance for puncture from a percutaneous transhepatic approach Rösch-Uchida needle into the SRS through the intervening liver parenchyma

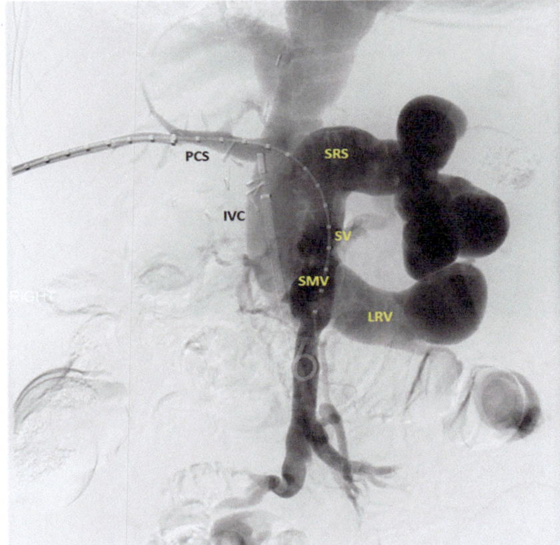

Fig. 41.6 DSA with pigtail catheter positioned within the proximal SMV, opacifying the PCS, SRS, left renal vein, and IVC

ence to the PV with flow redirection. Final angiogram confirmed hepatopetal flow through the stent (Fig. 41.7). Patient mentation status improved with normalization of the ammonia level. Follow-up portogram revealed continued hepatopetal flow with progressive enlargement of the portal venous branches (Fig. 41.8). Through 5 months follow-up, he remains free of encephalopathy episodes with a calculated Child-Turcotte-Pugh score of 4 (reduced from 7 at the time of the procedure).

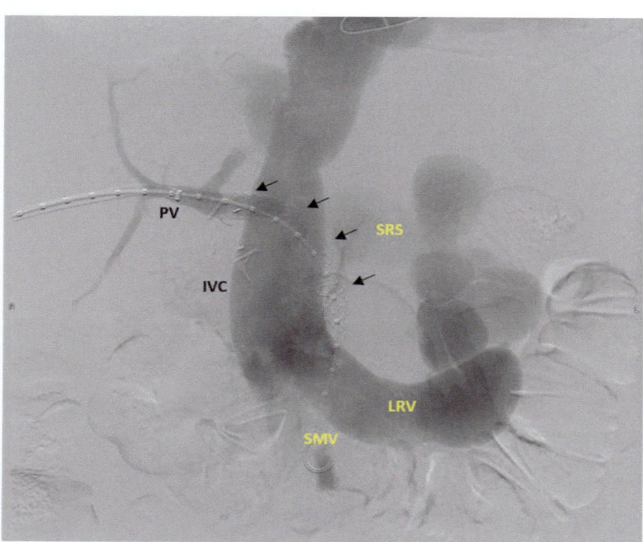

Fig. 41.7 DSA with pigtail catheter positioned within the SMV after deployment of a VIATORR endoprosthesis which extends from the distal confluence of the SMV and splenic vein into the transplant portal vein bypassing the portocaval anastomosis. There is now hepatopetal flow and flow through the splenorenal shunt

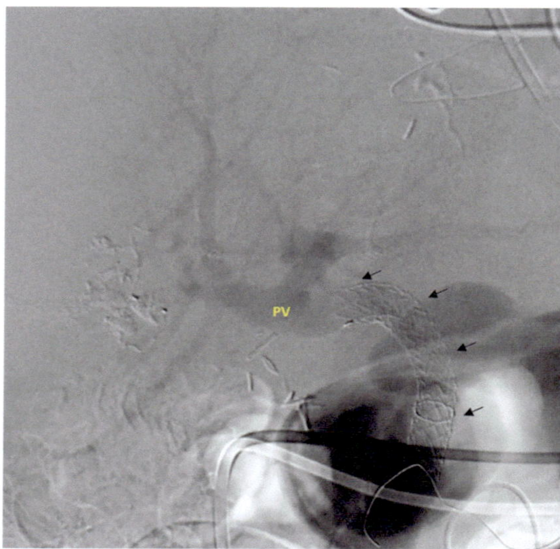

Fig. 41.8 Delayed DSA of the SMA shows hepatopetal flow through the VIATORR endoprosthesis (Gore, AR, USA) (arrows) into the transplant portal vein (PV) bypassing the portocaval anastomosis. There has been interval increase in size of the transplant PV and intrahepatic branches. There is still some persistent flow through the SRS after embolization; however, there has been significant clinical improvement in patient's encephalopathy with marked decrease of the ammonia levels

Mesocaval Shunt in Patient with Portocaval Transposition

42

Rahul S. Patel

An 18-year-old woman referred for management of medically refractory ascites after liver transplant. She had neuroblastoma at the age of 3 with a complicated treatment course leading to complete obstruction of mesenteric veins and biliary disease. Ultimately, she underwent orthotopic liver transplant with a failed surgical thrombectomy of the portal vein; a portocaval transposition was established to create portal inflow. The patient did well for many years until presenting with hypersplenism and refractory ascites. Diagnostic angiography (Fig. 42.1), venography (Fig. 42.2), and liver biopsy with pressure measurements were performed. After multidisciplinary discussion, we crafted a plan to create a percutaneous mesocaval shunt into the portocaval transposition.

Right transfemoral and trans-splenic (TS) vein approaches were established (Fig. 42.3). A 10 mm loop snare was placed at the spleno-superior mesenteric vein (SMV) confluence and a 20 mm snare within the IVC. Using a gunsight technique, a 20 g trans-abdominal needle was inserted through the both snares (Fig. 42.4) and ultimately exchanged for a V18 wire (Boston Scientific, Natick MA) which was externalized from both the common femoral and TS accesses. The tract was dilated, the guidewire upsized to an 0.035″ wire and a 7 × 19 mm VBX ePTFE stent-graft (W.L. Gore and Associates, Flagstaff AZ) was deployed across the tract (Fig. 42.5). Due to dense fibrous tissue from previous surgeries and radiation the VBX could not be initially expanded; it was ultimately enlarged to profile using a high pressure balloon. The stent graft was anchored with a 12 mm bare metal self-expanding stent. Final venography and angiography

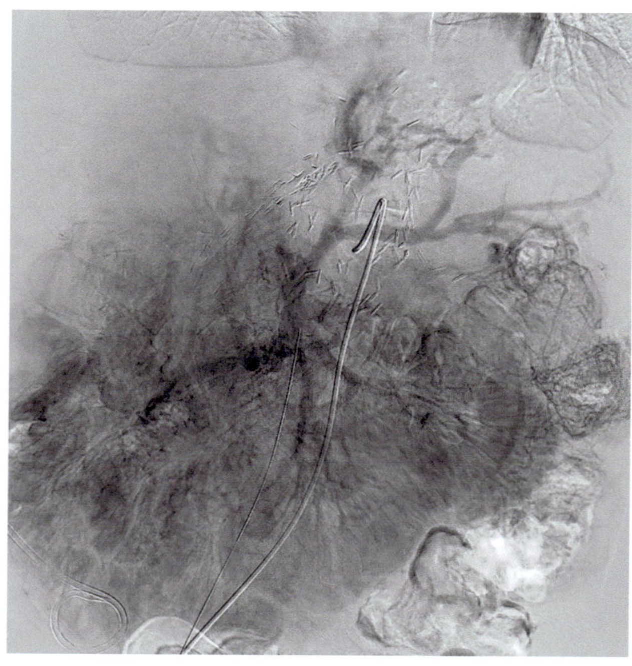

Fig. 42.1 Delayed imaging from SMA angiogram demonstrates no portal flow and retrograde flow through splenic vein and into perigastric varices

(Fig. 42.6) demonstrated brisk flow from mesenteric veins through shunt and into IVC. Sequential clinical and sonographic follow-up to 2 years showed a patent shunt and no notable ascites (Fig. 42.7).

R. S. Patel (✉)
Department of Radiology, Mount Sinai Medical Center, New York, NY, USA
e-mail: Rahul.patel@mountsinai.org

© The Author(s), under exclusive license to Springer Nature Switzerland AG 2023
Z. J. Haskal (ed.), *Extreme IR*, https://doi.org/10.1007/978-3-031-24251-9_42

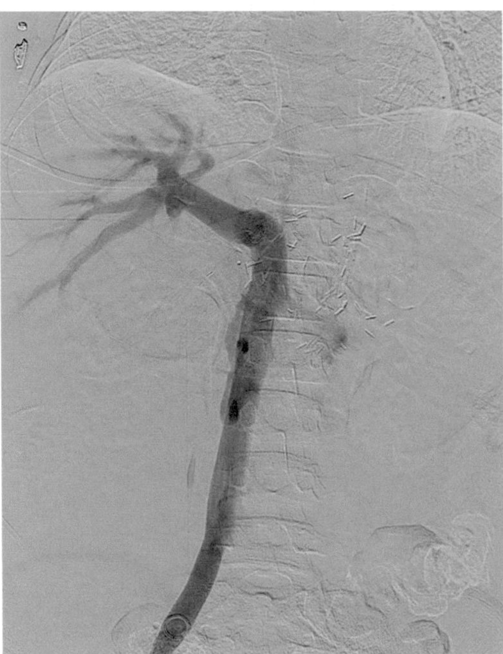

Fig. 42.2 Venogram from right common femoral vein injections demonstrates flow through IVC and into transplant portal vein consistent with patients known history of portocaval transposition

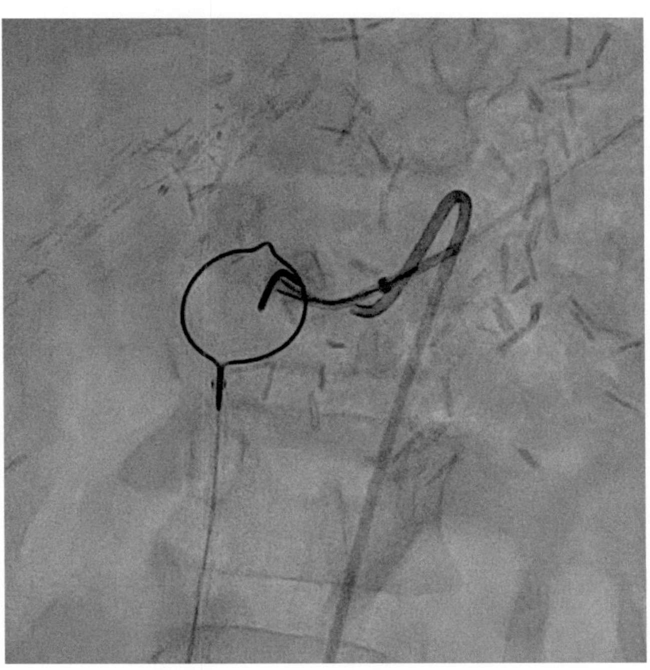

Fig. 42.4 A transabdominal 20G needle through the 10 mm mesenteric snare, which is cinched, and into the 25 mm IVC snare

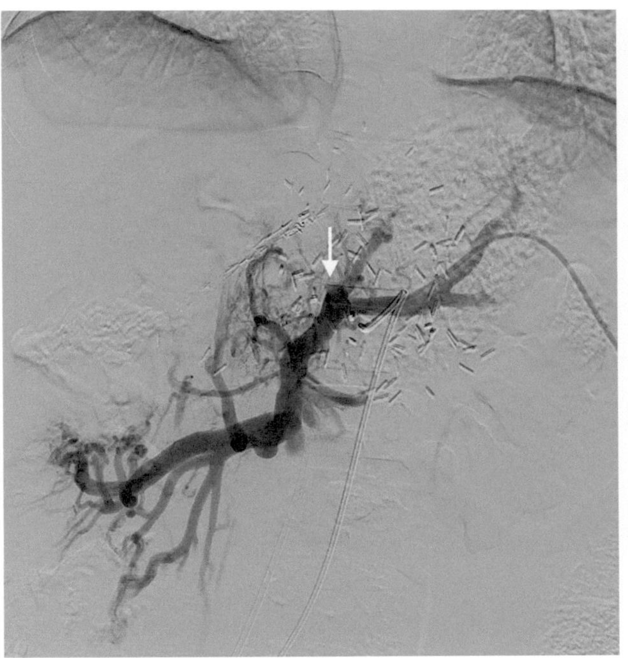

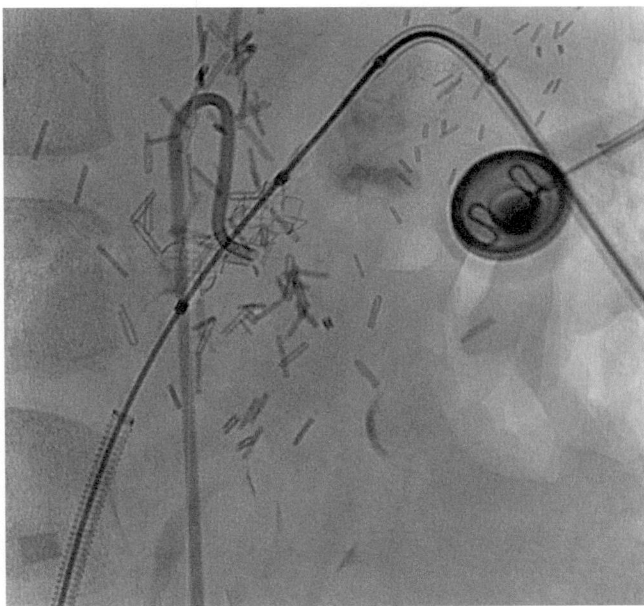

Fig. 42.5 VBX covered stent placed across the tract which is pinched due to dense fibrous tissue

Fig. 42.3 Injection of catheter in splenic vein demonstrates no portal flow. White arrow points to planned point of creation of mesocaval shunt. Based on pre-operative CT this spot was clear of the pancreas, duodenum, and the SMA

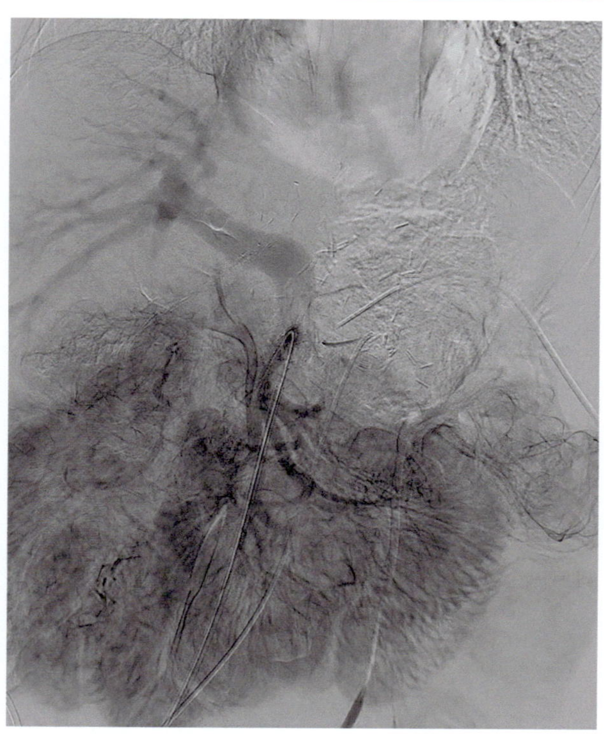

Fig. 42.6 Delayed SMA angiography demonstrates flow though the endovascular shunt and into the IVC and portal vein

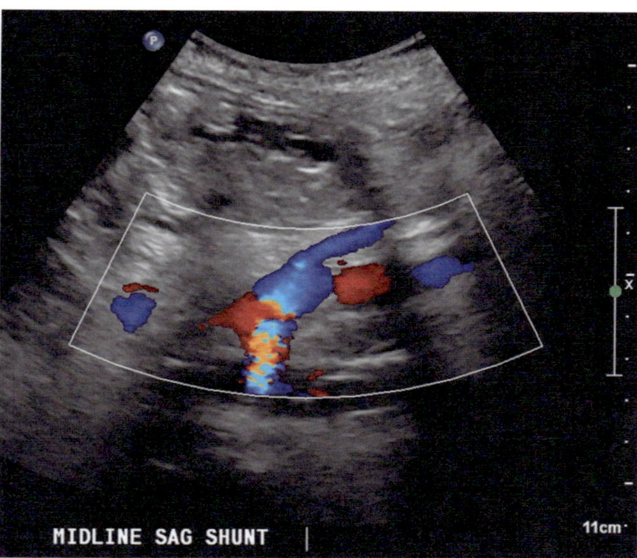

Fig. 42.7 Duplex US 2 years post-procedure demonstrates patent flow through the shunt with no ascites

Mohammad Arabi

A 49-year-old man with a history of hypercoagulability presented with recurrent intractable small bowel variceal hemorrhage. His portal, superior mesenteric, splenic veins, and inferior vena cava (IVC) were chronically thrombosed. Patient had a failed attempt at transjugular intrahepatic portosystemic shunt (TIPS) creation, and rethrombosis of reanalyzed IVC. His bleeding initially responded to proximal splenic artery and gastroduodenal artery embolization; however, it recurred 2 months later (Fig. 43.1). Fluoroscopy guided percutaneous trans-colonic (Fig. 43.2a) transhepatic access of a large varix in the porta hepatis (Fig. 43.2b) was performed by targeting a tri-loop snare in the IVC with a 22 G Chiba needle (Fig. 43.2c). The percutaneous 0.018″ wire was captured from the jugular access, and the parenchymal tract was predilated with a 7 mm balloon to allow for sheath introduction into the varix. A 10 mm × 36 mm balloon expandable stent (Valeo, Bard Inc., USA) was deployed. The percutaneous trans-colonic wire was removed, and final venography showed a widely patent shunt with effective decompression of the portal flow (Fig. 43.3). Perioperative antibiotic coverage was administered. The patient presented several times thereafter with GI bleeding that was addressed with shunt revision; the shunt remains patent 3 years after creation.

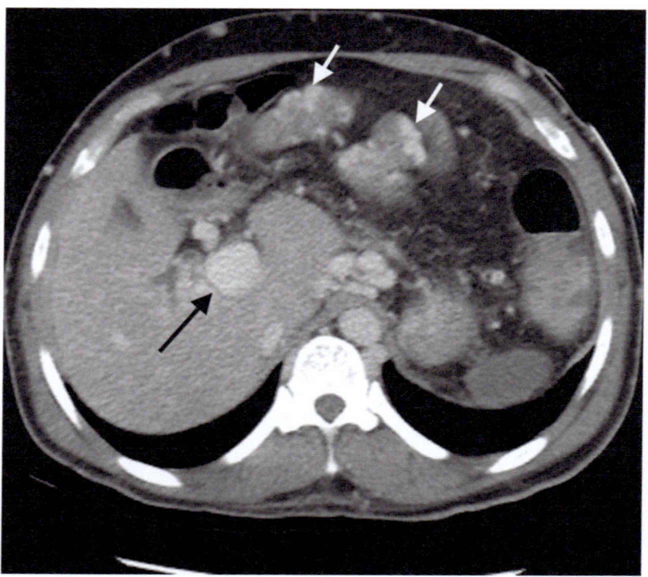

Fig. 43.1 Contrast-enhanced computed tomography of the abdomen demonstrates the submucosal small bowel varices (Short white arrows) and the cavernous transformation of the portal vein with a large varix in the porta hepatis (Black arrow)

M. Arabi (✉)
Vascular Interventional Radiology, Medical Imaging Department,
King Abdulaziz Medical City, National Guard Health Affairs,
Riyadh, Saudi Arabia

Z. J. Haskal (ed.), *Extreme IR*, https://doi.org/10.1007/978-3-031-24251-9_43

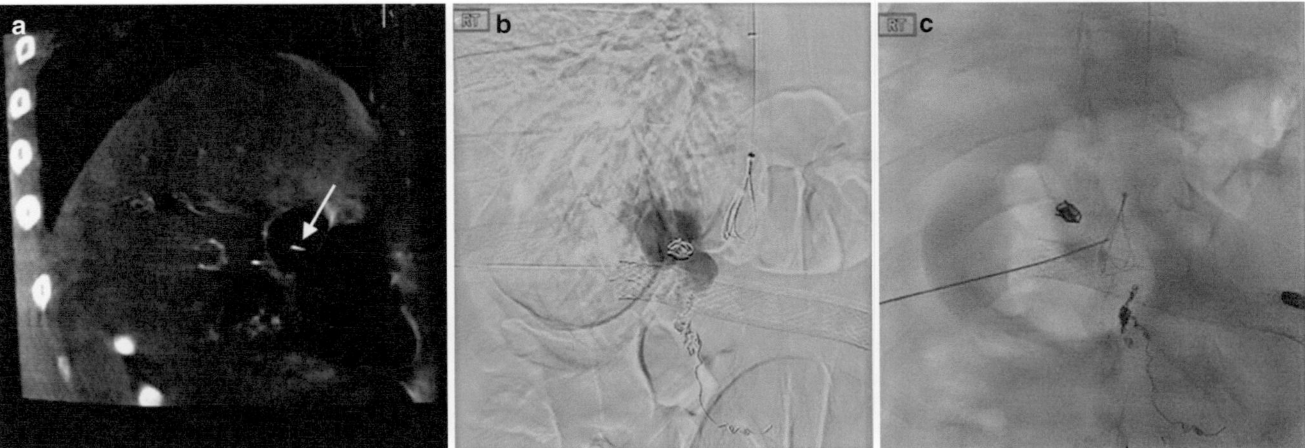

Fig. 43.2 (**a**) Cone-beam CT shows the trans-colonic course of the needle. (**b**) Contrast injection confirms opacification of the varix prior to targeting the snare in the IVC. (**c**) Chiba needle tip aiming at the IVC snare

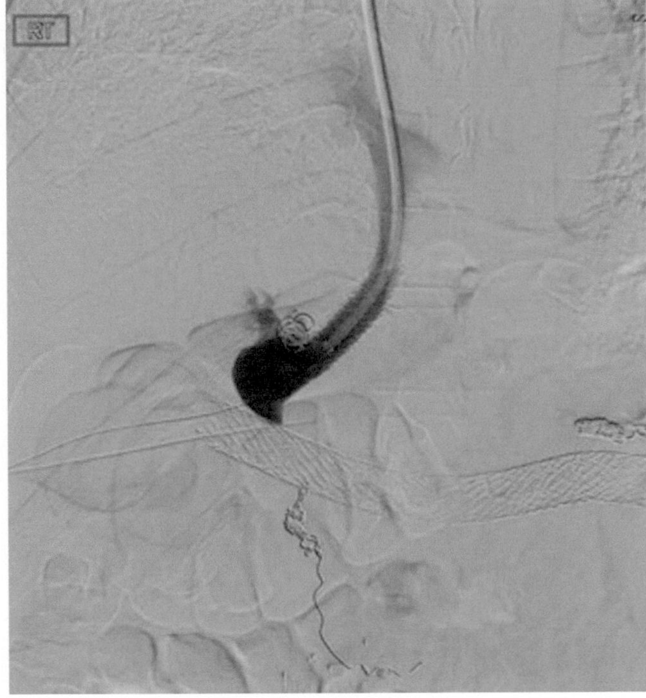

Fig. 43.3 Completion venography shows patent mesocaval shunt diverting flow from the varix into the IVC directly

Transcaval to Mesenteric Collateral Shunt Creation in a Patient with Chronic Spleno-Mesentero-Portal Thrombosis

Paul Haste and Maximilian Pyko

A 72-year-old woman with non-cirrhotic portal hypertension, MELD-Na 9, and cavernous transformation of the portal vein required multiple interventions and hospitalizations for recurrent GI bleeding secondary to hemobilia. CT scan showed extensive periportal collaterals surrounding the biliary tree (Fig. 44.1). Splenic vein occlusion precluded a trans-splenic approach and chronic occlusion of the intrahepatic portal veins was noted; however, a prominent mesenteric collateral vessel was identifiable anterior to the inferior vena cava (Fig. 44.2), allowing potential direct meso-caval shunt creation.

A 10F transjugular Rosch-Uchida access set was directed anteriorly from within the IVC into the dominant collateral vessel under transabdominal ultrasound guidance (Fig. 44.3). Desired target access was confirmed with contrast injection through the access cannula (Fig. 44.4). A hydrophilic cobra catheter and guidewire were advanced into the collateral vein, allowing for exchange to a Lunderquist wire. An 11 mm diameter × 39 mm long VBX stent graft (W.L Gore and Associates, Phoenix AZ) was deployed, extending from the target vein to the IVC (Fig. 44.5). Completion venogram demonstrated brisk flow through the stent (Fig. 44.6).

The patient's recurrent GI bleeding subsided and follow up CT scan obtained at 12 months after shunt creation showed a widely patent stent (Fig. 44.7).

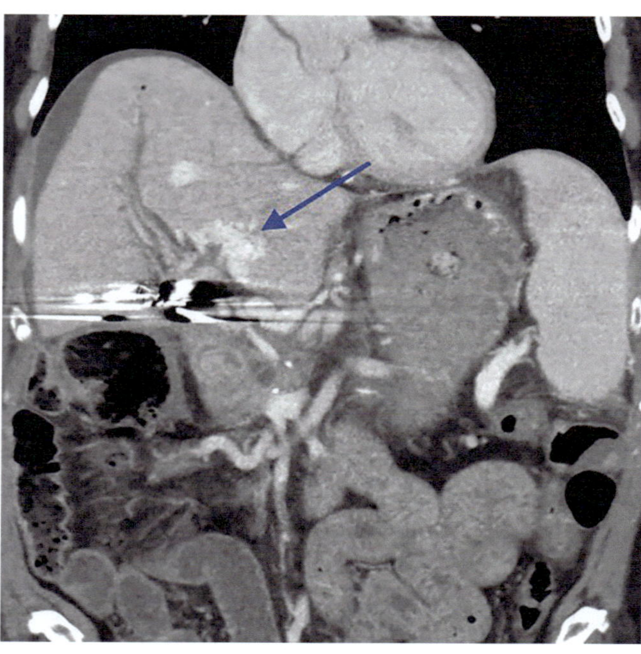

Fig. 44.1 Coronal contrast-enhanced CT demonstrating extensive cavernous transformation with abundant small veins surrounding the biliary tree (blue arrow)

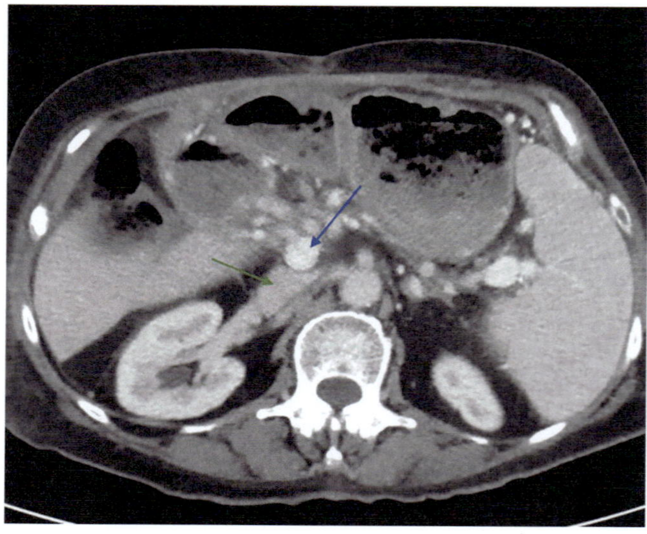

Fig. 44.2 Axial contrast-enhanced CT demonstrating the dominant draining collateral vein (blue arrow) immediately anterior to the IVC (green arrow)

P. Haste · M. Pyko (✉)
Department of Radiology and Imaging Sciences, Indiana University School of Medicine, Indianapolis, IN, USA
e-mail: phaste@iupui.edu; mpyko@iu.edu

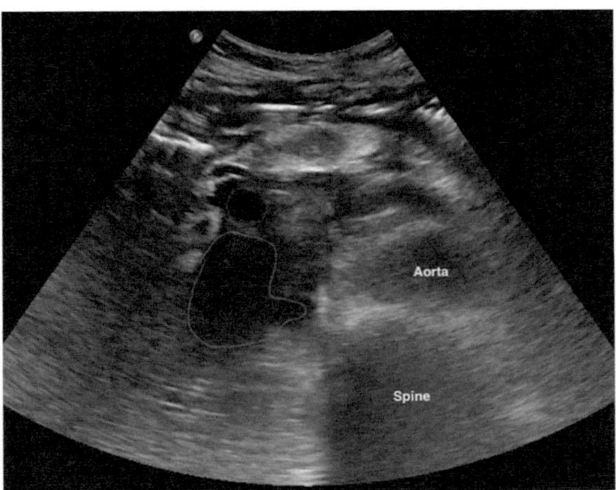

Fig. 44.3 Transabdominal ultrasound showing good visualization of the IVC (green outline) and the target vessel (blue outline)

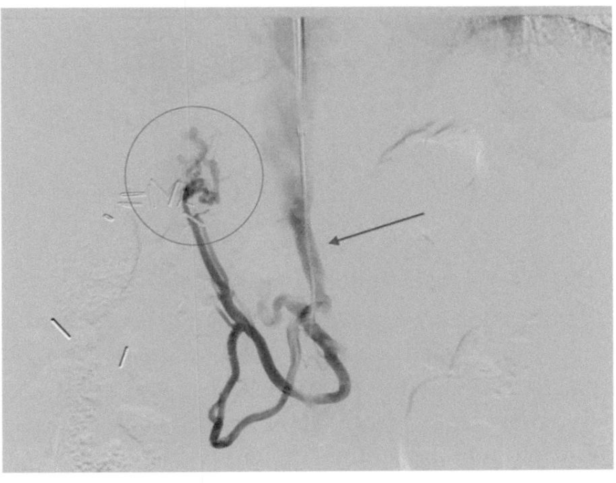

Fig. 44.6 Venogram from the mesenteric side showing brisk flow through the stent and into the IVC (blue arrow) with persistent (but decreased) flow to the liver (blue circle)

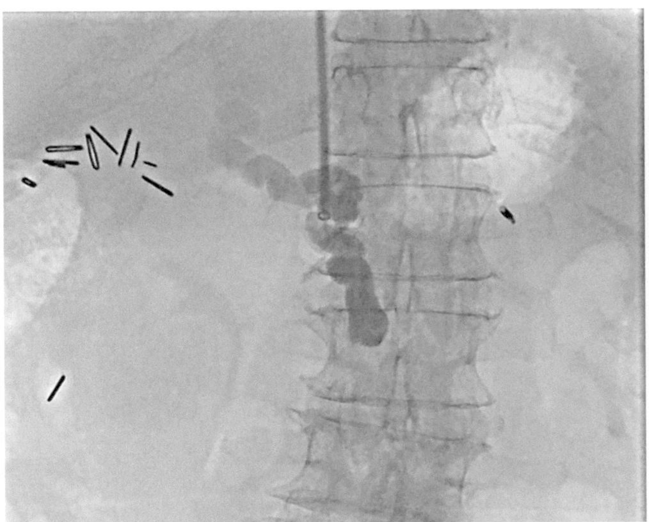

Fig. 44.4 Venogram through Rosch-Uchida cannula confirming access into the desired target vessel with flow towards the liver

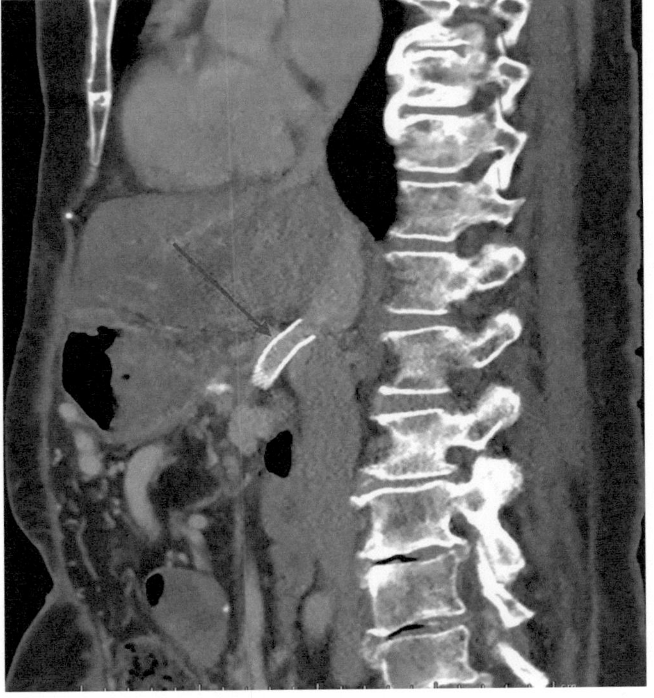

Fig. 44.7 Sagittal contrast-enhanced CT demonstrating a widely patent stent (blue arrow)

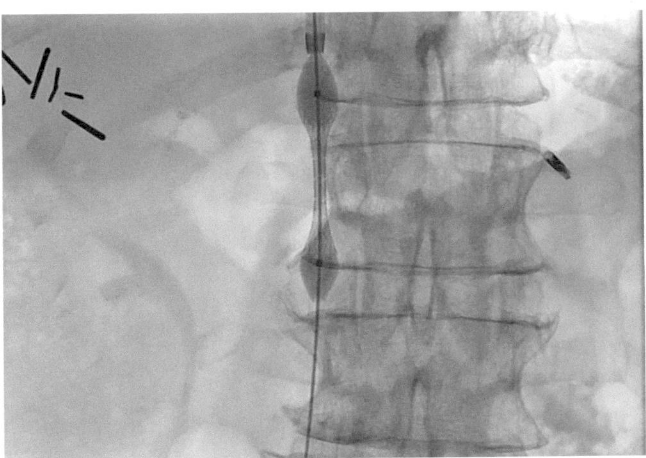

Fig. 44.5 Deployment of an 11 × 39 mm VBX stent

Mirror Mirror: TIPS in Situs Inversus with Transfemoral Transcaval Guidance

Jared Gans and Jacob Cynamon

An 18-year-old male with history of situs inversus and biliary atresia status post Kasai portoenterostomy in infancy presented with melena and syncope. Esophagogastroduodenoscopy demonstrated distal esophageal varices necessitating band ligation. His melena and transfusion requirement continued. A nuclear bleeding scan suggested a proximal small bowel bleed. CT demonstrated cirrhosis with small bowel varices and an interrupted left IVC (Fig. 45.1a–c). TIPS creation was considered. The anticipated obstacles included an absent intrahepatic IVC precluding potential intracardiac echocardiography (ICE) guidance, peripheral and posterior hepatic veins (HV) "far" from the portal vein (PV) target, and mirror image anatomy.

Using a right internal jugular approach and fluoroscopic guidance, a 16-gauge Colapinto needle could not be directed into the portal vein, thus another form of portal vein targeting was required. Poor acoustic ultrasound windows, and perisplenic varices complicated potential transhepatic, transplenic, and trans-mesenteric PV access [1]. However, CT did demonstrate the superior mesenteric vein (SMV) adjacent to the infrahepatic IVC (Fig. 45.1d). Based off of our transfemoral transcaval experience [2], a 7 Fr stiffened transjugular liver biopsy sheath (Argon) was advanced into the IVC from a right femoral access. Through this sheath, a coaxial 21-gauge Chiba needle was utilized to puncture the SMV, and a 0.018 wire advanced into the PV to be used as fiducial (Fig. 45.2a). The Colapinto needle was then directed into this PV target (Fig. 45.2b, c). The TIPS was completed using two overlapping 6 cm Viatorr CX endoprostheses (Gore) (Fig. 45.2d). The PV gradient dropped from 21 to 4 mmHg at procedure conclusion. The patient had no further melena or hepatic encephalopathy at discharge 2 days postprocedure or at 6-month follow-up. TIPS in situs inversus may be difficult. This case demonstrates the value of a transcaval PV wire in achieving a successful outcome.

J. Gans
Envision Healthcare, Fort Lauderdale, FL, USA

J. Cynamon (✉)
Department of Radiology, Montefiore Medical Center,
Bronx, NY, USA

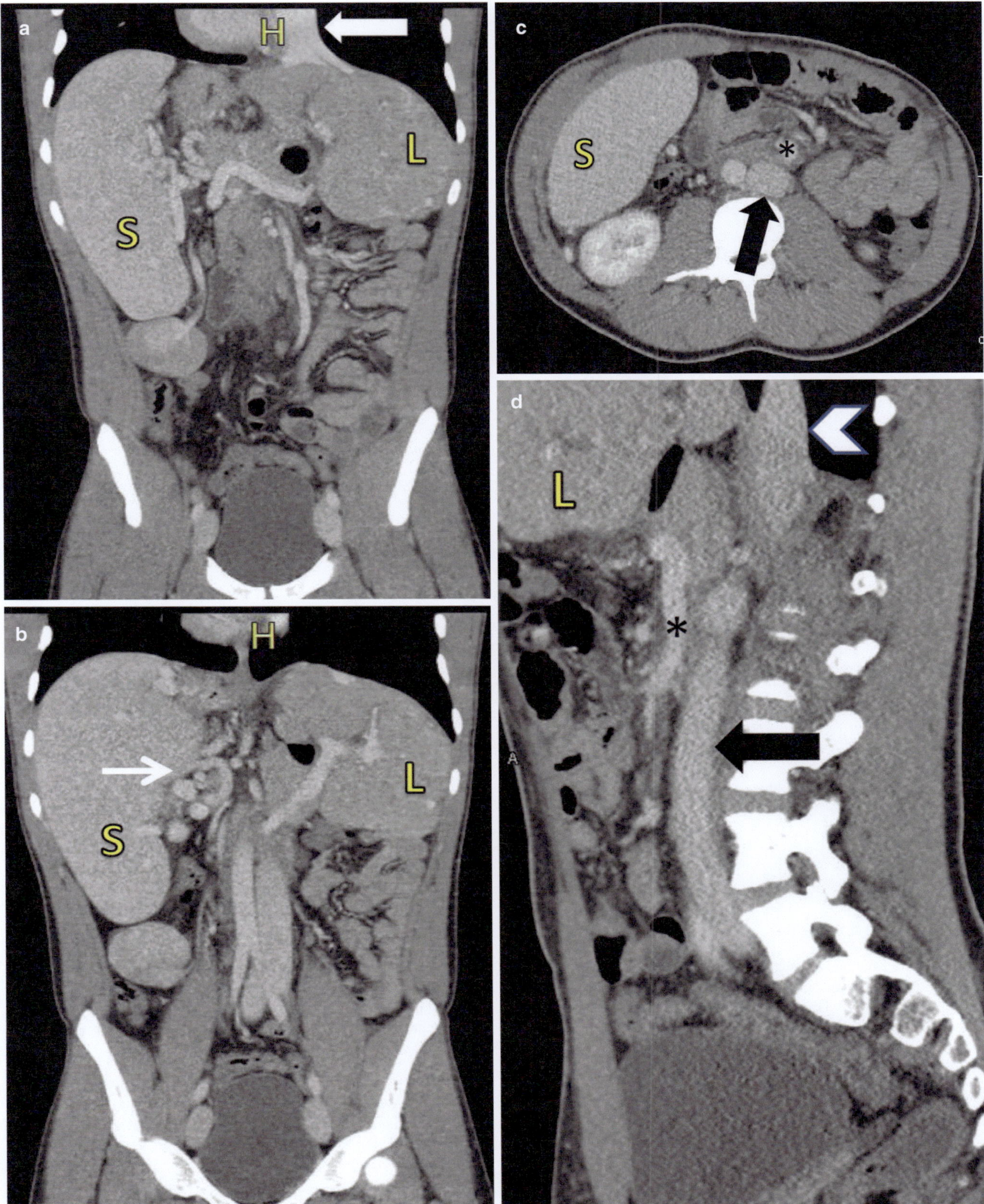

Fig. 45.1 (**a**) Coronal reformatted contrast-enhanced CT demonstrating situs inversus with spleen (S) on right and liver (L) on the left. There is an interrupted suprahepatic IVC (white arrow) entering the heart (H) with small peripheral hepatic veins. (**b**) More anterior coronal image demonstrates a cirrhotic liver (L) with a patent portal vein with tortuous perisplenic varices (dashed arrow). (**c**) Axial CT image shows the close relationship of the infrahepatic IVC (arrow) with the SMV (asterix). (**d**) Sagittal imaging demonstrates the discontinuous infrahepatic IVC (arrow) and large azygous vein (white arrowhead). Again note the adjacent infrahepatic IVC (arrow) and SMV (asterix)

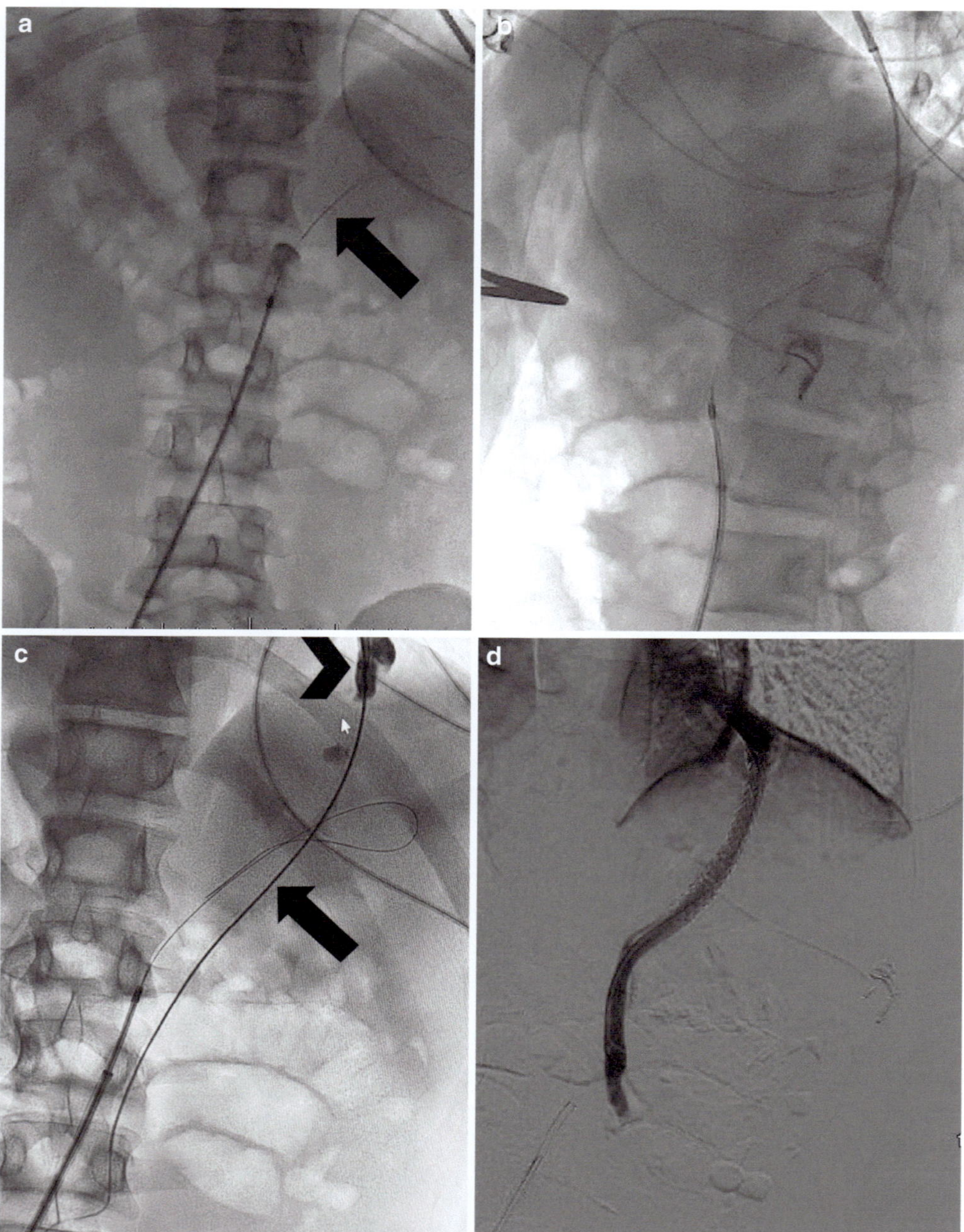

Fig. 45.2 Transfemoral transcaval portal vein fiducial guided TIPS. (**a**) Transfemoral transcaval portal access with a 0.018 guidewire (arrow) through a stiffened 7 Fr TLAB sheath. (**b**) Lateral fluoroscopic projection demonstrating use of the transcaval portal wire as a fiducial for transjugu- lar portal access. (**c**) Frontal projection with transjugular 0.035 wire in PV (arrow) and contrast opacifying the hepatic vein access (arrowhead). (**d**) Final portal venogram after placement of two overlapping endopros- theses demonstrates flow through the TIPS into the suprahepatic IVC

Bibliography

1. Knight GM, Clark J, Boike JR, et al. TIPS for adults without cirrho- sis with chronic mesenteric venous thrombosis and EHPVO refrac- tory to standard-of-care therapy. Hepatology. 2021;74(5):2735–44.

2. Peng R, Wattamwar K, Kuc N, Jagust M, Golowa Y, Cynamon J. Transjugular versus Transfemoral Transcaval liver biopsy: a single-center experience in 500 cases. J Vasc Interv Radiol. 2020;31(9):1394–400.

Ziv J Haskal

A 35-year-old woman autoimmune hepatitis, cirrhosis, MELD-NA 10, presented for TIPS for control of diuretic refractory ascites and previously bleeding esophageal and gastric varices. She had developed subacute thromboses of her splenic, mesenteric, main, and central right portal veins in the preceding year and was being treated with anticoagulation (Fig. 46.1).

A middle hepatic vein approach was used to puncture a segment 2 branch of the left lobe of the liver (Fig. 46.2), using a coaxial Colapinto needle and 21 g Chiba (Fig. 46.3). The circuitous route was negotiated using buddy wire techniques (Fig. 46.4), reaching the main portal vein. Progressively larger balloon was negotiated around the turns, together with "pre-paving" the liver tract with a self-expanding bare nitinol stent (Protégé, Medtronic, USA) (Fig. 46.5). This allowed sheath advancement and eventual deployment of Viatorr TIPS endoprostheses and portal thrombectomy (W.L. Gore and Associate, Flagstaff AZ) (Fig. 46.6).

Six-month computed tomographic images illustrate the serpentine course of the shunt in coronal and sagittal views and continued control of her ascites (Figs. 46.7 and 46.8). Her MELD-NA score was 13, she remained free of bleeding or detectable ascites and had regained over 10lbs in muscle mass.

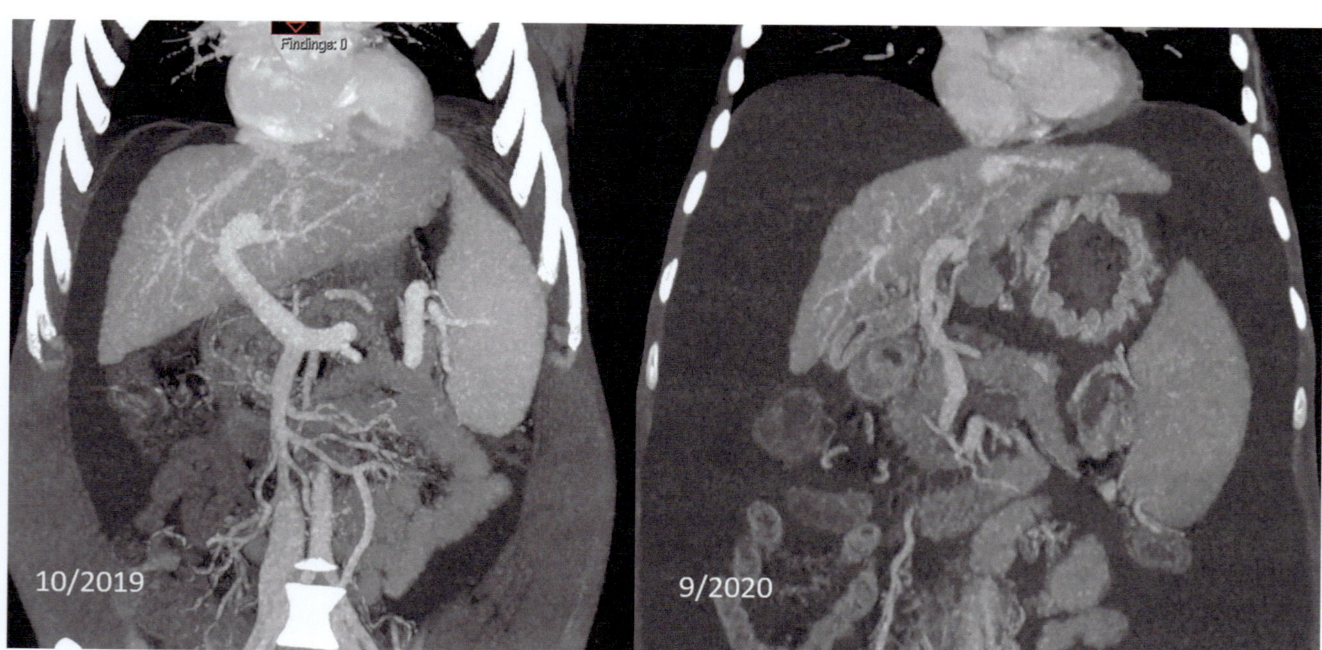

Fig. 46.1 Coronal CT images demonstrate a patent main portal vein in October 2019 and complete occlusion by September 2020. A large peri-portal collateral vein has developed, reconstituting intrahepatic portal veins in 2020. Mesenteric and splenic veins are occluded (not shown). Massive ascites has developed

Z. J Haskal (✉)

Department of Radiology and Medical Imaging, Interventional Division, University of Virginia, Charlottesville, VA, USA

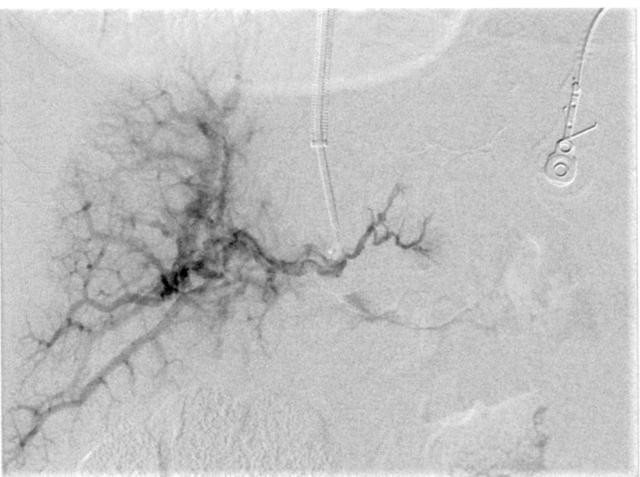

Fig. 46.2 A coaxial fine needle technique has been used to puncture a 2 mm diameter segment 2 branch of the left portal vein. Venography demonstrates intrahepatic collateral veins that cross the hilum to supply the peripherally patent native right portal vein branches

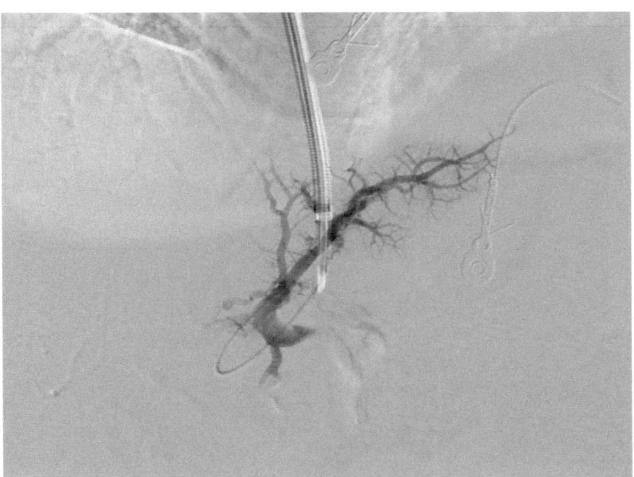

Fig. 46.3 An 0.018″ guidewire circles retrograde into segment 2. The Colapinto needle has been advanced forward over the fine needle so that its tip is at the portal vein entry

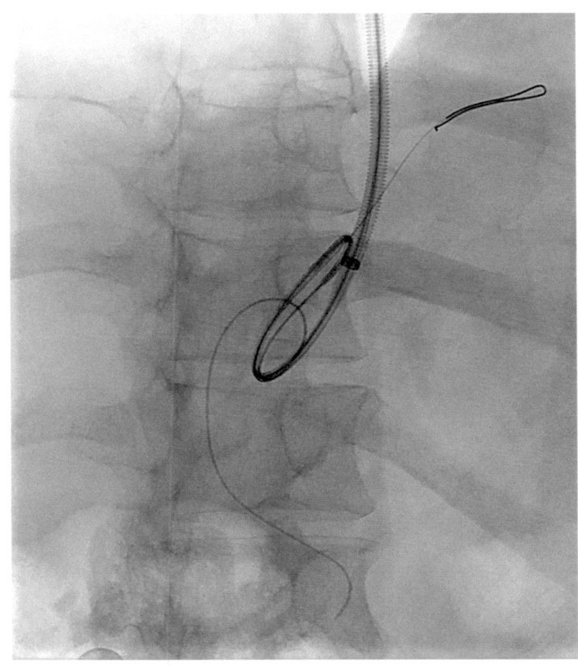

Fig. 46.4 An 0.018″ buddy wire remains in the peripheral left portal vein whilst a pra-axial 4 Fr catheter and hydrophilic wire are negotiated around the roundabout turn of the left portal vein and into the main portal vein

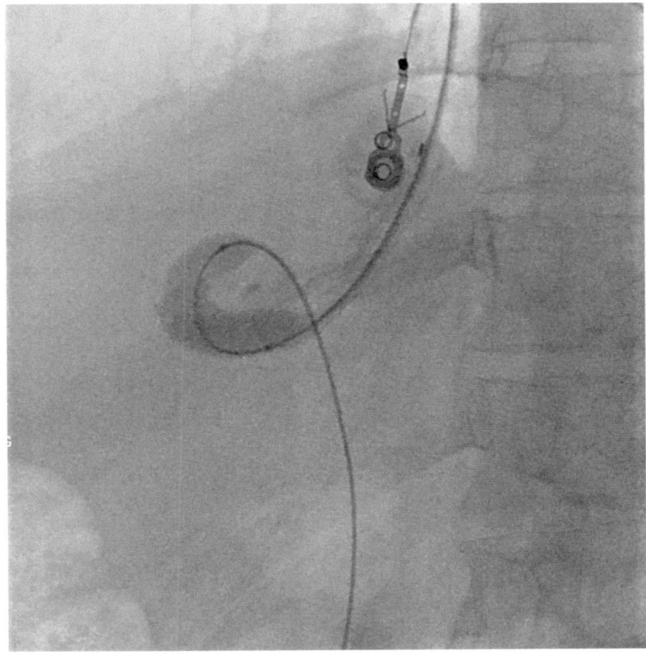

Fig. 46.5 A 10 mm self-expanding bare stent has been used to pave and stabilize the liver tract. An 8 mm diameter 4 cm long angioplasty balloon is inflated around the turn

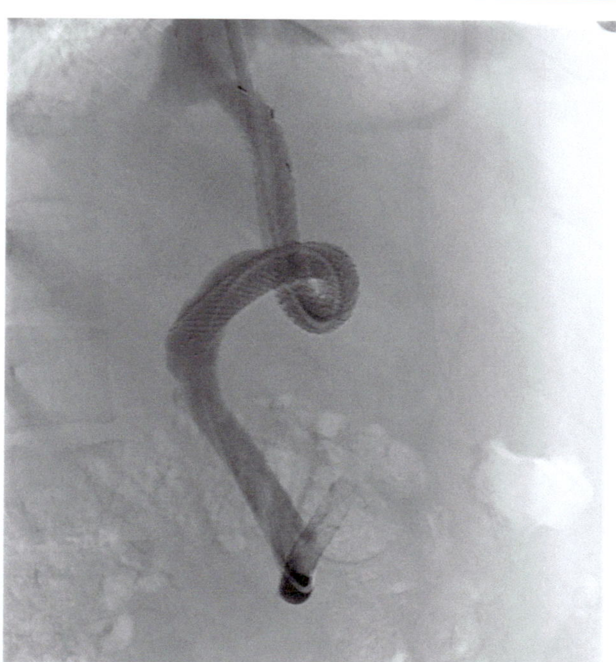

Fig. 46.6 Portal vein venography after TIPS creation with bare and covered stent deployments and main portal vein thrombectomy demonstrate flow through the shunt loop

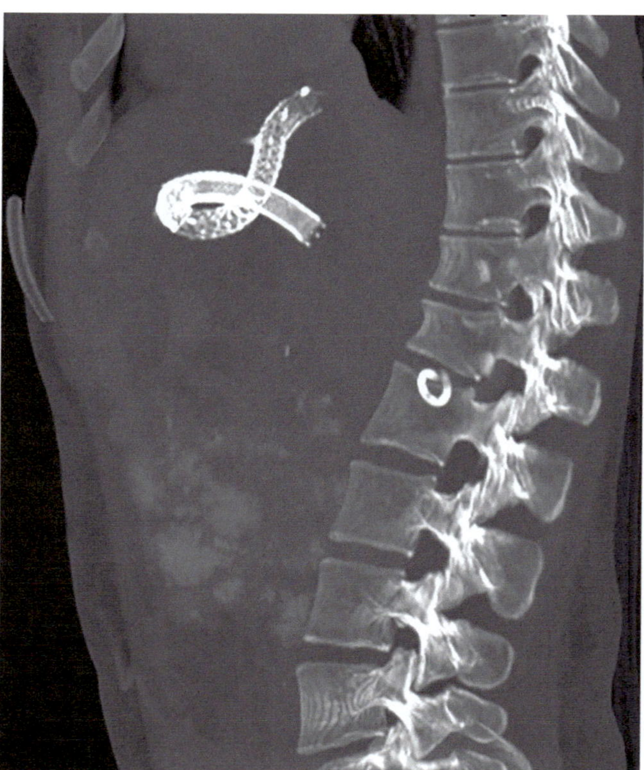

Fig. 46.8 Sagittal maximum intensity projection reconstruction image demonstrates the serpentine configuration of the TIPS

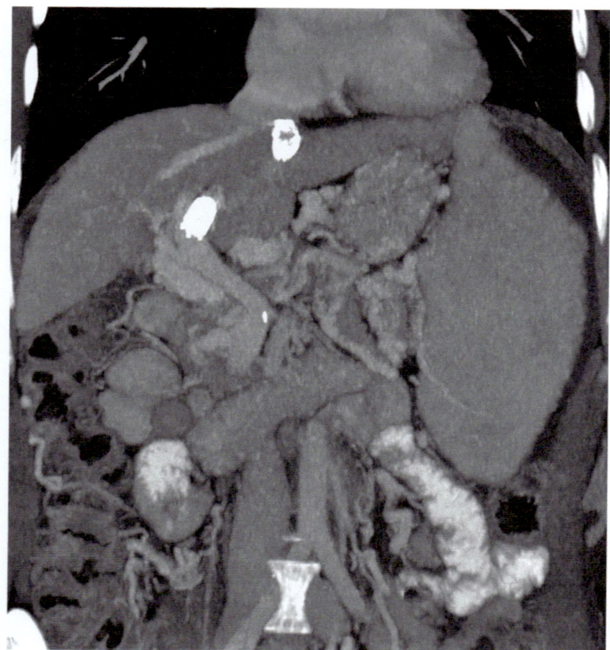

Fig. 46.7 6-month follow-up coronal CT image shows continued restored patency of the main portal vein and central superior mesenteric vein. Her ascites is absent

Explant of a VIATORR TIPS Endoprosthesis Misplaced into the Common Bile Duct

Adnan Hadziomerovic

A 76-year-old man with known cirrhosis presented with recurrent hemorrhage from rectal varices refractory to endoscopic treatment and inferior mesenteric vein embolization. He underwent urgent transjugular intrahepatic portosystemic shunt (TIPS) creation that was technically difficult resulting in an inadvertently misplaced 8-mm × 8-cm VIATORR TIPS Endoprosthesis (W.L. Gore and Associates, Inc., Flagstaff, Arizona) bridging the right hepatic vein to the common bile duct (Fig. 47.1). The patient's clinical condition deteriorated with increased serum bilirubin and recurrent hemorrhage.

An 18 Fr 40-cm long sheath (Cook Inc., Bloomington, Indiana) was advanced into the right atrium (RA) through a right internal jugular venous access. As the intrahepatic end of the VIATORR could not be engaged, percutaneous access into the stent was achieved with a 21G trocar needle (Fig. 47.2a) and a 0.018″ wire (AccuStick, Boston Scientific, Marlborough, MA), allowing snaring (15-mm Amplatz Goose Neck Snare, Medtronic, Minneapolis, MN) of the wire for a through-and-through access. A coaxial transjugular 7F 55-cm sheath (Ansel 2, Cook) was advanced through the VIATORR and into the common bile duct. The snare was preloaded on the shaft of an 8-mm × 4-cm balloon (Mustang, Boston Scientific) which was advanced over the wire and inflated within the stent (Fig. 47.3). As the snare would not encompass the leading edge of the stent, the entire system, with the balloon inflated, had to be pulled back into the right atrium. The snare was then advanced over the balloon and proximal stent where it was tightened as the balloon was deflated. The stent graft was collapsed into the 18F sheath (Fig. 47.4) and removed. A 7 Fr sheath was re-advanced into the hepatic parenchyma and a 10-mm Amplatzer 1 Vascular Plug (AGA Medical, Golden Valley, Minnesota) was deployed in the transhepatic tract (Fig. 47.5). The TIPS procedure was then redone (Fig. 47.6).

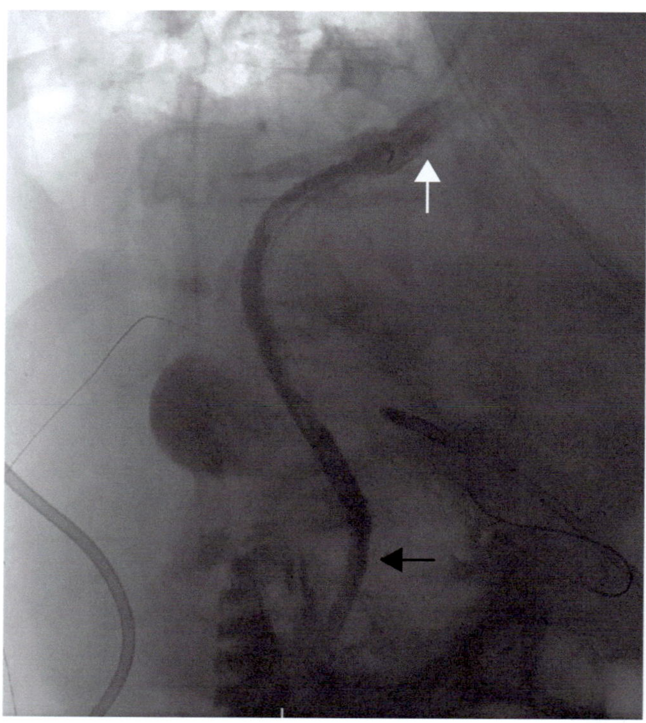

Fig. 47.1 Completion image following TIPS procedure demonstrating the VIATORR stent extending from the right hepatic vein (white arrow) to the common bile duct (black arrow)

A. Hadziomerovic (✉)
Department of Medical Imaging, The Ottawa Hospital,
Ottawa, ON, Canada
e-mail: ahadziomerovic@toh.ca

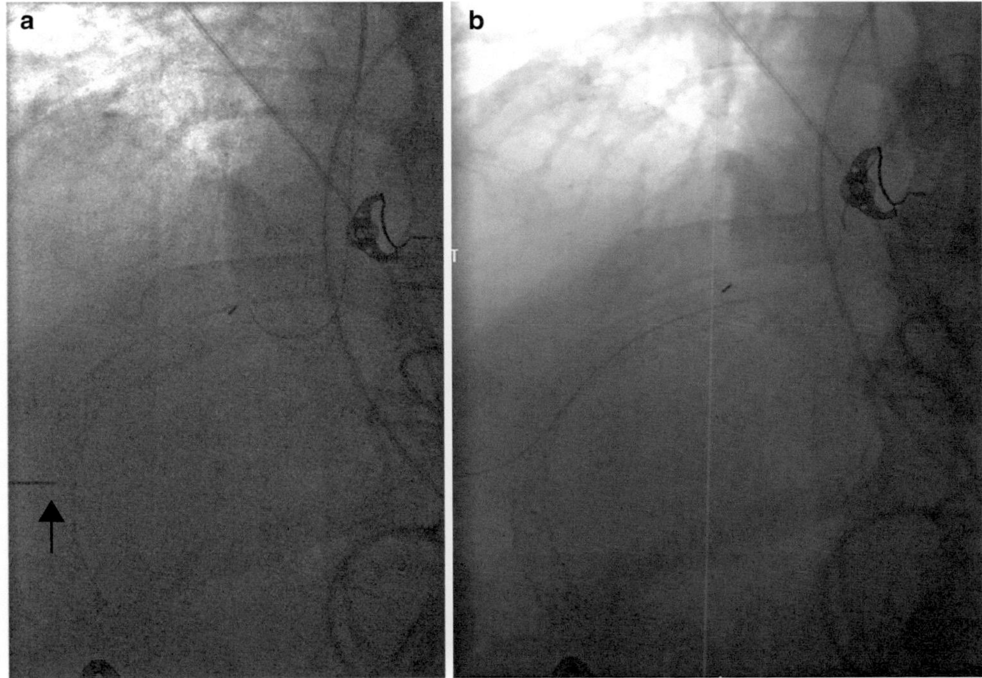

Fig. 47.2 Tip of a 21G needle (arrow) was advanced percutaneously into the stent (**a**) followed by advancement of a 0.018″ guidewire cephalad into the RA (**b**) where it was snared and externalized through the 18F sheath

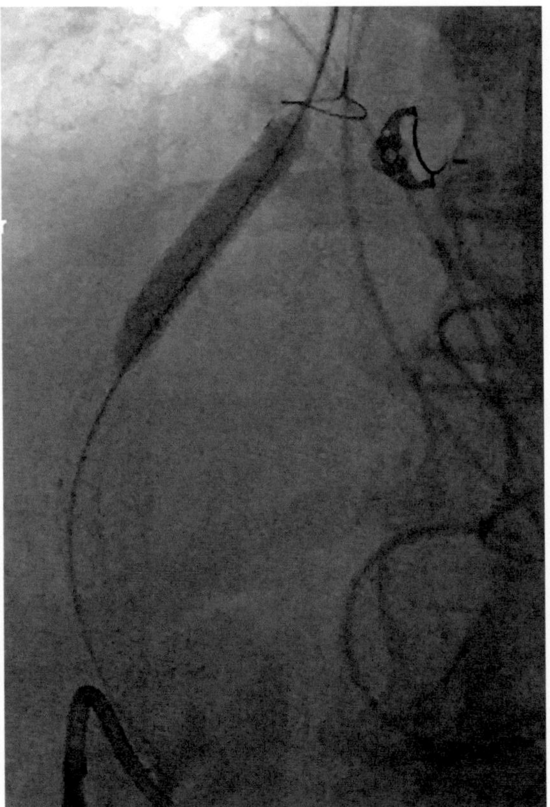

Fig. 47.3 An 8-mm × 4-cm balloon inflated in the cephalad portion of the sent with a goose neck snare preloaded on the shaft of the balloon

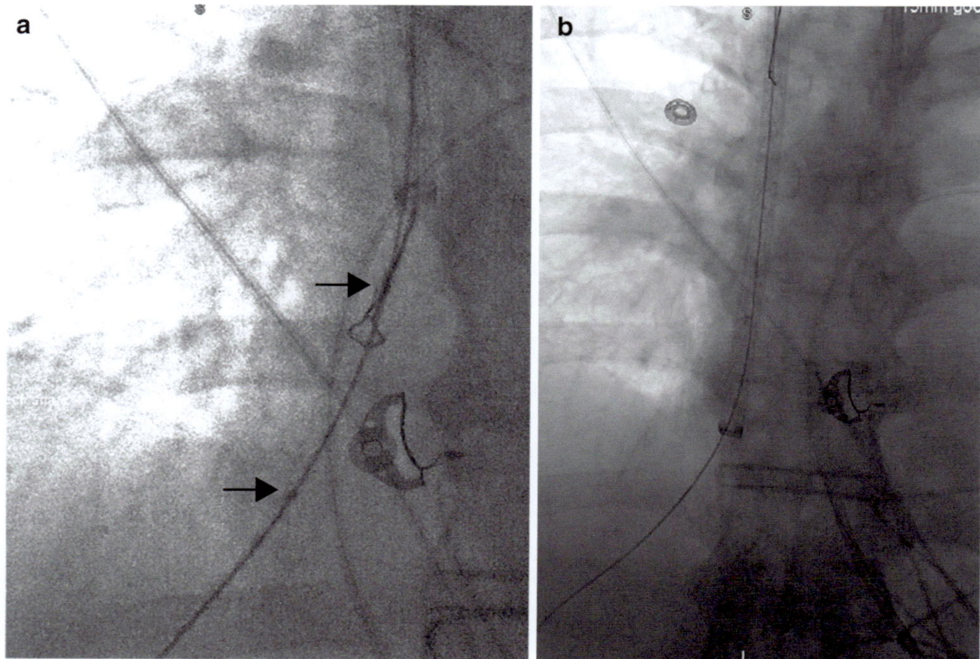

Fig. 47.4 (**a**) The snare collapsing the cephalad edge of the stent with the balloon deflated (Arrows identifying the balloon markers). VIATORR stent was then collapsed and withdrawn through the sheath (**b**)

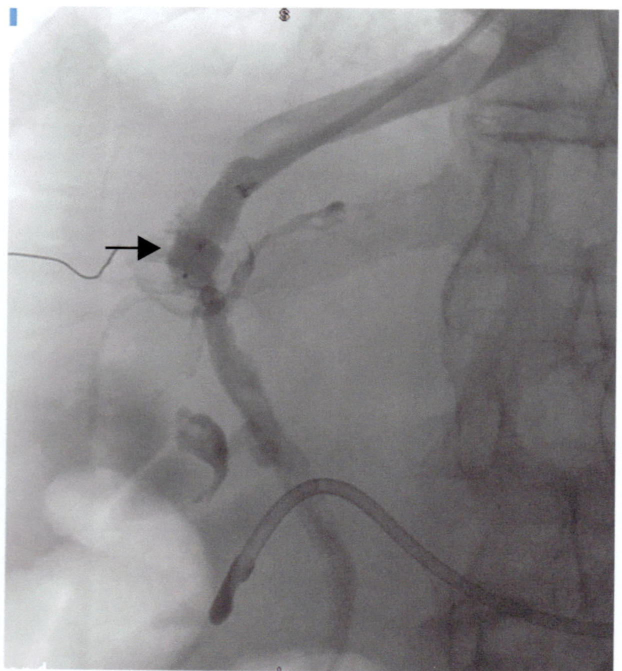

Fig. 47.5 A 10-mm AVP 1 (Arrow) deployed in the hepatic parenchyma between the confluence of intrahepatic biliary ducts and the hepatic vein

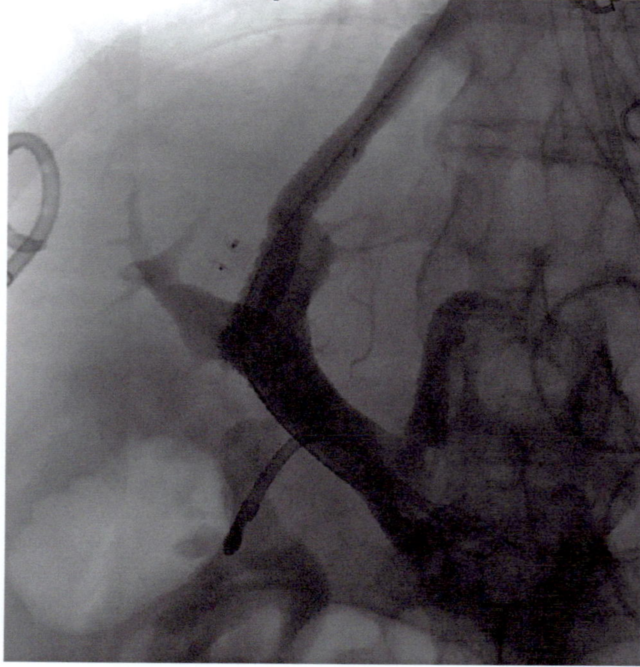

Fig. 47.6 A new TIPS was created between the right portal vein and the right hepatic vein

Antegrade Transmesenteric Stenting of a Kinked Portal Vein After Acute Liver Transplant

48

Jorge E. Lopera

A 54 year-old male with alcoholic cirrhosis and a previous liver transplant underwent second transplantation. Very low Doppler velocities were identified within the portal vein after surgery. At surgical re-exploration 3 days later, a kinked portal vein was identified; this improved after manually lifting and repositioning the liver. A surgical bypass was considered however his superior mesenteric vein was judged too small for a durable anastomosis. Diffuse oozing from acute portal hypertension was observed requiring multiple units of blood; this led to a severe coagulopathy. The patient returned to surgery a third time, the next day, and Interventional Radiology was consulted for emergent portal vein stent placement.

A mesenteric vein was accessed directly with a micro-puncture set. A wire was advanced antegrade into the portal vein and a 9 Fr sheath was placed (Fig. 48.1). Direct portography demonstrated a severe kink of the portal vein at the prior anastomosis with hepatofugal filling of esophageal varices (Fig. 48.2). A 14 mm × 4 cm self-expandable stent was deployed and dilated to 14 mm (Fig. 48.3). Portography showed resolution of the kink and decompression of the varices (Fig. 48.4). Portal vein velocities improved immediately and the diffuse oozing in the abdominal cavity resolved.

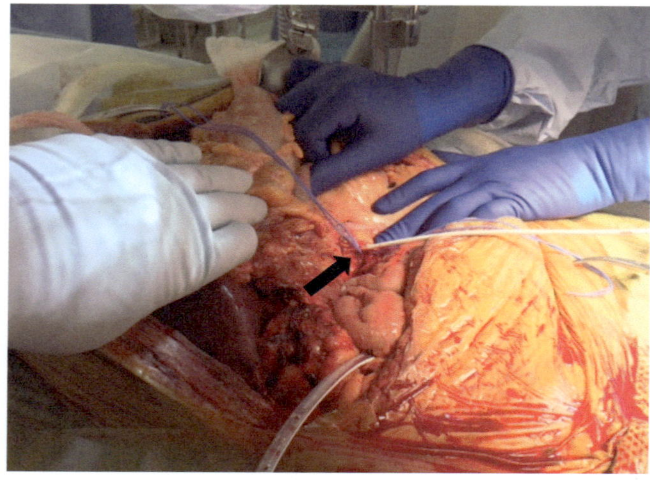

Fig. 48.1 Intraoperative photograph shows access into a mesenteric vein and a catheter through the vascular sheath (arrow)

He later developed hepatic artery thrombosis and biliary necrosis that has been managed with percutaneous articulated biliary stents that are exchanged every 3 months. His liver function is normal and the portal vein stent is patent 4 years after the transplantation (Fig. 48.5).

J. E. Lopera (✉)
Department of Radiology, UT Health San Antonio,
San Antonio, TX, USA
e-mail: Lopera@uthscsa.edu

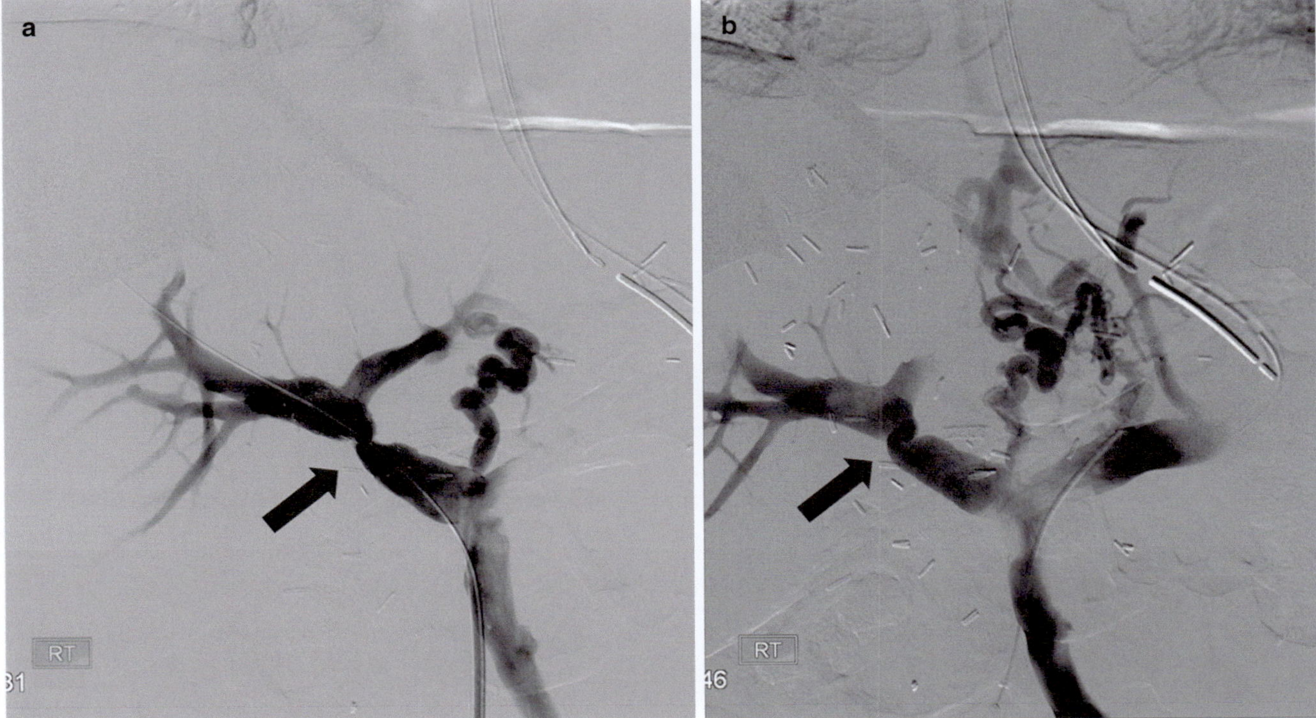

Fig. 48.2 Direct portography, early (**a**) and delayed phases (**b**), show the anastomotic kink in the portal vein (arrows). Note the esophageal varices

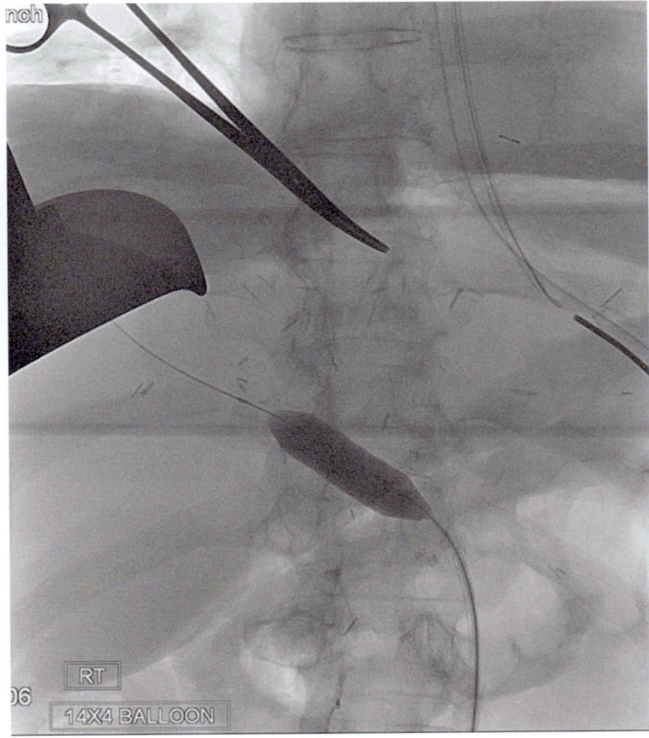

Fig. 48.3 Spot radiograph shows the inflated balloon dilating the stent at low pressures

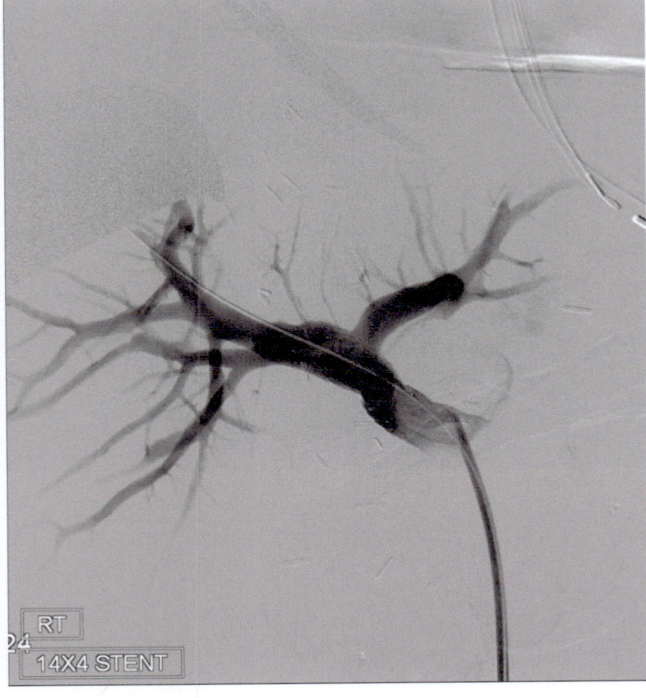

Fig. 48.4 Final portogram shows resolution of the kink of the portal vein after stent placement and dilation

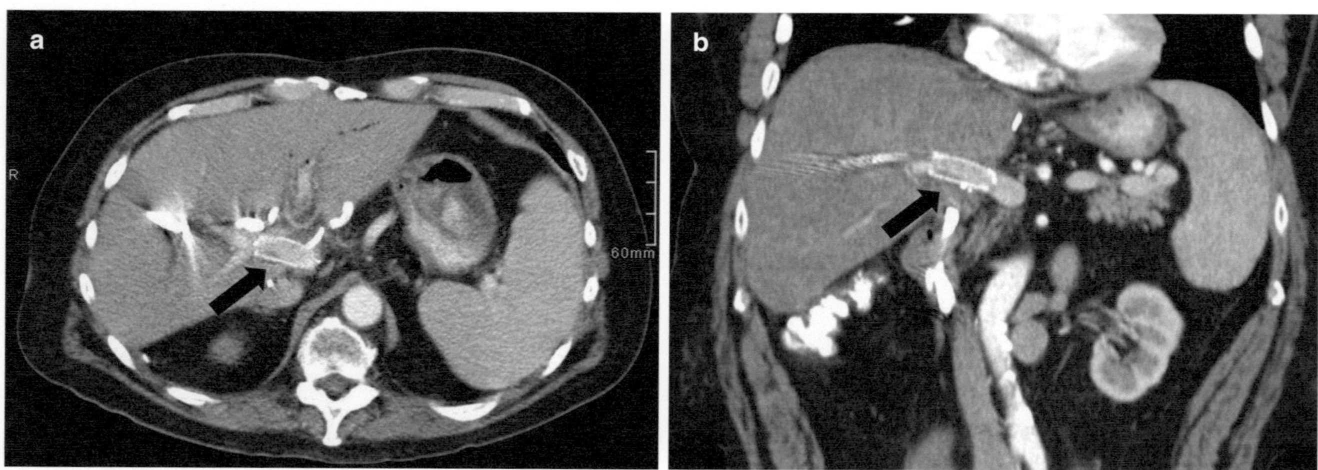

Fig. 48.5 Contrast enhanced CT images in axial (**a**) and coronal (**b**) planes 4 years after the procedure, show the patent portal vein stent with minimal intimal hyperplasia (arrows)

Transcatheter Thrombolysis for Acute Massive Portal and Mesenteric Vein Thrombosis in the Postpartum Period

Keigo Osuga and Kaishu Tanaka

A healthy 38-year-old female, gravida 4, para 3 presented with severe epigastric pain 8 days after an uneventful spontaneous transvaginal delivery. Serum liver function tests were within normal limits. Contrast-enhanced CT (Fig. 49.1a, b) revealed extensive thrombosis of the main, right, and left portal veins (PV) extending from the superior mesenteric vein (SMV). Considering the scope of clot and uncertain and unlikely efficacy of anticoagulation therapy alone, catheter-directed thrombolysis was undertaken using an ultrasound-guided transhepatic approach. Using a thrombosed left PV approach, a 6-Fr guide catheter was inserted into main PV. A 4-Fr multiple-side hole catheter was coaxially advanced into SMV and a continuous infusion of urokinase of 120,000–240,000 U/day was initiated, with concomitant systemic heparinization (Fig. 49.2a). Aspiration thrombectomy and balloon venoplasty were performed daily for the next 4 days (Fig. 49.2b), resulting in gradual decrease in thrombus and relief of her abdominal pain (Fig. 49.2c, d). The catheter was removed with liver tract coil embolization after 1 week. Her hypercoagulability workup revealed protein S deficiency, thus human antithrom-

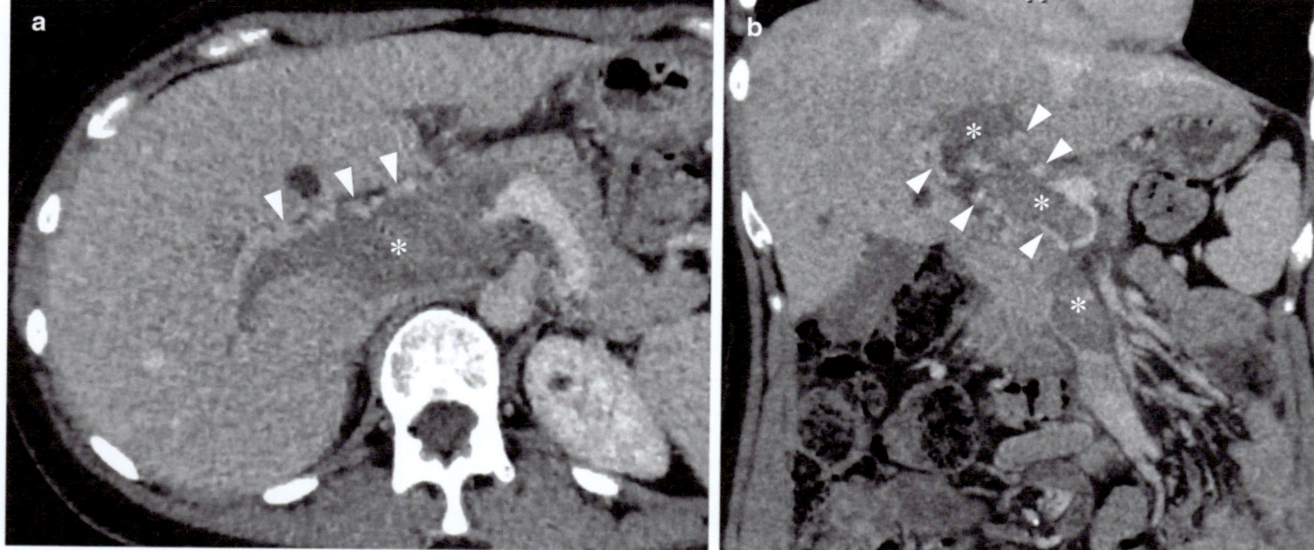

Fig. 49.1 (**a**, **b**) Contrast-enhanced CT images show massive thrombosis (asterisks) extending from the dilated portal veins to the superior mesenteric vein. Small collateral veins (arrowheads) are seen around the main portal vein

K. Osuga (✉)
Department of Diagnostic Radiology,
Osaka Medical and Pharmaceutical University, Takatsuki,
Osaka, Japan
e-mail: osuga@ompu.ac.jp

K. Tanaka
Department of Diagnostic and Interventional Radiology,
Osaka University Graduate School of Medicine, Suita,
Osaka, Japan
e-mail: k-tanaka@radiol.med.osaka-u.ac.jp

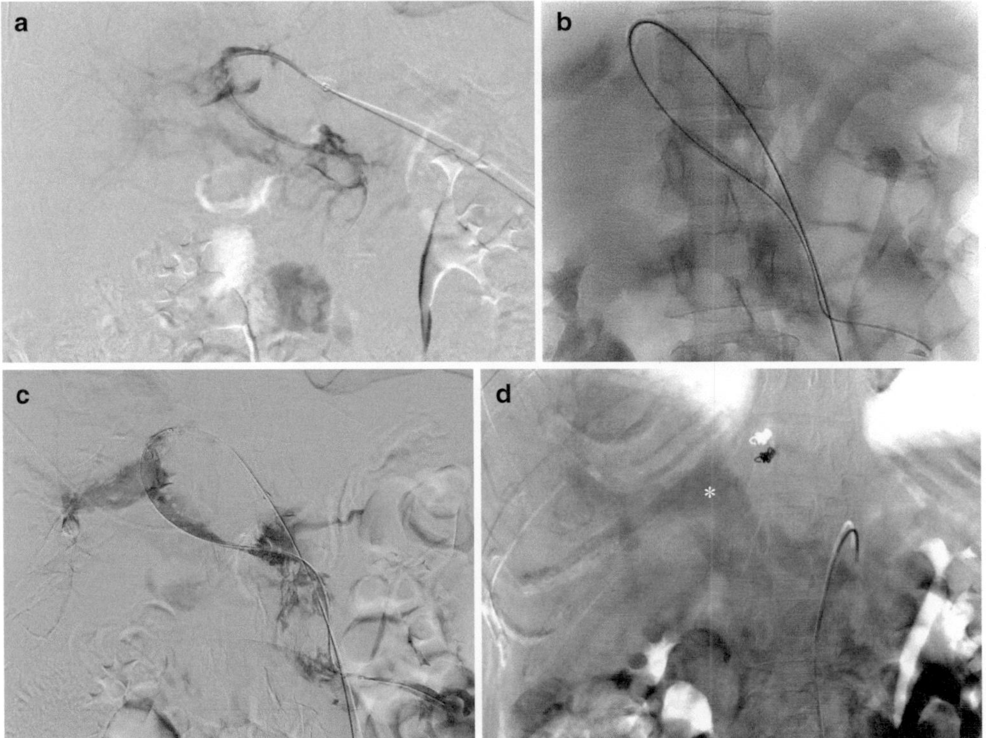

Fig. 49.2 (**a**) Transhepatic venography shows filling defects in the portal veins with collateral formation toward intrahepatic branches. Aspiration thrombectomy and local thrombolysis were performed. (**b**) Balloon venoplasty was used to macerate the clot within the SMV and PV. (**c**) Transhepatic venography after four sessions shows decrease of PV thrombus. (**d**) The venous phase of the superior mesenteric arteriogram shows recanalization of the enlarged portal vein (asterisk)

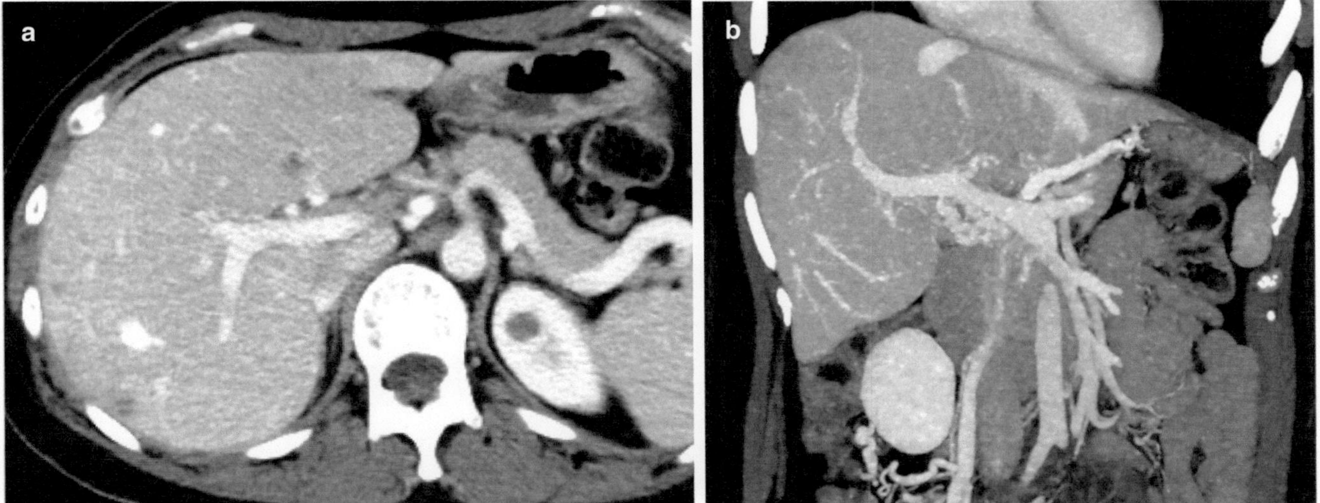

Fig. 49.3 (**a**, **b**) Contrast-enhanced CT images after 1 year show nearly complete resolution of the thrombus and normalization of the PV diameter

bin III agent was intravenously administered for two additional weeks, and oral warfarin was continued after discharge. One-year follow-up CT showed nearly complete resolution of the PV and SMV thrombosis (Fig. 49.3a, b).

Although pregnancy itself is associated with hypercoagulability, acute massive PV and SMV thrombosis is a rare complication in the postpartum period [1]. This case highlights the effectiveness of transcatheter thrombolysis combined with anticoagulation for reducing thrombus burden and improving venous flow to prevent intestinal ischemia or symptomatic portal hypertension with risk of variceal bleeding. However, the benefits must be weighed against the procedural and hemorrhagic risks [2, 3].

Conflict of Interest None of the authors have identified a conflict of interest.

Bibliography

1. Dasari P, Balusamy S. Portal vein thrombosis during pregnancy. BMJ Case Rep. 2013;2013:bcr2012008325. https://doi.org/10.1136/bcr-2012-008325.
2. Charlie CC. Direct thrombolytic therapy in portal and mesenteric vein thrombosis. J Vasc Surg. 2012;56:1124–6.
3. Hollingshead M, Burke CT, Mauro MA, et al. Transcatheter thrombolytic therapy for acute mesenteric and portal vein thrombosis. J Vasc Interv Radiol. 2005;16:651–61.

Rendezvous Recanalization of an Occluded Hepatic Artery Stent Via Percutaneous Transhepatic Access

Justin Kwan and Sundeep Punamiya

A 57-year-old male with a locally advanced pancreatic malignancy underwent a Whipple's procedure and portal vein reconstruction. In the immediate post-operative period, the patient suffered acute hematemesis and hypotension due to a pseudoaneurysm arising from the gastroduodenal artery (GDA) stump, successfully excluded by placement of a hepatic artery (HA) stent-graft.

Three months later, the patient presented with abdominal pain and abnormally elevated serum liver function tests. Contrast-enhanced computed tomography revealed extensive thrombosis of the reconstructed portal vein and occlusion of the HA stent-graft (Fig. 50.1), with biochemical and clinical features of hepatic ischemia. The multi-disciplinary team judged an endovascular approach for restoring liver reperfusion to be the preferred route.

Recanalization of the HA stent-graft was attempted from a transfemoral approach but proved unsuccessful as guidewires could not traverse the occlusion (Figs. 50.2). Using ultrasound guidance, an intrahepatic branch of the left HA was percutaneously accessed with a 21G micropuncture needle (Fig. 50.3). The occluded HA stent-graft was crossed retrogradely with an 0.014-inch Command ES wire (Abbott Vascular, Santa Clara, CA), through a 2.7F Progreat (Terumo, Somerset, NJ) microcatheter and 4F angled catheter. The wire was manipulated into the aorta and snared from the femoral access (Figs. 50.4, 50.5 and 50.6). The occluded HA stent-graft was balloon dilated

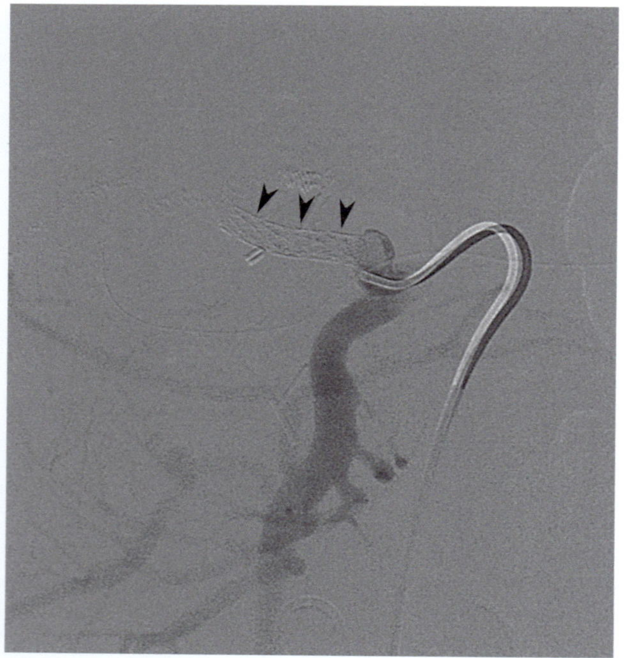

Fig. 50.1 Mesenteric angiogram showing complete occlusion of the previously deployed HA stent-graft (LifeStream balloon expandable vascular covered stent, Bard Peripheral Vascular, Tempe, AZ) (*arrowheads*)

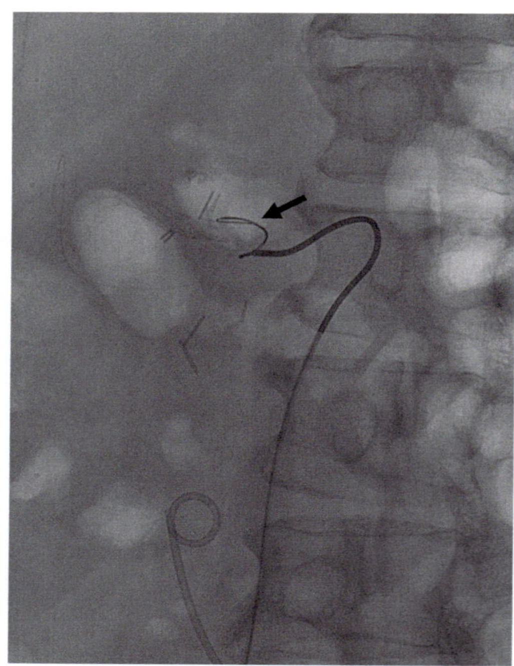

Fig. 50.2 Failed attempt at antegrade crossing of the occluded stent-graft with a microcatheter system (Progreat, Terumo, Somerset, NJ) (*black arrow*) buckling alongside the proximal end of the occluded HA stent-graft. This was likely related to the chronicity of the occlusion as well as a lack of catheter support at the hepatic artery ostium

J. Kwan · S. Punamiya (✉)
Department of Diagnostic and Interventional Radiology,
Tan Tock Seng Hospital, Singapore, Singapore
e-mail: justin_kwan@ttsh.com.sg;
sundeep_punamiya@ttsh.com.sg

(Fig. 50.7) and re-lined with bare metal stents, re-establishing satisfactory antegrade flow (Fig. 50.8). Unfortunately, this was not enough to improve the patient's clinical condition and the patient eventually passed away.

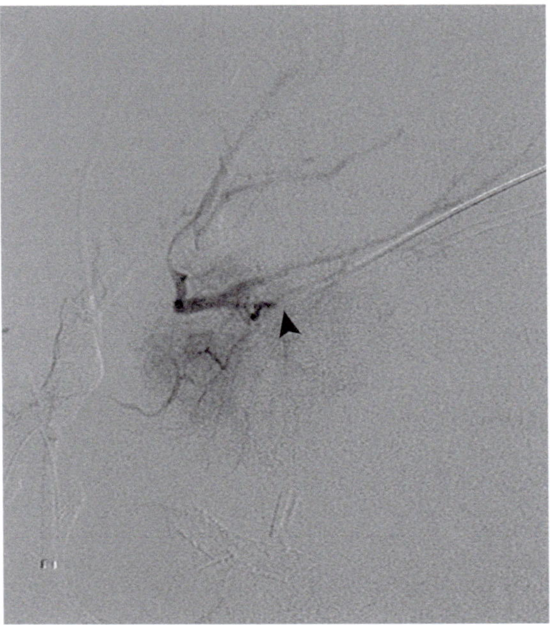

Fig. 50.3 Using sonographic guidance, an intrahepatic branch of the left HA was identified and punctured using a 21G micropuncture needle. Angiogram obtained via the needle shows the tip of the needle (*black arrowhead*) within a tiny branch of the left HA, with opacification of left intrahepatic arterial branches

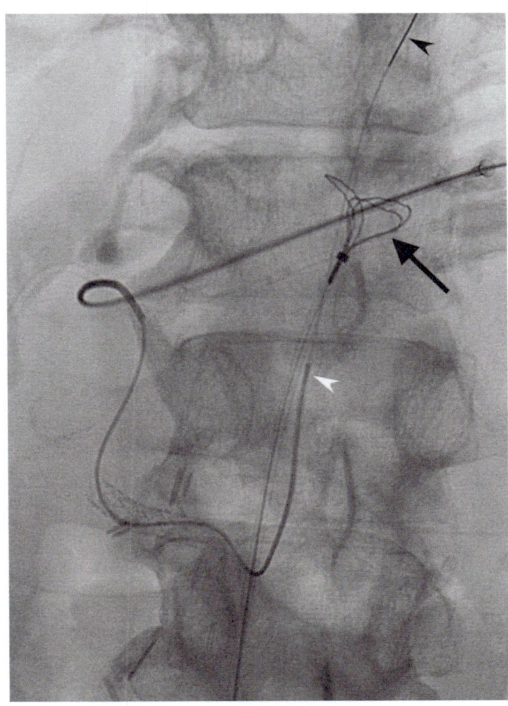

Fig. 50.5 The needle was replaced for a triaxial system comprising of a 4F Berenstein catheter, 2.7F Progreat microcatheter, and 0.014-inch Command ES wire. The wire (*black arrowhead*) and microcatheter (*white arrowhead*) were successfully manipulated across the occluded HA stent-graft into the aorta, and captured by a snare (EN Snare, Merit Medical System, South Jordan, UT) (*arrow*) introduced from the femoral access

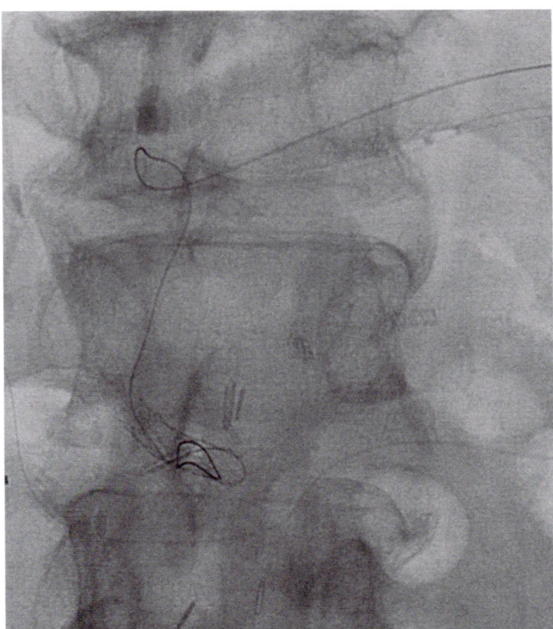

Fig. 50.4 Through the 21G needle, a 0.014-inch wire (Command ES, Abbott Vascular, Santa Clara, CA) was advanced retrograde into the occluded stent-graft, but unable to cross it without catheter support

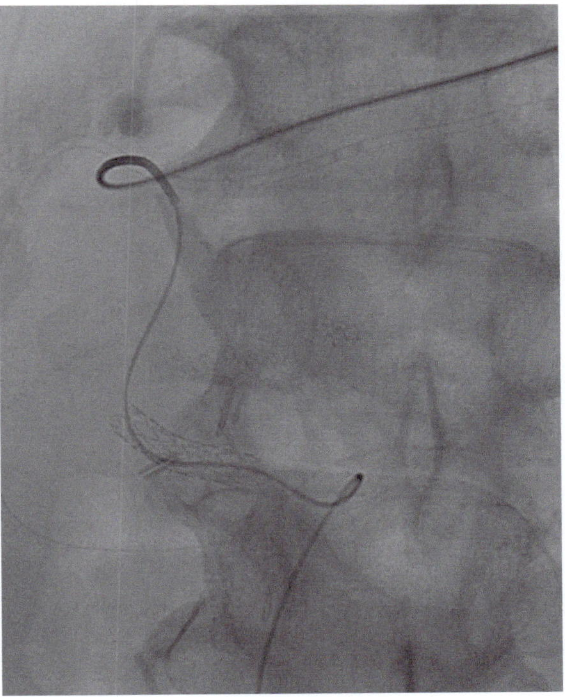

Fig. 50.6 The wire was exteriorized to obtain through-and-through access, providing sufficient support for the subsequent passage of the angioplasty balloon and stents

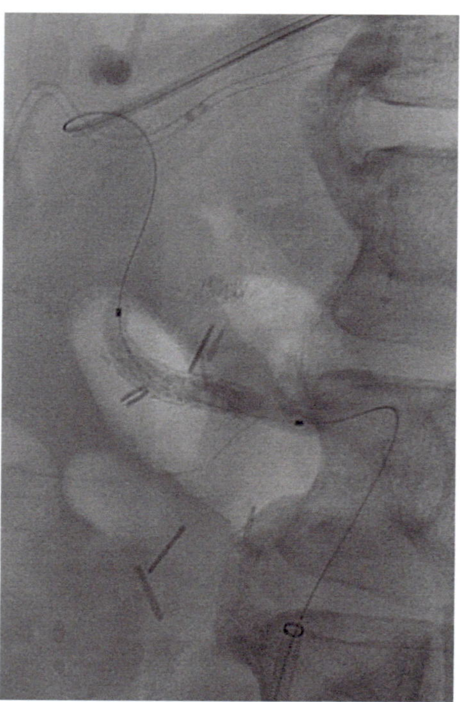

Fig. 50.7 The occluded HA stent-graft was dilated with a 4 mm × 40 mm angioplasty balloon

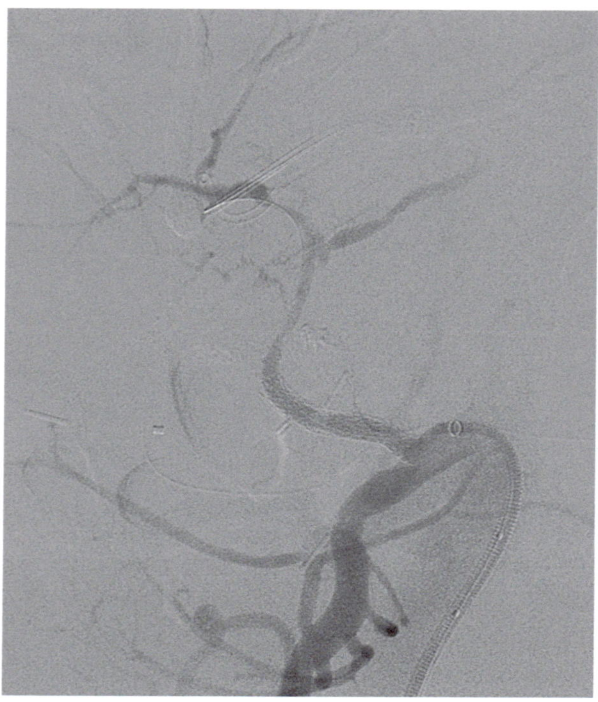

Fig. 50.8 Final angiogram shows re-established antegrade flow through the stent-graft after relining and extending with a 5 mm stent distally, and a 7 mm stent proximally (Herculink stents, Abbott Vascular, Santa Clara, CA)

Percutaneous Trans-Needle Glue Embolization of an Isolated Visceral Aneurysm

Dhara Kinariwala, Daniel Sheeran and Ziv J Haskal

A 65-year-old female presented with acute epigastric pain and nausea suggesting pancreatitis. Shortly after admission, she developed hypotension, a drop in hemoglobin from 12.6 to 6.9 g/dL. CTA demonstrated an approximately 1.5 cm diameter ruptured pancreaticoduodenal artery (PDA) branch aneurysm (Fig. 51.1).

Superior mesenteric arteriography demonstrated its supply from a distant, peripheral PDA branch, with retrograde flow into the gastroduodenal, hepatic, and splenic arteries (Fig. 51.2). Despite use of multiple specialized microcathe-

ters and guidewires, the aneurysm could not be reached and focal dissection and rupture of a 2 mm feeding vessel developed (Fig. 51.3). Two microcoils were deployed: at this rupture site and within the outflow vessel. Repeat angiography

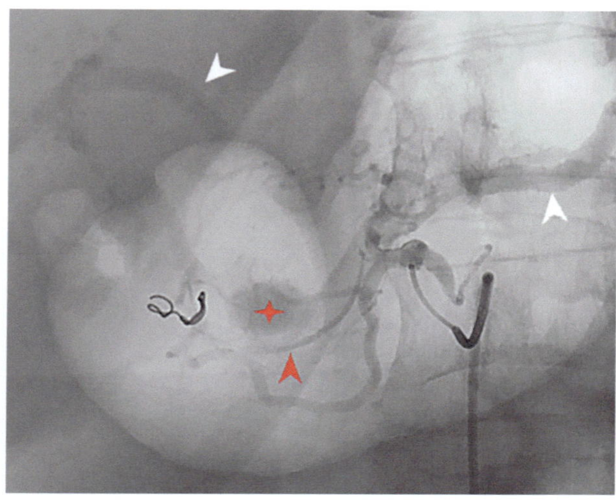

Fig. 51.2 Superior mesenteric artery angiography demonstrates filling of an oval-shaped aneurysm (red asterisk) arising from a small pancreaticoduodenal branch (red arrow), with marked retrograde filling of the hepatic and splenic artery branches (white arrows), secondary to celiac artery stenosis

Fig. 51.1 Axial CTA demonstrates a pancreaticoduodenal artery aneurysm (red arrow) with surrounding inflammation and high density perihepatic fluid (white arrow) indicative of rupture

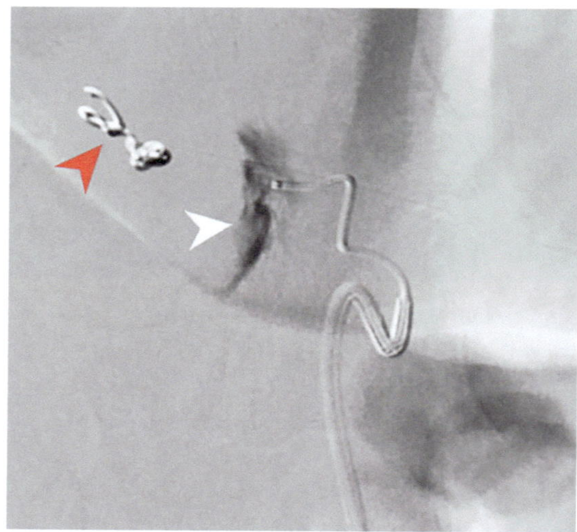

Fig. 51.3 Digital subtraction angiography (DSA) demonstrating focal PDA branch dissection and rupture (white arrow). Previously placed microcoil in an outflow PDA branch is also present (red arrow)

D. Kinariwala
Department of Radiology and Medical Imaging, University of Virginia, Charlottesville, VA, USA
e-mail: djk4x@virginia.edu

D. Sheeran
Department of Radiology, University of Virginia, Charlottesville, VA, USA
e-mail: dps7u@hscmail.mcc.virginia.edu

Z. J Haskal (✉)
Department of Radiology and Medical Imaging, Interventional Division, University of Virginia, Charlottesville, VA, USA

Z. J. Haskal (ed.), *Extreme IR*, https://doi.org/10.1007/978-3-031-24251-9_51

suggested some persistent filling of the vessel supplying the aneurysm (Fig. 51.4); this was confirmed by CTA the next day (Fig. 51.5).

Using a combined angiographic/CT room, the aneurysm was identified and punctured directly using a 21-gauge (Fig. 51.6). Pulsatile blood emerged from its hub; angiography affirmed its position within the aneurysm (Fig. 51.7). Using fluoroscopic guidance, 2 cc of a 1:2 dilution of ethiodized oil and N-butyl cyanoacrylate (Trufill, Johnson & Johnson) was injected through the needle until the aneurysm was filled and stasis of flow demonstrated. Non-contrast CT affirmed that glue filled the entire aneurysm without surrounding hemorrhage or other complication (Fig. 51.8). She was discharged symptoms-free, 2 days hence; she remained well through 1-year follow-up. PDA aneurysms have long been associated with celiac artery stenosis and occlusion, as has percutaneous coil embolization. This case expands upon these with the safe, efficient, and definitive use of relatively dense glue delivered directly through a small caliber needle.

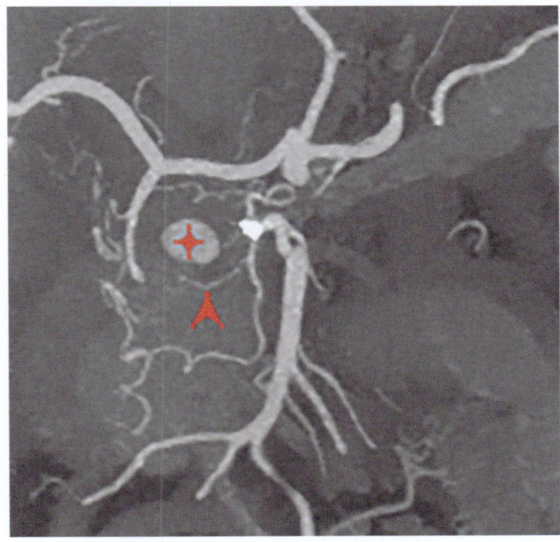

Fig. 51.5 Coronal CTA with maximum intensity projection (MIP) 1 day following coil embolization demonstrates decreased but persistent filling of the feeding branch vessel (red arrow) and aneurysm (red asterisk)

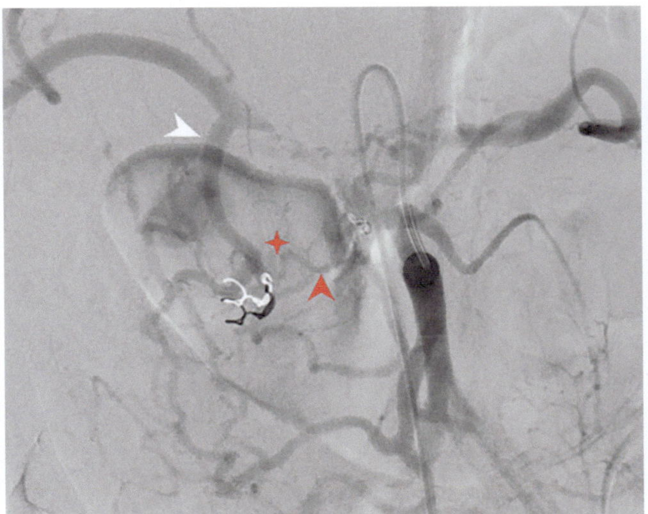

Fig. 51.4 Post-coiling SMA angiography demonstrates persistent flow in the feeding PDA branch vessel (red arrow) and suggestive faint filling of the aneurysm (red asterisk). There is continued retrograde flow through the gastroduodenal artery (white arrow)

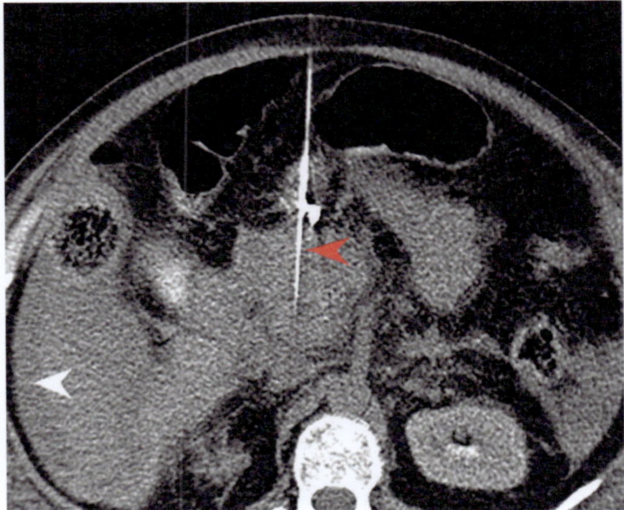

Fig. 51.6 Axial non-contrast CT demonstrates direct puncture into the aneurysm with a 22-gauge needle (red arrow). Perihepatic hemorrhage remains (white arrow)

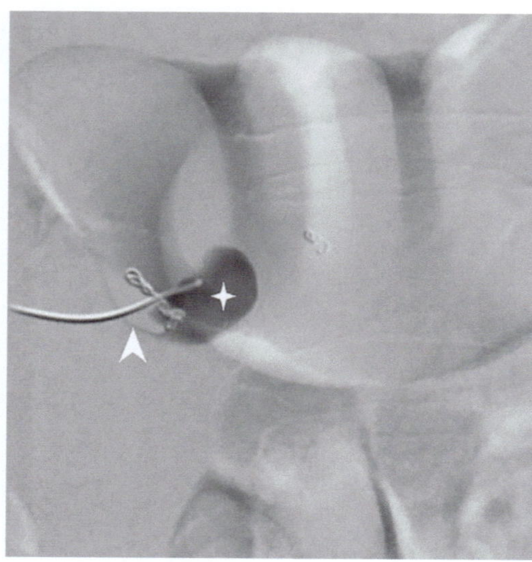

Fig. 51.7 DSA through the 22-gauge needle demonstrates appropriate position of the needle with opacification of the aneurysm (white asterisk) as well as the outflow arterial branch (white arrow)

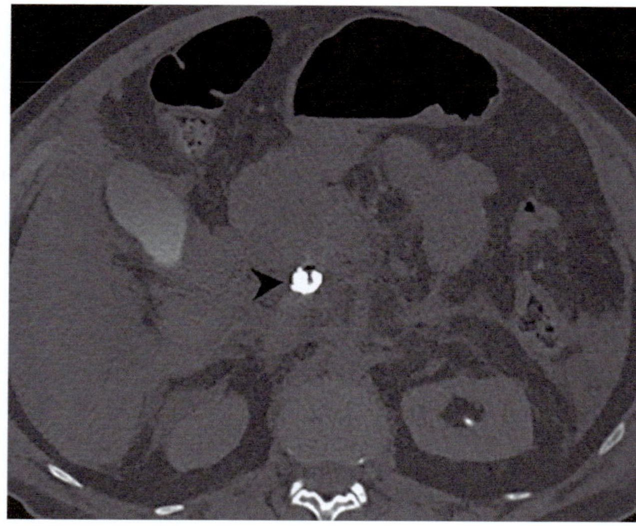

Fig. 51.8 Post-intervention non-contrast CT demonstrates presence of the embolic agent in the aneurysm cavity (black arrow) without extravasation or nontarget embolization

Vascular Ehlers-Danlos Syndrome Complicated by Ruptured Hepatic Artery Pseudoaneurysm

M. Gonsalves and Robert Morgan

A 35-year-old male with no prior past medical history, presented to a district general hospital with left flank pain; he was provisionally diagnosed with renal colic. He deteriorated acutely, suffered cardiorespiratory arrest, and following resuscitation, was transferred to our unit for ongoing management. Triple phase CT demonstrated a ruptured hepatic artery pseudoaneurysm (Fig. 52.1) and extensive hemoperitoneum (Fig. 52.2). There was a left main renal artery pseudoaneurysm, occlusion of the anterior division, and extensive acute renal cortical infarction (Fig. 52.3). The right kidney was severely atrophic with focal dissections and stenoses of the right renal artery.

Emergency embolization of the hepatic artery pseudoaneurysm was performed using a 0.027″ microcatheter and detachable Ruby microcoils (Penumbra Inc.) (Figs. 52.3 and 52.4). The patient stabilized promptly and was extubated the following morning. The left renal artery pseudoaneurysm was embolized during the same admission (Fig. 52.5). CT angiogram of the cerebral arteries showed several dissections, stenoses, and pseudoaneurysms. After discharge, genetic analysis found COL3A1 genotype mutation confirming vascular Ehlers-Danlos syndrome (vEDS). At 3-month follow-up, the patient remained well and symptom free.

Vascular Ehlers-Danlos syndrome is a rare (1:50000 to 1:25000 people) autosomal dominant condition resulting from mutations in the COL3A1 gene-encoding type 3 collagen [1]. Up to 50% of cases are sporadic. Patients are at risk

M. Gonsalves
Department of Interventional Radiology,
St. George's University Hospitals NHS Foundation Trust,
London, UK
e-mail: michaelgonsalves@nhs.net

R. Morgan (✉)
Department of Interventional Radiology,
St. George's University Hospitals NHS Foundation Trust,
London, UK

Cardiovascular Clinical Academic Group, Molecular and Clinical Sciences Research Institute, St. George's University of London and St George's University Hospitals NHS Foundation Trust,
London, UK
e-mail: rmorgan@sgul.ac.uk

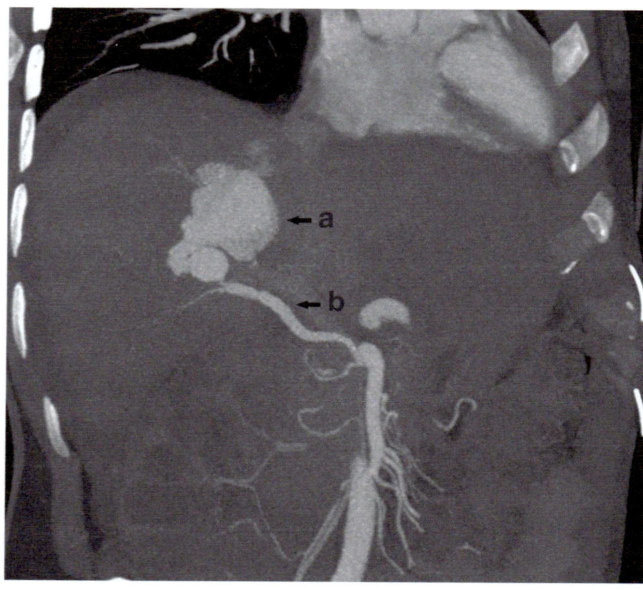

Fig. 52.1 MIP of arterial phase CT showing hepatic artery pseudoaneurysm (**a**). Note variant anatomy with replaced right hepatic artery arising from the SMA (**b**)

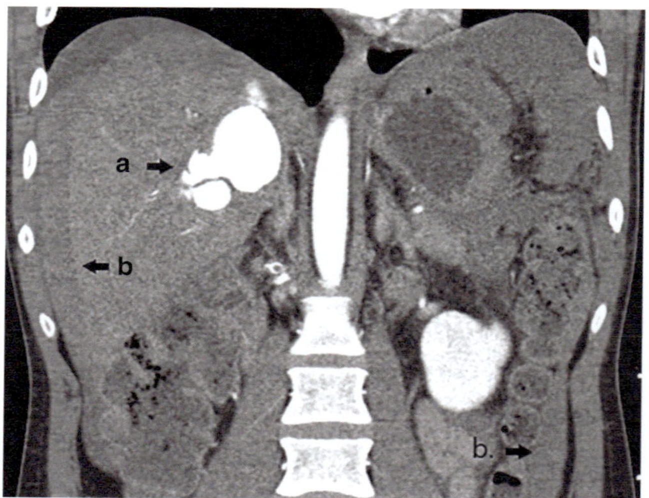

Fig. 52.2 Coronal reformat of arterial phase CT showing pseudoaneurysm (**a**) and hemoperitoneum (**b**)

of arterial dissection and vascular rupture with a median life expectancy of 40–50 years. Caution is required with arterial puncture in vEDS with major morbidity reported in up to 67% of patients [2]. Surgical buttress of the common femoral artery should be considered prior to puncture [2].

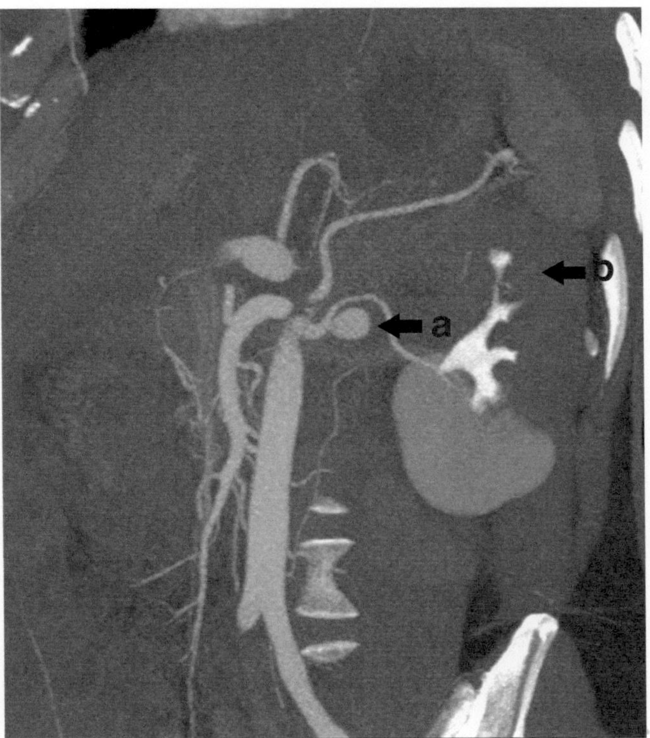

Fig. 52.3 MIP of arterial phase CT showing left main renal artery pseudoaneurysm (**a**) and extensive renal cortical infarction (**b**)

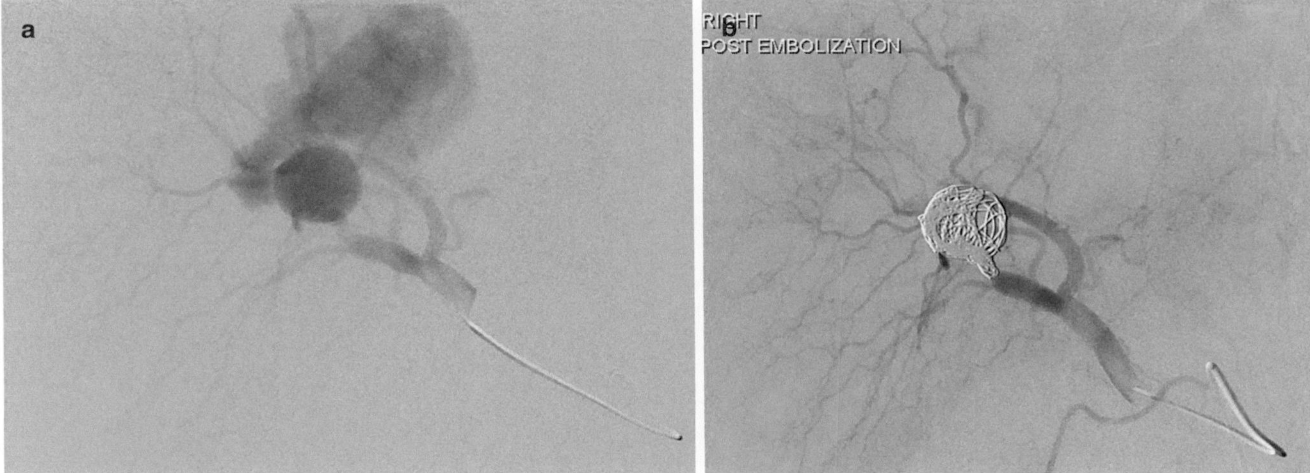

Fig. 52.4 Images, Pre- (**a**) and post- (**b**) micro coil embolization of hepatic artery pseudoaneurysm. Note improved filling of intra hepatic arterial branches post-embolization

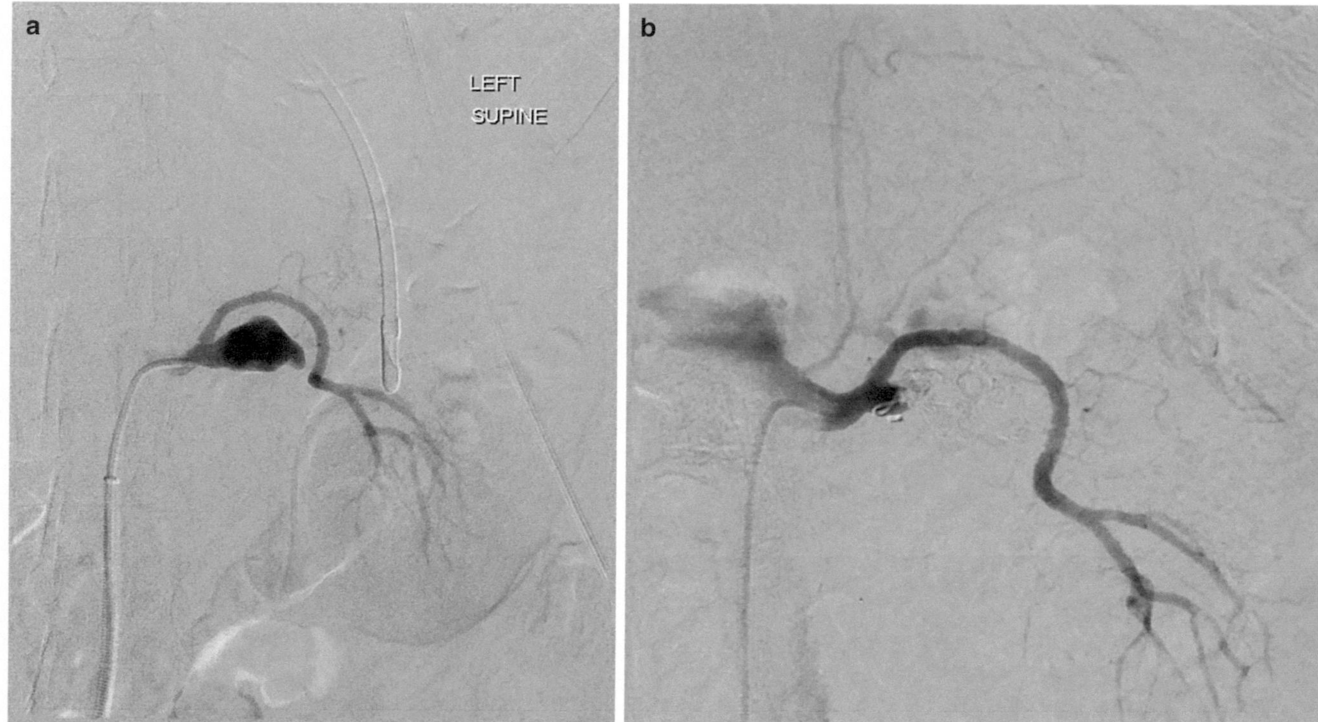

Fig. 52.5 Images, Pre- (**a**) and post- (**b**) embolization of left renal artery pseudoaneurysm

Bibliography

1. Malfait F, Francomano C, Byers P, Belmont J, Berglund B, Black J, et al. The 2017 international classification of the Ehlers–Danlos syndromes. Am J Med Genet C Semin Med Genet. 2017;175C:8–26. https://doi.org/10.1002/ajmg.c.31552.
2. Eagleton J. Arterial complications of vascular Ehlers-Danlos syndrome. J Vasc Surg. 2016;64(6):1869–80. https://doi.org/10.1016/j.jvs.2016.06.120.

Endovascular Recanalization of Hepatic Artery Thrombosis After Liver Transplantation

Tiago Bilhim

A 55-year-old man with alcoholic chronic hepatic disease, Child-Pugh C (C-P score, 11), sodium model for end-stage liver disease (MELD Na$^+$) score of 22, presented with ascites and spontaneous bacterial peritonitis. Hepatic transplantation was performed, followed by a re-transplantation 3 months later due to graft failure. CT angiography (CTA) 5 days after re-transplantation showed hepatic artery thrombosis (Fig. 53.1). Immediate transfemoral endovascular revascularization was undertaken using a 6-French 45 cm-long sheath placed in the celiac trunk (Fig. 53.2). After aspiration thrombectomies using the 6-French Indigo catheter (Penumbra), persistent hepatic artery thrombosis remained (Fig. 53.3). A 6-French catheter was placed in the hepatic artery and thrombolysis was initiated with alteplase

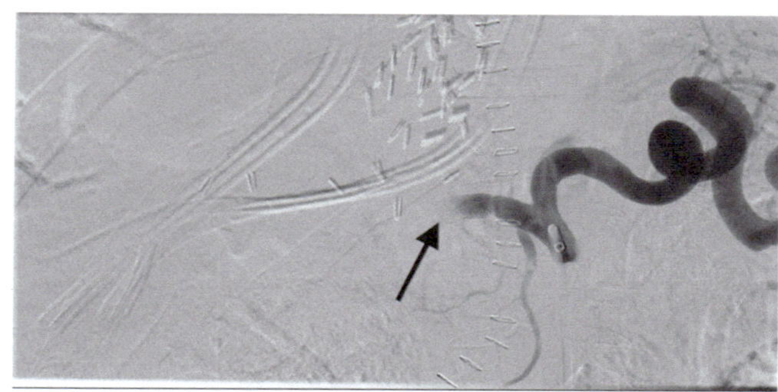

Fig. 53.2 Digital subtraction angiography (DSA) of the celiac artery confirms hepatic artery thrombosis (arrow)

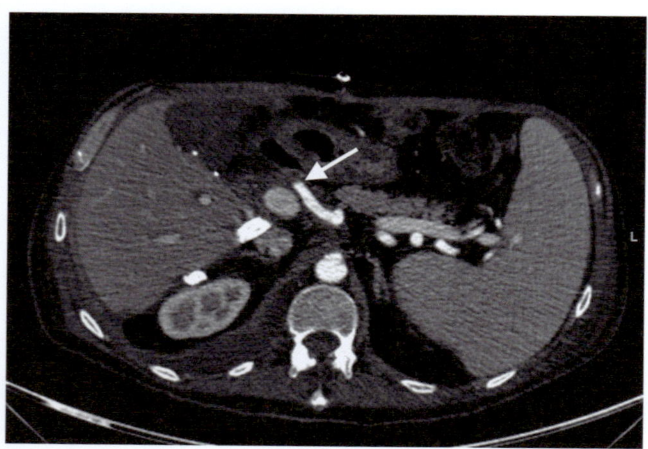

Fig. 53.1 CT angiography (CTA) 5 days after re-transplantation. Axial image shows the hepatic artery thrombosis (arrow)

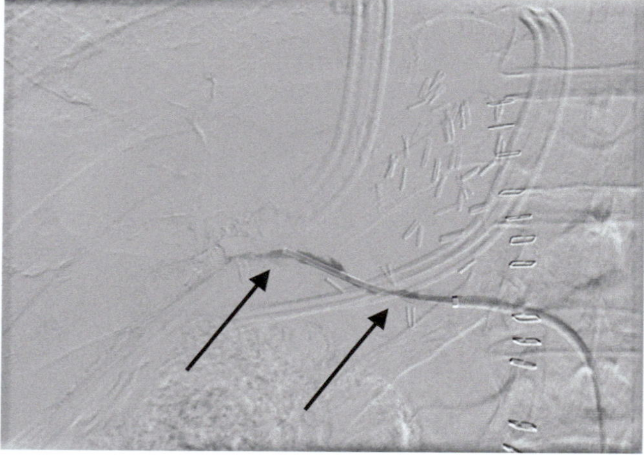

Fig. 53.3 Digital subtraction angiography shows persistent hepatic artery thrombosis (arrows) after multiple aspiration thrombectomies

T. Bilhim (✉)
Department of Interventional Radiology, Curry Cabral Hospital, Centro Hospitalar Universitário de Lisboa Central (CHULC), Lisbon, Portugal
e-mail: tiago.bilhim@chlc.minsaude.pt

(Actilyse, Boehringer Ingelheim) using a 10 mg intra-arterial bolus, and 1.5 mg/h 18 h infusion. Follow-up DSA showed partial revascularization. Intra-arterial alteplase 1 mg/h continued for another 24 h. Fibrinogen levels were 1.67 g/L before and 1.63 g/L after thrombolysis. DSA revealed residual stenosis of the anastomosis (Fig. 53.4); this was addressed with a 6 mm diameter × 2.5 cm long ePTFE stent graft (Viabahn, Gore) (Fig. 53.5). CTA at 2 days (Fig. 53.6) and Doppler sonography at 3 months confirmed patency of the hepatic artery (Fig. 53.7). Four months later, he presented with pruritus, jaundice, and total bilirubin of 7.7 mg/dL. MR cholangiography showed a biliary anastomotic stricture (Fig. 53.8). Re-hepaticocoledocostomy was performed, followed by graft dysfunction and hepatic artery thrombosis. The patient received a third liver transplant and is currently well.

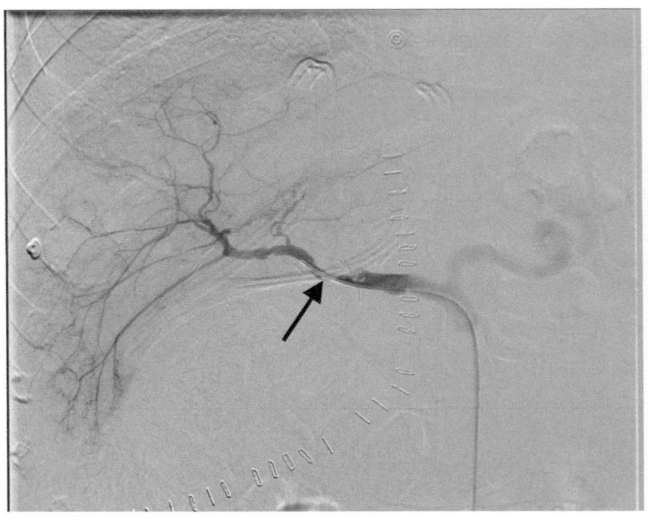

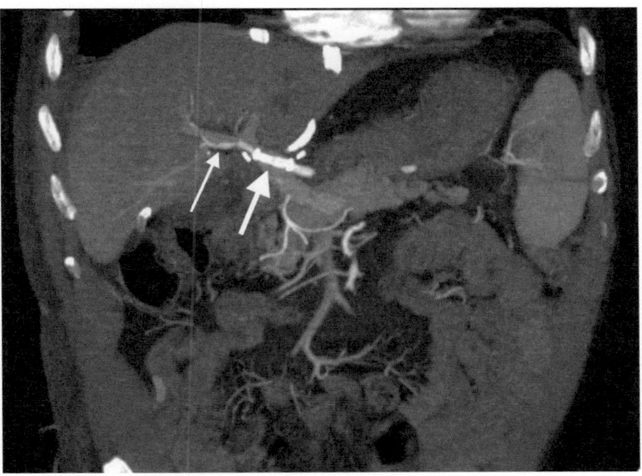

Fig. 53.6 CTA 2 days later depicts stent and hepatic artery patency (arrows)

Fig. 53.4 Control digital subtraction angiography after thrombolysis shows revascularization of the hepatic artery with a residual underlying stenosis of the surgical anastomosis (arrow)

Fig. 53.5 Immediate CT scan after placement of the self-expanding covered stent (arrow) in the hepatic artery affirms stent patency

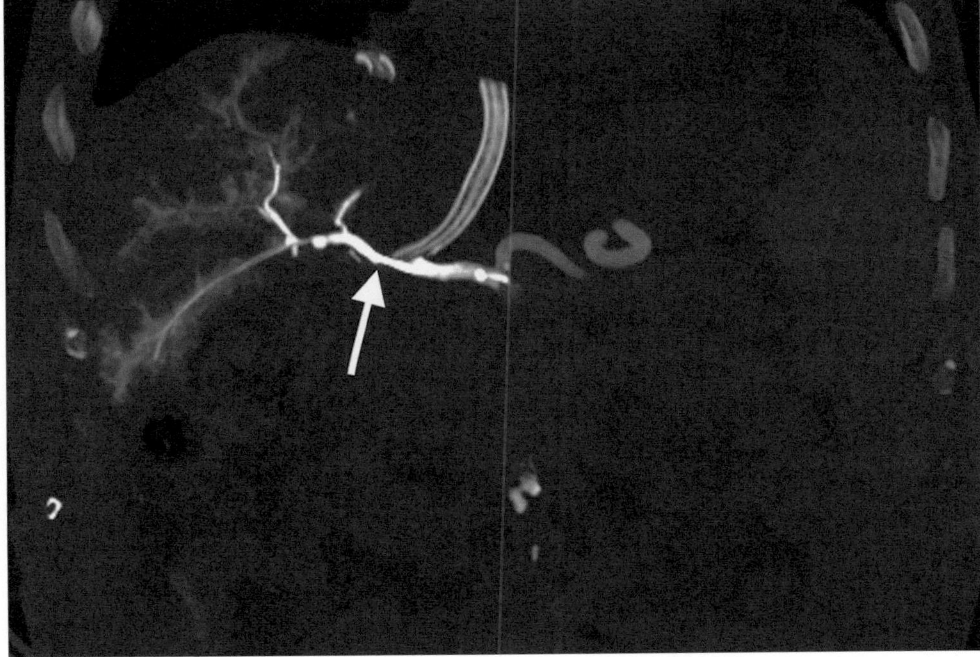

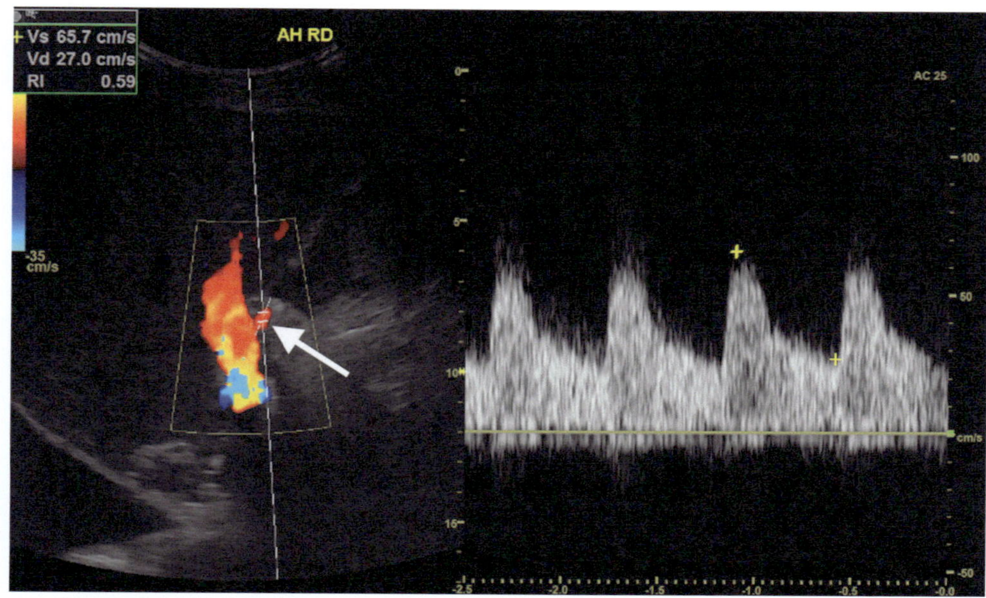

Fig. 53.7 Doppler ultrasound 3 months afterwards confirms patency of the hepatic artery (arrow)

Fig. 53.8 MR cholangiography demonstrates the biliary anastomotic stricture (arrow)

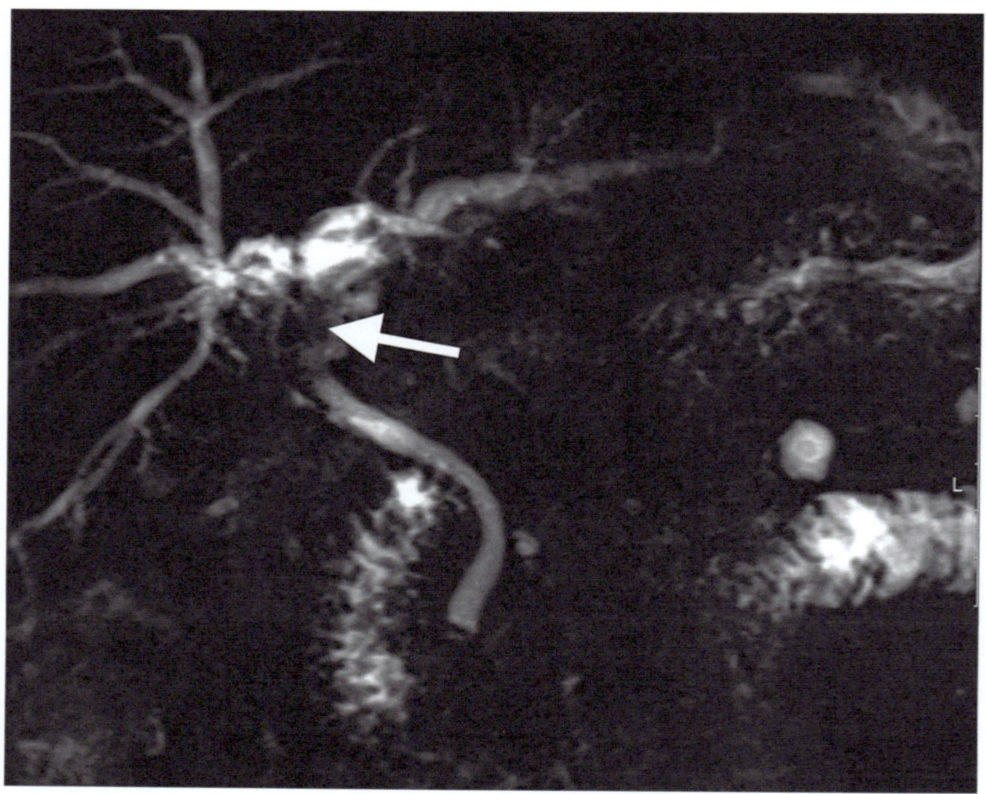

Celiac Trunk Avulsion Treated with Endograft and Embolization During Open Cardiac Massage

Abdul Rehman Mustafa and R. Torrance Andrews

A 45-year-old motor vehicle trauma patient with a hostile surgical abdomen presented with celiac trunk avulsion (Figs. 54.1 and 54.2). The bleeding was not successfully controlled in the operating room, so the patient was transferred to the interventional suite. Whilst the patient underwent open cardiac massage, an aortic endograft extension was placed over the origin of the avulsed celiac artery (Fig. 54.3), and coil embolization of the splenic, left gastric, and common hepatic arteries was performed through the pancreaticoduodenal arcade to prevent retrograde flow (Figs. 54.4 and 54.5). The bleeding ceased and the celiac trunk avulsion was successfully treated (Fig. 54.6). However, the patient died 24 h later from multi-organ system failure related to the severe initial trauma.

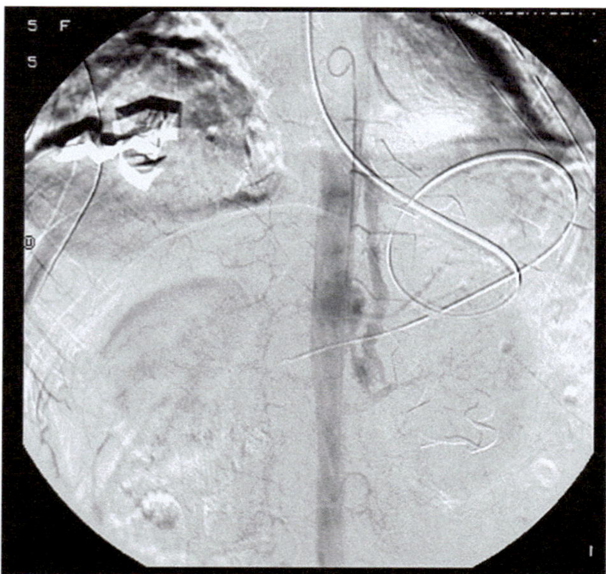

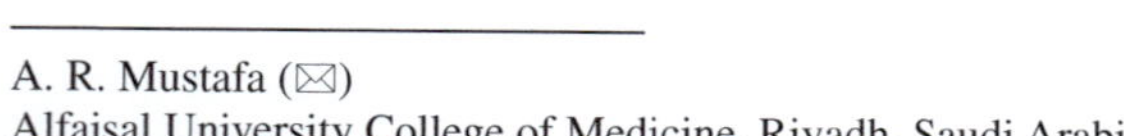
Fig. 54.2 Delayed image showing the extent of the extravasation

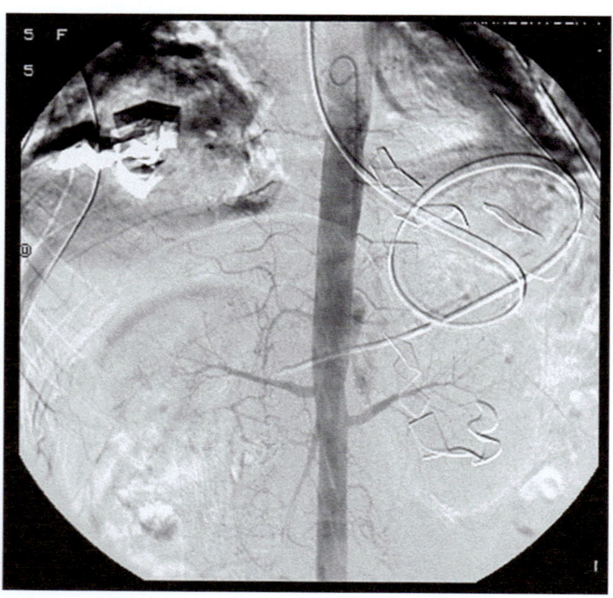
Fig. 54.1 Nonselective aortogram demonstrating diffuse vasospasm and extraluminal contrast to the left of the celiac origin

A. R. Mustafa (✉)
Alfaisal University College of Medicine, Riyadh, Saudi Arabia

R. T. Andrews
Department of Interventional Radiology, Swedish Medical Center, First Hill Campus, Seattle, WA, USA
e-mail: randrews@radiax.com

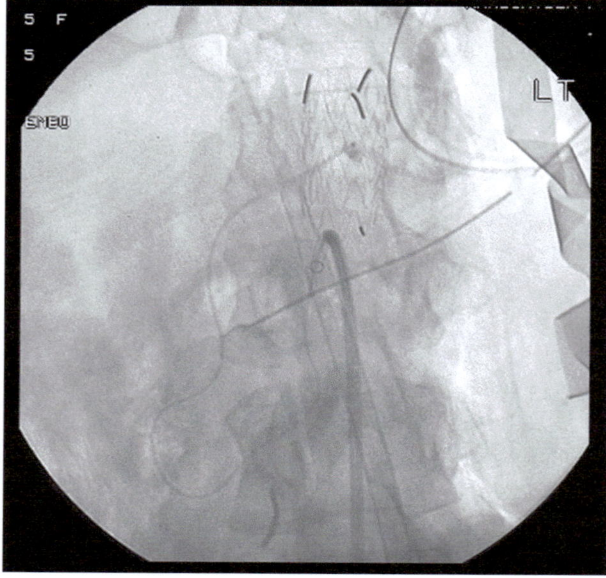
Fig. 54.3 Following placement of an endograft across the origin of the celiac, a microcatheter is advanced from the superior mesenteric artery and the pancreaticoduodenal arcade to the celiac trunk

© The Author(s), under exclusive license to Springer Nature Switzerland AG 2023
Z. J. Haskal (ed.), *Extreme IR*, https://doi.org/10.1007/978-3-031-24251-9_54

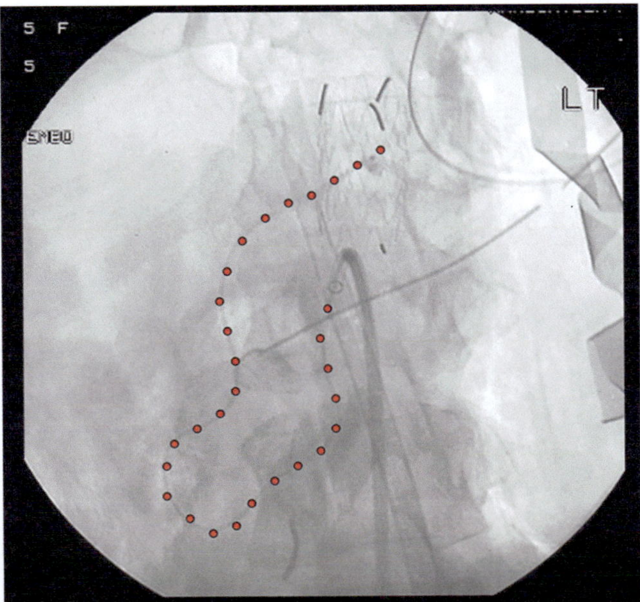

Fig. 54.4 Microcatheter course delineated by red dots

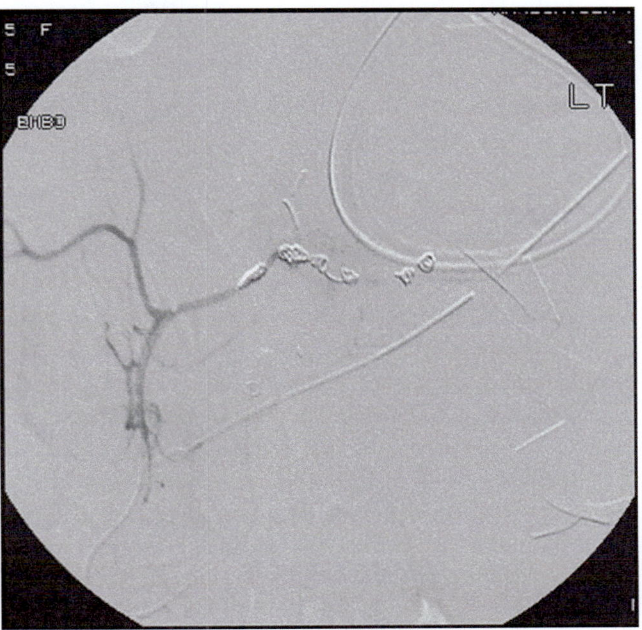

Fig. 54.5 Coils placed across the celiac trunk, spanning from the splenic artery to the common hepatic, to prevent backbleeding through the avulsed celiac trunk

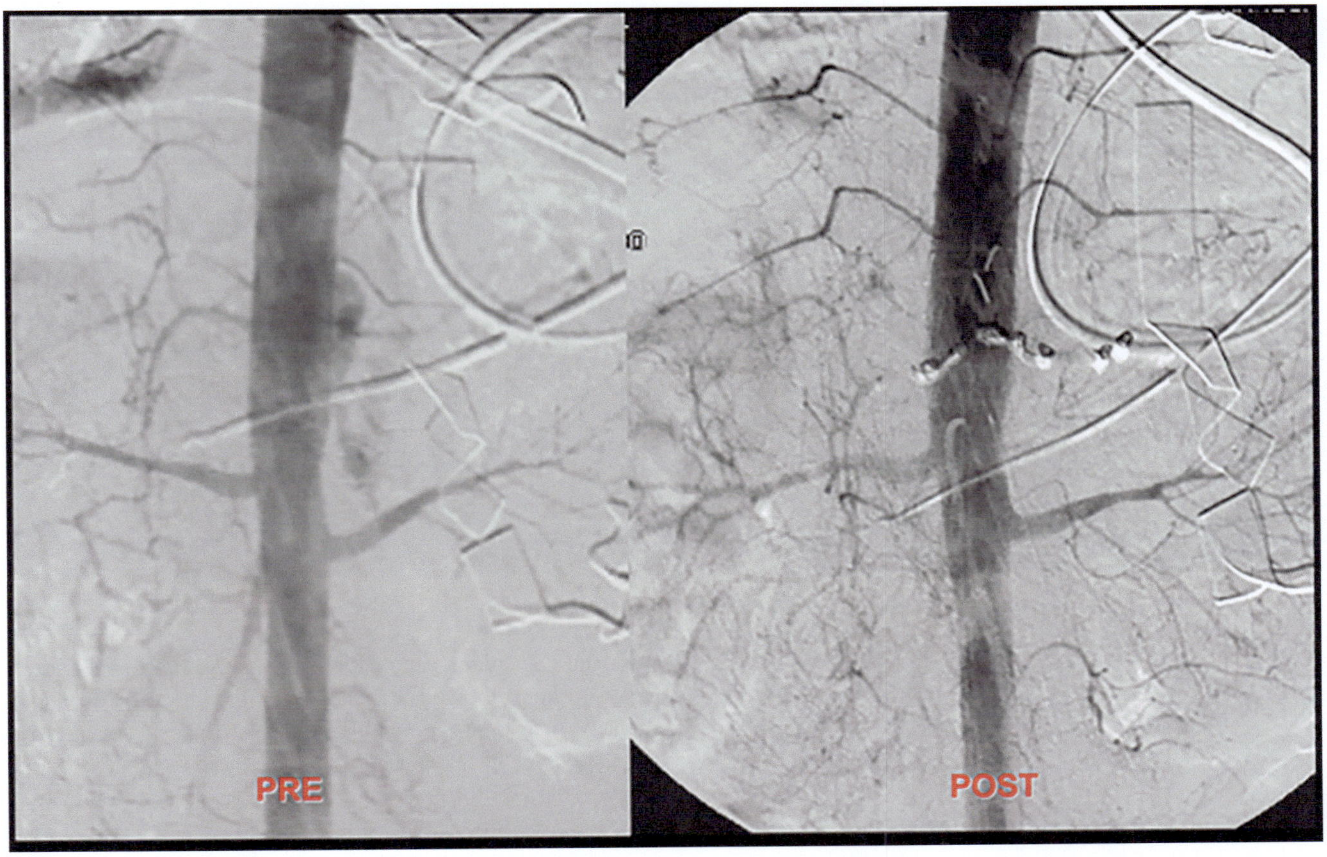

Fig. 54.6 Images before and after intervention demonstrate control of extravasation

Pancreas Transplant Anastomotic Breakdown Treated with Stents and Thrombin

Abdul Rehman Mustafa and R. Torrance Andrews

A patient with a pancreas transplant presented with an arterial pseudoaneurysm involving the anastomosis of the right common iliac artery and the pancreatic transplant artery (Fig. 55.1). Using a transfemoral approach, as SOS selective catheter was advanced into the pseudoaneurysm (Fig. 55.2). A self-expanding 10 mm × 40 mm bare-metal stent was deployed within the common iliac artery (Fig. 55.3), extending across anastomosis. The SOS catheter was reintroduced into the transplant pancreatic artery through the interstices of the bare stent (Fig. 55.4), followed by an Ansel sheath. A 5 × 26 mm balloon-expandable endograft was then deployed, spanning from the iliac stent across the pseudoaneurysm and

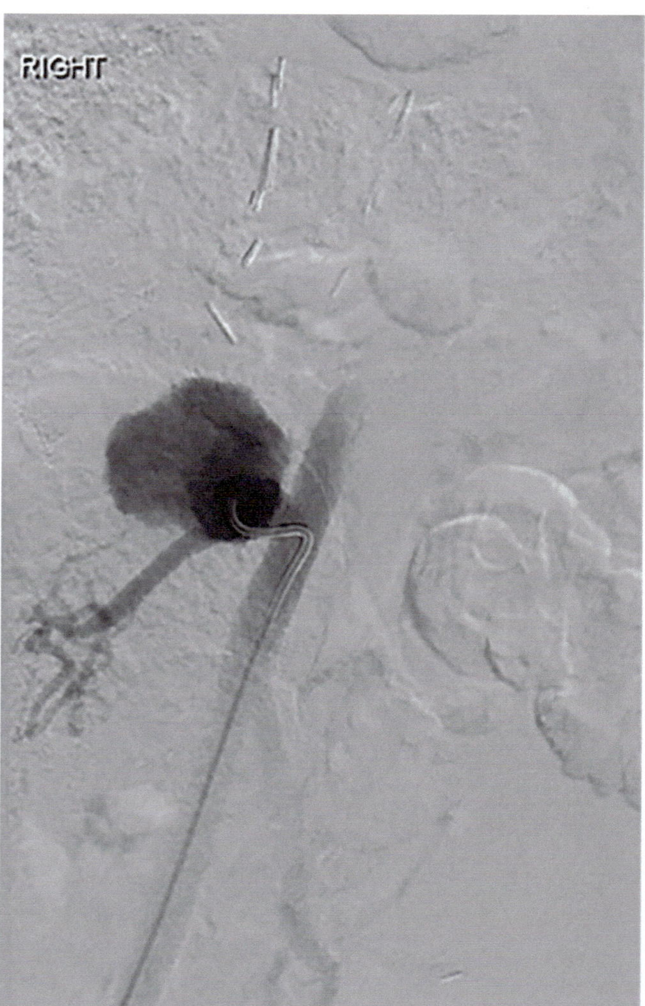

Fig. 55.2 Selective arteriogram showing anastomotic disruption with a large pseudoaneurysm

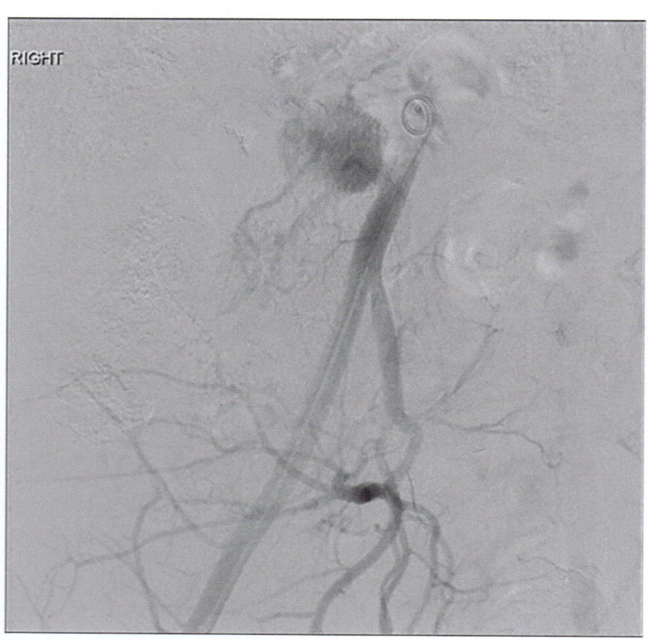

Fig. 55.1 Right common iliac arteriogram demonstrating a large volume of extraluminal contrast at the pancreatic artery anastomosis

into the transplant pancreatic artery (Fig. 55.5). Post-stent arteriography showed residual opacification of the pseudoaneurysm, so a Kumpe catheter was introduced through the interstices of the bare-metal stent and into the pseudoaneurysm. This was followed by transcatheter thrombin injection into the pseudoaneurysm (Fig. 55.6).

Subsequent iliac arteriography demonstrated excellent flow through the transplant pancreatic artery and minimal

A. R. Mustafa (✉)
Alfaisal University College of Medicine, Riyadh, Saudi Arabia

R. T. Andrews
Department of Interventional Radiology, Swedish Medical Center, First Hill Campus, Seattle, WA, USA
e-mail: randrews@radiax.com

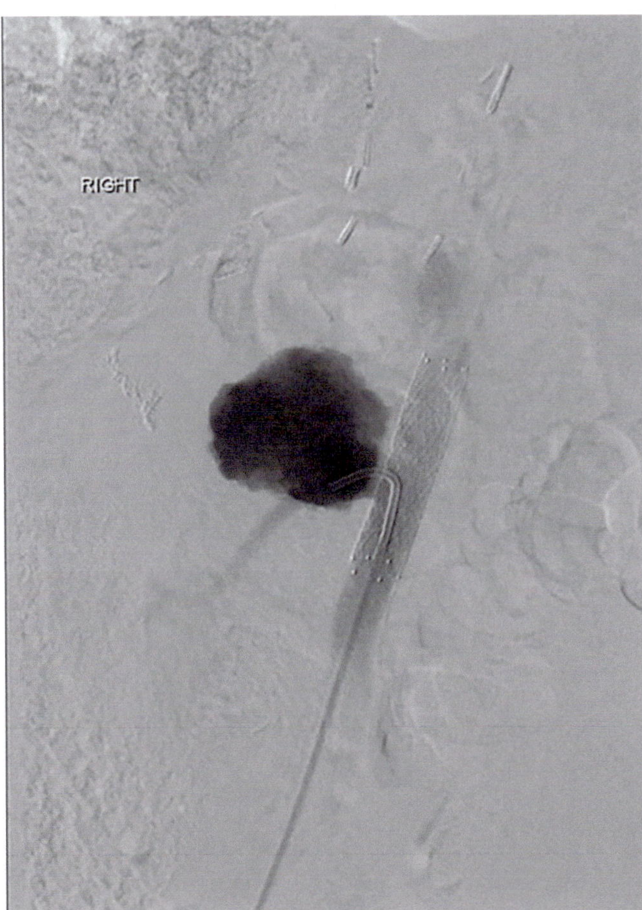

Fig. 55.3 Bare stent placed across the anastomotic origin; pseudoaneurysm is still filling

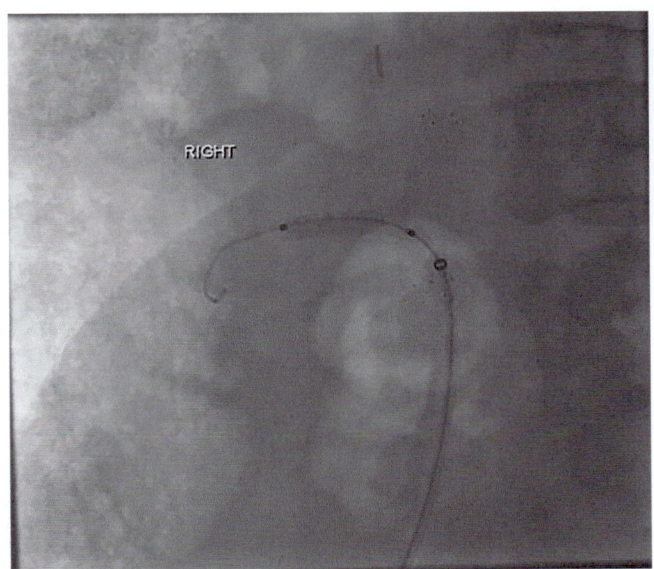

Fig. 55.4 Placement of a covered endograft through the interstices of the bare stent

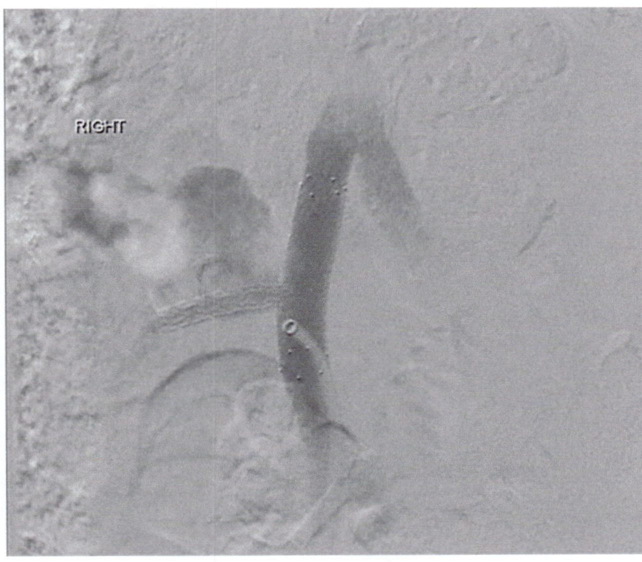

Fig. 55.5 Markedly reduced opacification of the pseudoaneurysm after endograft placement

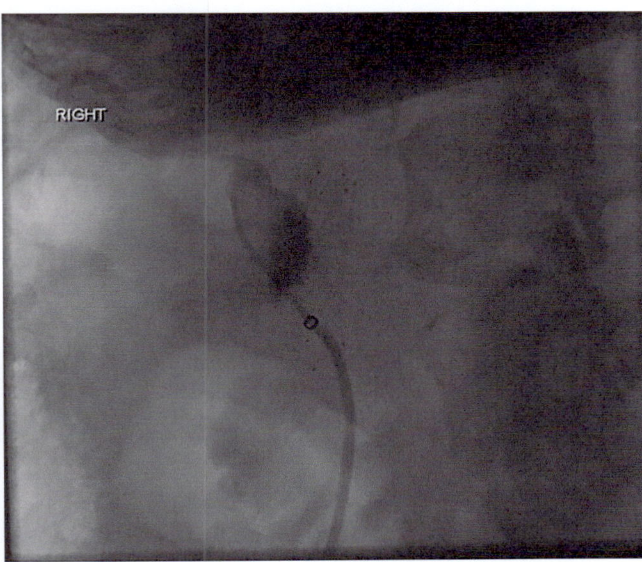

Fig. 55.6 Delivery of thrombin directly into the lumen of the pseudoaneurysm

flow in the pseudoaneurysm (Fig. 55.7). At follow-up, the anastomotic pseudoaneurysm was without perfusion and stable in size (Fig. 55.8). This appearance was unchanged on serial examination over 4 years of follow up, and the pancreas has remained functional.

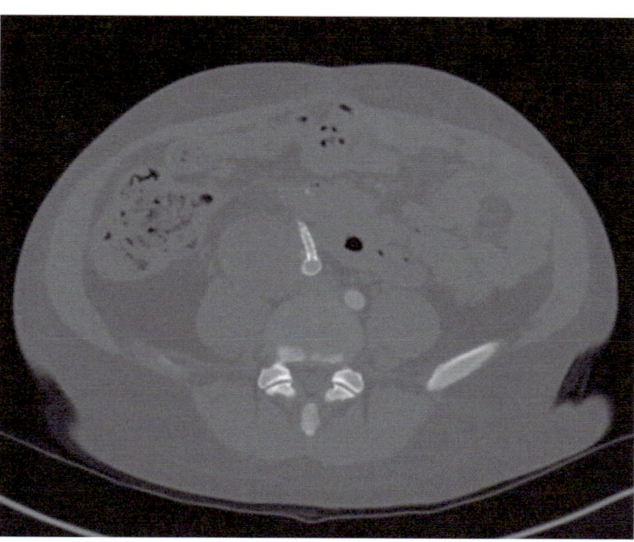

Fig. 55.8 Representative image from a contrast-enhanced CT showing the relationship between the stents and thrombosis of the large pseudoaneurysm immediately to the right of the stents

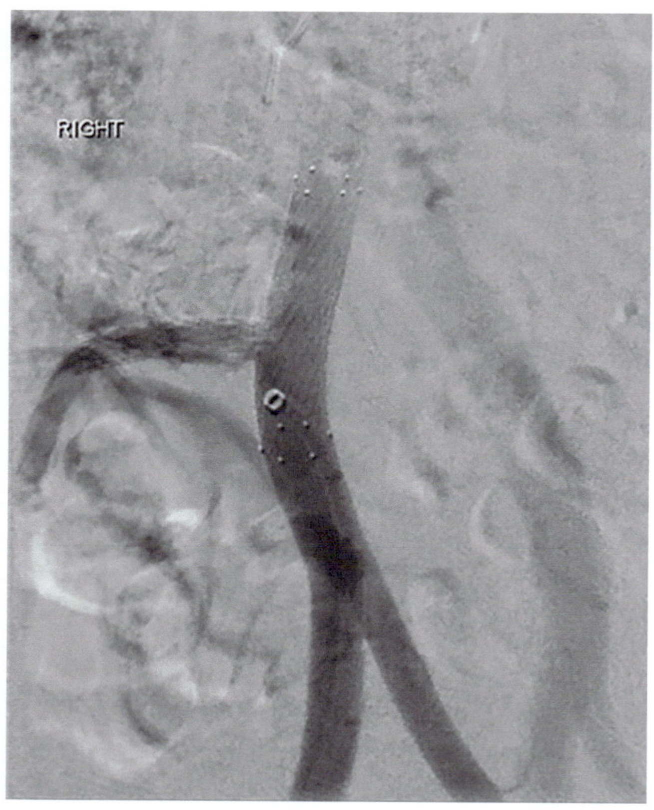

Fig. 55.7 Final result shows no opacification of the pseudoaneurysm with preservation of flow into the pancreatic artery

A Challenging High Flow Renal AVF with Giant Venous Aneurysm

R. Garcia-Monaco, O. Peralta and M. Rabellino

A 63-year-old hemodynamically stable male with diarrhea, abdominal distention, and a palpable mass in the right flank associated with bilateral lower limb edema. No history of trauma or abdominal surgery. CT scan showed a high flow renal arteriovenous fistula (AVF) with a giant aneurysmal vein compressing the inferior vena cava (Fig. 56.1). Aortic angiography confirmed the CT findings (Fig. 56.2).

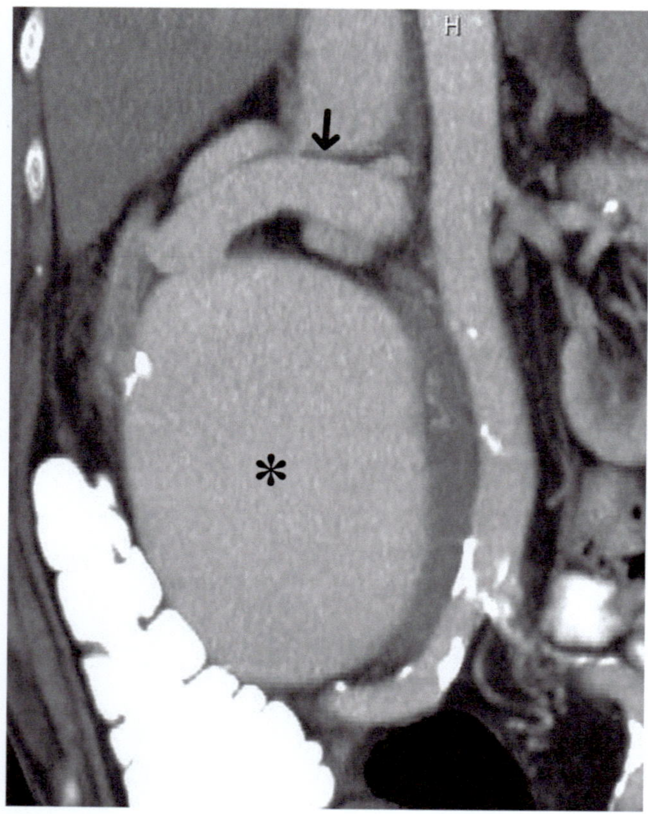

Fig. 56.1 Contrast-enhanced CT (coronal view) shows a high flow right renal AVF supplied by an enlarged inferior polar artery (arrow) draining to a giant renal vein aneurysm (asterisk). The venous aneurysm displaces and compresses the right colon and the IVC. Notice enlarged suprarenal IVC due to venous hypertension and poor flow in the compressed infrarenal segment of the IVC. *AVF* Arteriovenous fistula, *IVC* Inferior Vena Cava

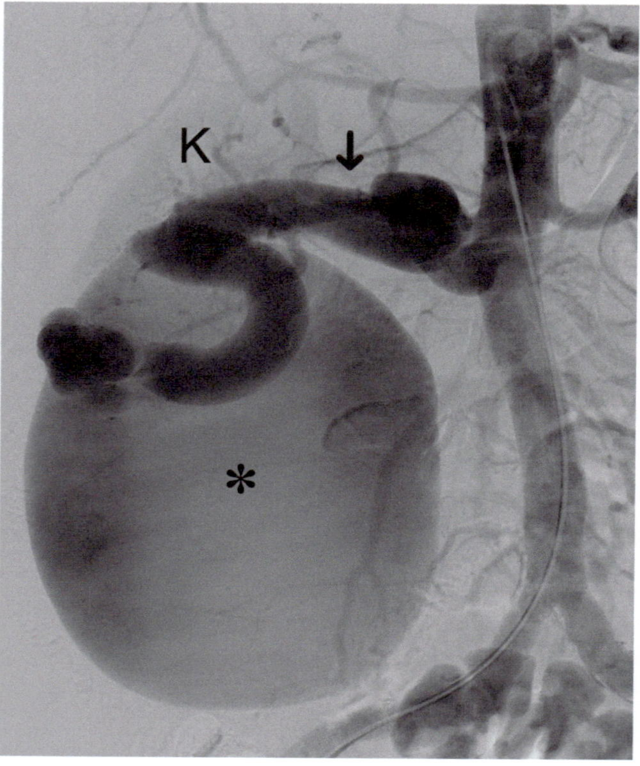

Fig. 56.2 Aortic angiography shows a high flow right renal AVF from an inferior polar artery (arrow) to a giant dilated renal vein (asterisk). Notice the enlargement and tortuosity of the inferior renal polar artery (compared to the aorta or contralateral renal artery) typical of a high flow angiopathy consistent with a chronic AVF. *AVF* Arteriovenous fistula, *K* right kidney

R. Garcia-Monaco (✉) · O. Peralta · M. Rabellino
Department of Vascular and Interventional Radiology,
Hospital Italiano de Buenos Aires,
Ciudad de Buenos Aires, Argentina
e-mail: ricardo.garciamonaco@hospitalitaliano.org.ar;
oscar.peralta@hospitalitaliano.org.ar;
martin.rabellino@hospitalitaliano.org.ar

Using a right transfemoral approach, a 20 mm Amplatzer Vascular Plug (AVP II) (AGA, USA) was placed in the polar renal artery, but proving unstable because of the high flow, was not deployed. Thus, a 5F catheter was additionally introduced and eighteen 14 mm Nester coils (Cook, USA) were placed parallel to the AVP to decrease the flow (Fig. 56.3). During coiling, the non-liberated AVP migrated forward in the renal artery because of the high flow. After coil placements, a 16 mm AVP II was placed proximal to the previous one (Fig. 56.4). Because the flow has slowed down at this point, the proximal 16 mm AVP was released and, subsequently, the formerly placed 20 mm AVP. As the AVF was still patent, embolization was continued with modified 0.35 guide wire coils, and ultimately completed with glue (Fig. 56.5). At the end of the procedure, there was still a subtle flow that was assumed that would occlude spontaneously. At 24 h follow-up, symptoms improved and CT showed 90% venous sac thrombosis, still with a subtle flow (Fig. 56.6). At 1-month follow-up, limb edema completely disappeared, and CT showed complete AVF closure (Fig. 56.7). Follow-up was uneventful at 5 years (Fig. 56.8).

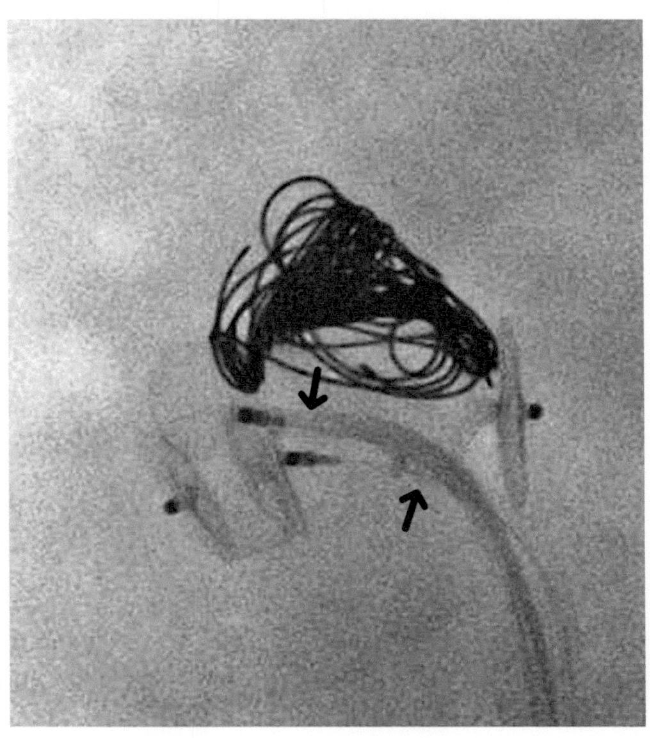

Fig. 56.4 Oblique plain film shows the 18 coils and both AVP plugs. Notice two 7F sheaths in the artery (arrows), both holding the plug system before release

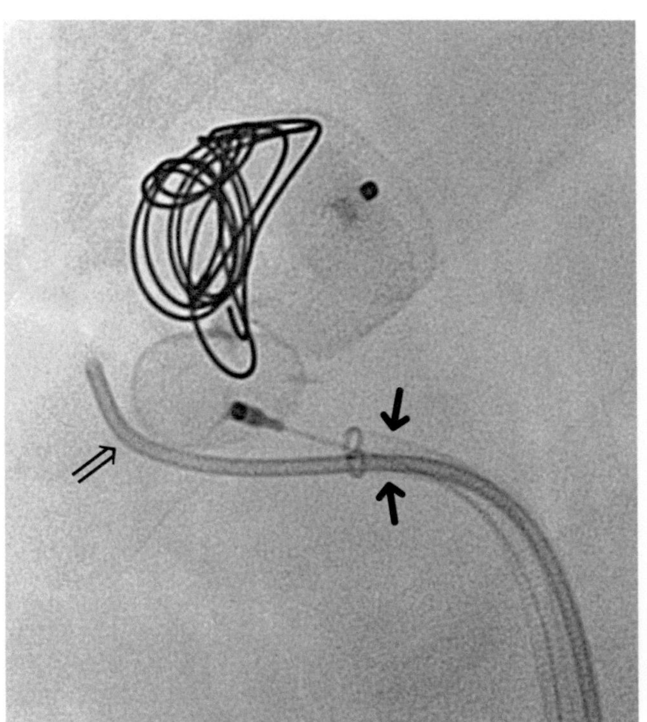

Fig. 56.3 Plain film during coiling in the inferior polar artery parallel to the non-liberated 20 mm AVP. Notice two 7 F sheaths in the polar artery (arrows), one with a coaxial 5F catheter (open arrow) to introduce the coils and the other holding the plug system

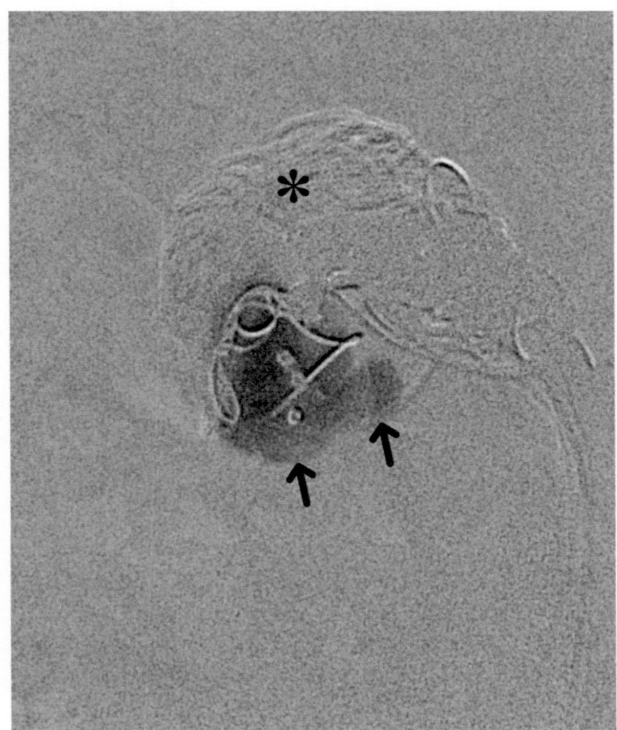

Fig. 56.5 Subtraction angiography during glue embolization (arrow) to supplement the previous placed AVP and mesh of coils (asterisks). The glue is radiopaque because of its mixture with Lipiodol, therefore shown in black in this picture

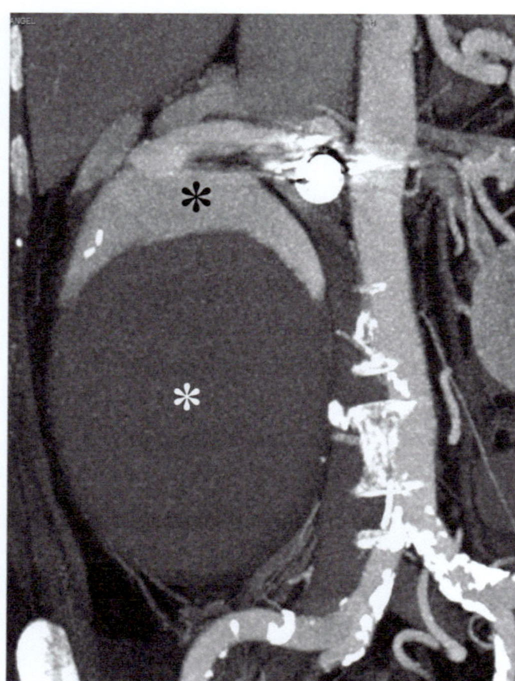

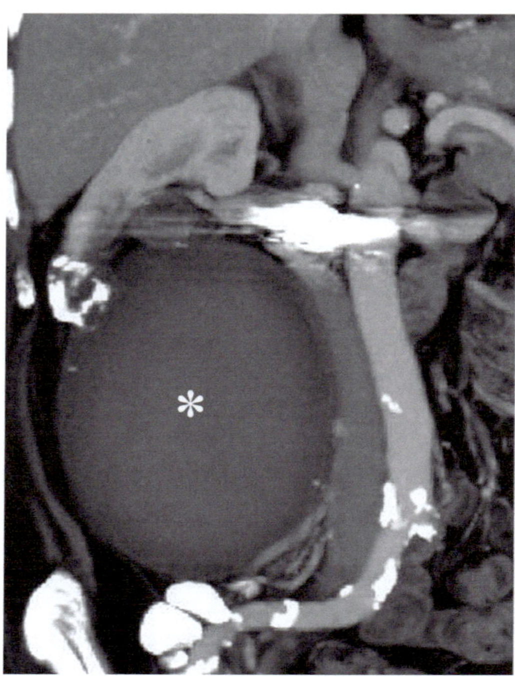

Fig. 56.6 Contrast-enhanced CT (coronal view) at 24 h follow-up shows almost complete thrombosis of giant renal vein aneurysm (white asterisk) but still subtle patent flow (black asterisk) from the polar renal artery (arrow)

Fig. 56.7 Contrast-enhanced CT (coronal view) at 1-month follow-up shows complete spontaneous thrombosis of the residual flow in the giant renal vein aneurysm (asterisk) reflecting total occlusion of the AVF. Notice certain shrinkage of the venous aneurysm with flow restoral in the IVC leading to complete disappearance of lower limb edema (not shown). Metallic artifacts by plugs and coils in the polar renal artery. Round calcification in the distal polar artery presumably due to a calcified aneurysm whose rupture may have caused the AVF. *AVF* Arteriovenous fistula, *IVC* Inferior Vena Cava

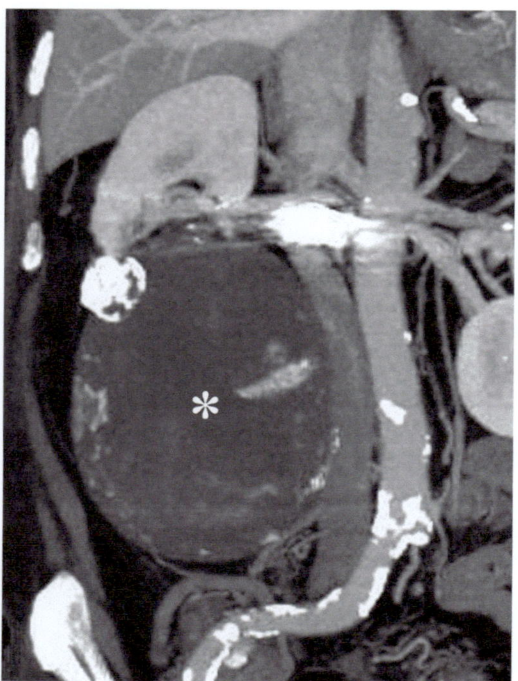

Fig. 56.8 Contrast-enhanced CT (coronal view) at 5 years follow-up confirms persistent thrombosis with certain shrink of the thrombosed venous aneurysm in an otherwise asymptomatic patient. (Compare with figs. 56.1 and 56.6) Metallic artifacts by plugs and coils in the polar renal artery. Round calcification in the distal polar artery presumably due to a calcified aneurysm whose rupture may have caused the AVF. *AVF* Arteriovenous fistula

Renal Artery Graft Anastomosis Gone Wrong: Bowel Ischemia

57

John Matson, Tyler Lee Smith, and Auh Whan Park

A 79-year-old woman underwent open thoracoabdominal aortic aneurysm repair of a ruptured aortic aneurysm with branch grafts to the superior mesenteric artery (SMA), celiac artery, and both renal arteries. Three months later, she presented with abdominal pain, hypotension, hemoglobin of 5.6 g/dL, worsening kidney function (creatinine 3.5 mg/dL), and elevated lactic acid (3.5 mmol/L). CTA (Figs. 57.1 and 57.2) showed an 8 cm pseudoaneurysm arising from the right renal graft caused by anastomotic breakdown. It compressed the mesenteric vessels, causing visceral malperfusion and acidosis. These findings were confirmed with emergent (Figs. 57.3 and 57.4): the pseudoaneurysm severely narrowed the celiac artery, SMA, and grafts (Fig. 57.5). An 8 mm diameter 40 cm long self-expanding bare stent (Protege, Medtronic USA) was used to restore the SMA lumen and normal bowel perfusion (Fig. 57.6).

To prevent catastrophic rupture, we chose to sacrifice the right kidney and embolize its branch graft in entirety. The right renal artery graft was first propped open with a 10 mm diameter Protege stent to provide scaffolding for embolization. The vessel was then occluded with a 12 mm Amplatzer II plug and detachable microcoils (Penumbra, CA) (Fig. 57.7).

The patient's elevated lactate rapidly normalized to 2.0 mmol/L after procedure conclusion. Her oliguric acute kidney injury required transient hemodialysis; her dialysis catheter was removed by day 4. She was treated with an indefinite course of antibiotics for presumed mycotic breakdown of the right renal artery graft anastomosis.

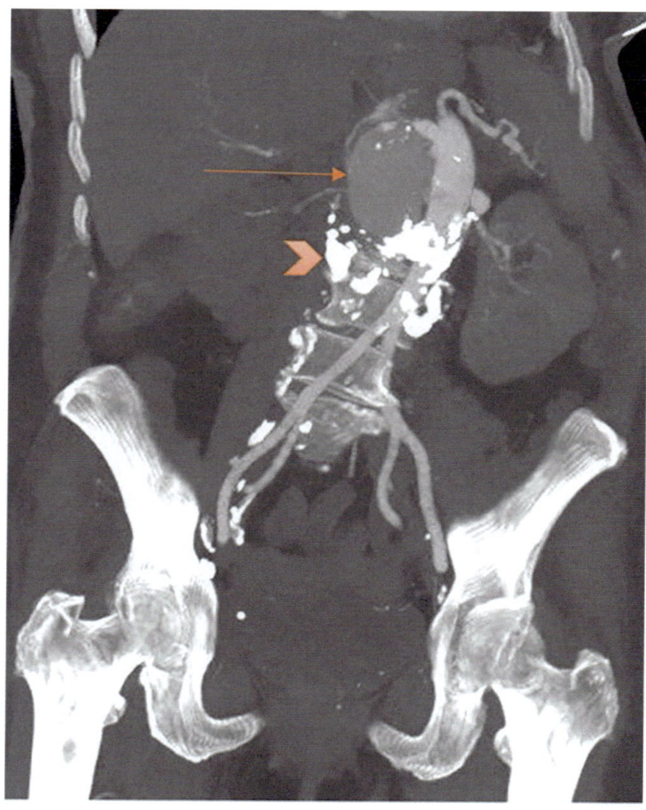

Fig. 57.1 Thick slice maximum intensity projection reconstruction of the pre-procedure CTA centered on the branched aortic graft. Hyperdense material within the retroperitoneum (chevron arrow) represents Lipiodol and glue from a prior lymphangiogram and lymphatic leak embolization. The large pseudoaneurysm (thin arrow) is seen along the right side of the aortic graft

J. Matson (✉) · T. L. Smith
Department of Radiology and Medical Imaging, University of Virginia Health System, Charlottesville, VA, USA
e-mail: jtm9sk@hscmail.mcc.virginia.edu

A. W. Park
Department of Radiology, University of Texas Southwestern, Dallas, TX, USA
e-mail: AP7WV@hscmail.mcc.virginia.edu

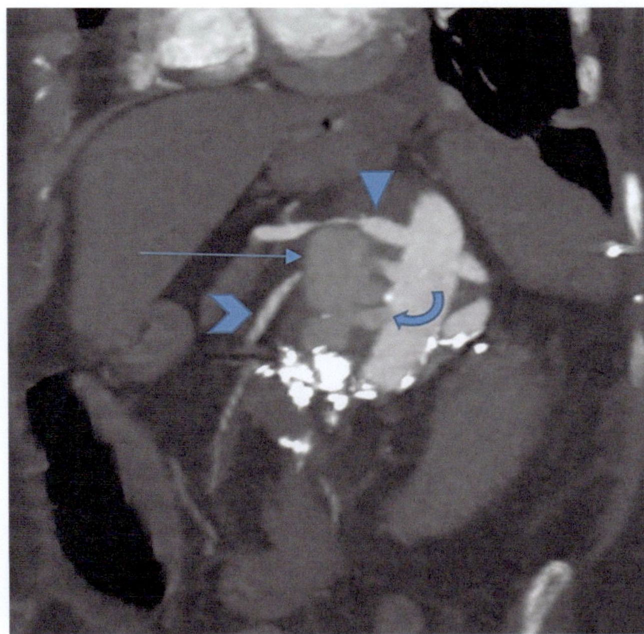

Fig. 57.2 Single image from a 3D reconstruction of the pre-procedure CTA demonstrating the large pseudoaneurysm (thin arrow) measuring 8 cm arising from the right renal artery branch graft (curved arrow). Additionally, mass effect from the pseudoaneurysm results in external compression of the celiac artery (arrow head) and superior mesenteric artery (chevron arrow), raising concern for visceral malperfusion given the abdominal pain and elevated lactic acid

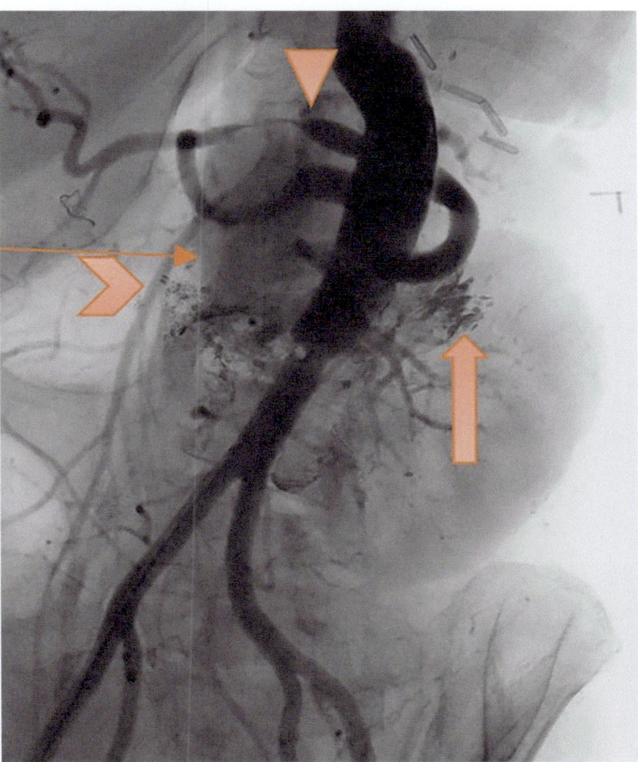

Fig. 57.4 Maximum intensity projection of the initial aortogram with anatomic reference shows severe narrowing of the celiac artery graft (arrow head) and complete effacement of the proximal superior mesenteric artery graft (chevron arrow) caused by the large pseudoaneurysm arising from the distal right renal graft (thin arrow). Note that the right kidney does not enhance with contrast. Also seen is the high density material in the retroperitoneum (thick arrow) from prior lymphangiogram and lymphatic leak embolization

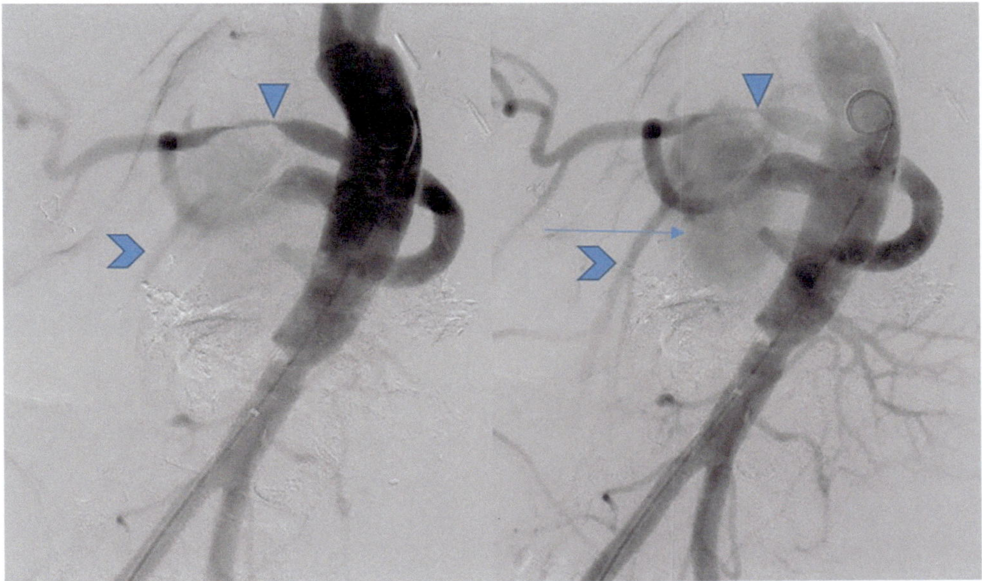

Fig. 57.3 Two sequential frames from the initial digital subtraction aortogram show severe narrowing of the celiac artery graft (arrow head) as well as delayed filling and complete effacement of the proximal superior mesenteric artery graft (chevron arrow). Visceral vessel narrowing is caused by mass effect from the late filling, large pseudoaneurysm (thin arrow) arising from the distal right renal artery branch graft

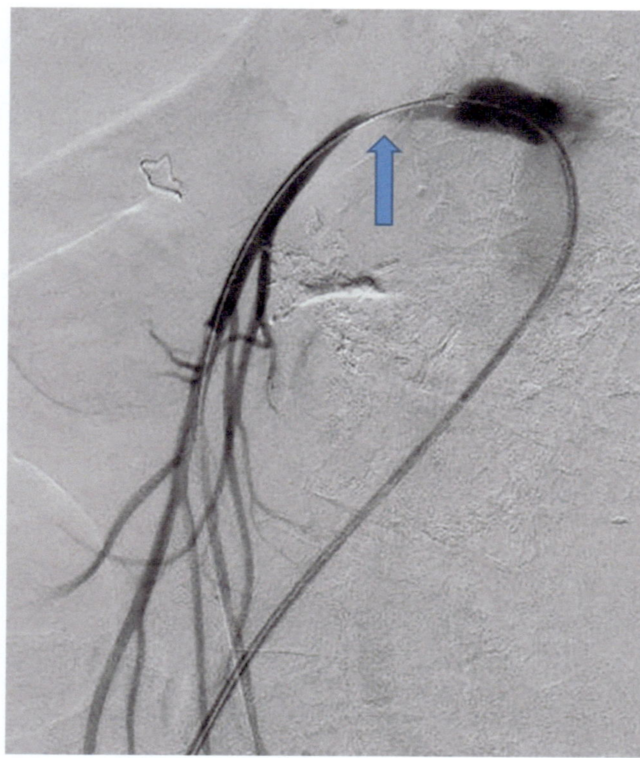

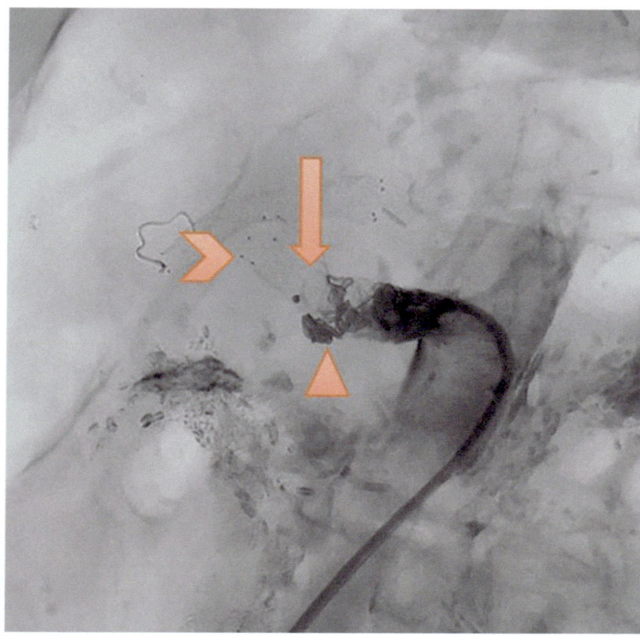

Fig. 57.7 The right renal artery branch graft was stented using a non-covered self-expanding stent (chevron arrow) to provide scaffolding within the graft and then embolized using an Amplatzer plug (arrow) and microcoils (arrowhead) until no residual filling of the pseudoaneurysm was seen

Fig. 57.5 Selective SMA angiogram demonstrating severe compression of the proximal SMA (arrow) secondary to mass effect from the pseudoaneurysm

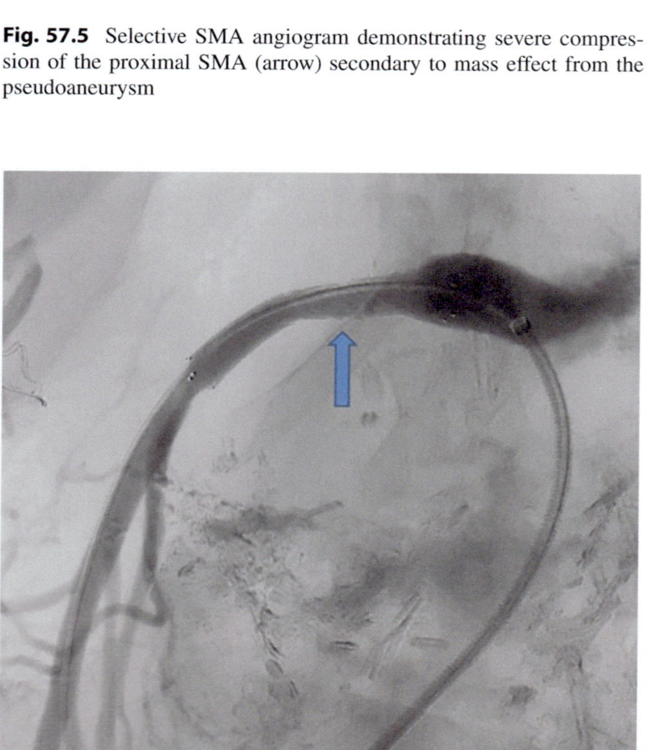

Fig. 57.6 A non-covered, self-expanding stent (Protege, Medtronic USA) (arrow) was placed within the proximal SMA to facilitate bowel perfusion

Complex Right Renal Artery Aneurysm Treatment with a Stent-Graft After Migration of an Intra-Aneurysmal Bare Stent

58

Hideyuki Torikai, Masanori Inoue, Seishi Nakatsuka, and Masahiro Jinzaki

A 30-year-old man with a wide-necked 2 cm main right renal artery aneurysm presented for endovascular repair (Fig. 58.1). Coil embolization with a stent-assisted technique had failed at an outside hospital. The proximal edge of the bare stent had migrated into the aneurysmal sac and was abutting its wall, raising a risk of aneurysm rupture (Figs. 58.2 and 58.3). Therefore, exclusion of the aneurysm using a stent-graft through the cells of the migrated stent was planned. A guiding sheath was placed in the proximal aneurysm. A stiff guidewire was advanced distally through the stent cells, followed by a balloon-expandable stent-graft; unfortunately, the tip of its delivery system caught on the edge of the stent strut and could not be passed through the stent mesh, even after balloon dilation of the stent cells. After exchanging the stiff guidewire for a thinner flexible one, it was advanced through the wall cell because of a change in the angle between the stent and guidewire (Fig. 58.4). The stent-graft was successfully deployed. Although aneurysm exclusion was achieved, flow stagnation due to an ostial renal artery stenosis was seen, and hence, an additional stent-graft was placed. Final angiography confirmed patency of the vascular reconstruction and exclusion of the aneurysm (Figs. 58.5 and 58.6). At 8-month follow-up, computed tomography angiography confirmed patency of the renal stents and continued thrombosis of the aneurysm.

Fig. 58.1 A volume rendering computed tomography angiography image demonstrating a saccular aneurysm at the right main renal artery, along with ostial stenosis

H. Torikai
Department of Radiology and Medical Imaging, University of Virginia Health System, Charlottesville, VA, USA
e-mail: HT4AZ@hscmail.mcc.virginia.edu

M. Inoue (✉) · S. Nakatsuka · M. Jinzaki
Department of Radiology, Keio University School of Medicine, Tokyo, Japan
e-mail: inomasa@rad.med.keio.ac.jp;
nakatsuka@rad.med.keio.ac.jp; jinzaki@rad.med.keio.ac.jp

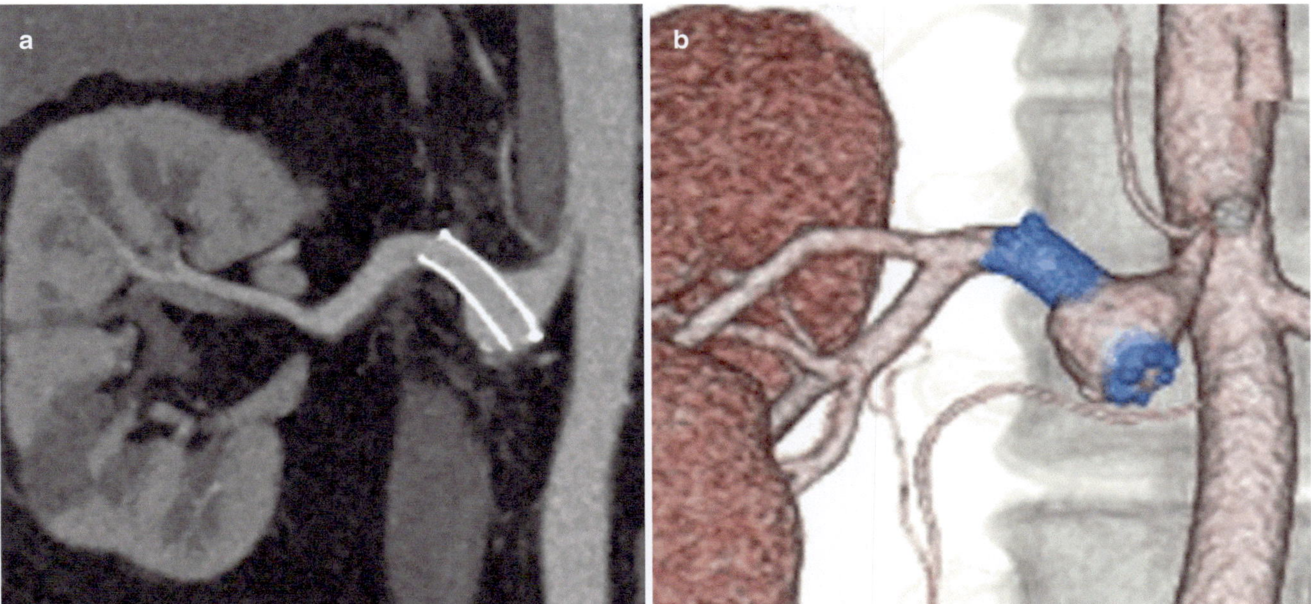

Fig. 58.2 (**a, b**) An oblique coronal image (**a**) and volume rendering computed tomography angiography image (**b**) showing migration of the stent into the aneurysm

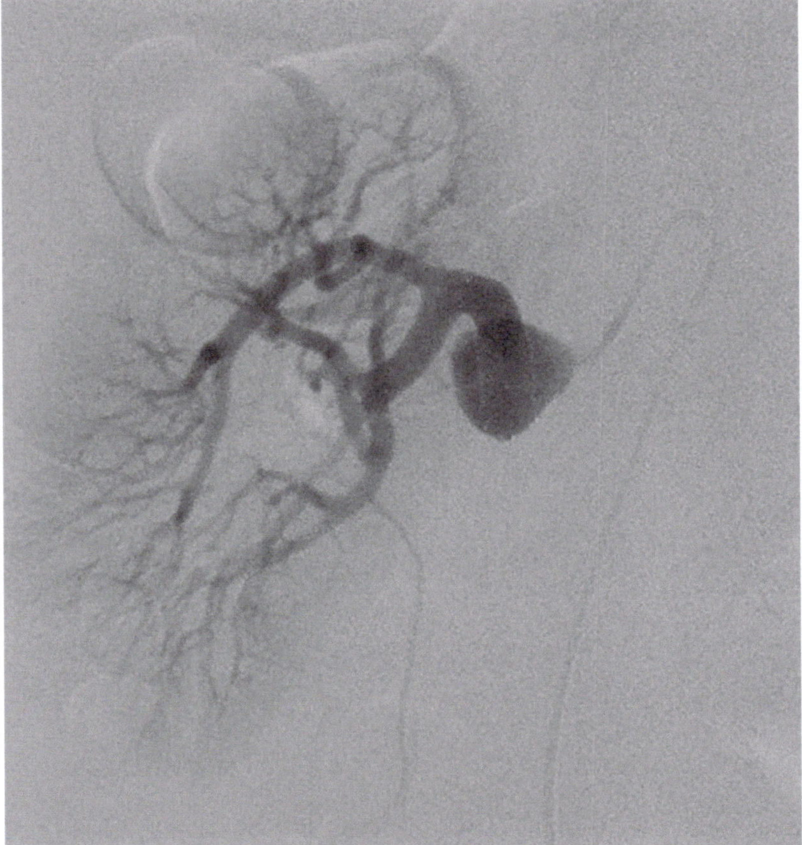

Fig. 58.3 Digital subtraction angiography from the right renal artery demonstrating the renal artery aneurysm and the migrated stent in the dome of the aneurysm

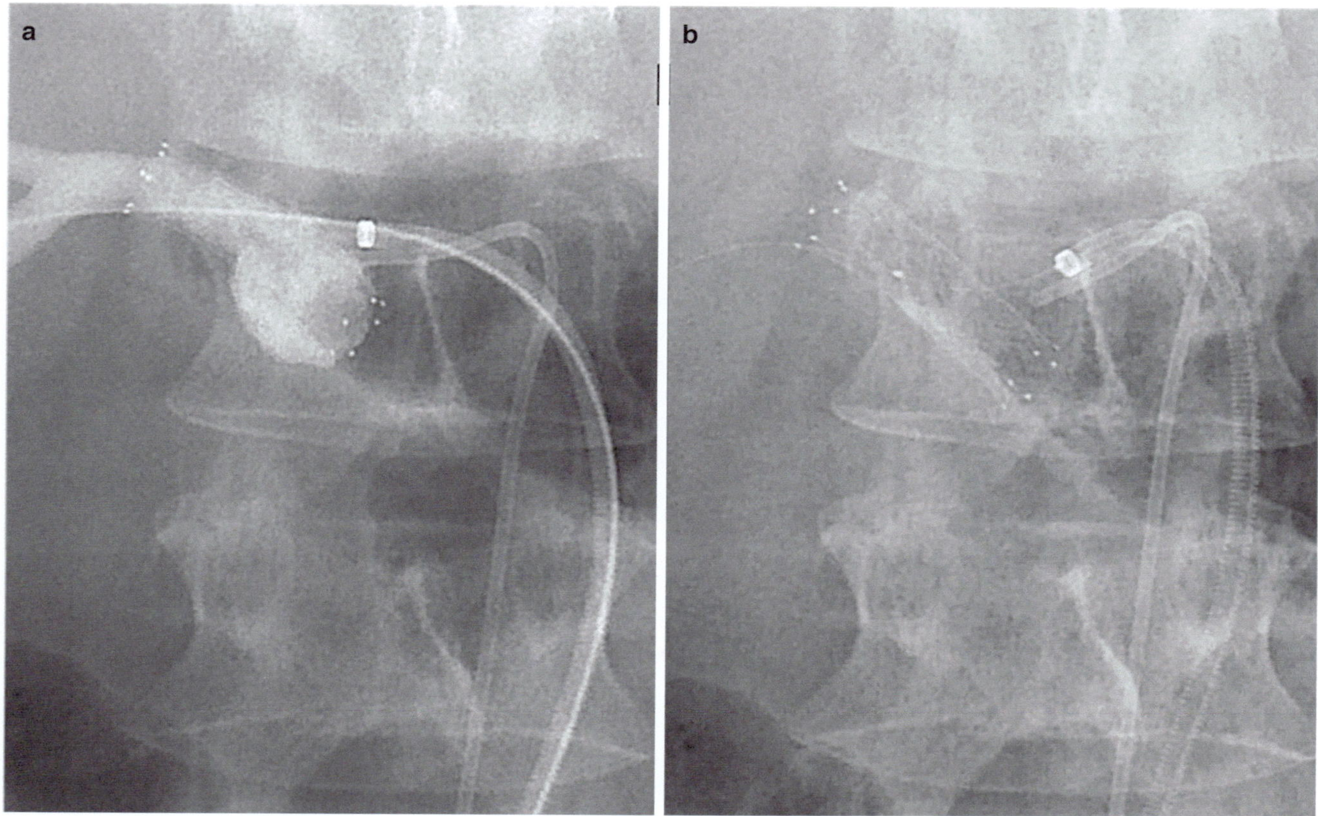

Fig. 58.4 (**a, b**) A 0.035-inch stiff guidewire passed the stent cell (**a**), and a 0.014-inch guidewire passed the same stent cell (**b**). The 0.014-inch guidewire passed the stent cell vertically compared to the 0.035-inch guidewire

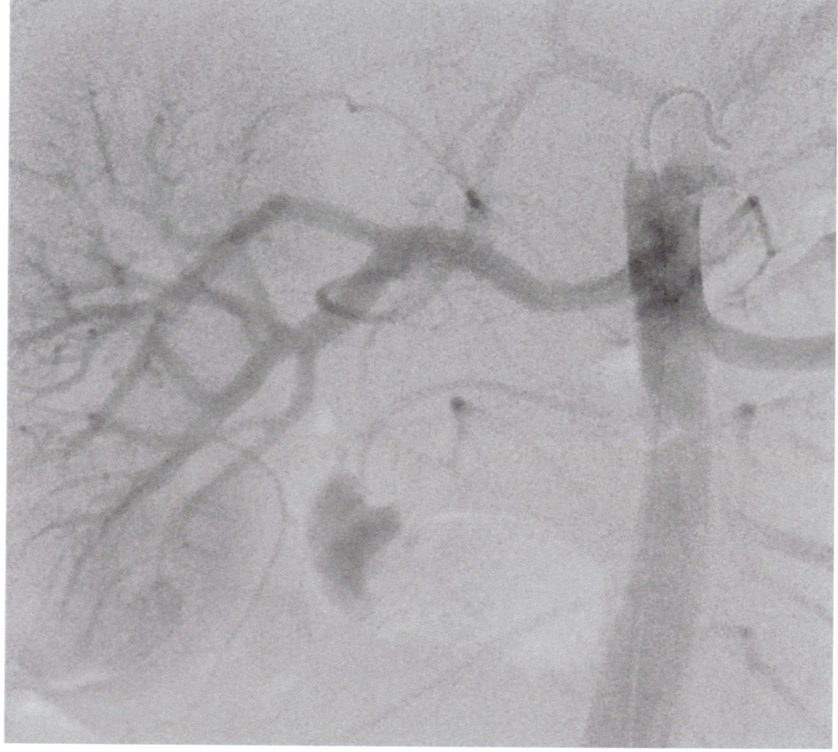

Fig. 58.5 Post-procedure aortography demonstrating exclusion of the aneurysm and patency of the right main renal artery

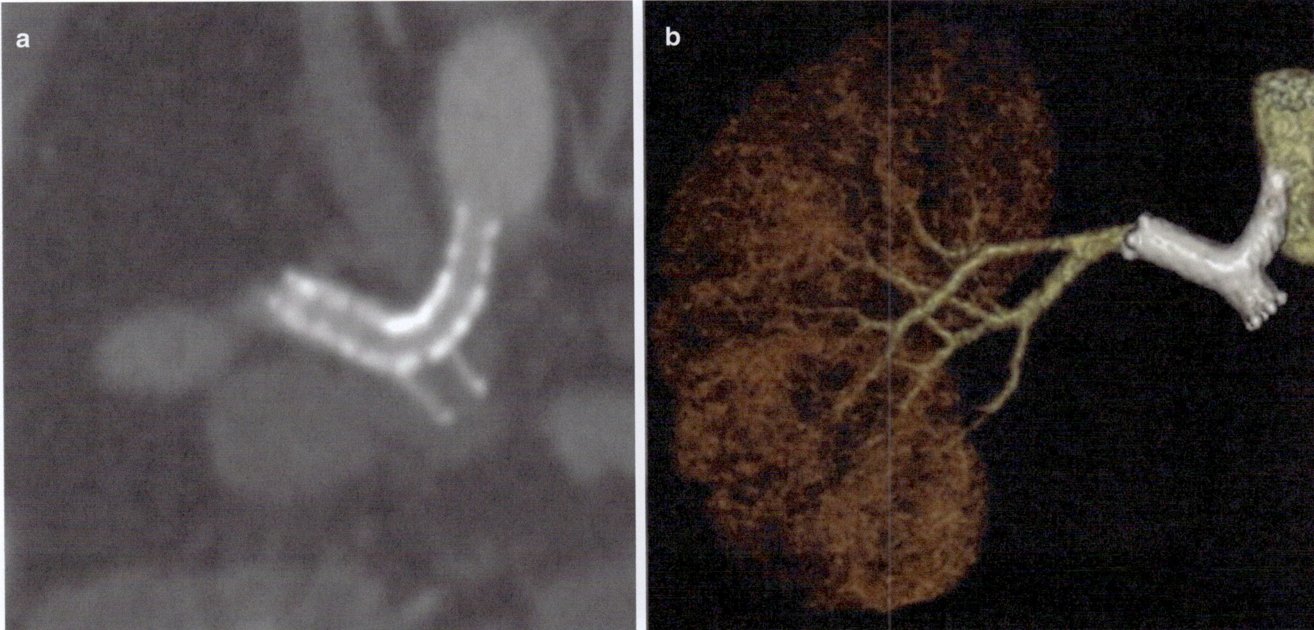

Fig. 58.6 (**a, b**) Visualization of the patent stent grafts and the thrombosed aneurysm without renal infarction on an oblique coronal image (**a**) and volume rendering image (**b**) of computed tomography angiography

Endovascular Treatment of a Wide-Necked Proximal Celiac Artery Aneurysm

John Matson, Marc C. Kryger, Margaret C. Tracci, and Luke Wilkins

A 74-year-old woman with remote superior mesenteric artery (SMA) stent placement for chronic mesenteric ischemia presented with an incidental 2.6 cm diameter broad-based celiac aneurysm (Figs. 59.1 and 59.2).

To exclude the wide-necked aneurysm, the distal celiac artery was occluded with a 10 mm diameter Amplatzer II Vascular Plug (Abbott Vascular, Chicago IL), after which a 25 mm diameter Endurant aortic endograft (Medtronic, Dublin, Ireland) was deployed across the celiac origin (Fig. 59.3). A concomitant 6 French 55 cm long sheath was kept within the SMA to prevent inadvertent encroachment of the endograft upon its origin, and a 5Fr catheter and Progreat (Terumo, Tokyo, Japan) microcatheter within the celiac for additional embolization (temporarily jailed by the endograft).

Angiography showed persistent antegrade flow into the left gastric artery, distal to the celiac aneurysm (Fig. 59.4). To prevent retrograde perfusion of the aneurysm, an additional 10 mm Amplatzer II Vascular Plug and a 10 mm diameter 19 cm long Azur detachable coil (Terumo, Tokyo, Japan) were deployed within the celiac. Thereafter, angiography showed successful isolation of the aneurysm, (Fig. 59.5). Finally, the aneurysm sac was filled with 6 cc of ethylene–vinyl alcohol copolymer (Onyx, Medtronic, Dublin, Ireland) (Fig. 59.6) injected through the microcatheter. Final angiography showed exclusion of the celiac aneurysm and embolization of the proximal celiac artery (Fig. 59.7). The downstream hepatic continued filling via the pancreaticoduodenal arcade. She was discharged on post-operative day 2. At 1-month follow-up, she was doing well, denying postprandial pain or changes in bowel movements. While increasing reports describe endovascular approaches to celiac artery aneurysms, broad based ones can present unique challenges.

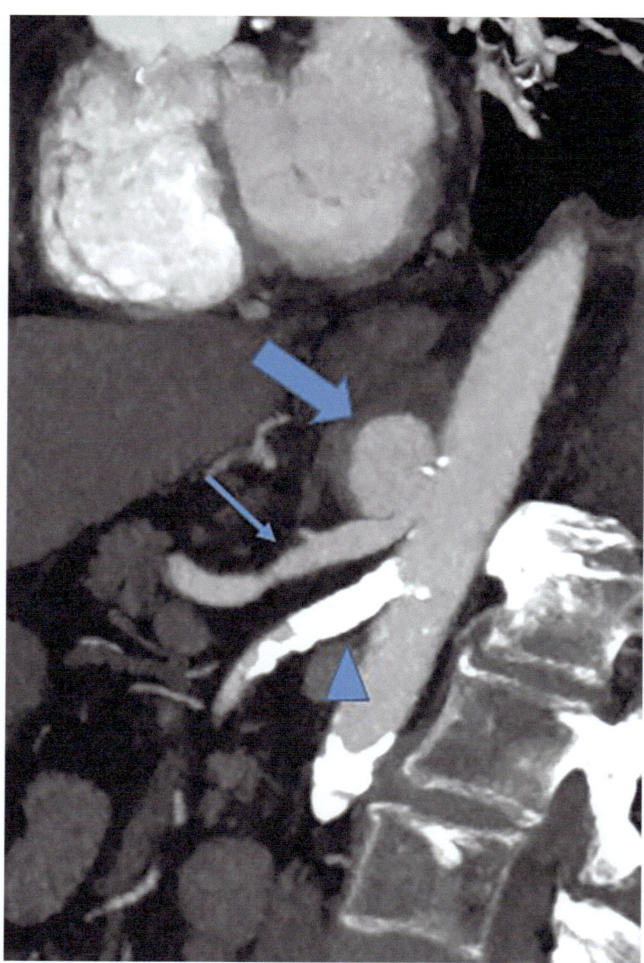

Fig. 59.1 Maximum intensity projection CT image of the aorta centered on the origin of the celiac artery highlighting the wide neck of the celiac artery aneurysm, thick arrow, arising from the celiac artery origin. The proximity to the celiac origin limits the ability to exclude the aneurysm and preserve flow to the celiac artery. Note the existing stent in the proximal superior mesenteric artery, arrowhead

J. Matson (✉) · M. C. Tracci · L. Wilkins
University of Virginia Health System, Charlottesville, VA, USA
e-mail: JTM9SK@hscmail.mcc.virginia.edu

M. C. Kryger
Department of Radiology and Medical Imaging, University of Virginia Health System, Charlottesville, VA, USA

Z. J. Haskal (ed.), *Extreme IR*, https://doi.org/10.1007/978-3-031-24251-9_59

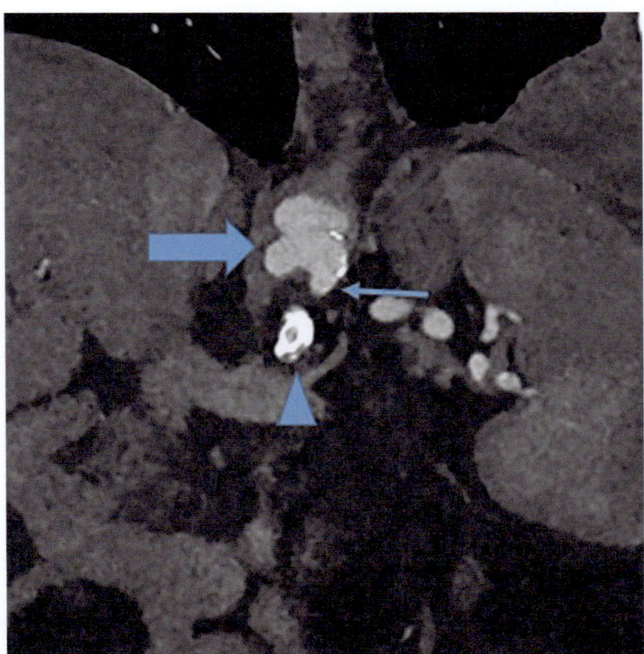

Fig. 59.2 Multiplanar CT reconstruction centered on the proximal celiac artery, thin arrow, highlighting the wide neck of the lobulated and irregular celiac artery aneurysm, thick arrow. Again note the existing stent in the proximal superior mesenteric artery, arrowhead

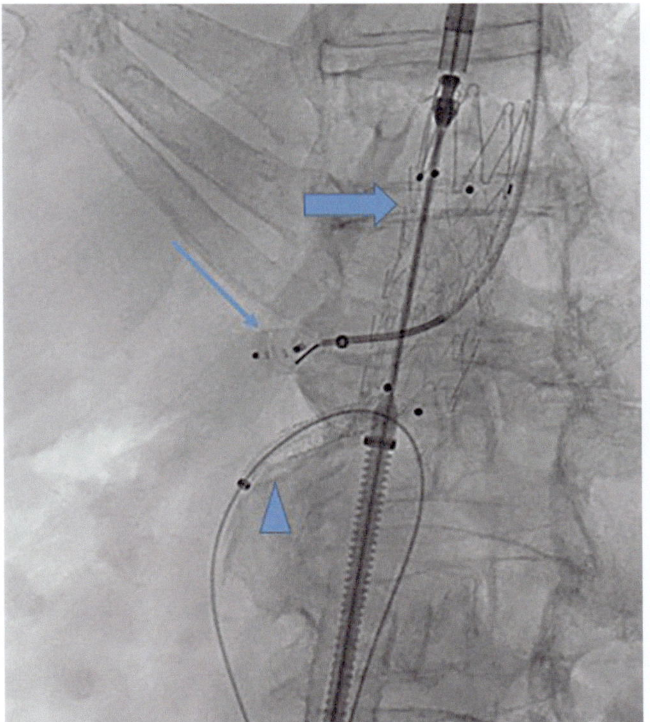

Fig. 59.3 Fluoroscopic spot film during stent exclusion of the celiac artery using an Endurant aortic endograft (Medtronic, Dublin, Ireland), thick arrow. A sheath and catheter, excluded by the stent graft, remain selective within the celiac artery which has been embolized by an Amplatzer II Vascular Plug (Abbott Vascular, Chicago IL), thin arrow. A sheath, arrowhead, has also been placed within the SMA to protect the SMA from coverage during stent exclusion of the celiac artery

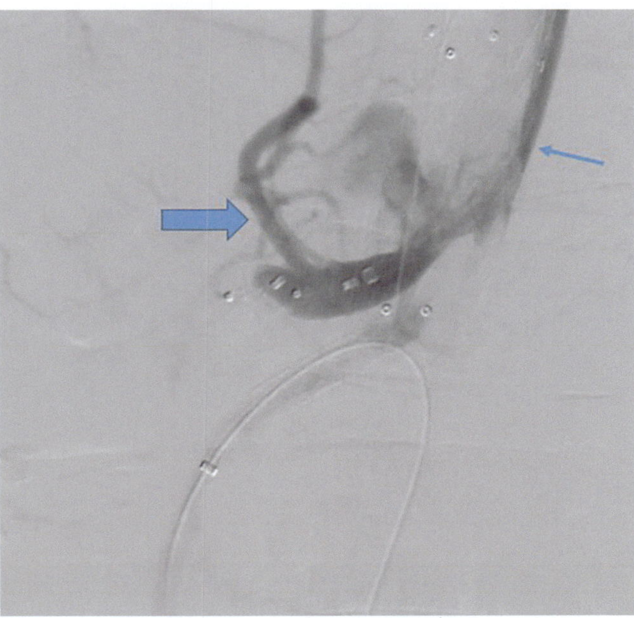

Fig. 59.4 Celiac artery digital subtraction angiogram following stent exclusion of the celiac artery origin demonstrates successful plug embolization of the distal celiac artery and successful coverage of the celiac artery origin. There remains flow within a prominent left gastric artery, thick arrow. There is also a gutter leak alongside the celiac artery sheath, thin arrow

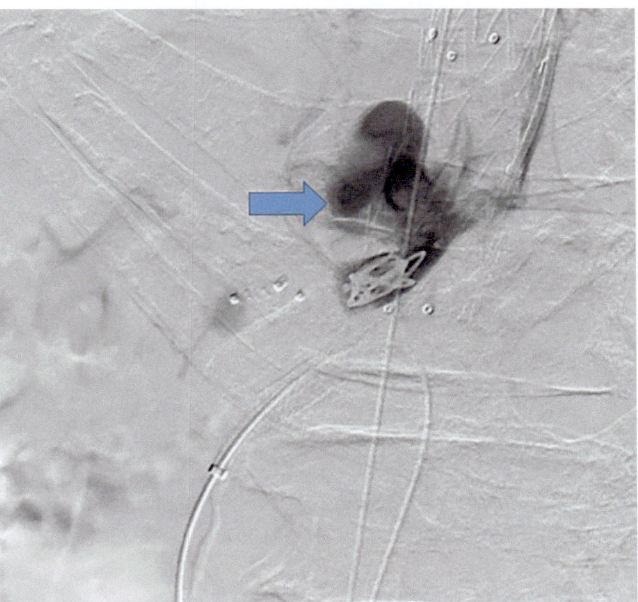

Fig. 59.5 Digital subtraction angiography of the celiac artery following successful coil embolization of the proximal celiac artery Azur detachable coil (Terumo, Tokyo, Japan). There is filling of the celiac artery aneurysm, thick arrow. There is no residual filling of the celiac artery peripheral to the aneurysm origin following plug and coil embolization

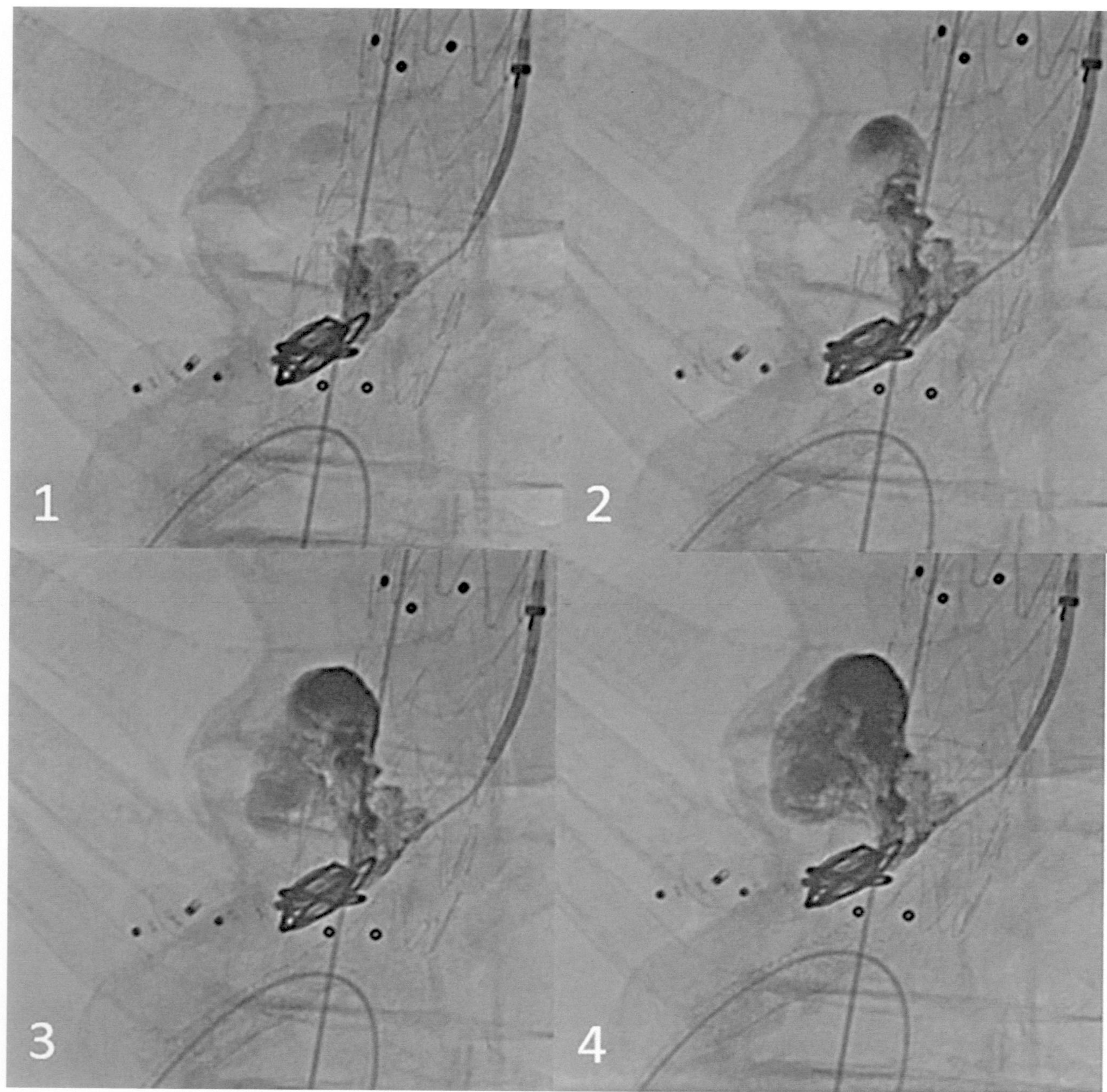

Fig. 59.6 Multiple fluoroscopic spot film taken during progressive filling of the excluded celiac artery aneurysm with Onyx (Medtronic, Medtronic, Dublin, Ireland)

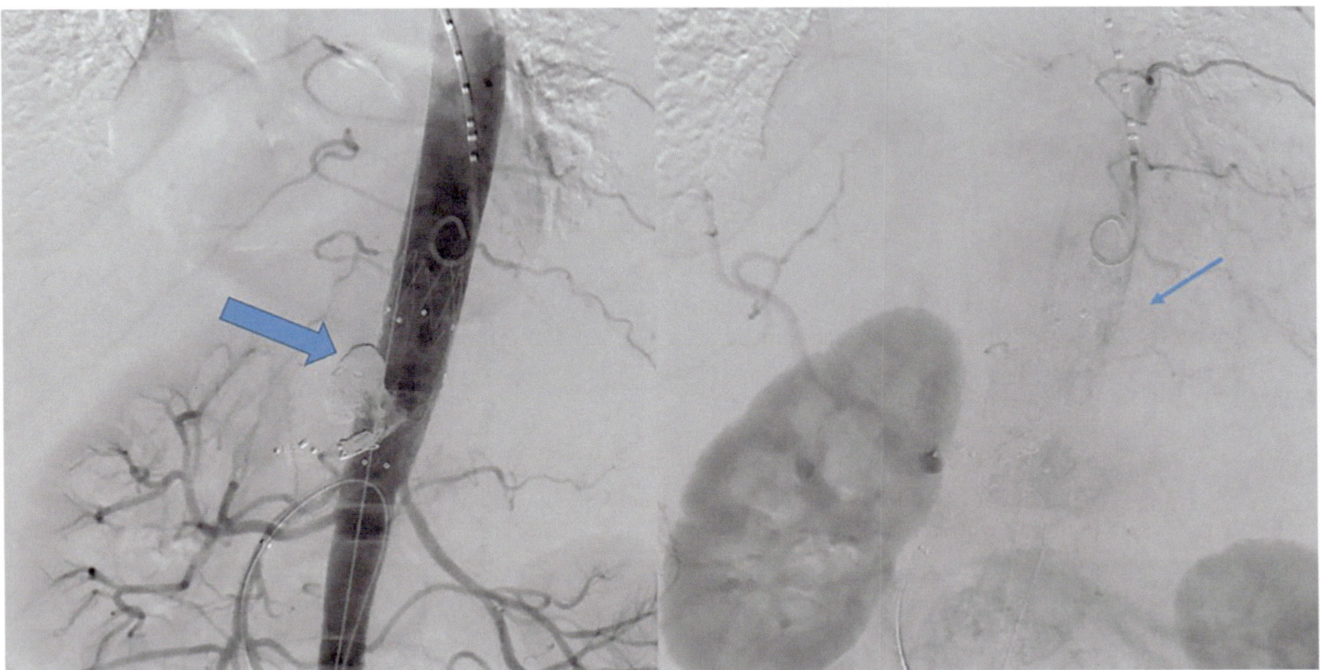

Fig. 59.7 Completion aortography demonstrating the successful excluded and embolized celiac artery aneurysm with no residual flow, thick arrow. There is no residual flow through the celiac artery. On delayed images, filling of the hepatic vasculature, thin arrow, can be seen filling via collateral blood flow through the pancreaticoduodenal arcade

Bibliography

1. Zhang W, Fu YF, Wei PL, Bei E, Li DC, Xu J. Endovascular repair of celiac artery aneurysm with the use of stent grafts. J Vasc Interv Radiol. 2016;27(4):514–8. PMID: 26922007

2. Nzekwu E, Wang AY, Mirakhur A, Halliwell O, Bakshi D. Technical considerations and clinical outcomes in the endovascular management of celiac arterial aneurysms. J Vasc Interv Radiol. 2019;30(11):1743–9. PMID: 31521454

Ziv J Haskal and Allen R. Goode

A 31-year-old G2P1 healthy pregnant woman was diagnosed with adjacent left 3.8 × 3 × 3 cm and 2 × 2.8 × 1.8 cm uterine artery aneurysms posterior to the lower uterine segment, during asymptomatic prenatal sonography at 12 weeks (Fig. 60.1). At the outside hospital, a thin section contrast CT was performed, approximately 26 mGy (Fig. 60.2); they appeared connected by a 2 mm vessel. At her request, we provided outside consultation regarding definitive therapy and potential fetal radiation dose in addition to the dose already delivered by CT.

At 27 weeks, left uterine artery angiography confirmed the findings and suggested that the smaller aneurysm might be venous (Fig. 60.3). The procedure was performed using 2.5fps pulsed fluoroscopy in a Siemens Pheno room at least magnification, highly coned, keeping conceptus out of the field, and two DSA runs, at start and finish at 0.5fps. The venous aneurysm was catheterized, packed densely with detachable 45–60 cm long Ruby coils (Penumbra Inc) (Fig. 60.4). A coil was extended across the bridging vessel and the arterial aneurysm densely packed with similar 45–60 cm coils. Finally, 2 5-cm coils were placed in the normal distal uterine artery at the entry to the aneurysm (Figs. 60.5 and 60.6). The estimated fetal dose was less

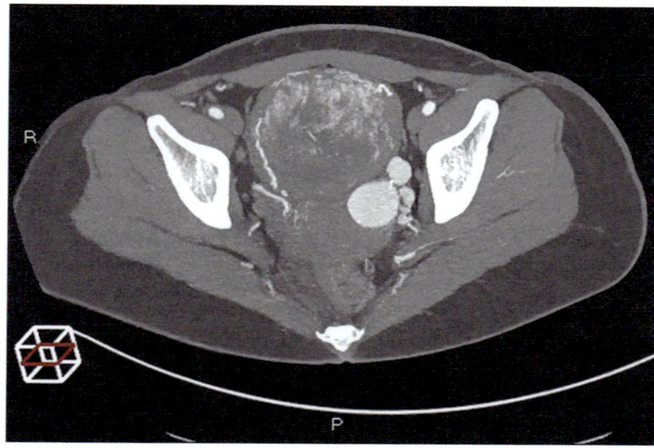

Fig. 60.2 Axial maximum intensity projection image from contrast-enhanced CT obtained at outside hospital at 14 weeks pregnancy demonstrates the larger 3.8 × 3 × 3 cm aneurysm

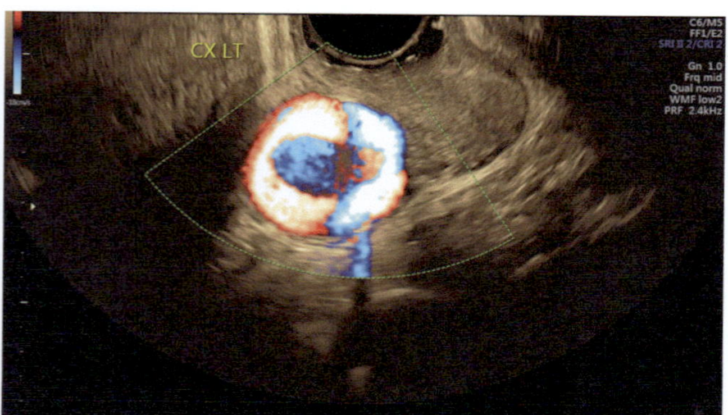

Fig. 60.1 Twelve-week prenatal sonography demonstrates the larger aneurysm

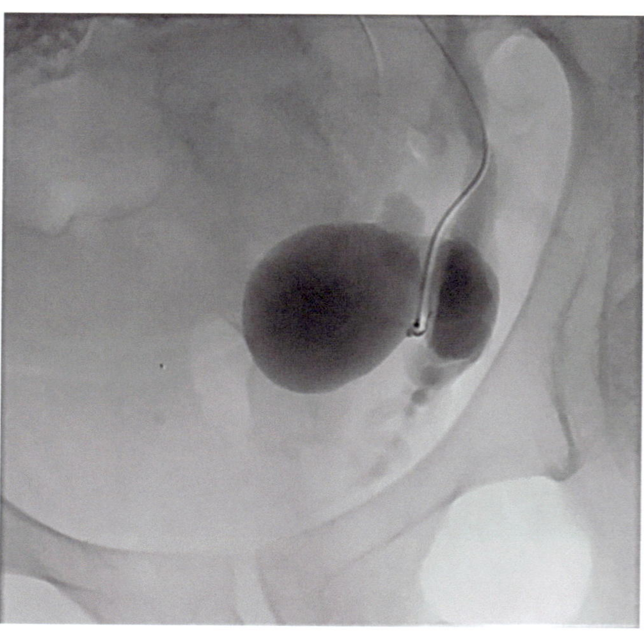

Fig. 60.3 Angiogram demonstrates the larger medial uterine artery aneurysm and adjacent venous aneurysm. Outflow from second aneurysm is through the left gonadal vein

Z. J Haskal (✉)
Department of Radiology and Medical Imaging, Interventional Division, University of Virginia, Charlottesville, VA, USA

A. R. Goode
Department of Radiology and Medical Imaging, University of Virginia Health System, Charlottesville, VA, USA
e-mail: agoode@virginia.edu

© The Author(s), under exclusive license to Springer Nature Switzerland AG 2023
Z. J. Haskal (ed.), *Extreme IR*, https://doi.org/10.1007/978-3-031-24251-9_60

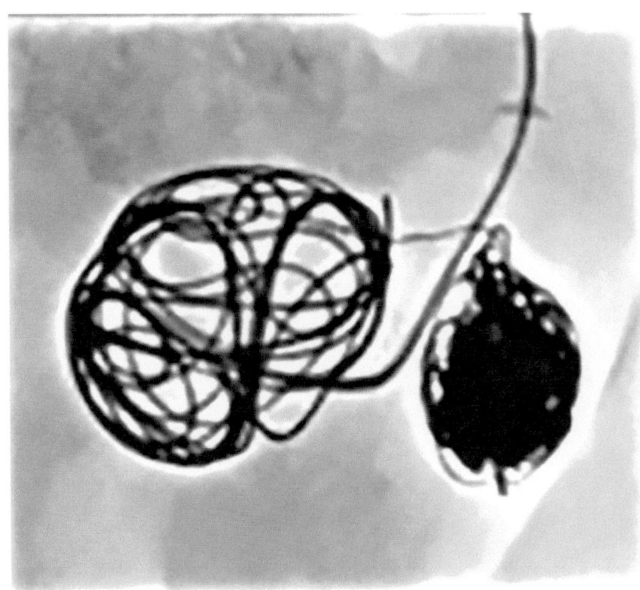

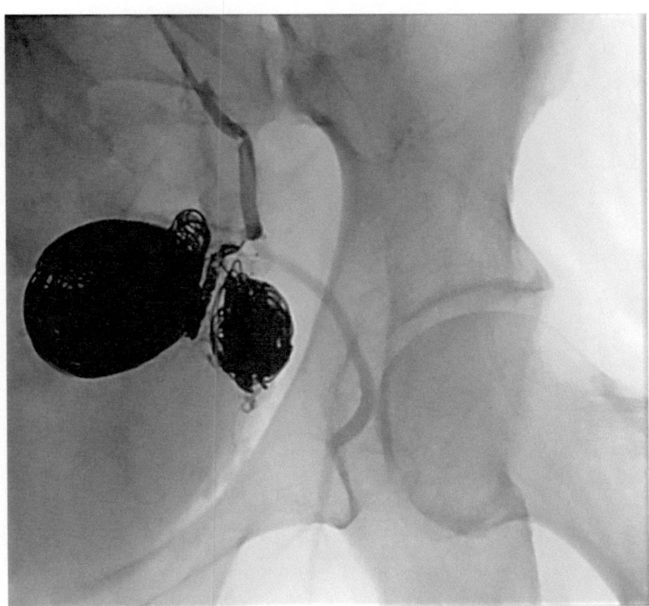

Fig. 60.4 Fluoro screen saver image after coil packing of the smaller distal aneurysm and start of packing of the arterial aneurysm. A horizontal coil limb intentionally bridges the two aneurysms to fill the ~2 mm bridging vessel

Fig. 60.6 Final angiogram shows the normal left uterine artery is seen, absent perfusion of the aneurysms

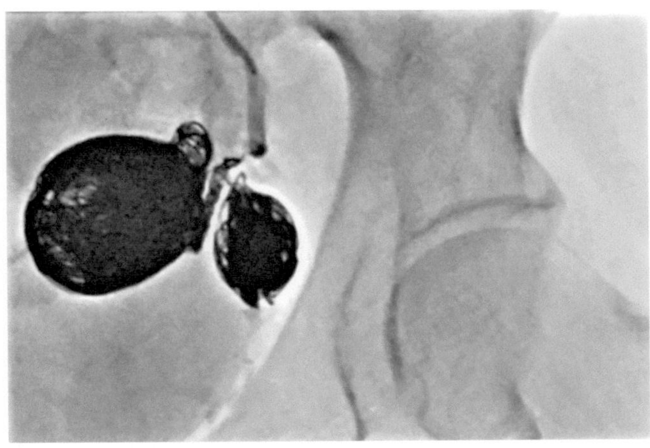

Fig. 60.5 Radiograph demonstrates final dense packing of both aneurysms and the distal normal uterine artery in between them

than 10.5 mGy, associated with low or negligible risk. 13.15 m (1315 cm) of coils were used to assure permanent occlusion, high packing density, and lowest possible lifelong likelihood of recanalization as sonography (or MRI) would be otherwise unable to detect reperfusion amidst the coils. Next day, sonography suggested normal uterine perfusion with no detectable aneurysms, excepting echos from the coils.

Uterine artery aneurysms are extremely rare and mostly likely caused by vessel trauma during caesarean section. They primarily present with massive life-threatening during pregnancy, delivery or post-partum hemorrhage. Elective embolotherapy during pregnancy, absent hemorrhage is extremely rare. Dose reduction strategies and timing, for example, beyond first trimester, can allow definitive therapy, avoiding subsequent hemorrhage.

Part VI

Biliary

Reconnecting the Bile Duct: Percutaneous Hepatico-Cholecysto-Enterostomy

Sundeep Punamiya

A 60-year-old woman with an invasive colonic tumor underwent en bloc tumoral resection, right hemicolectomy and pancreatico-duodenectomy, Roux-en-Y gastro-jejunostomy, cholecysto-jejunostomy, and pancreatico-gastrostomy. Postoperatively, the patient developed sepsis and jaundice, with CT scan showing common bile duct (CBD) obstruction and abdominal fluid collections.

Due to a suspected bile leak, a percutaneous transhepatic biliary drainage was placed, confirming common bile duct (CBD) stump blowout leaking into a pancreatic bed collection (Fig. 61.1). The intended biliary outflow through the cholecysto-jejunostomy was interrupted, likely from inadvertent CBD ligation cephalad to an unrecognized low cystic duct insertion (Fig. 61.2). A revision hepatico-jejunostomy was not feasible. Since the gallbladder was adjacent to the pancreatic bed collection, and there was an existing cholecysto-jejunostomy, bridging the CBD to the gallbladder was considered.

The collapsed gallbladder was accessed percutaneously with a micropuncture set and distended with iodinated contrast (Fig. 61.3). Using the existing percutaneous biliary access, a 5F Berenstein catheter containing an Amplatz gooseneck snare was advanced through the CBD stump blowout and positioned within the pancreatic bed collection. A transhepatic 21G needle was advanced under fluoroscopic guidance through the gallbladder and directed toward the snare loop in the collection (Fig. 61.4). A guidewire was inserted through this needle, captured by the snare, and exteriorized through the biliary access (Fig. 61.5). The wire was reversed into the gallbladder lumen through a support microcatheter (Fig. 61.6). Finally, the tract was balloon-dilated and lined with Niti-S fully covered stents (Taewoong Medical, Gimpo-Si, South Korea), restoring biliary continuity through the hepatico-cholecysto-enterostomy neo-anastomosis (Fig. 61.7).

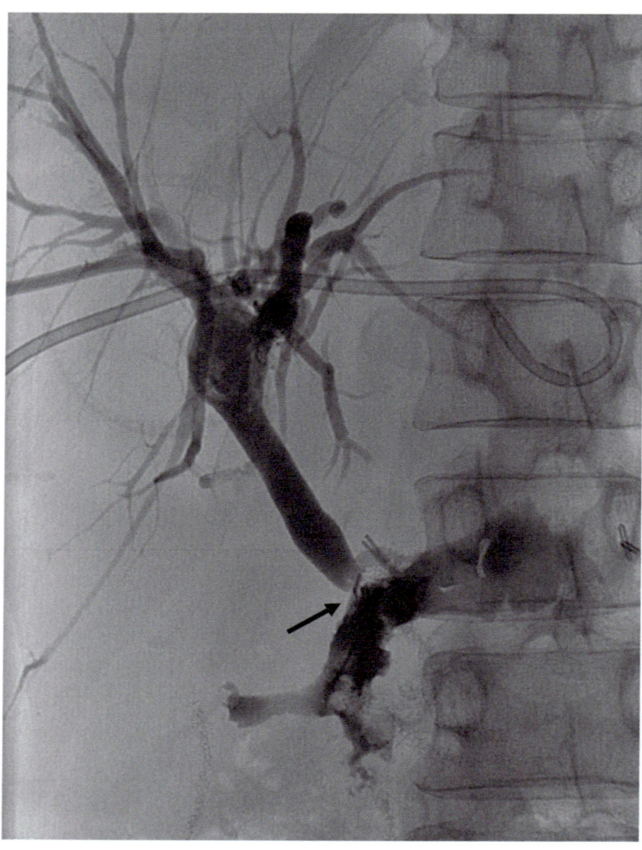

Fig. 61.1 Cholangiogram after percutaneous transhepatic biliary drainage reveals a blowout from the CBD stump (*arrow*), with contrast leaking into the pancreatic bed collection. The cystic duct and rest of the biliary outflow via cholecysto-jejunostomy is not opacified

The sepsis resolved and all drains were removed. The patient was discharged to hospice care and died after 6 weeks from advanced metastatic disease.

S. Punamiya (✉)
Department of Diagnostic and Interventional Radiology, Tan Tock Seng Hospital, Singapore, Singapore
e-mail: sundeep_punamiya@ttsh.com.sg

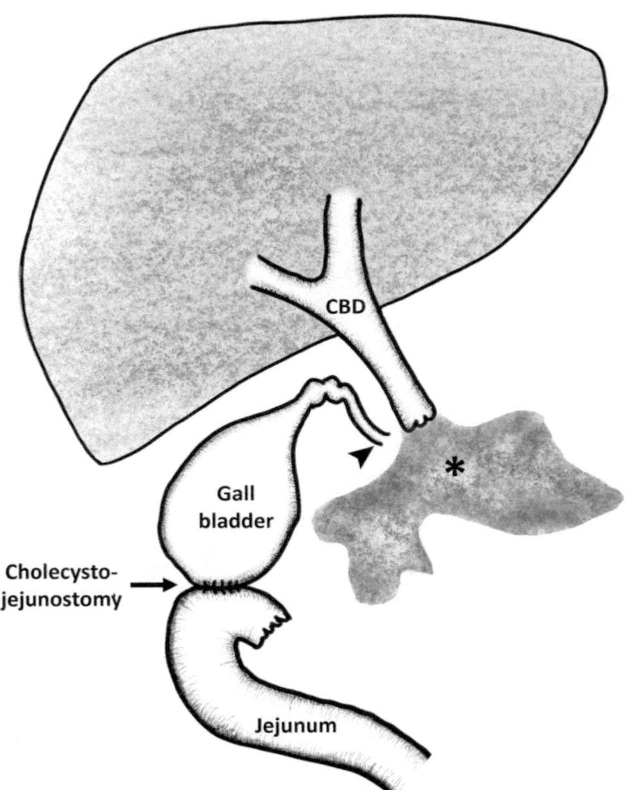

Fig. 61.2 Schematic diagram of surgical anastomoses and site of biliary disconnection from CBD ligation and cystic duct transection (*arrowhead*), resulting in CBD stump blowout into the pancreatic bed collection (*asterisk*)

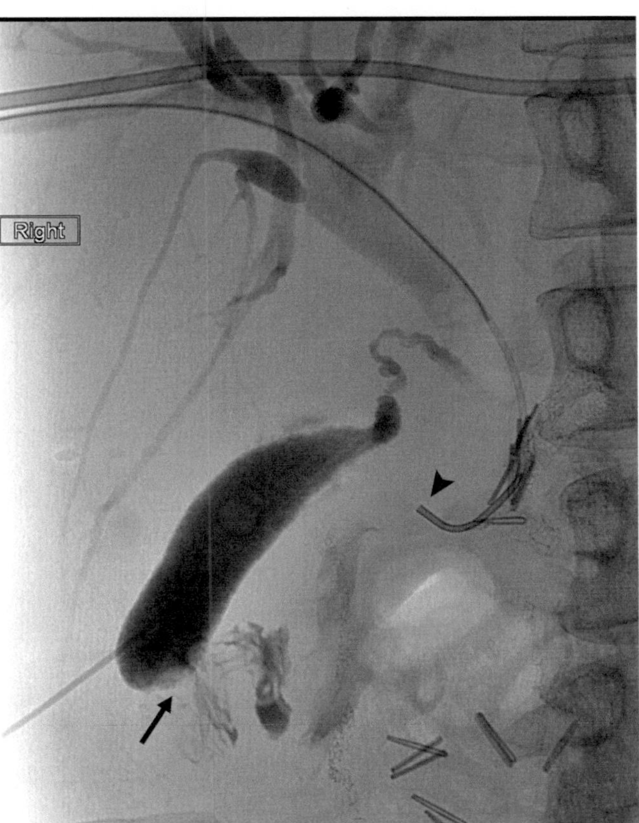

Fig. 61.3 Gallbladder was accessed with a micropuncture set under US guidance and distended with contrast, demonstrating a patent cholecysto-jejunostomy (*arrow*). From the existing biliary access, a 5F Berenstein catheter was advanced through the CBD blowout, and tip positioned within the lateral recess of the collection (*arrowhead*)

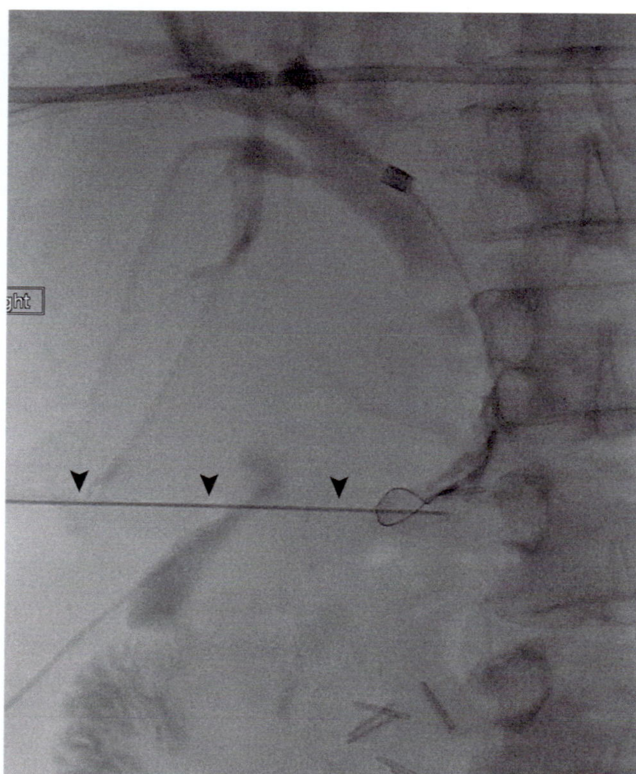

Fig. 61.4 The loop of a 10 mm snare (Amplatz gooseneck snare, ev3 Inc., Plymouth, MN) was opened within the collection, following which a 21G AccuStick needle (*arrowheads*) was inserted and advanced under fluoroscopic guidance from a lateral transhepatic approach. The needle was directed toward the snare, traversing the gallbladder lumen en route

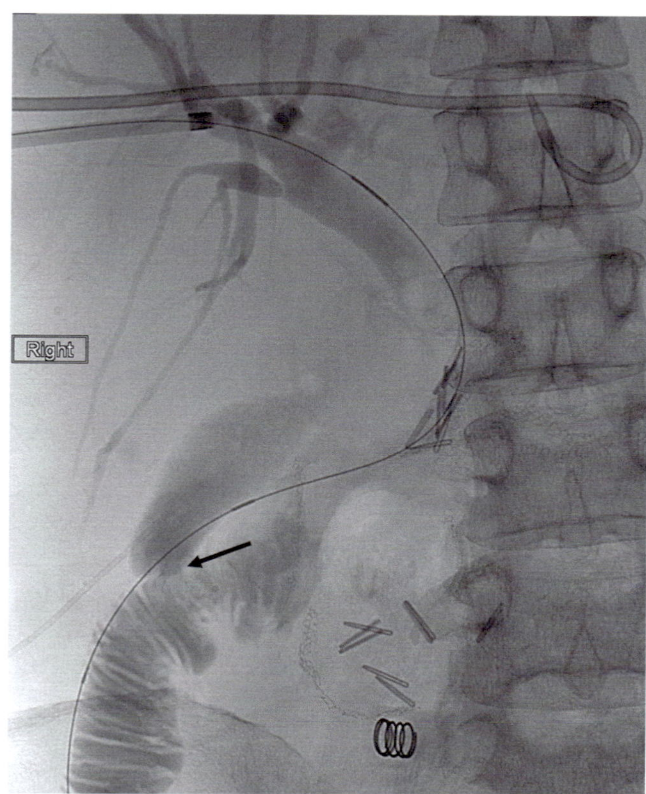

Fig. 61.6 From the biliary access, a 2.6F catheter (CXI support catheter, Cook Incorporated, Bloomington, IN) was advanced over the V18 wire. When the tip of the support catheter approached the gallbladder, the wire was removed and reversed to enter the gallbladder lumen, then advanced across the cholecysto-jejunostomy (*arrow*) into the afferent jejunal loop

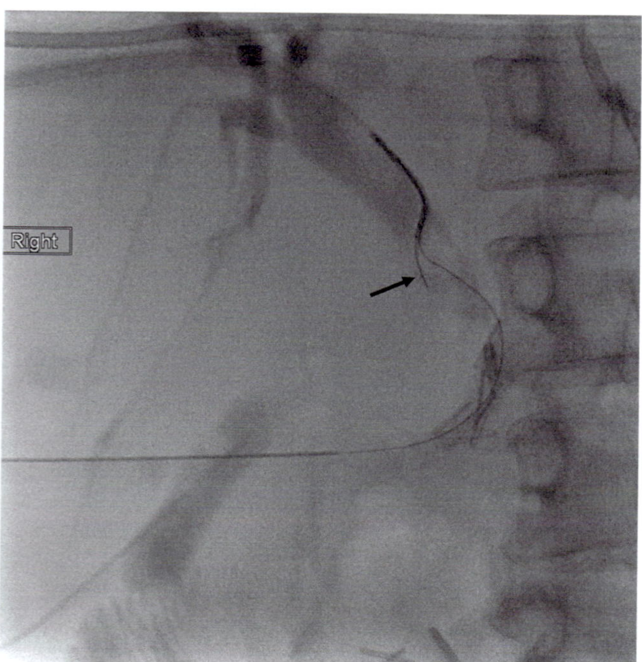

Fig. 61.5 Once the needle was within the snare loop, a 0.018″ guidewire (V18, Boston Scientific, Heredia, Costa Rica) (*arrow*) was inserted, captured, and exteriorized by the snare

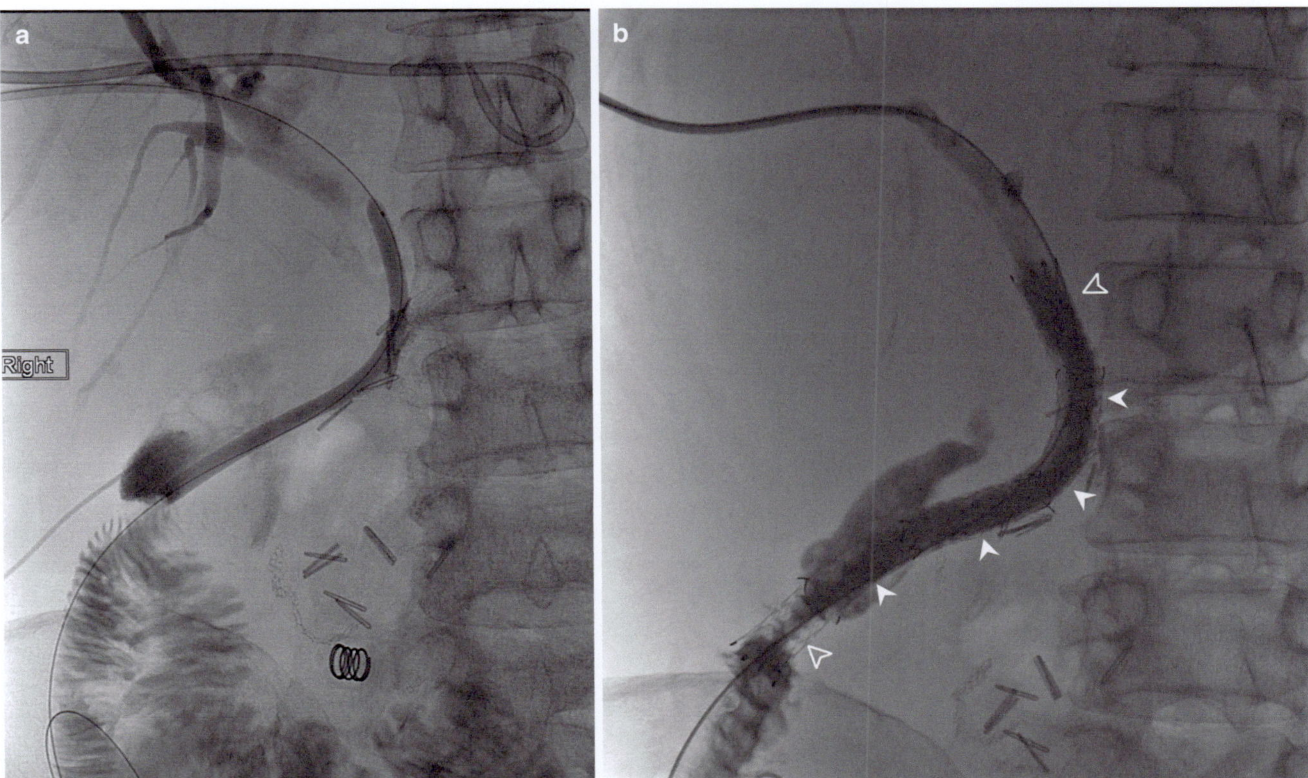

Fig. 61.7 The tract between the CBD stump and gallbladder was (**a**) dilated with a 5 mm × 100 mm angioplasty balloon, then (**b**) lined with stents: two overlapping covered stents (*arrowheads*) (10 mm × 60 mm Niti-S, Taewoong Medical, Gimpo-si, Korea), anchored by a long bare stent (*blank arrowheads*) (10 mm × 120 mm E-Luminexx, Angiomed GmbH & Co., Karlsruhe, Germany), ensuring stent coverage from CBD through the cholecysto-jejunostomy anastomosis. Cholangiogram after stenting shows restoration of biliary outflow via the neo-anastomosis with no further leak

Mina S. Makary and Hooman Khabiri

A 60-year-old male with cirrhosis and primary sclerosing cholangitis status post orthotropic liver transplantation complicated by biliary strictures requiring placement of bilateral percutaneous biliary drains. The patient's left-sided external-only biliary drain was problematic resulting in bile leakage, suboptimal drainage, electrolyte imbalances, and multiple attempts at internalization using conventional guidewire and catheter approaches had been unsuccessful.

Left-sided intrahepatic neobiliary formation was pursued to potentially convert the external left biliary drain to an internal-external drain. Following cholangiography (Fig. 62.1a) and placement of a right-sided safety wire through the hepaticojejunostomy (Fig. 62.1b), a catheter was advanced via the right-sided sheath towards the left biliary tree and positioned near the point of obstruction. Cone-beam CT was used to define the relation of the left-sided access and hepatic structures (Fig. 62.1c). Using fluoroscopy, the left-directed radiofrequency (RF) wire (Baylis Medical, Canada) was aligned with a right-sided snare (Fig. 62.1d). The RF wire was used to create a new tract, to the target snare, followed by balloon dilation (Fig. 62.1e). The left-sided wire was next internalized through patent central ducts beyond the left-sided obstruction, and a left-sided internal-external biliary drainage catheter was placed thereafter (Fig. 62.1f). The presenting biliary issues resolved and have remained so, at 4 years follow-up.

M. S. Makary (✉)
Department of Radiology, Division of Vascular and Interventional Radiology, The Ohio State University Wexner Medical Center, Columbus, OH, USA
e-mail: mina.makary@osumc.edu

H. Khabiri
Section of Interventional Radiology, Washington DC VA Medical Center, Washington, DC, USA

© The Author(s), under exclusive license to Springer Nature Switzerland AG 2023
Z. J. Haskal (ed.), *Extreme IR*, https://doi.org/10.1007/978-3-031-24251-9_62

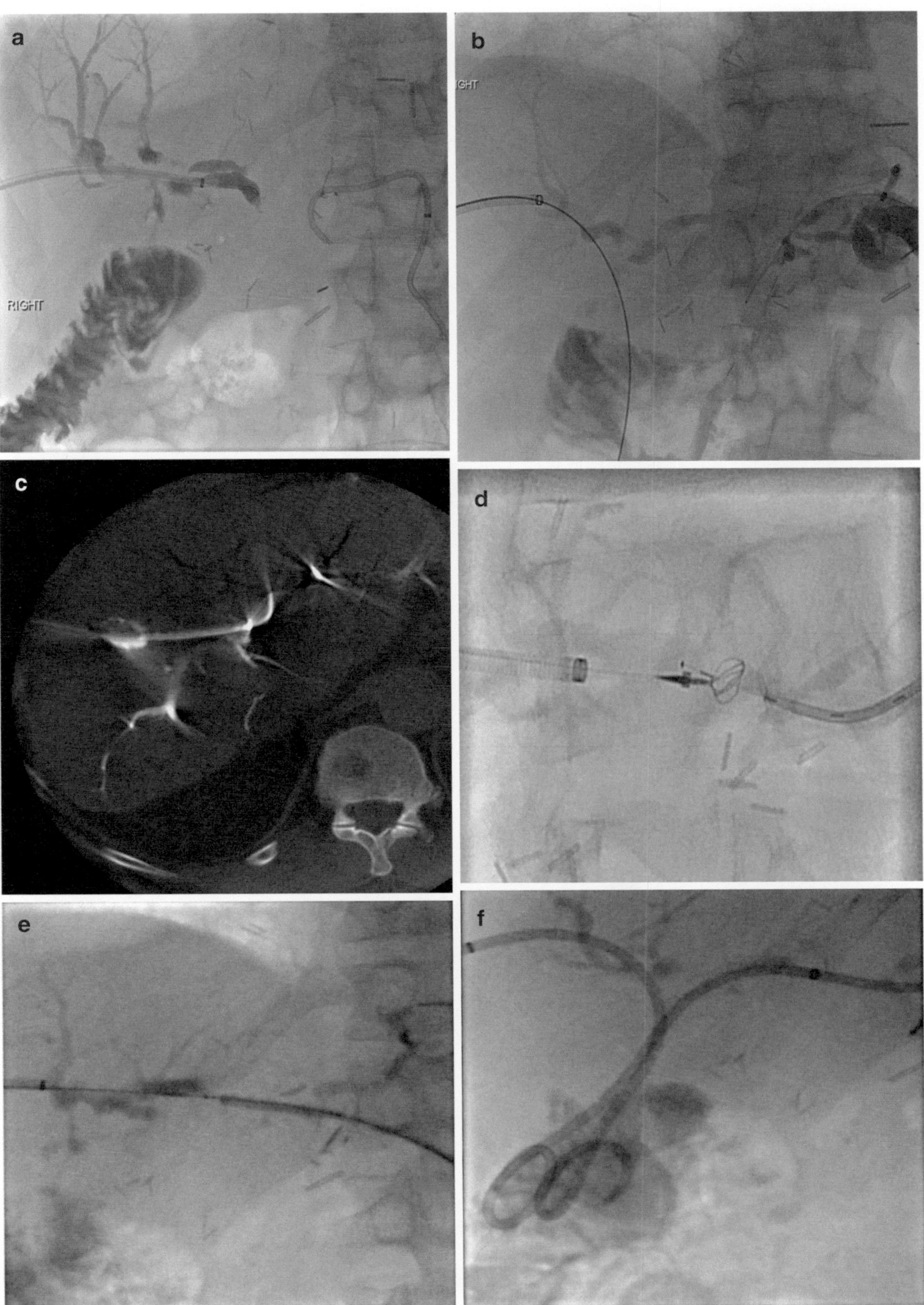

Fig. 62.1 (**a**) Diagnostic cholangiography demonstrating contrast central occlusion with lack of opacification of the left-sided biliary tree. (**b**) Placement of a wire through the right-sided access and into the hepaticojejunostomy as well as a second wire through the left-sided access terminating at the level of the occlusion. (**c**) Placement of a right-sided catheter towards the left-sided tree to the level of the blockage and use of cone-beam CT to confirm catheter location in relation to the left-sided access wire and hepatic structures. (**d**) Targeting a snare placed via the right-sided approach by a left-sided radiofrequency (RF) wire utilizing fluoroscopic guidance, and followed by tract plasty (**e**). (**f**) Internalization of the left-sided wire and successful placement a left-sided internal-external biliary drainage catheter, along with the pre-existing right-sided catheter

Radiofrequency-Wire Guided Reconstruction and Neo-Duct Creation for Complete Right Extrahepatic Bile Duct Ligation after Robotic Cholecystectomy

Ziv J Haskal

A 51-year-old female underwent robotic cholecystectomy (Fig. 63.1), complicated by complete ligation of the extrahepatic right hepatic duct at the liver surface (Fig. 63.2). An externally draining right biliary catheter was placed; mechanical attempts to traverse the ligated duct proved fruitless. Using a retrograde endoscopic approach, a balloon was placed in the common bile duct (CBD) (Fig. 63.3). A deflectable sheath (Oscor) was used to point an angled radiofrequency wire (Bayliss) which was activated and advanced toward the balloon (Fig. 63.4), across the 2 cm extrahepatic gap, and into the distal CBD. This was followed by a 5Fr catheter. A customized transampullary biliary catheter was

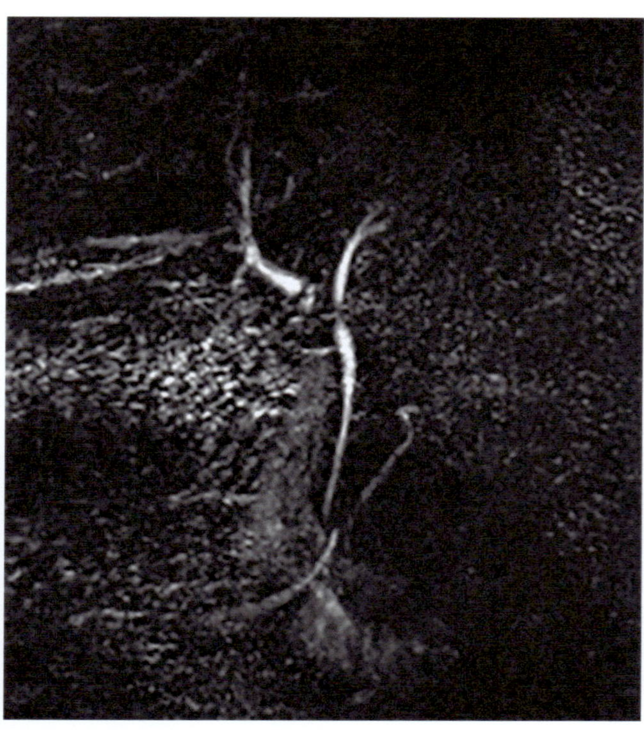

Fig. 63.2 Magnetic resonance cholangiopancreatography (MRCP) demonstrates the isolated right ducts; the gap from right duct to common bile duct measured 2 cm. The left duct is incompletely seen but was normal throughout

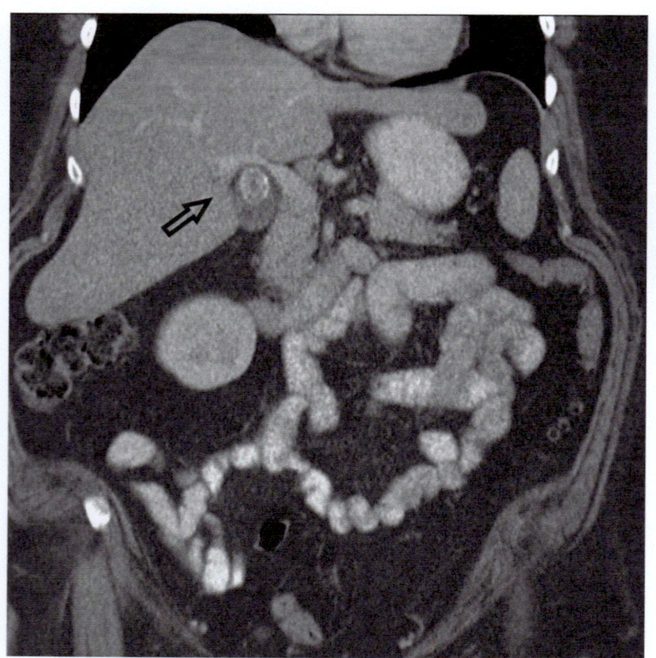

Fig. 63.1 Coronal CT image demonstrates a normal liver and gallstone (arrow)

constructed, with measured sideholes cut to reside within the CBD and right ducts, and a "skip" segment (no sideholes) in the extrahepatic portion.

Over the next 4 months, the catheter was increased to 12Fr and the neo-duct tract dilated to 6 mm and beyond (Fig. 63.5). Despite long-term intubation and dilation with larger catheters and balloons, the neo-duct failed to reach a self-sustaining caliber allowing complete tube removal (Figs. 63.6 and 63.7).

Z. J Haskal (✉)
Department of Radiology and Medical Imaging, Interventional Division, University of Virginia, Charlottesville, VA, USA

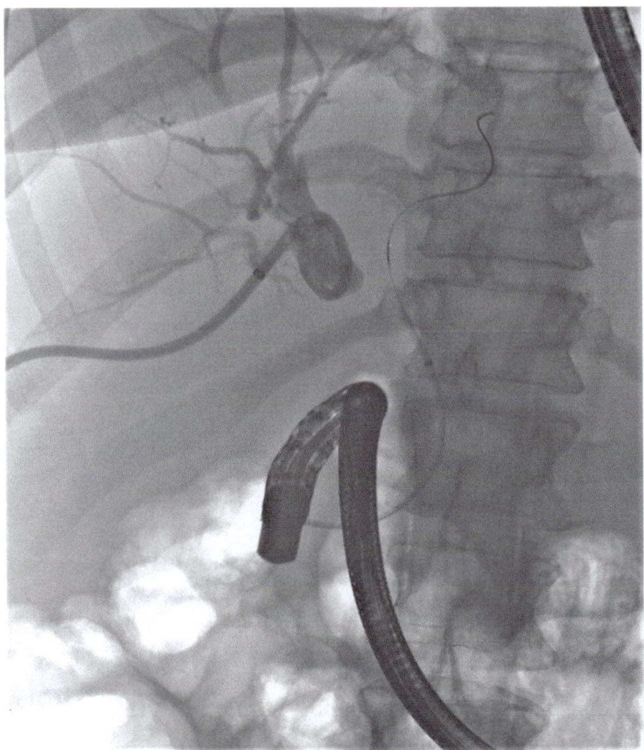

Fig. 63.3 Cholangiogram demonstrates the 2 cm long extrahepatic right duct occlusion due to inadvertent surgical ligation. The retrograde endoscopic CBD catheter and wire are seen. The wire tip is in the left biliary tree

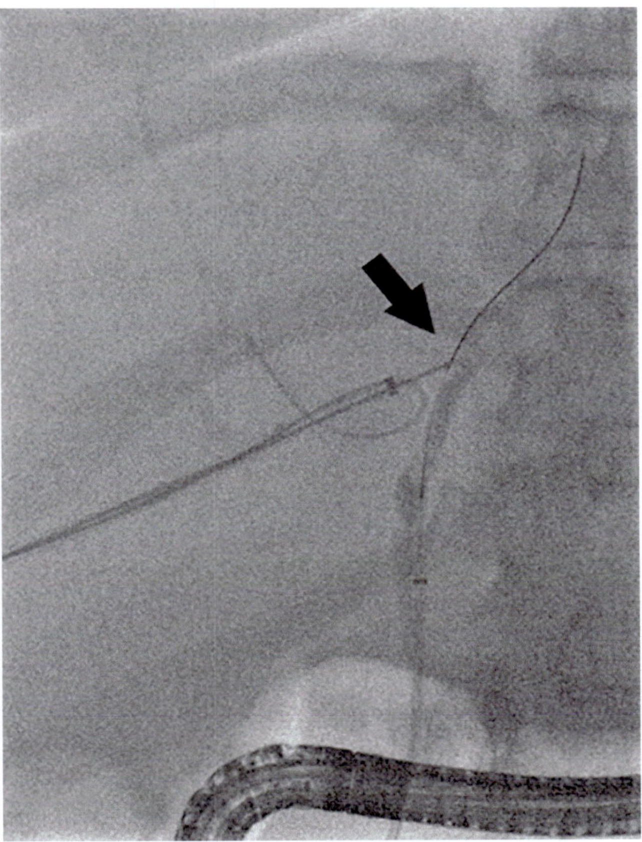

Fig. 63.4 The radiofrequency wire has been activated and advanced toward the endoscopic balloon target (arrow), whilst directed by the deflectable biliary sheath

At 4 years follow-up, she remains asymptomatic, with a capped biliary catheter, and normal liver function. Because of the original inadvertent ligation at the liver surface, a surgical reconstruction was deemed unfeasible (and right hepatectomy was reserved).

Sharp, and now radiofrequency (thermal) assisted neo-anastomosis creation has been increasingly described in scenarios of ureterovesical and biliary anastomotic occlusions. The ability to create durable tube-free neo-anastomoses has been variable. This case demonstrates a more unusual use of the technique—to span a 2 cm long extrahepatic right duct occlusion.

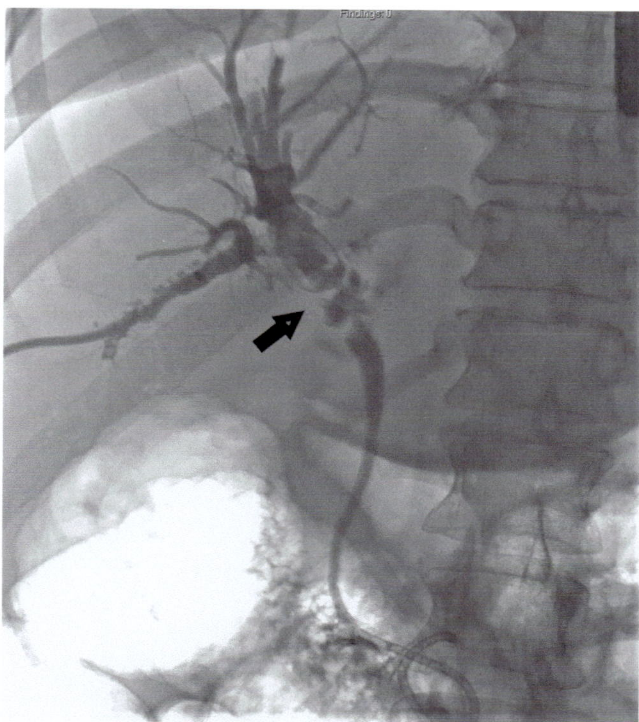

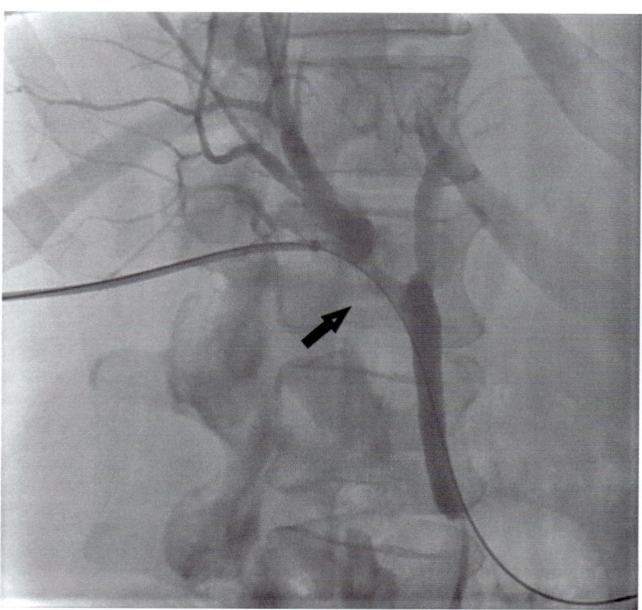

Fig. 63.7 At 6 months of intubation with a large caliber tube and repeated 6 mm dilations, the stable neo-duct is visible (arrow), but proved insufficient to sustain antegrade flow (during capping trials of external biliary catheters and manometry)

Fig. 63.5 Cholangiography after placement of the internal external transampullary biliary catheter with a skip-zone of sideholes in the extrabiliary tract. Irregularity across that zone reflects the contrast leaking in the area uncircumscribed by duct (arrow)

Bibliography

1. Close ON, Akinwande O, Varma RK, Santos E, Kim HS. Percutaneous hepaticojejunostomy using a radiofrequency wire for management of a postoperative bile leak. Cardiovasc Intervent Radiol. 2017;40(1):139–43. https://doi.org/10.1007/s00270-016-1468-1.
2. Mansueto G, Contro A, Zamboni GA, De Robertis R. Retrograde percutaneous transjejunal creation of biliary Neoanastomoses in patients with complete Hepaticojejunostomy dehiscence. J Vasc Interv Radiol. 2015;26(10):1544–9. https://doi.org/10.1016/j.jvir.2015.06.009. s
3. Kloeckner R, Dueber C, dos Santos DP, Kara L, Pitton MB. Fluoroscopy-guided hepaticoneojejunostomy in recurrent anastomotic stricture after repeated surgical hepaticojejunostomy. J Vasc Interv Radiol. 2013;24:1750–2.
4. Guimaraes M, et al. Successful recanalization of bile duct occlusion with a radiofrequency puncture wire technique. J Vasc Interv Radiol. 2010;21(2):289–94.

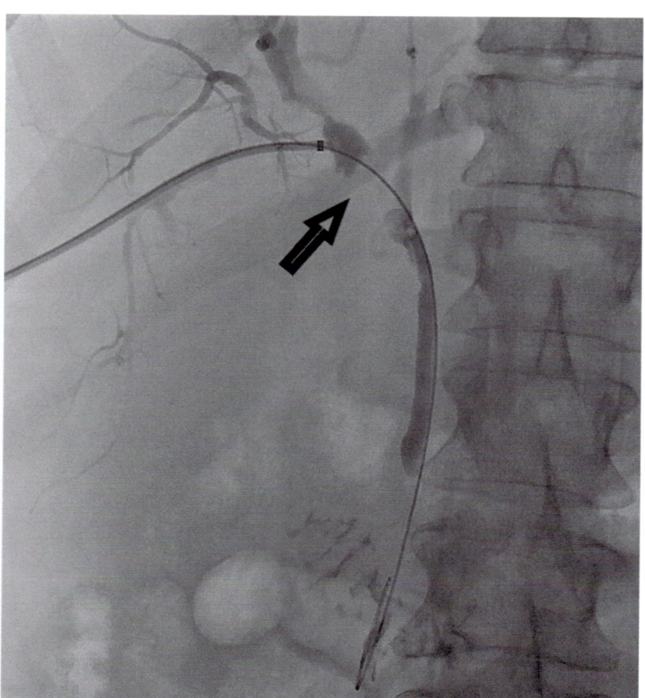

Fig. 63.6 Three weeks after creation of the neo passage, cholangiography demonstrated no extravasation of bile, and no antegrade passage of contrast (arrow)

Hilar Biliary Obstruction Treated with Extraordinary Extra-Anatomical Endoprostheses

Yasuaki Arai, Miyuki Sone, and Shunsuke Sugawara

A 70-year-old female presented with obstructive jaundice caused by hepatic hilar cholangiocarcinoma (Bismuth IV); she underwent placement of a nasoenteric biliary catheter by an endoscopist. This provided insufficient improvement of her jaundice as only segment 3 was drained. Whilst outpatient chemotherapy was being planned, she strongly wished to be tube-free at home. The tumor was located mainly within the right lobe of her liver, and the anterior segment had already atrophied (Fig. 64.1). Percutaneous transhepatic biliary drainage (PTBD) was performed via B6 and B3 segments of the biliary tree (Fig. 64.2). Though the left duct to common bile duct (CBD) stricture was traversed, the stricture spanning B6 to the CBD could not be, because of the hard tumor (Fig. 64.3).

Using a 17G hand-bent needle (Fig. 64.4), B6 was punctured via a B3 route through the tumor, and a 0.035-inch guidewire was pulled through from B3 to B6, through the tumor, using a loop snare (Fig. 64.5 and 64.6). After balloon dilatation of this route, covered stents (8 mm diameter × 6 cm long) were placed from the posterior bile duct to B3, and two covered stents (8 mm × 6 cm) from B3 to CBD (Fig. 64.7). The bile from the posterior segment could flow to B3 through the stent connecting the posterior bile duct and B3, then flow to CBD through the stent connecting B3 and CBD (Fig. 64.8).

Ten days later, all biliary catheters were removed and coil embolization of the tracts was performed. At 5 months of follow-up, she was undergoing intended chemotherapy without any biliary obstruction or cholangitis.

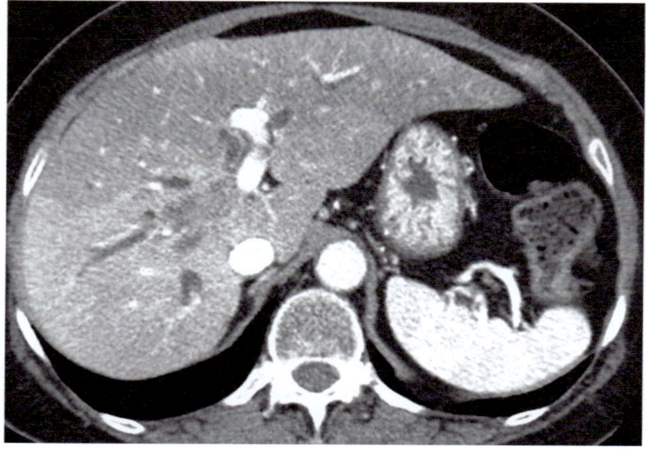

Fig. 64.1 The hepatic hilar cholangiocarcinoma located mainly in the right side of the liver and the anterior segment (*) was already atrophied

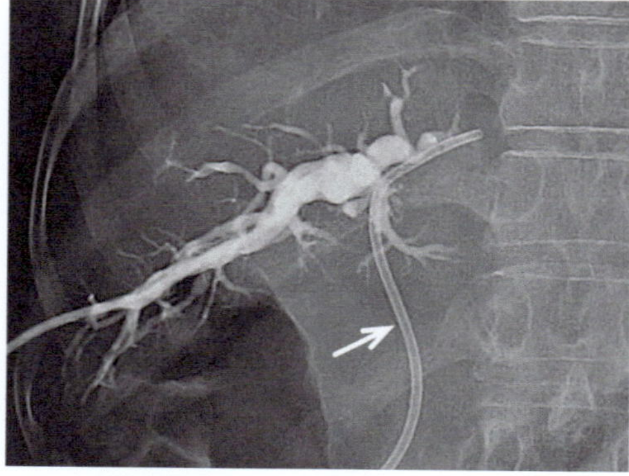
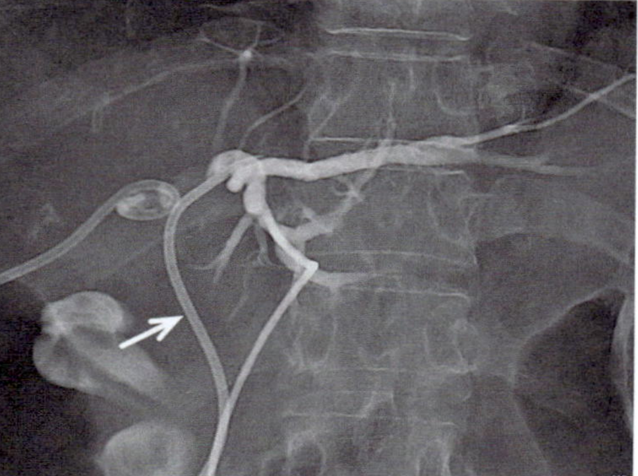

Fig. 64.2 PTBDs were performed to B6 and B3. The endoprosthesis tube (arrows) inserted by endoscopists was removed later

Y. Arai (✉) · M. Sone · S. Sugawara
Department of Diagnostic Radiology, National Cancer Center, Tokyo, Japan
e-mail: arai-y3111@mvh.biglobe.ne.jp; shsugawa@ncc.go.jp

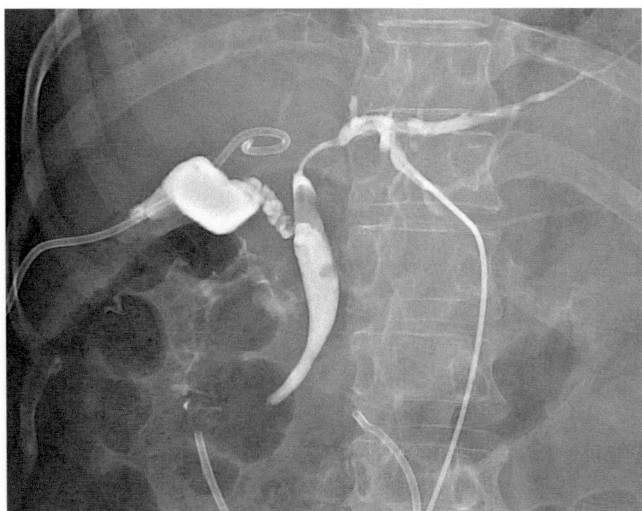

Fig. 64.3 The transverse of stricture from the left bile duct to CBD was successfully done. However, the transverse of the stricture from B6 to CBD was impossible because of hard tumor

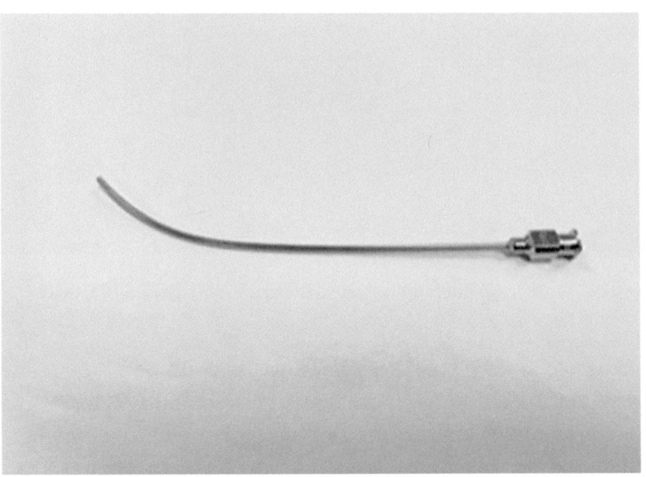

Fig. 64.4 A 17G hand-bent needle

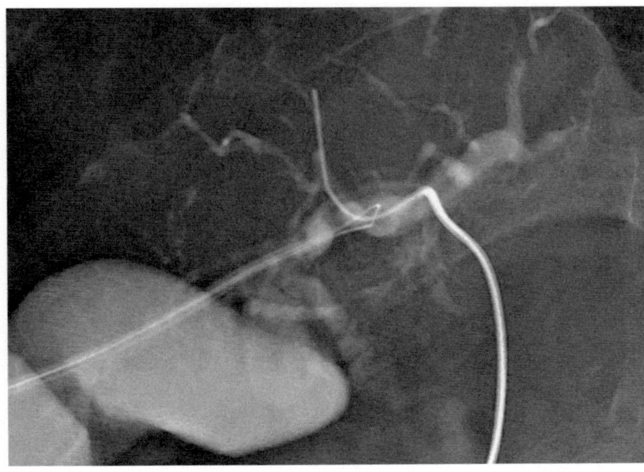

Fig. 64.5 B6 was punctured with a hand-bended needle via B3, and an inserted guidewire was grasped a loop snare inserted from B6

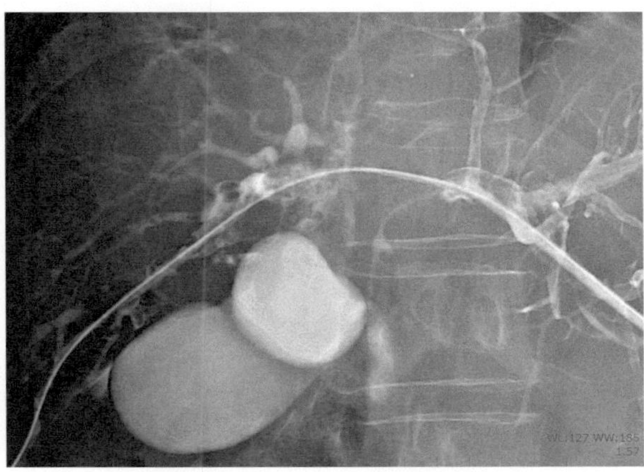

Fig. 64.6 A 0.035 inch guidewire was pulled through from B3 to B6

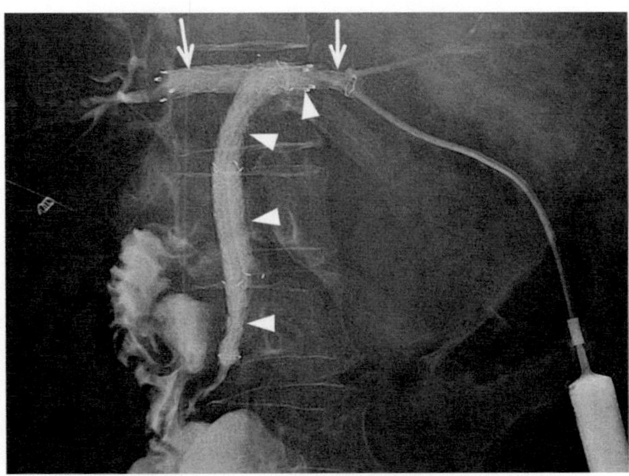

Fig. 64.7 A covered stents (8 mm × 6 cm) were inserted from the posterior bile duct to B3 through the tumor (arrows), and two covered stent (8 mm × 6 cm) was inserted from B3 to CBD (arrow heads)

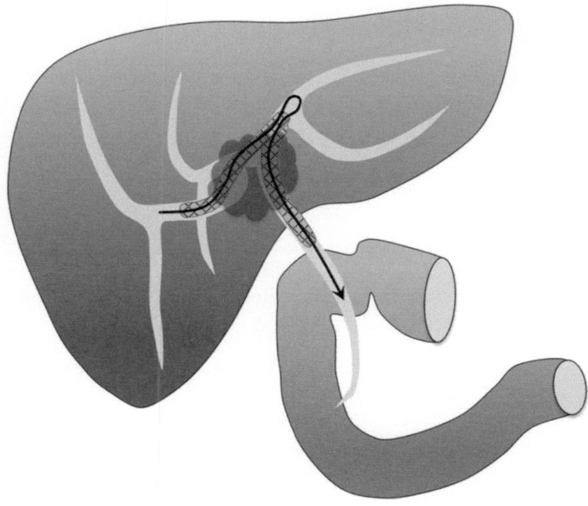

Fig. 64.8 The bile of the posterior segment could flow to B3 through the stent connecting the posterior bile duct and B3, then flow to CBD through the stent connecting B3 and CBD. (Yasuaki Arai, M.D. Shunske Sugawara, M.D., Miyuki Sone, M.D.)

Leave Only Liquid: Prophylactic Liquid Embolization of a Chronic Transpleural Biliary Drain Tract

Marc C. Kryger and Ziv J Haskal

A 79-year-old man presented for preoperative removal of a 1-month-old transpleural biliary drain placed for an obstructive pancreatic adenocarcinoma. The intent was to prevent of a post-Whipple procedure biliopleural fistula. The malpositioned right biliary drain was found secured in the proximal common bile duct (Fig. 65.1). Cholangiography showed adequate transampullary prograde drainage through an endoscopically placed metallic common bile duct stent (Fig. 65.2). The catheter was exchanged for a long 6 French vascular sheath and 0.018″ nitinol safety wire. An adjacent Progreat microcatheter (Terumo) was advanced through the sheath and used to deploy an oversized 6 × 12 cm Ruby coil as an

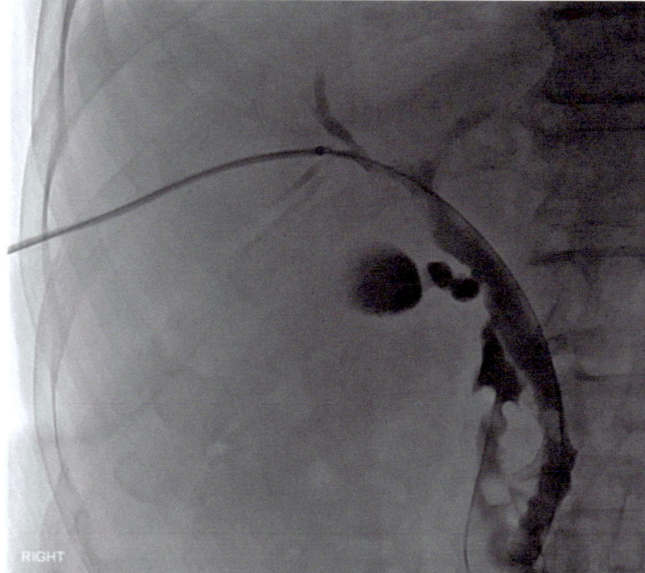

Fig. 65.2 Sheath cholangiogram demonstrating patent CBD stent

intratract safety plug peripheral to the bile duct entry site (Fig. 65.3). The safety wire was removed and EVOH (Onyx 34, Medtronic) was injected against the coil into the hepatic tract, filling the transpleural passage and cutaneous tract (Figs. 65.4 and 65.5). No material embolized central to the coil (into the biliary tree). All wires, catheters, and sheath were removed. Subsequent chest CT demonstrated no pneumothorax or effusion, and the patient was discharged the next morning (Fig. 65.6). The patient returned 2 weeks with fever, no pneurothorax nor pleural effusion. As small hepatic abscess was identified and resolved treated with antibiotics and drainage. Unfortunately, due to progressive cognitive and performance status decline since his cancer diagnosis, the patient and surgeon decided against resection or systemic treatment, and the patient retired home with hospice care.

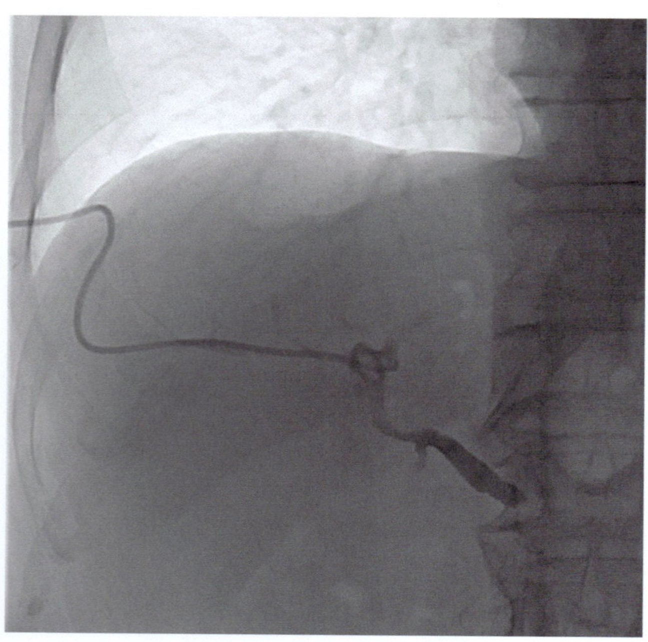

Fig. 65.1 Transpleural right biliary drain entering at the seventh to eighth interspace. Inspiratory radiograph

M. C. Kryger
Department of Radiology and Medical Imaging, University of Virginia Health System, Charlottesville, VA, USA
e-mail: MK9ZV@hscmail.mcc.virginia.edu

Z. J Haskal (✉)
Department of Radiology and Medical Imaging, Interventional Division, University of Virginia, Charlottesville, VA, USA

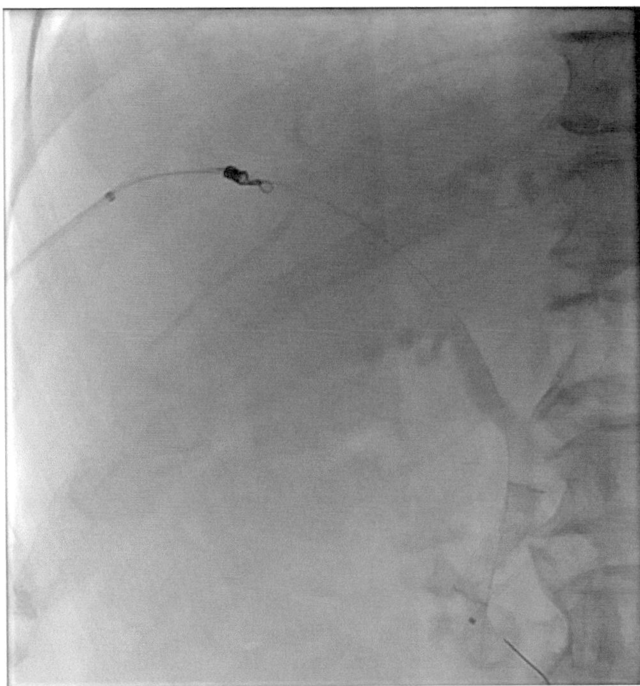

Fig. 65.3 Post deployment of 6 mm × 12 cm Ruby coil just proximal to ductotomy

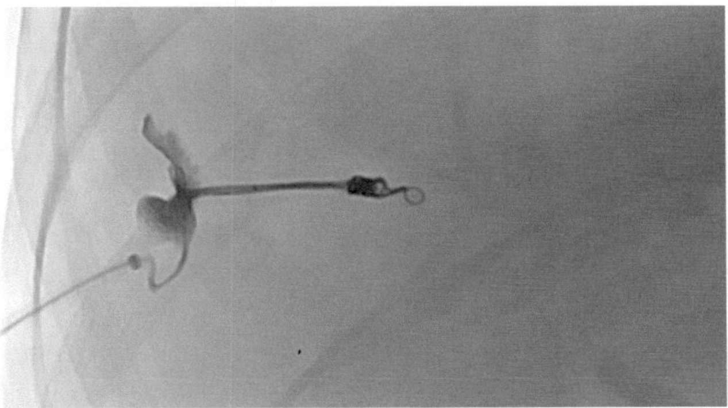

Fig. 65.4 Post injection of Onyx 34 into hepatic tract. Note no embolization material central to the coil

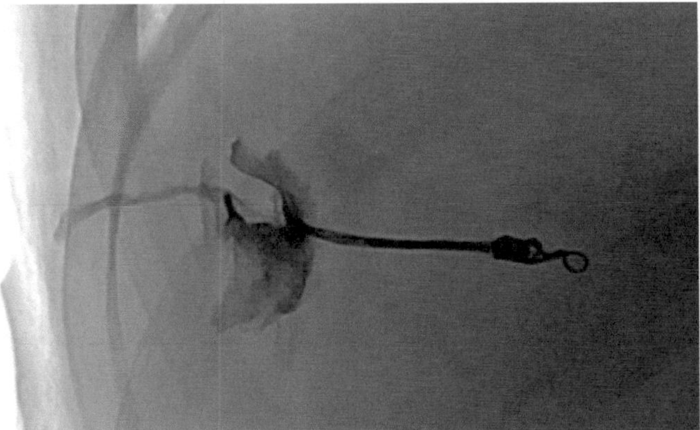

Fig. 65.5 Post injection of Onyx 34 into the cutaneous tract and removal of all instruments. Note some material in the pleural space

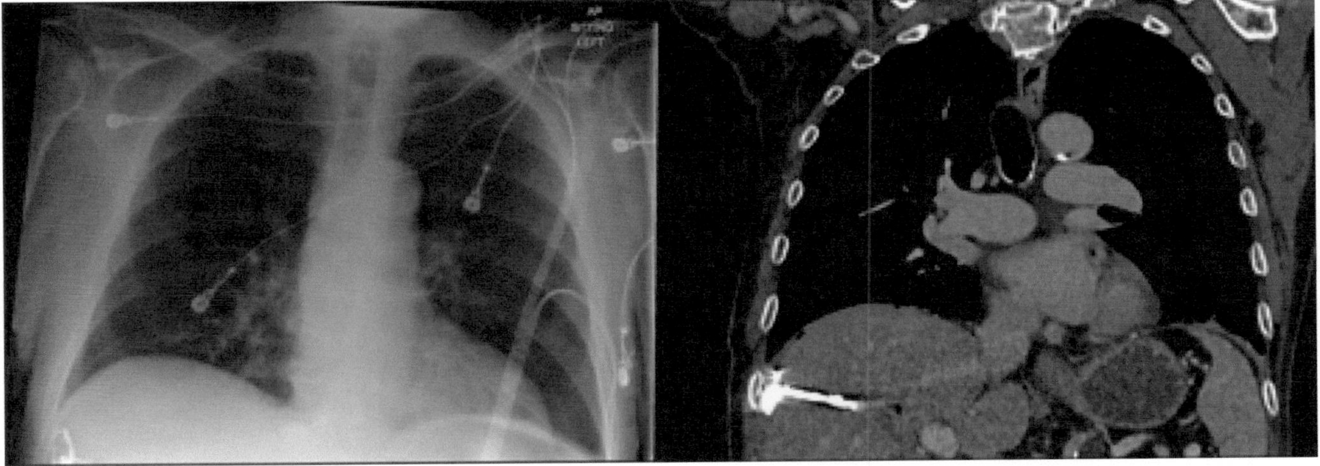

Fig. 65.6 Post-procedure AP chest radiograph and coronal CT image demonstrating no pleural effusion or pneumothorax

Bibliography

1. Kortes N, Gnutzmann D, Konietzke P, Mayer P, Sumkauskaite M, Kauczor HU, Radeleff BA. Occlusion of a long-term Transpleural biliary drainage tract using a gelatin Pledget (Hep-plug™). Cardiovasc Intervent Radiol. 2017;40(11):1800–3. https://doi.org/10.1007/s00270-017-1695-0.
2. Saad WE, Wallace MJ, Wojak JC, Kundu S, Cardella JF. Quality improvement guidelines for percutaneous transhepatic cholangiography, biliary drainage, and percutaneous cholecystostomy. J Vasc Interv Radiol. 2010;21(6):789–95. https://doi.org/10.1016/j.jvir.2010.01.012.
3. Strange C, Allen ML, Freedland PN, Cunningham J, Sahn SA. Biliopleural fistula as a complication of percutaneous biliary drainage: experimental evidence for pleural inflammation. Am Rev Respir Dis. 1988;137(4):959–61. https://doi.org/10.1164/ajrccm/137.4.959.
4. Turkington RC, Leggett JJ, Hurwitz J, Eatock MM. Cholethorax following percutaneous transhepatic biliary drainage. Ulster Med J. 2007;76(2):112–3.

Glue Embolization of a High Output Biliary Fistula After RFA

66

Jorge E. Lopera

A 74-year-old male with small bowel carcinoid tumor and multiple liver metastases underwent radiofrequency ablation of a segment 6 liver tumor. He developed high fevers thereafter and was admitted with sepsis 1 week after the ablation. Contrast-enhanced CT imaging demonstrated a large abscess in the right lobe with an air -fluid level (Fig. 66.1). A percutaneous drain was placed in the collection and the infection was controlled. The drain had a persistent daily bilious output of 100–200 cc for the preceding 10 days. A contrast abscessogram showed that the cavity communicated with biliary radicles (Fig. 66.2). Cone beam CT demonstrated a biliary fistula to the segment 6 radicles with no communication with the central bile ducts (Fig. 66.3).

The drain was exchanged for a 10Fr sheath, through which an angled catheter was advanced into the biliary tree

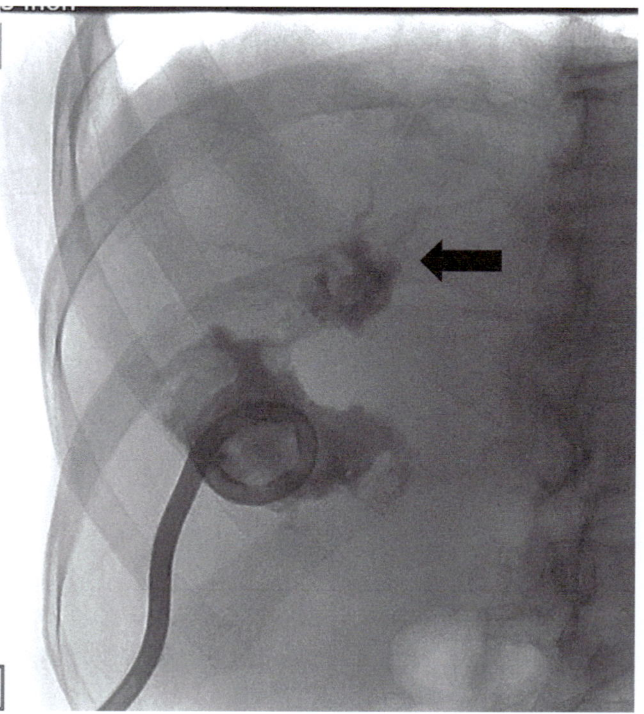

Fig. 66.2 Fluoroscopic abscess study shows communication of the cavity with multiple biliary radicles in the right lobe (arrow)

(Fig. 66.4). nBCA cyanoacrylate glue mixed with Lipiodol (Trufill, Codman, Raynham, MA) in a 1:2 ratio was injected until all the biliary radicles were casted full of glue (Fig. 66.5). The bilious output ceased and the drain was removed 3 days later. MRI obtained 2 years later showed atrophy of the segment 6 (Fig. 66.6). The patient's carcinoid disease progressed to his death 4 years later.

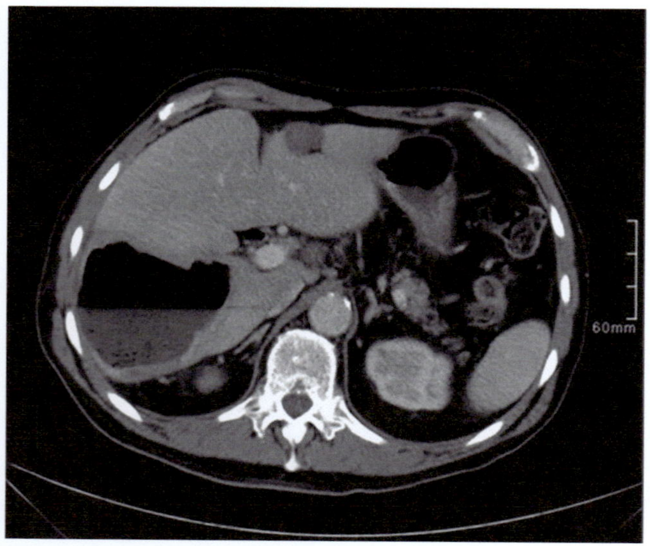

Fig. 66.1 Axial contrast-enhanced CT scan shows a large abscess in the right lobe with an air-fluid level

J. E. Lopera (✉)
Department of Radiology, UT Health San Antonio,
San Antonio, TX, USA
e-mail: Lopera@uthscsa.edu

Z. J. Haskal (ed.), *Extreme IR*, https://doi.org/10.1007/978-3-031-24251-9_66

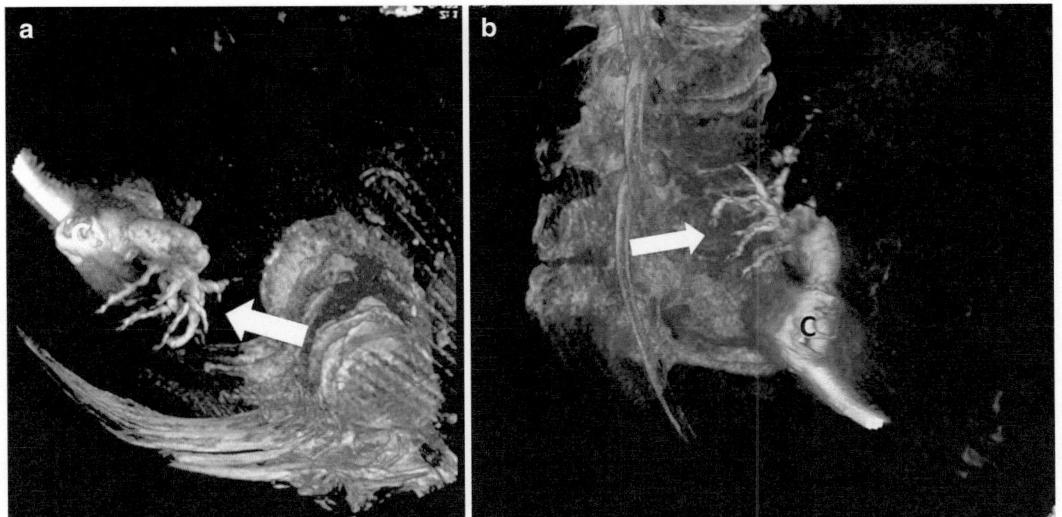

Fig. 66.3 Cone beam CT images in axial (**a**) and sagittal (**b**) projections show the cavity (**c**) in communication with segment 6 biliary radicles (arrows)

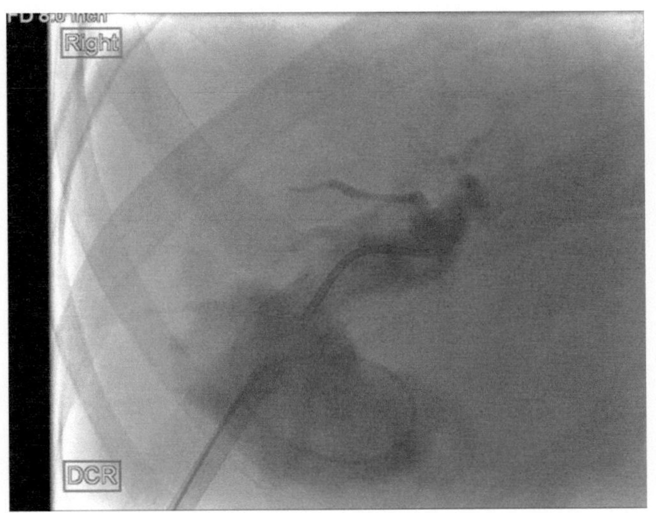

Fig. 66.4 Spot radiograph shows a safety wire placed inside the abscess cavity, a 10 Fr sheath and a 5 Fr angled catheter within the biliary system

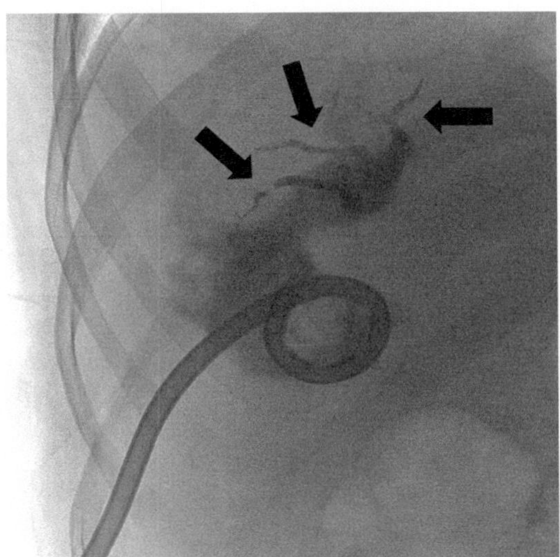

Fig. 66.5 Spot radiograph shows multiple biliary radicles now filled with glue. A new drainage catheter was placed over the safety wire

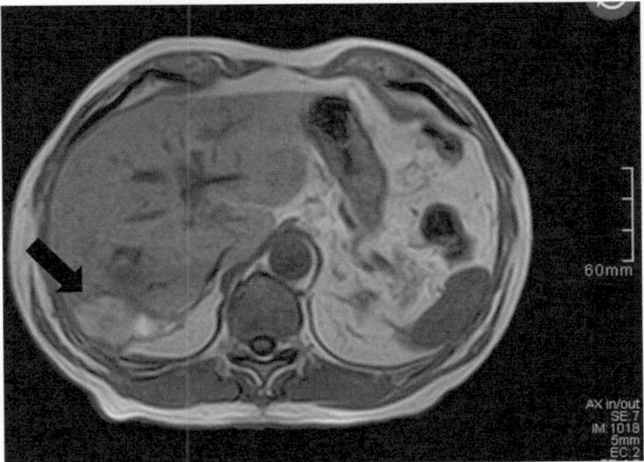

Fig. 66.6 Axial MRI obtained 2 years later shows abnormal signal and atrophy of segment 6 (arrow)

67

EVOH Embolization of a Subtle Arterio-Biliary Fistula: From Artery into the Bile Duct

Ziv J Haskal

A 71-year-old man underwent left hepatectomy and chemo-radiation for cholangiocarcinoma 2 years prior. Since then he had increasing intermittent episodes of fever, chills, and night sweats attributed to recurrent cholangitis. Imaging showed air in the biliary tree due to his roux anastomosis and focal ductal obstruction in the anterior margin of the residual liver (Fig. 67.1). He underwent US and fluoroscopic-guided biliary drainage of the affected segment (Fig. 67.2 Cholangiogram). One week later, he developed hemobilia requiring transfusion; hepatic angiography (with tube withdrawal) did not reveal a cause (Fig. 67.3), and the catheter was upsized; he was discharged 4 days later. He returned emergently 4 days later with recurrent hemobilia, anemic.

Hepatic arteriography was performed in multiple projections whilst filming at 7.5fps revealing a suspected irregular narrowing and subtle enlargement of an artery traversing the tube (Fig. 67.4a, b). Because of the need to assure of embolization beyond, across, and proximal to this potential pseudoaneurysm (PSA), EVOH (18 concentration) was slowly

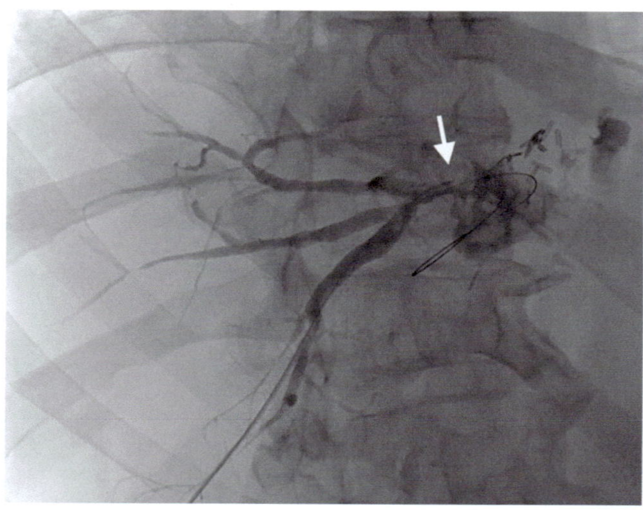

Fig. 67.2 Cholangiography during initial drain placement demonstrates several isolated obstructed ducts converging upon a narrowed bilioenteric anastomosis (arrow)

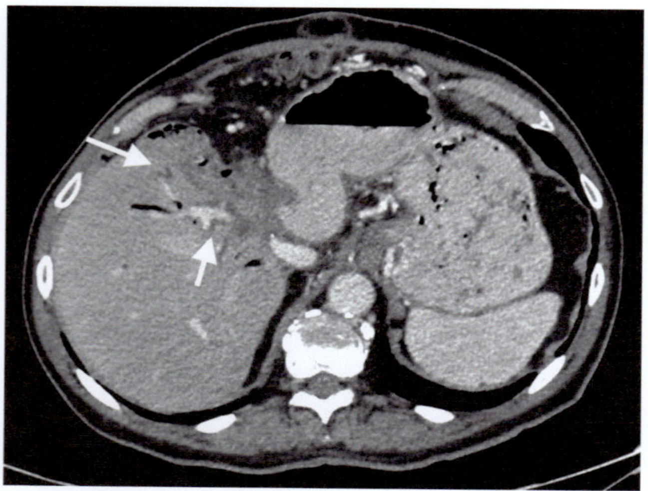

Fig. 67.1 Contrast-enhanced abdominal CT shows the left hepatectomy and subtle area of ductal dilation near anterior surface of the liver at the resection margin (arrows)

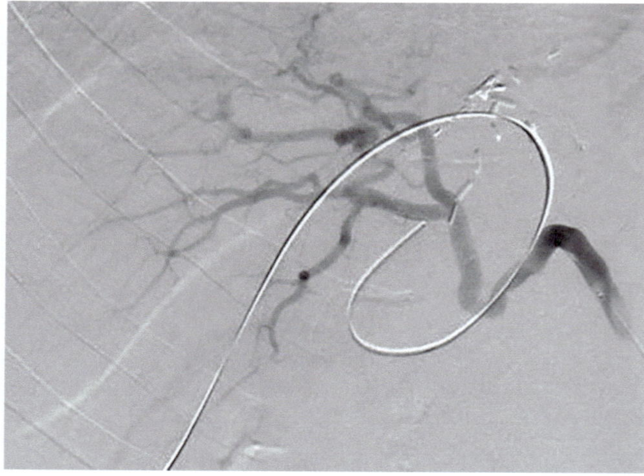

Fig. 67.3 Single images from first multi-view hepatic angiography during transient over-the-wire removal of the biliary catheter showed no contrast entering the biliary tree (or catheter path); no hepatic artery injury was diagnosed by the operator

injected over >5 min, casting the artery beyond, the evident PSA across the tube, and proximal artery (Fig. 67.5). During injection, EVOH was seen entering the biliary tree, defini-

Z. J Haskal (✉)
Department of Radiology and Medical Imaging, Interventional Division, University of Virginia, Charlottesville, VA, USA

Z. J. Haskal (ed.), *Extreme IR*, https://doi.org/10.1007/978-3-031-24251-9_67

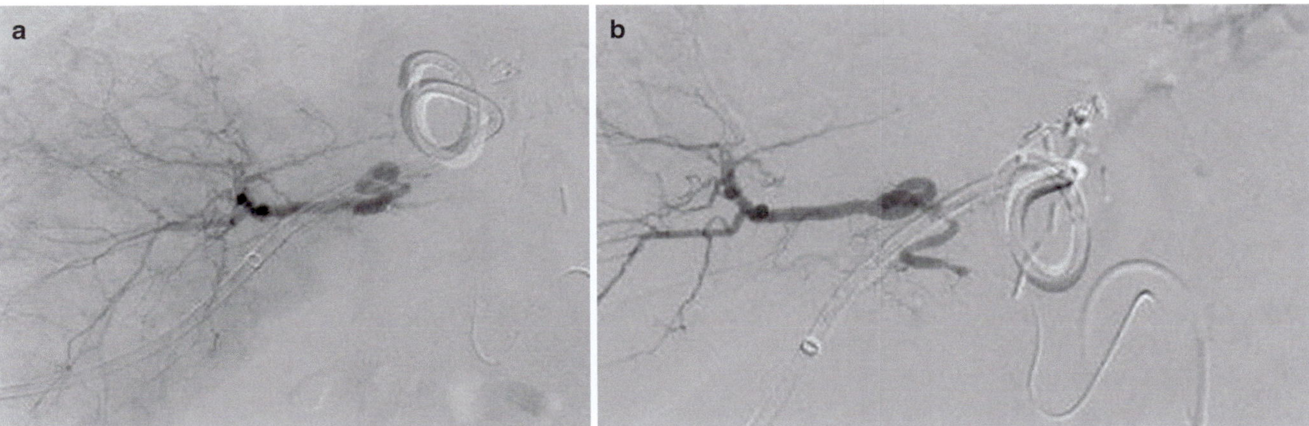

Fig. 67.4 Two images from hepatic angiography at the second session. (**a**) one of the multiple obliquities which did not directly reveal an abnormality. (**b**) Another projection, in the best of multiple obliquities, showed a subtle suggestion of narrowing, irregularity, and enlargement across the catheter

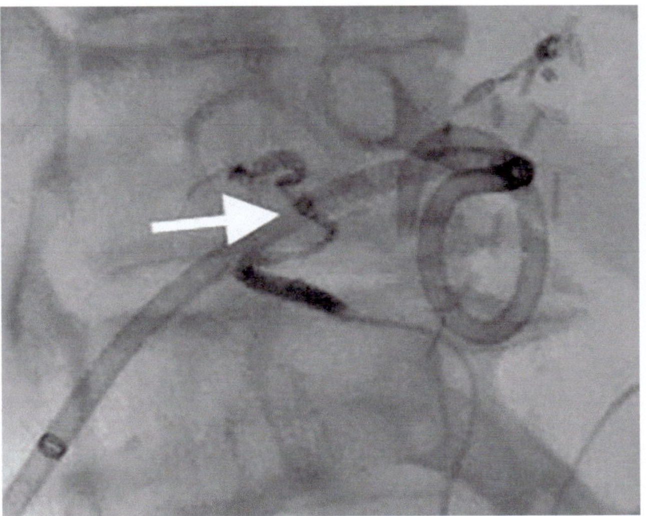

Fig. 67.5 EVOH casting of the affected artery traversing the biliary catheter fills the artery proximal, across the catheter and beyond, the so-called front and back doors. Filling of the suspected pseudoaneurysm is affirmed

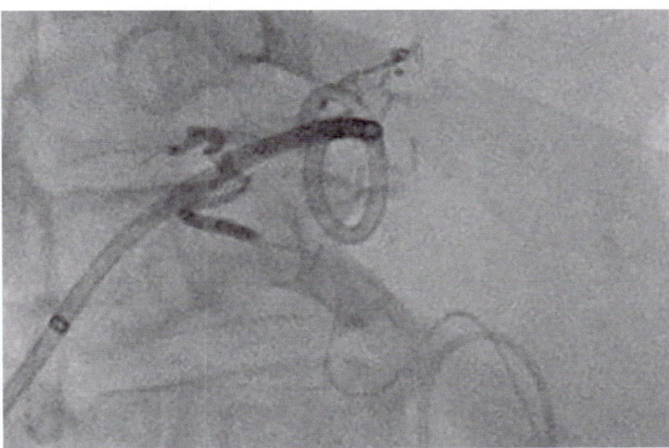

Fig. 67.6 Spot radiograph at end of EVOH injection shows the radio-opaque embolic within the leading end of the biliary catheter confirming the arterio-biliary connection

tively affirming the PSA a the source of the arterio-biliary fistula (Fig. 67.6). The biliary catheter was exchanged and EVOH and the endobiliary EVOH was removed, adherent to the catheter (Fig. 67.7). His bile cleared immediately after the procedure and remained so at several weeks follow-up.

Arterial injuries due to percutaneous hepatic interventions may prove elusive. Extravasation of contrast (and blood) along the partly removed biliary drain cannot be expected in every case. High suspicion and high-speed filming, with many DSA masks, may be needed to identify subtle culprit lesions.

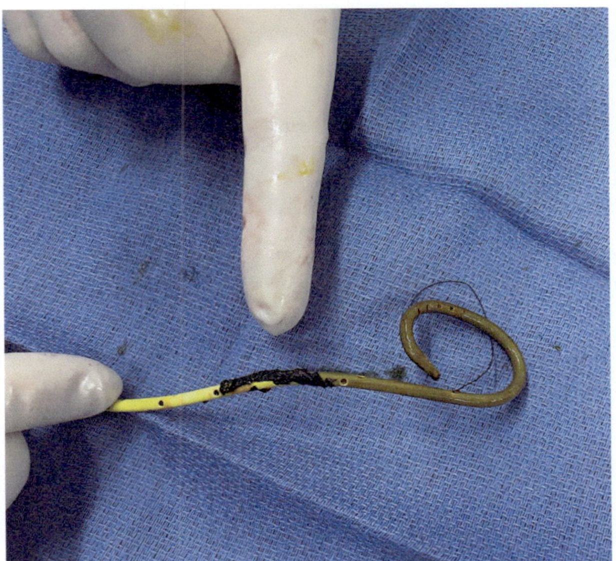

Fig. 67.7 Table top image of the biliary catheter immediately after its exchange at the end of the procedure demonstrates the black EVOH agent on the catheter, further affirming the arterio-biliary fistula

Use of a Ventricular Septal Defect Device to Seal a Post-Ablation Gallbladder Wall Injury

68

Ziv J Haskal and Dylan Suttle

A 57-year-old man with hepatitis C cirrhosis presented with segment 2 and 5 hepatocellular carcinoma (Fig. 68.1). His MELD score was 11, alpha-fetoprotein level 36. The segment 2 tumor was successfully chemoembolized; however, the 4 cm segment 5 tumor vessels could not be isolated from cystic arteries (Fig. 68.2). He underwent microwave ablation of that mass 2.5 weeks later with two microwave antennae (Neuwave) activated for 9 min at 65 W (Fig. 68.3); the antennae were positioned back from the GB wall.

On day 3, he developed fever, leukocytosis, and elevation of liver function tests. CT demonstrated that the ablation zone had encompassed the gallbladder (GB) wall (Fig. 68.4); an externally draining cholecystostomy catheter was placed, he improved, and was discharged with antibiotics. Catheter

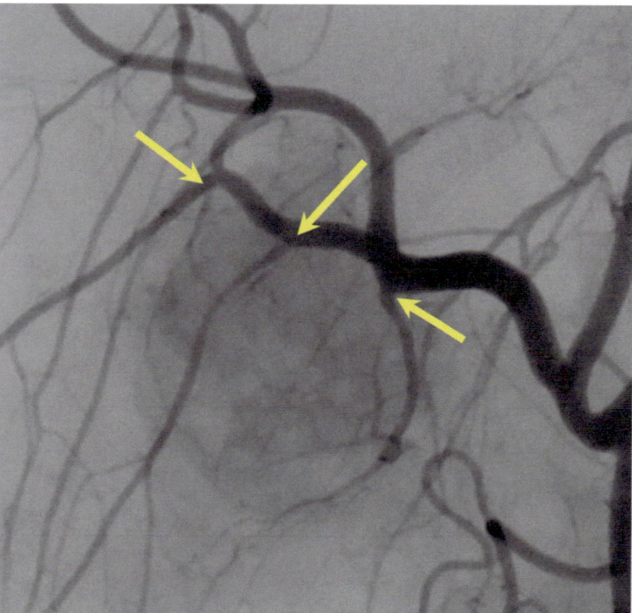

Fig. 68.2 Cropped image from a digital subtraction common hepatic angiogram demonstrates the tumor and near imperceptible small arteries supplying it (yellow arteries). Catheterization of several of these demonstrated dual supply to both tumor and gallbladder (not shown)

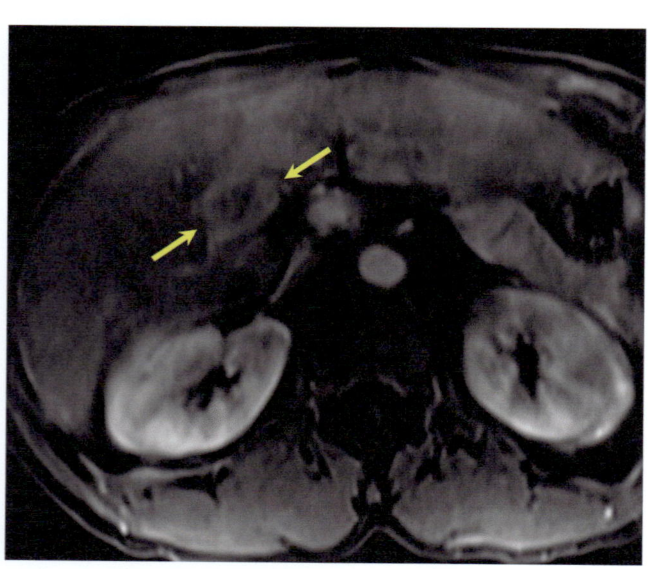

Fig. 68.1 Axial image from an MRI demonstrates the mass (yellow arrows). This abutted the gallbladder

studies at 1, 2, and 3 months demonstrated no cystic duct; however, output persisted at >50 cc/day. At 4 months, a large GB wall defect and fistula into the ablation cavity was first demonstrated (Fig. 68.4). Open cholecystectomy was dismissed as too high a risk.

A 10 mm × 7 mm muscular ventriculoseptal defect closure device (Amplatzer) was deployed across the GB wall defect. Immediate 1- and 2-month contrast studies showed a complete seal of the fistula. After a capped asymptomatic period of 2 months, the GB catheter was removed (Fig. 68.5). He remained asymptomatic at 1-year follow-up (Fig. 68.6).

Whilst juxta-gallbladder thermal ablations have been reported as safe and accomplishable, there remain uncertainties about predicted vs. achieved ablation zones, especially with heat, compared with cryoablation wherein the iceball might potentially be monitored and controlled. This nonvascular use of a cardiologic occluder in this setting is new; however, other atypical uses have been described, such as aortic pseudoaneurysms.

Z. J Haskal (✉)
Department of Radiology and Medical Imaging, Interventional Division, University of Virginia, Charlottesville, VA, USA

D. Suttle
Greensboro Radiology, Greensboro, NC, USA
e-mail: Dylan.suttle@radpartners.com

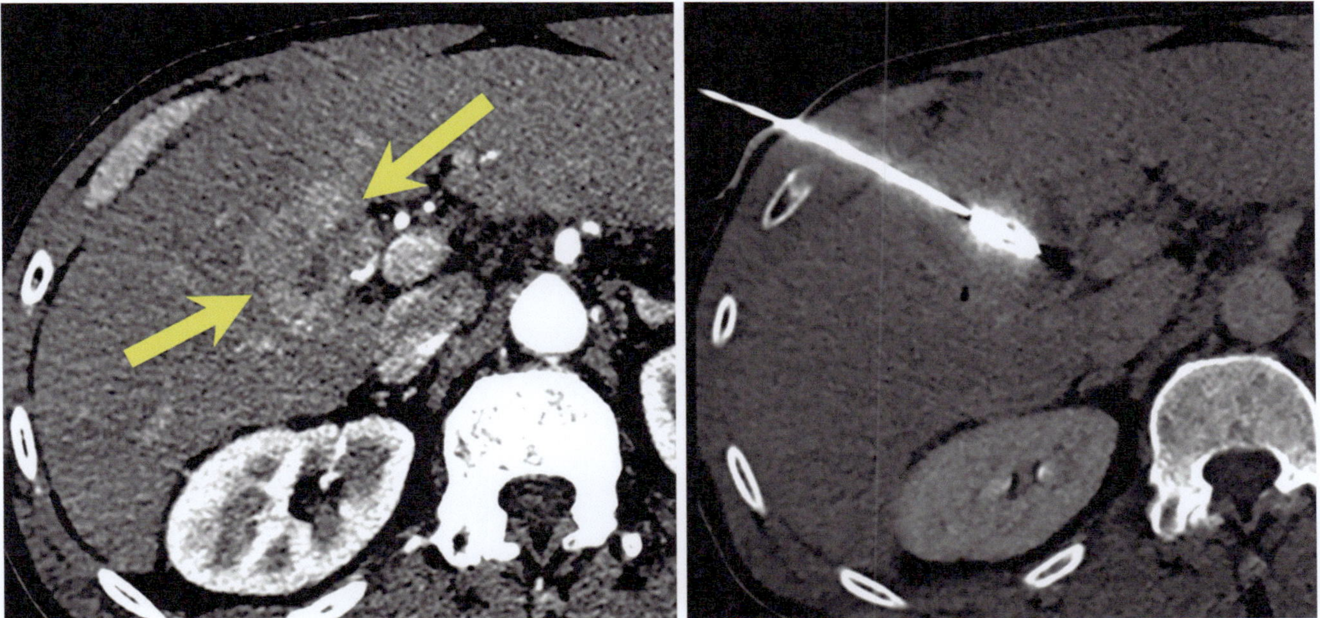

Fig. 68.3 Intraprocedural CT images during ablation show the enhancing mass (arrows, left) and position of one of the two MWA antenna (right)

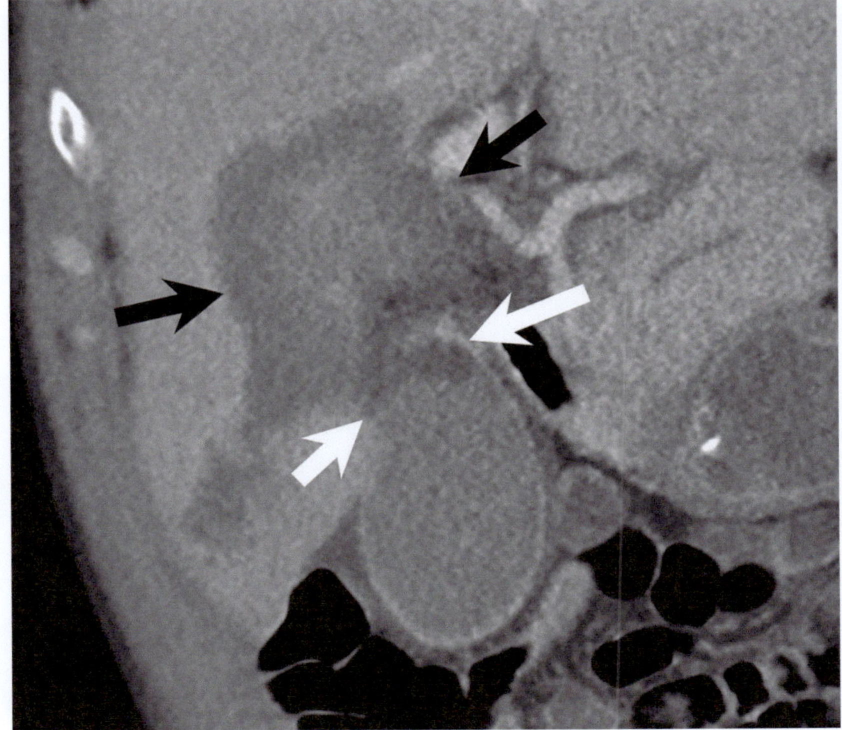

Fig. 68.4 Post-ablation coronal CT image 3 days after ablation demonstrates the defect in the GB wall (white arrows) in contact with the ablation cavity (black arrows)

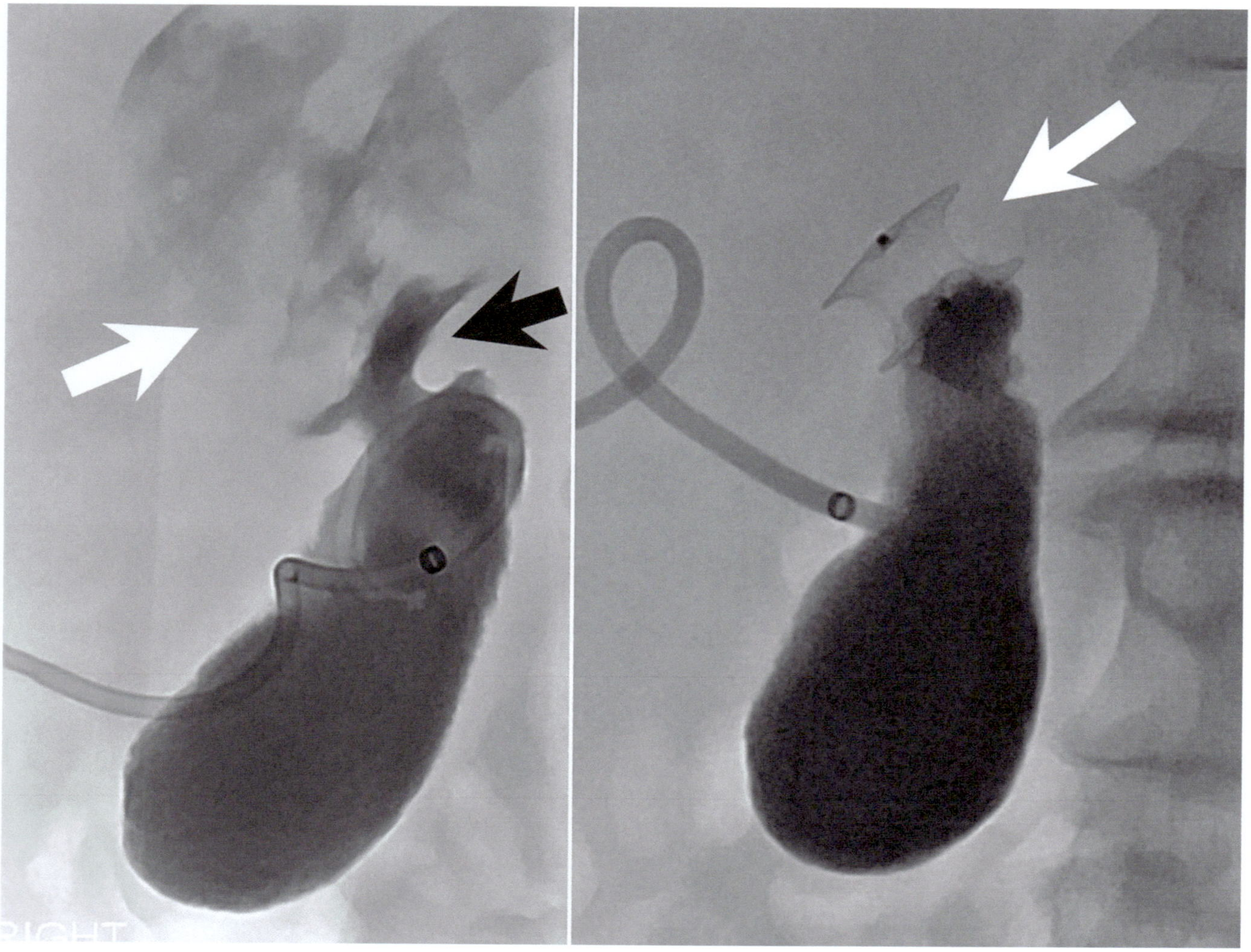

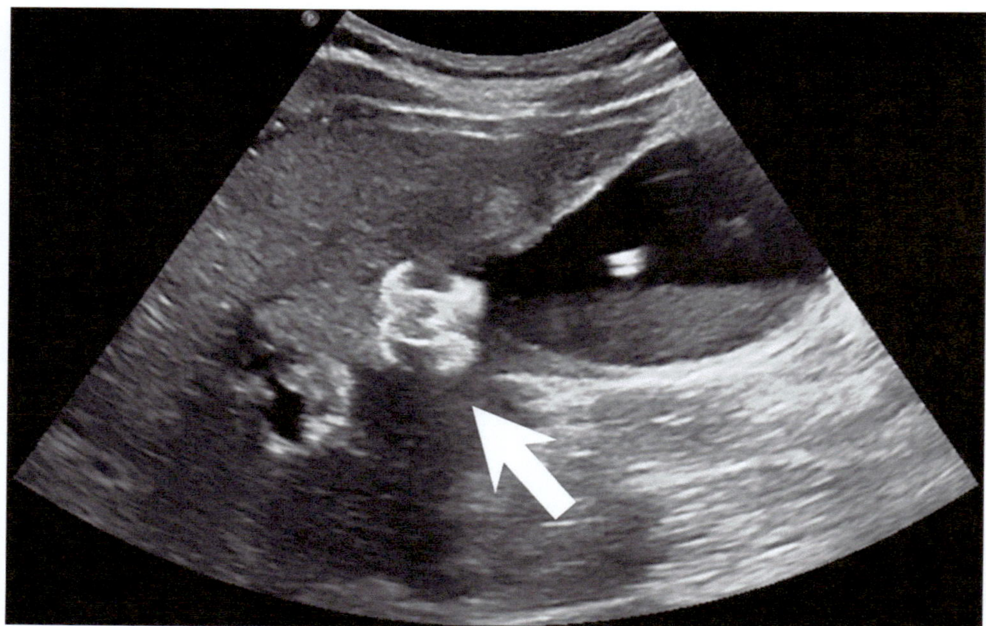

Fig. 68.5 The GB fistula (black arrow) into the ablation cavity (white arrow) is demonstrated (left). The deployed muscular VSD device has been deployed and no further leak is present (white arrow)

Fig. 68.6 Follow-up sonogram demonstrates the VSD device adjacent to the partly sludge-filled thin-walled gallbladder

Complete Response to Intra-arterial Therapy of an Infiltrative Hepatocellular Carcinoma with Extensive Parasitization

Daniel Y. Sze

A 60-year-old man with fatty liver and obesity reported unintentional weight loss, early satiety, postprandial pain, and asthenia resulting in disability from employment. Tests showed normal liver function and alpha fetoprotein (AFP) of 22,131 ng/mL. Computed tomography (CT) revealed a 17 cm infiltrative mass occupying the left lobe with mass effect on the stomach (Fig. 69.1). At the time of mapping angiography for radioembolization, conventional transarterial chemoembolization (cTACE) was performed on parasitized branches of the right gastric artery (Fig. 69.2). The left lobe was treated with glass microspheres at a dose of 190 Gy.

Two months later, the mass was smaller, pain had improved, and AFP was 9648, but new portal vein tumor invasion was diagnosed (Fig. 69.3). In 3 treatments over the following 3 months, additional cTACE was performed on parasitized branches of the right gastroepiploic artery

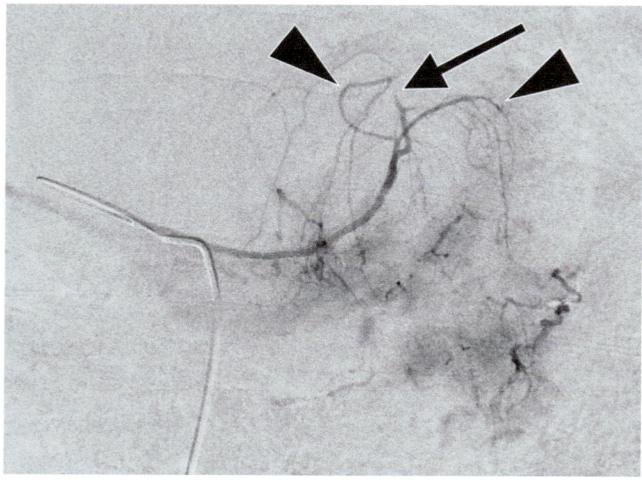

Fig. 69.2 Digital subtraction angiogram (DSA) of the right gastric artery confirmed parasitization of two branches (arrowheads) by the tumor, which was treated with conventional transarterial chemoembolization (cTACE). Note competitive flow from the left gastric artery (arrow). The main tumor was treated with radioembolization

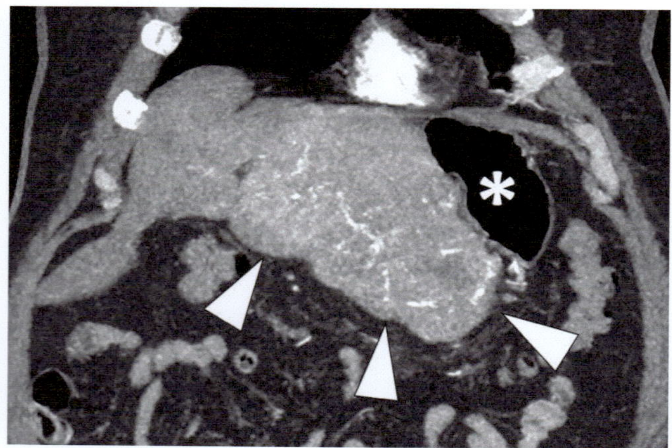

Fig. 69.1 Oblique coronal reformat of arterial phase computed tomography (CT) showed an exophytic 17 cm hepatocellular carcinoma in the left lobe (arrowheads), displacing the stomach (asterisk)

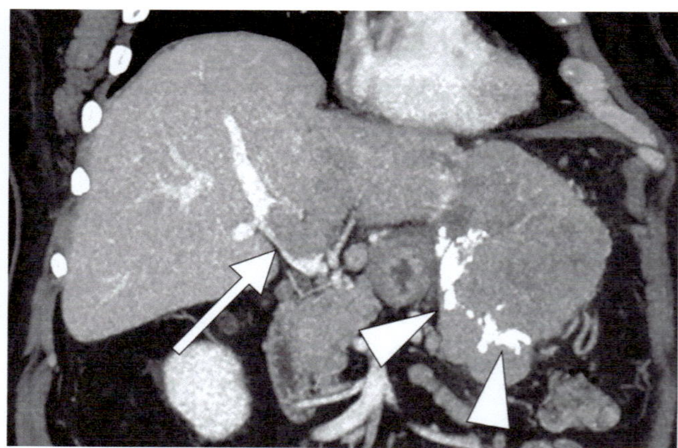

Fig. 69.3 Oblique coronal reformat of portal phase CT showed new left and main portal vein tumor invasion (arrow). Note retained lipiodol from previous right gastric artery branch cTACE (arrowheads)

(Fig. 69.4), right inferior phrenic artery (Fig. 69.5), left superior epigastric artery, left musculophrenic artery (Fig. 69.6), right superior epigastric artery, and additional branches of the right gastroepiploic artery.

This case was presented in the Extreme IR session at the Society of Interventional Radiology Annual Scientific Meeting in Austin, TX, March, 2019.

D. Y. Sze (✉)
Division of Interventional Radiology, Stanford University, Stanford, CA, USA
e-mail: dansze@stanford.edu

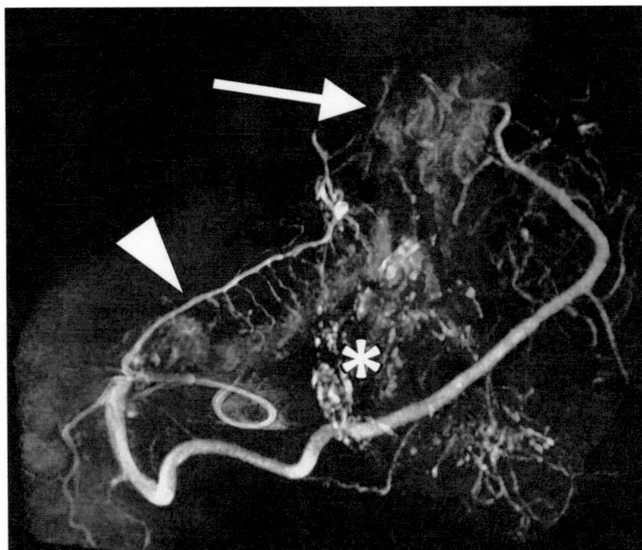

Fig. 69.4 Right anterior oblique maximum intensity projection of a cone beam CT with injection of contrast medium into the gastroduodenal artery (GDA) confirmed parasitized supply to the tumor from the right gastroepiploic artery (arrow), which was treated with cTACE after coil embolization of branches supplying normal stomach. The right gastric artery (arrowhead) no longer supplied the tumor after previous cTACE of parasitized branches, resulting in retained lipiodol (asterisk)

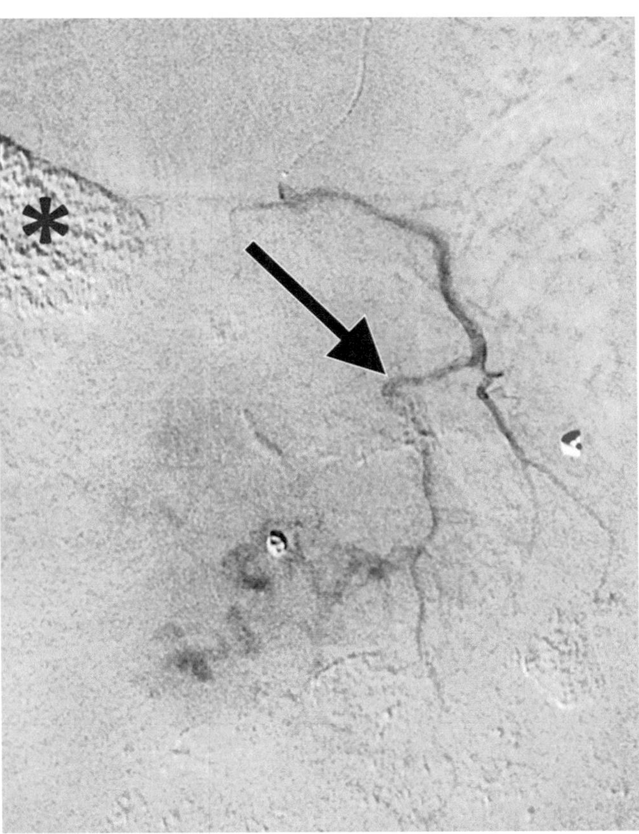

Fig. 69.6 DSA of the left musculophrenic artery (arrow) showed parasitized supply to the anterior aspect of the mass, which was treated with cTACE after application of ice to the abdominal wall to limit cutaneous nontarget deposition. Branches of the left and right superior epigastric arteries were also treated (not shown), all from left radial artery access. Note retained lipiodol from treatment of vena caval branch (asterisk) and small embolization coils from previous treatment of the gastroepiploic artery

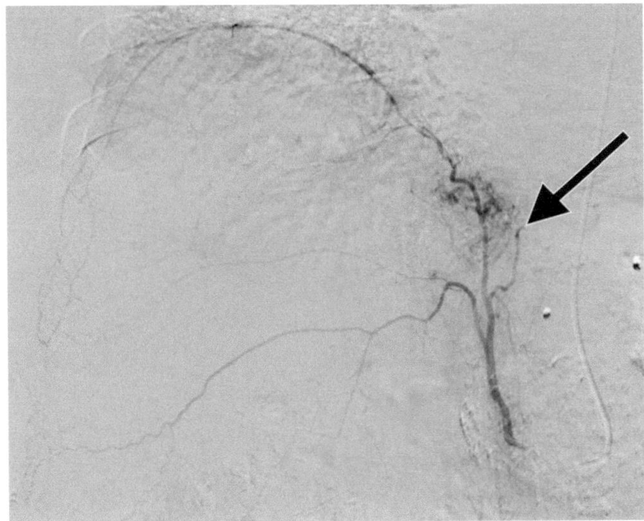

Fig. 69.5 DSA of the right inferior phrenic artery confirmed parasitized supply to the paracaval subsegment of segment 1 from the vena caval branch (arrow), which was treated with cTACE

AFP dropped to 3287, tumor thrombus was devitalized and stained with lipiodol, but a large portion of the tumor remained viable. CT angiography identified parasitization of the superior mesenteric artery; the posterior leaf omental branch of the middle colic artery (Fig. 69.7) was treated with cTACE. Two months later, AFP was 2.4 and CT showed a patent main portal vein and no residual viable tumor.

The patient regained performance status of 0, intentionally lost 31 kg, and returned to employment. AFP has remained <2 for 49 months since the last cTACE (Fig. 69.8).

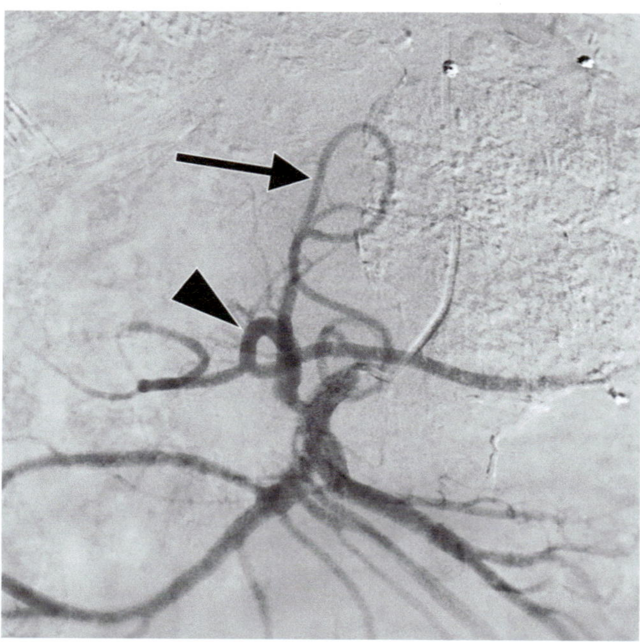

Fig. 69.7 DSA of the superior mesenteric artery showed the middle colic artery (arrowhead) giving rise to a tortuous posterior leaf greater omental artery (arrow), parasitized to supply the tumor, which was treated with cTACE

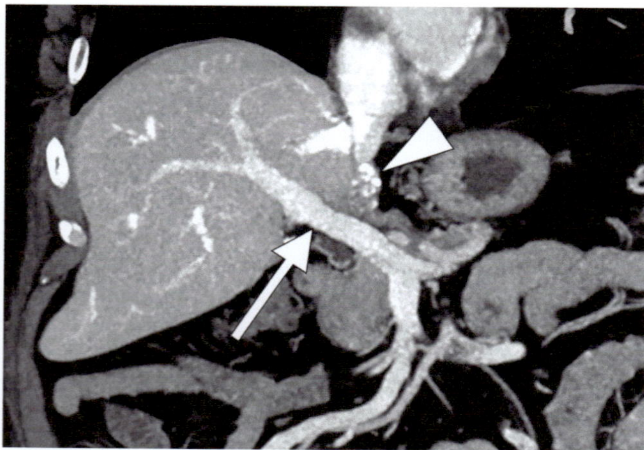

Fig. 69.8 Oblique coronal reformat of portal phase CT performed 17 months after last cTACE treatment showed resolution of main portal venous invasion (arrow). Note retained lipiodol in paracaval subsegment of segment 1 (arrowhead). Residual 7 cm nonviable tumor was situated anterior to the gastric fundus, out of plane and not depicted

Bibliography

1. Chung JW, Kim HC, Yoon JH, Lee HS, Jae HJ, Lee W, Park JH. Transcatheter arterial chemoembolization of hepatocellular carcinoma: prevalence and causative factors of extrahepatic collateral arteries in 479 patients. Korean J Radiol. 2006;7:257–66.

Leigh Casadaban and Siddharth A. Padia

A 65-year-old male with hepatitis C virus, Child-Pugh A cirrhosis, hepatocellular carcinoma (HCC), and three prior chemoembolizations at an outside facility, presented with tumor recurrence. Imaging showed multifocal HCC without vascular invasion or extrahepatic disease (Fig. 70.1).

Celiac angiography showed hepatic artery atresia and minimal perfusion of a 5.8 cm arterially enhancing segment 2 tumor (Fig. 70.2). Angiography of the thoracic and lumbar arteries, right and left inferior phrenic arteries, right coronary and left anterior descending artery failed to show perfusion of tumor. Finally, catheterization of the right and left internal mammary arteries (RIMA and LIMA) demonstrated a single branch from each supplying the segment 2 hypervascular tumor, confirmed with cone-beam CT (Figs. 70.3, 70.4, 70.5, and 70.6).

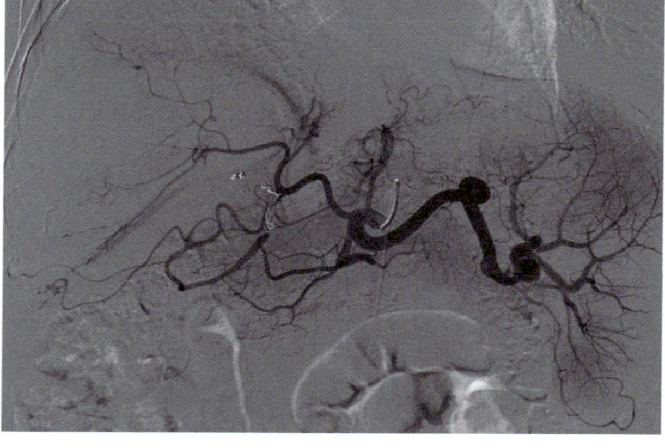

Fig. 70.2 Digital subtraction angiography from the celiac artery demonstrates irregular and pruned hepatic arteries and patchy parenchymal filing of the liver. Notably, there is minimal perfusion of the subcapsular hepatic segment 2 lesion

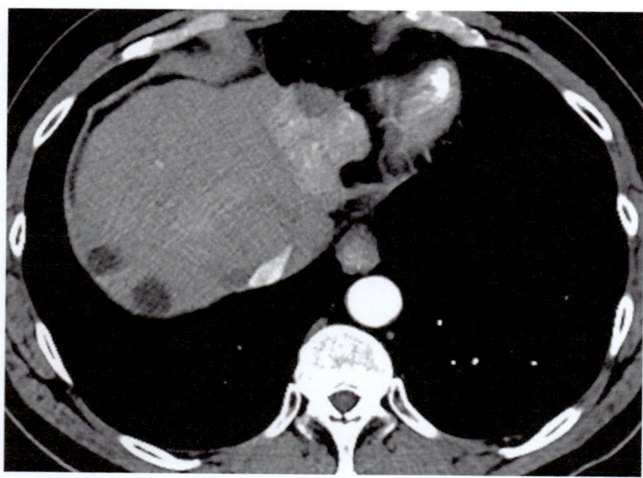

Fig. 70.1 Pre-procedural contrast-enhanced MRI demonstrates infiltrative tumor in hepatic segment 2, adjacent to the diaphragm, anterior abdominal wall and right ventricle

L. Casadaban
University of Colorado Anschutz Medical Campus,
Aurora, CO, USA
e-mail: Leigh.Casadaban@cuanschutz.edu

S. A. Padia (✉)
Division of Interventional Radiology, Department of Radiology,
David Geffen School of Medicine at University of California,
Los Angeles, CA, USA
e-mail: spadia@mednet.ucla.edu

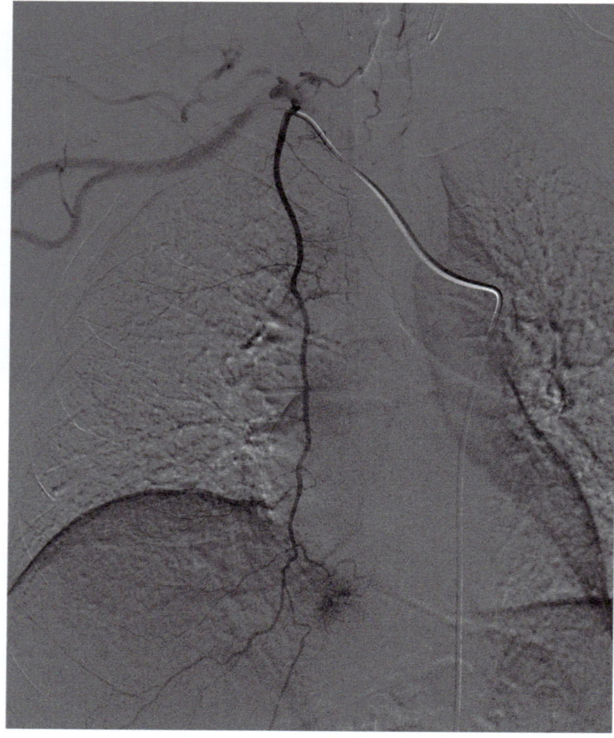

Fig. 70.3 Right internal mammary artery (RIMA) digital subtraction angiography demonstrates perfusion of hypervascular hepatic segment 2 tumor. Superselective catheterization of a single medial branch (arrow) is performed for ^{90}Y administration

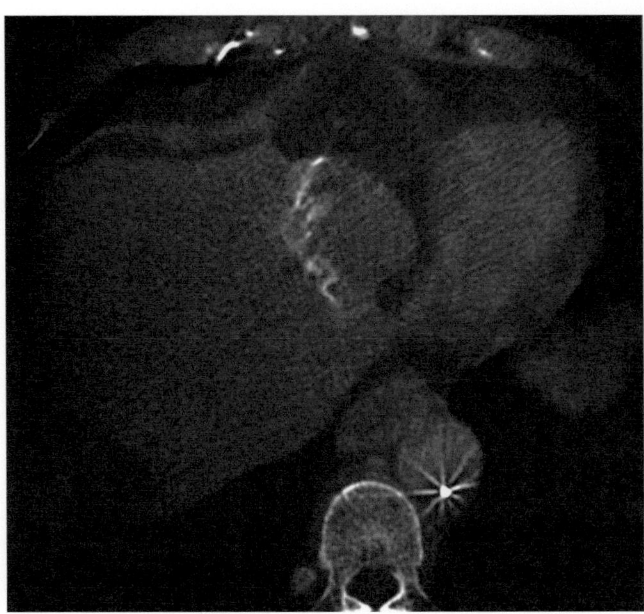

Fig. 70.4 Intra-procedure cone-beam CT of the abdomen with contrast injection into the RIMA confirms extrahepatic arterial supply to segment 2 tumor

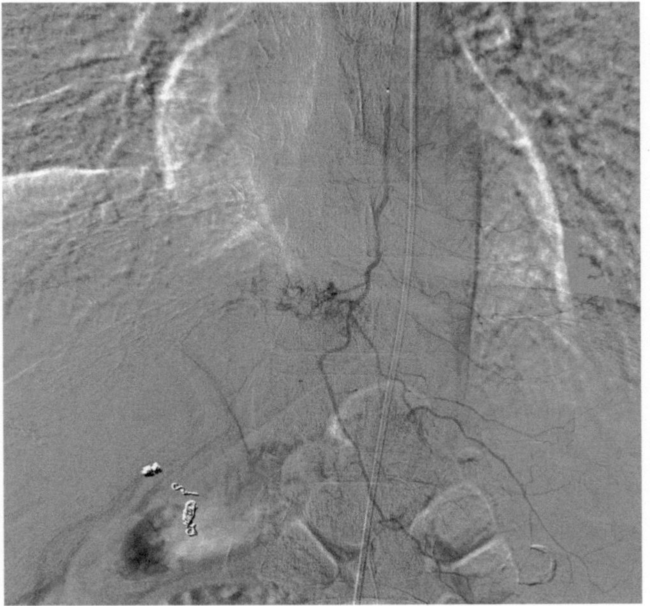

Fig. 70.5 Left internal mammary artery (LIMA) angiography demonstrates additional extrahepatic arterial supply to the hepatic segment 2 lesion. Superselective catheterization is performed for ^{90}Y administration (arrow)

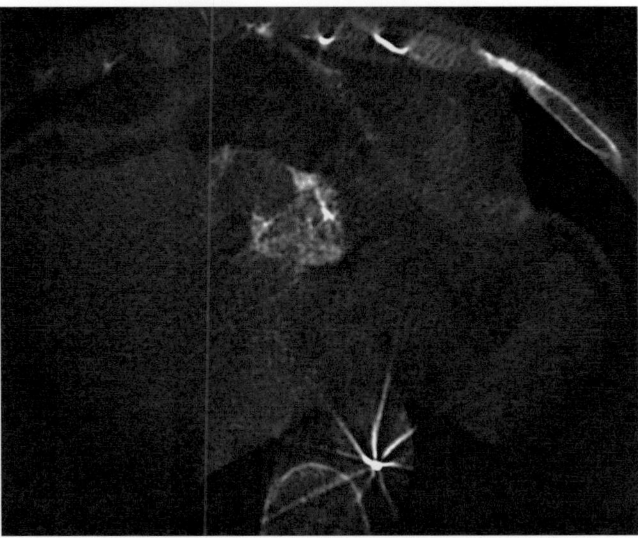

Fig. 70.6 Intra-procedure cone-beam CT of the abdomen with contrast injection into the LIMA confirms extra-hepatic arterial supply to segment 2 tumor

Superselective transarterial radioembolization with ^{90}Y was performed using 0.82 GBq doses of TheraSphere, (Boston Scientific Corporation, Marlborough, MA; 3 GBq vial of first week calibration) delivered into the RIMA, LIMA, and replaced left hepatic artery sharing a common trunk with the left gastric artery. Given the overlap in the treatment areas, the delivered dose to the tumor was approximately 800 Gy. The patient developed self-limiting superficial skin ulcerations over the epigastric region from non-target embolization 2 weeks later, which required no treatment (Fig. 70.7). Three- and 12-month post-procedure imaging demonstrated complete mRECIST response (Fig. 70.8).

Cutaneous injury from treating extrahepatic tumor supply via the RIMA and LIMA has been documented from other types of embolization [1–3]. Protective skin ice cooling and superselective catheterization can be used to minimize off-target effects.

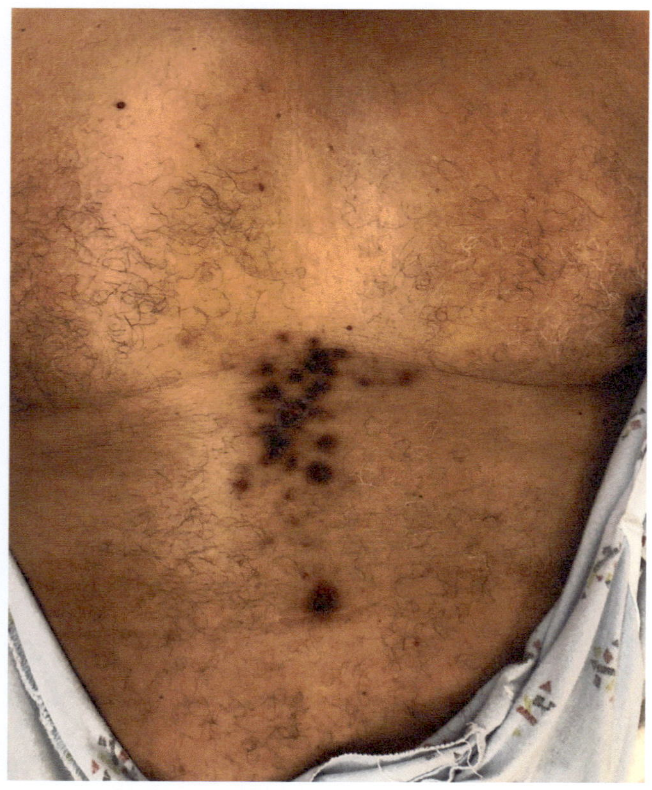

Fig. 70.7 Sub-centimeter cutaneous ulcerations and eschars from focal necrosis after radioembolization via the RIMA and LIMA

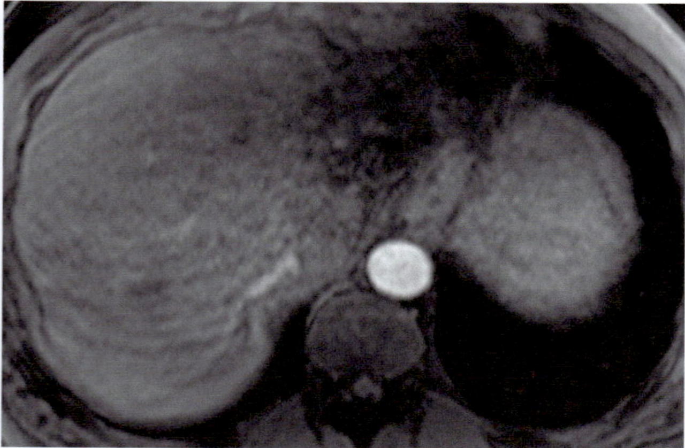

Fig. 70.8 Follow-up contrast-enhanced MR demonstrates complete mRECIST response

Bibliography

1. Miyayama S, Matsui O, Taki K, Minami T, Ryu Y, Ito C, et al. Extrahepatic blood supply to hepatocellular carcinoma: angiographic demonstration and transcatheter arterial chemoembolization. Cardiovasc Interv Radiol. 2006;29(1):39–48. https://doi.org/10.1007/s00270-004-0287-y.
2. Kajiwara K, Kakizawa H, Takeuchi N, Toyota N, Hieda M, Ishikawa M, et al. Cutaneous complications after transcatheter arterial treatment for hepatocellular carcinoma via the internal mammary artery: how to avoid this complication. Jpn J Radiol. 2011;29(5):307–15.
3. Kim H-C, Chung JW, Choi SH, Yoon J-H, Lee H-S, Jae HJ, et al. Hepatocellular carcinoma with internal mammary artery supply: feasibility and efficacy of transarterial chemoembolization and factors affecting patient prognosis. J Vasc Interv Radiol. 2007;18(5):611–9. quiz 620

Neoadjuvant TACE for IVC Leiomyosarcoma with Non-target Embolization

Lawrence Lin, Amanda Smolock, and William S. Rilling

A 50-year-old male presented with leiomyosarcoma of the IVC with hepatic invasion (Fig. 71.1). He did not respond to chemotherapy or radiation and was referred to IR for TACE. Right adrenal arteriography identified supply to the posterior portion of the tumor and chemoembolization was performed with doxorubicin, mitomycin C, and ethiodized oil (Figs. 71.2 and 71.3). Right testicular arteriography identified supply to the anterior portion of the tumor and a second TACE was performed with the same agents after coil protection of the proximal vessel (Figs. 71.4, 71.5, and 71.6). Despite this, there was non-target embolization to the scrotum through intercostal and lumbar collaterals, which was recognized immediately (Fig. 71.7). Fortunately, he had no adverse outcome from this event. After downstaging, the patient went on to have successful *en bloc* resection of this tumor with IVC reconstruction 4 months after his second TACE (Fig. 71.8). He lived for four and a half years after resection. This case demonstrates novel treatment of a rare malignancy, the variability in tumor vascular anatomy, and the constant vigilance needed during embolization.

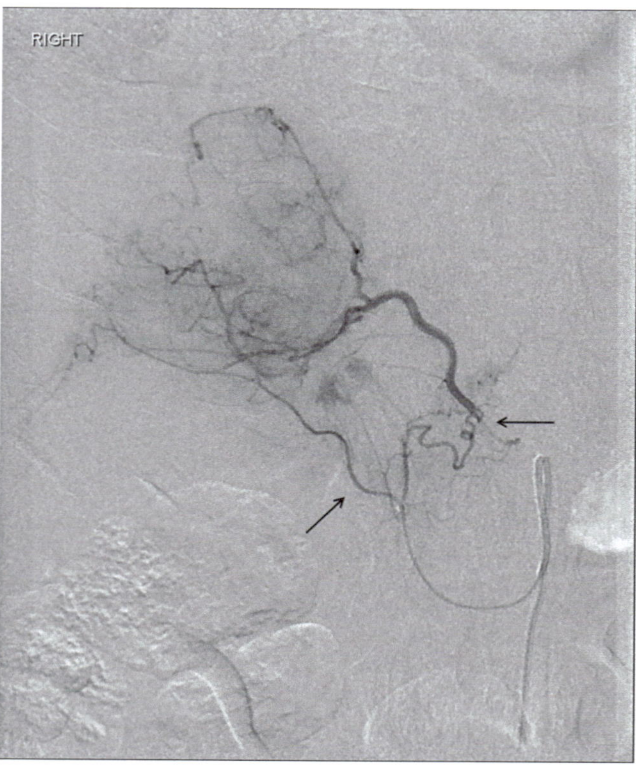

Fig. 71.2 Right adrenal arteriography demonstrates tortuous vessels supplying the posterior portion of the tumor (arrows). This was confirmed with cone beam CT. A non-target adrenal branch was coil-protected prior to chemoembolization (not shown)

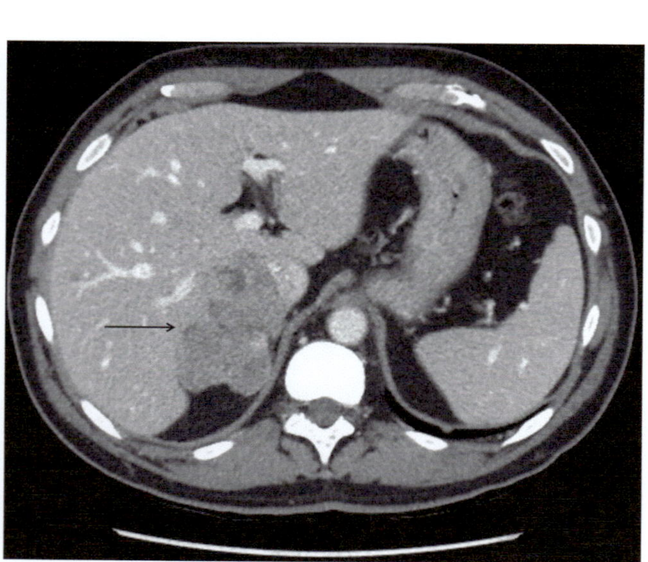

Fig. 71.1 Axial contrast-enhanced CT image demonstrates a large caval mass with hepatic invasion (arrow)

L. Lin · A. Smolock · W. S. Rilling (✉)
Division of Vascular and Interventional Radiology, Department of Radiology, Medical College of Wisconsin, Milwaukee, WI, USA
e-mail: lalin@mcw.edu; asmolock@mcw.edu; wrilling@mcw.edu

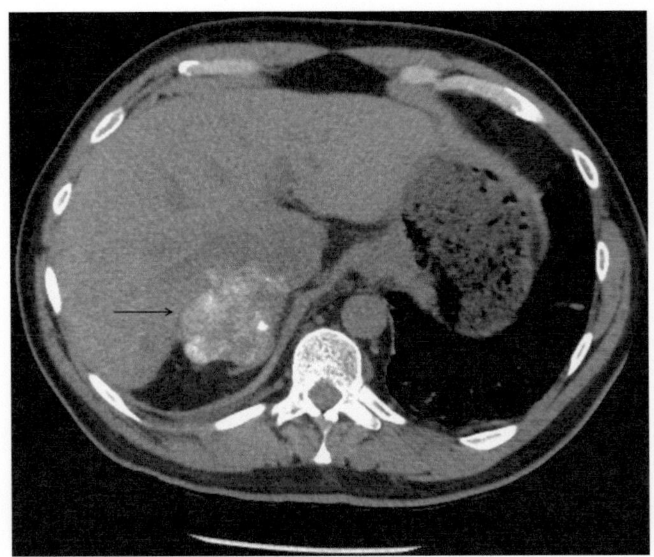

Fig. 71.3 Axial noncontrast CT image demonstrates ethiodized oil deposition in the posterior portion of the tumor (arrow)

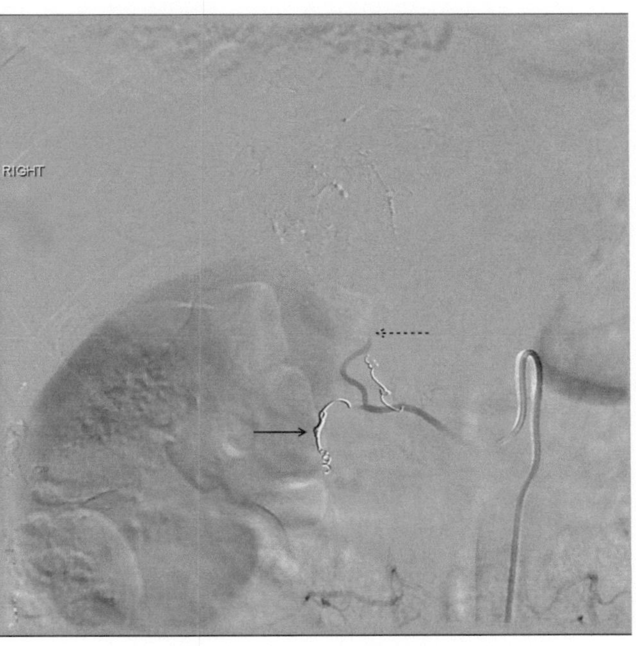

Fig. 71.5 Right testicular arteriography after coil protection of the proximal testicular branch vessel (solid arrow) and chemoembolization of the anterior portion of the tumor. There is pruning of tumor vascularity (dashed arrow)

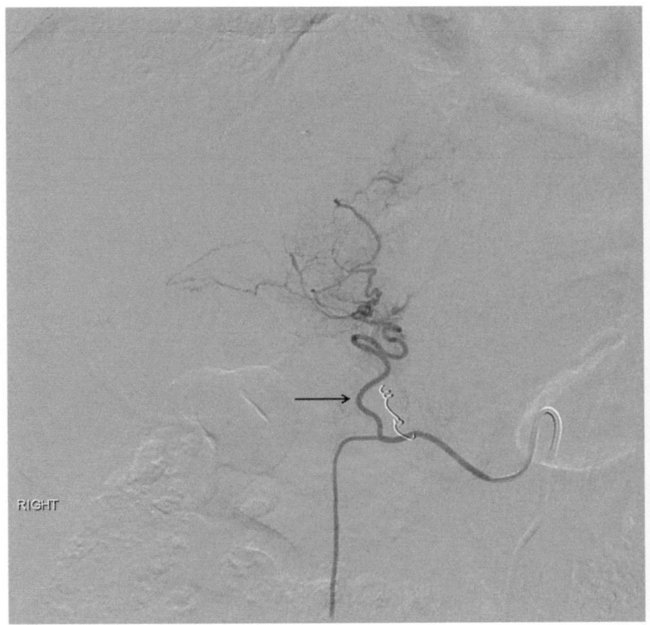

Fig. 71.4 Right testicular arteriography demonstrates a large superiorly directed parasitized branch vessel supplying the anterior portion of the tumor (arrow). This was confirmed with cone beam CT. Coil in a right adrenal artery branch from prior treatment is seen

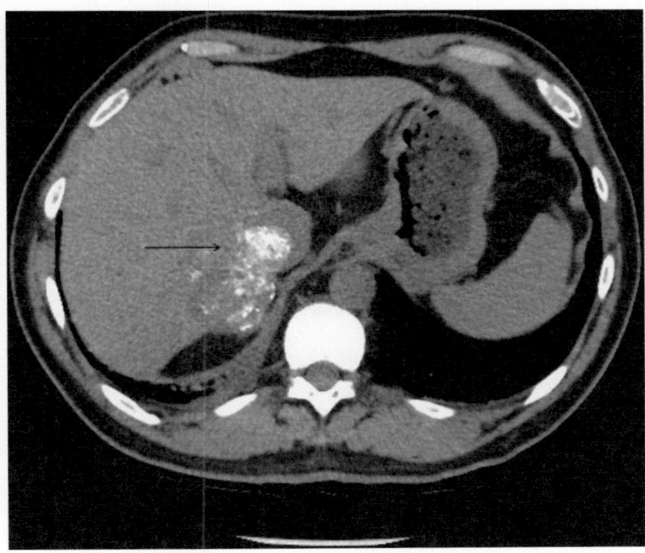

Fig. 71.6 Axial noncontrast CT image demonstrates ethiodized oil deposition in the anterior portion of the tumor (arrow)

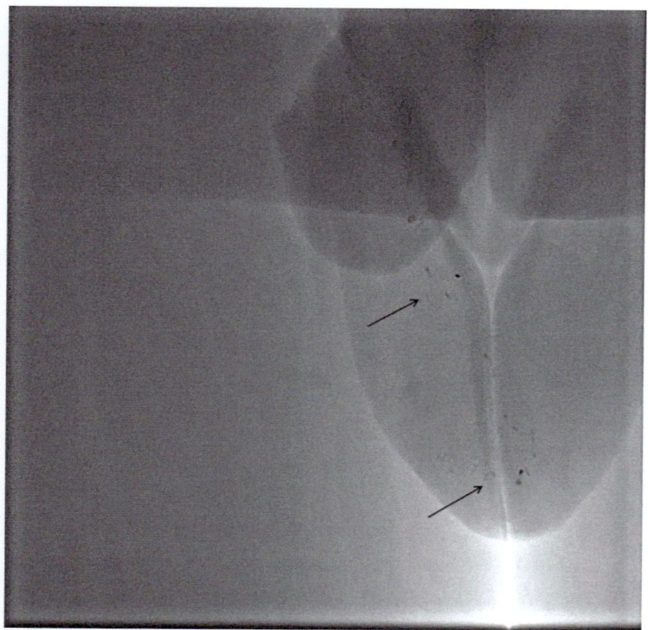

Fig. 71.7 Fluoroscopic image demonstrates ethiodized oil droplets in the scrotum from non-target embolization (arrows)

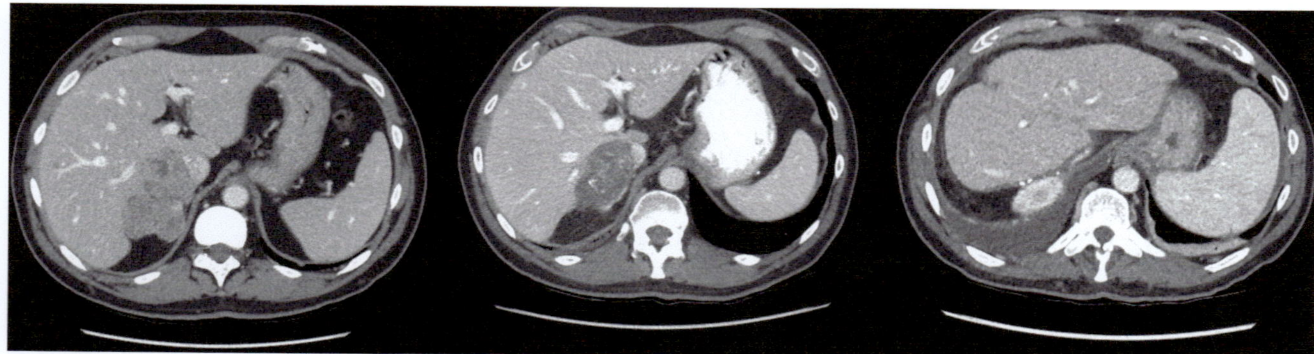

Fig. 71.8 Summary images including pre-treatment (left panel), three and a half months post-TACE (middle panel), and one and a half months post-resection (right panel)

Janesh Lakhoo and Daniel B. Brown

A 57-year-old female initially diagnosed with a sacral chordoma at age 54 was initially treated with primary resection, followed by adjuvant radiation. She had local recurrence at age 56 and underwent neoadjuvant radiation therapy and repeat resection. She was started on Erlotinib adjuvant chemotherapy in the setting of positive resection margins. She unfortunately presented once again at age 57 with local progression into the right hemi-pelvis measuring 9.0 × 9.3 × 4.0 cm (Fig. 72.1a, b). The mass involved the right hip joint with marked destruction of the acetabulum and ischium and extended into the right sacroiliac joint. She presented with severe pain and spent much of the day in the left lateral decubitus position. Our team was consulted for debulking cryoablation for symptomatic management.

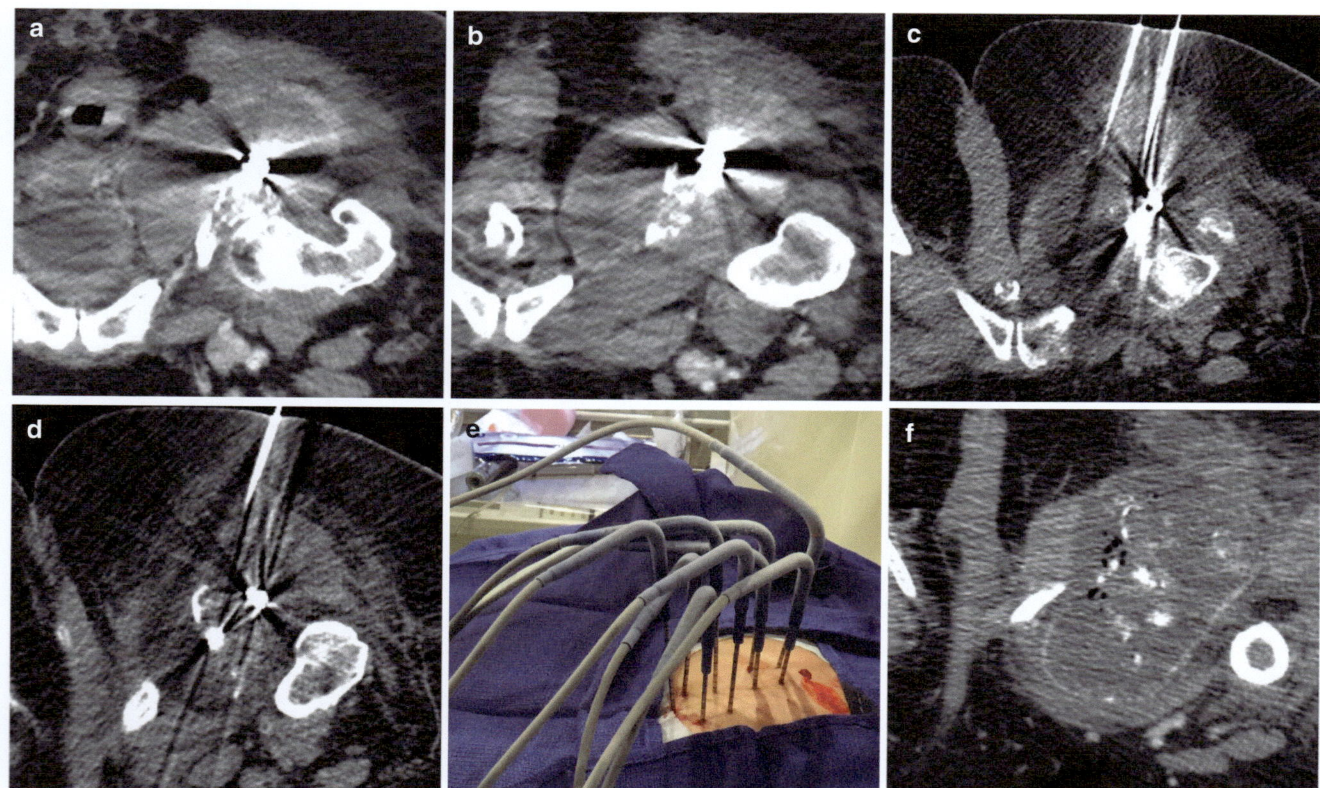

Fig. 72.1 (**a, b**) Recurrent chordoma measuring 9.0 × 9.3 × 4.0 cm presented with the patient in prone position for diagnostic scanning. (**c, d**) The mass was treated with nine IceEdge™ (Boston Scientific) cryoablation needles. Images c, d demonstrate the resulting 9.6 cm ice ball which covered the majority of the mass. (**e**) The cryoprobe array is shown in situ. (**f**) Follow-up imaging demonstrates necrotic changes with dystrophic calcification

J. Lakhoo · D. B. Brown (✉)
Department of Radiology, Vanderbilt University Medical Center, Nashville, TN, USA
e-mail: daniel.b.brown@vumc.org

Nine IceEdge™ (Boston Scientific, Watertown, MA) needles were placed into the mass extending from the inferior margin of the ischial tuberosity to the sciatic notch (Fig. 72.1c–e). Cryoablation was performed with two 10-min ablations with an interval 5-min passive thaw. The ice ball covered the entire ischial tuberosity during this period with a 9.6 cm maximal diameter. Following the freeze, a 15-min active thaw was performed. At 1 month imaging follow-up, the mass continued to progress although the debulking procedure improved her pain enough to allow her to sit upright (Fig. 72.1f).

Shockingly Cold: Irreversible Electroporation and Cryoablation of Periportal Nodal and Serosal Metastases

Uei Pua

A 73-year-old woman underwent mastectomy for right breast carcinoma 9 years earlier, with subsequent chemotherapy for lung metastases, liver metastasectomies, and peripancreatic metastatic nodal resection. She presented with induced oligometastases with a large 4.5 × 4 cm periportal lymph node (Fig. 73.1, circle) and a 3.8 × 3.6 cm serosal metastasis on the ascending colon (Fig. 73.1, arrow).

The periportal lymph node was first ablated using four cryoablation probes (IceFORE, Boston Scientific, Marlborough, MA) under ultrasound and CT guidance (Fig. 73.2). For the serosal metastasis, decision was made to perform irreversible electroporation (IRE) to the portion of the tumor adjacent to the bowel loop with a 5 mm safety distance (Fig. 73.3, curved arrow), followed by cryoablation of the bulk of the tumor (Fig. 73.3, curved arrow)), overlapping into the IRE ablation zone. Two IRE probes (Nanoknife, Angiodynamics Inc., Netherlands) were positioned in the cranio-caudal direction and ablation performed using 3 cm tip exposure with 2000 V delivered for 120 pulses. With the IRE probes left in place as markers. Two cryoablation probes (ICEFORCE) was then inserted in the bulk of the tumor and ablation performed with real-time monitoring to ensure ice ball overlap into the IRE probes but not encroach into the colon (Fig. 73.4 curved arrow and Fig. 73.5). The patient was discharged well with no complications.

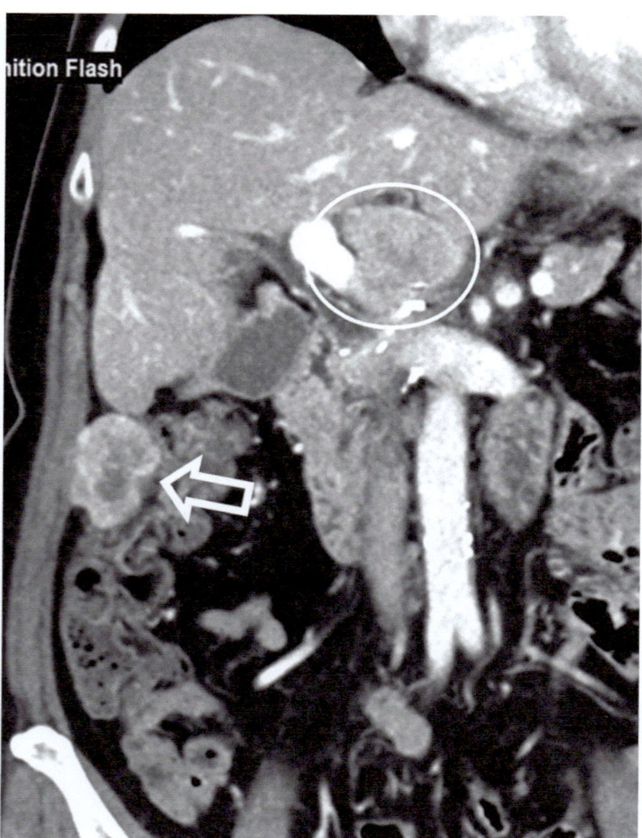

Fig. 73.1 Induced oligometastasis, in the form of periportal lymphadenopathy (circle) and serosal metastasis along the ascending colon (arrow)

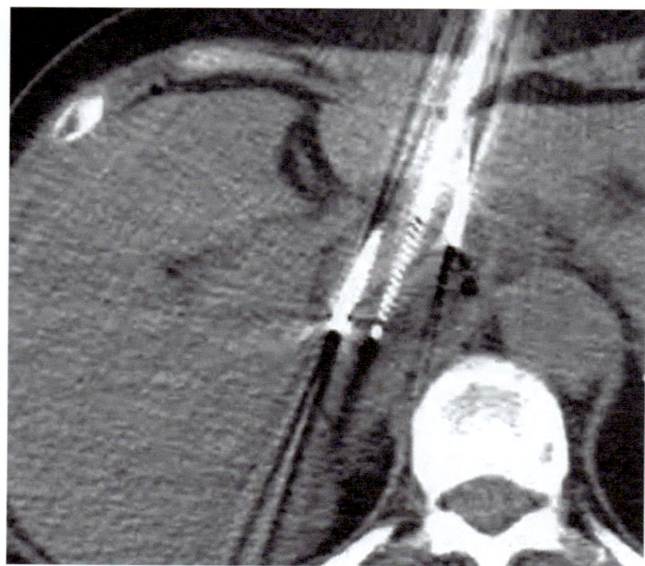

Fig. 73.2 CT image of the cryoprobes within the periportal lymph node with ice ball formation

U. Pua (✉)
Department of Diagnostic Radiology, Tan Tock Seng Hospital, Singapore, Singapore

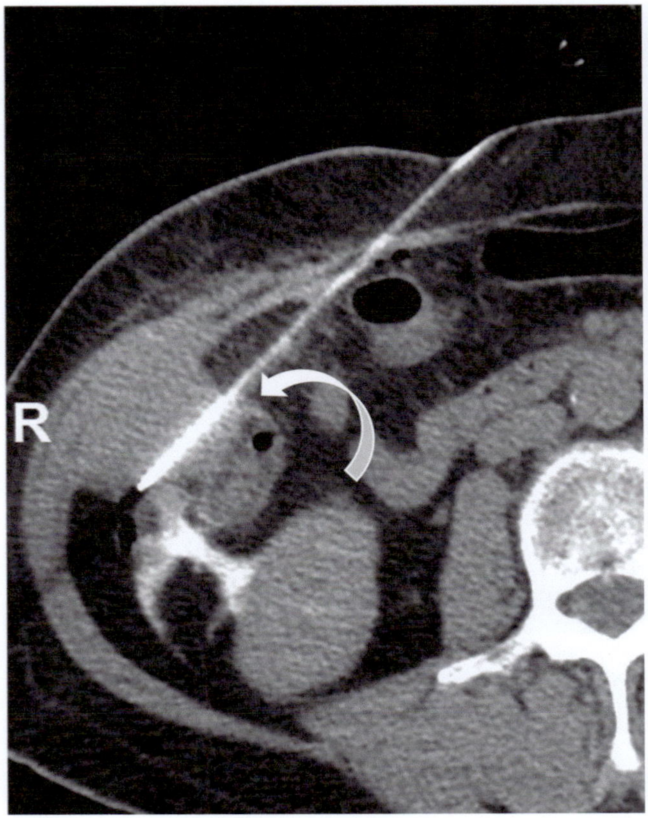

Fig. 73.3 CT image of one of the IRE probes inserted into the serosal metastasis with 5 mm safety margin from the colonic wall (curved arrow)

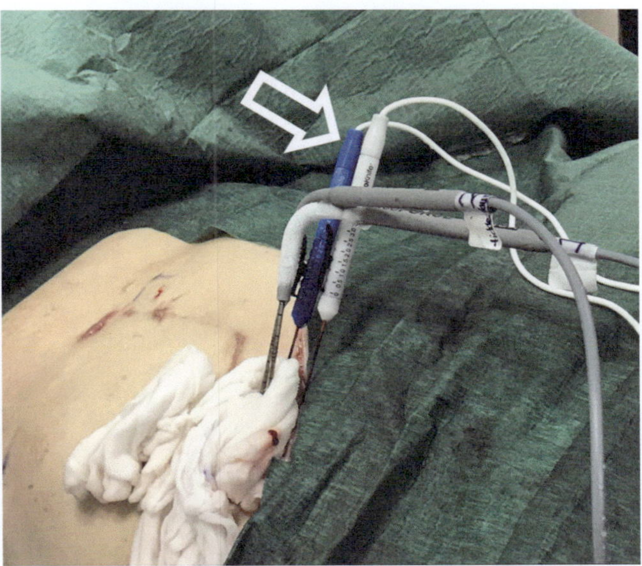

Fig. 73.5 Photo of the position of the IRE probes (medial and superior, white arrow) and the cryoablation probes. Note the presence of warm gauze for skin protection during cryoablation

The patient remained well at 24 months with non-enhancement and significant reduction in size of the periportal lymph node (Fig. 73.6, left pre and right 24 months) and near-complete involution of the serosal metastasis (Fig. 73.7, left pre- and right 24 months) save for a subcentimeter enhancing nodule in the paracolic region which was kept on surveillance.

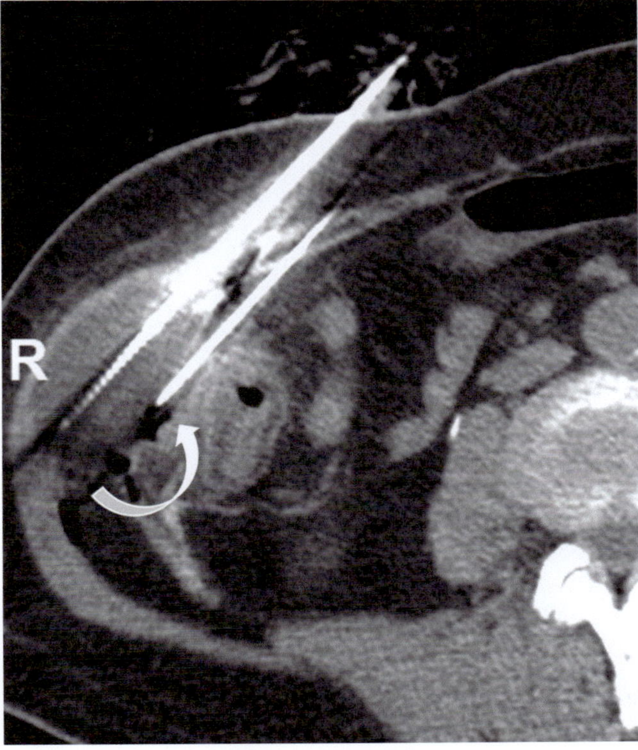

Fig. 73.4 CT image of overlap of the ice ball into the IRE probe but not onto the colonic wall (arrow)

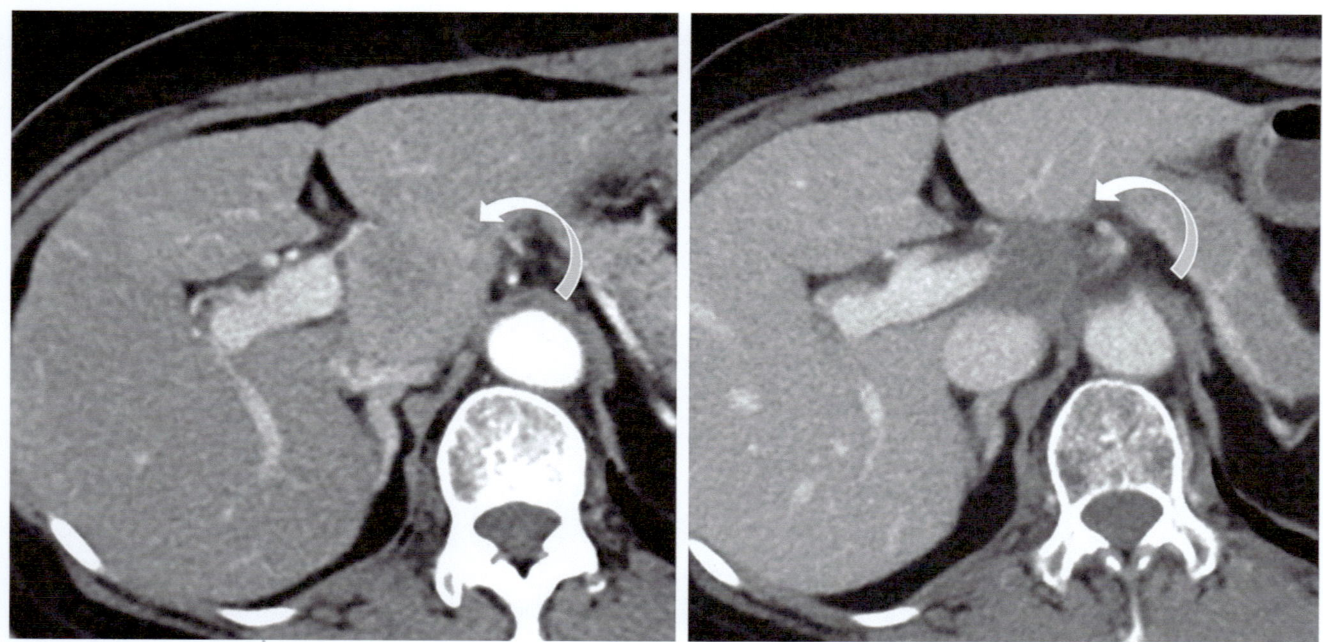

Fig. 73.6 CT of the periportal mass (arrows): left (pre-ablation), right (24 months), showing non-enhancement with significant size reduction

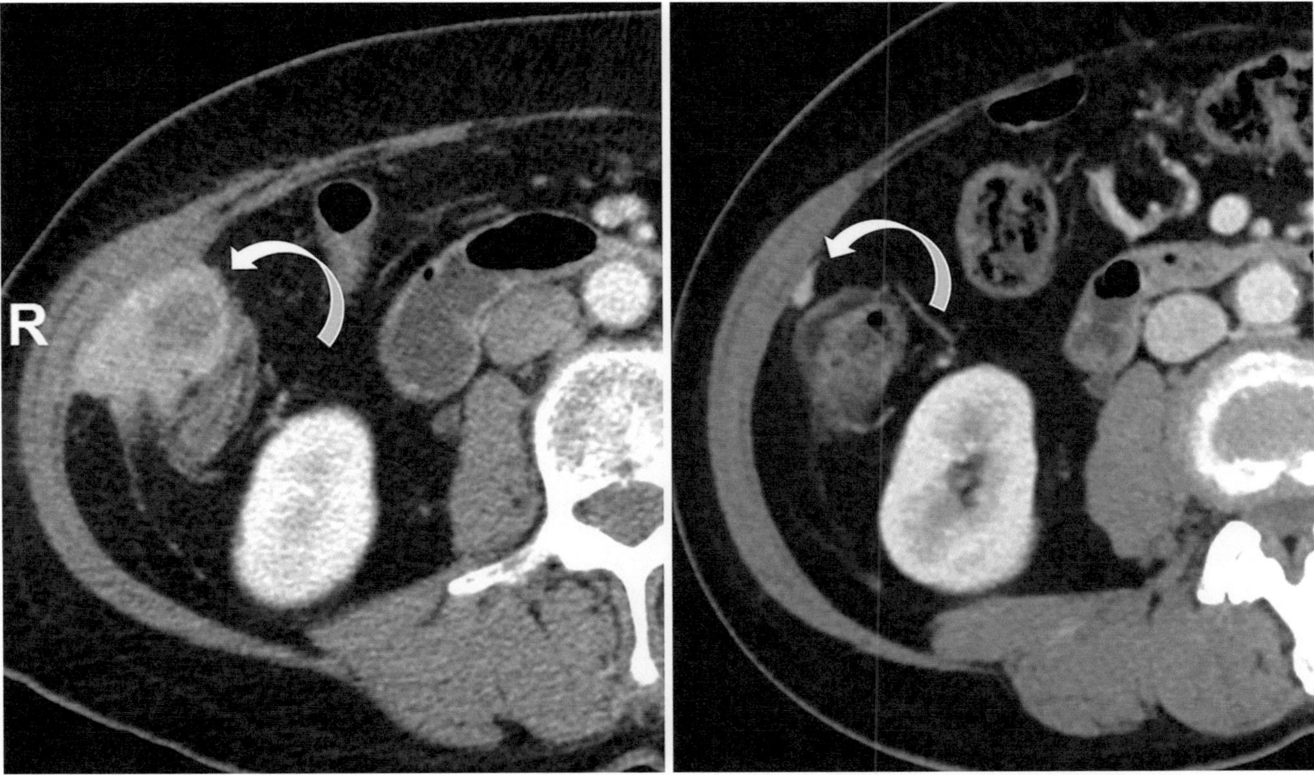

Fig. 73.7 CT of the serosal metastasis (arrows): left (pre-ablation), right (24 months), showing near-complete involution of the metastasis with a subcentimeter residual nodule which was kept on surveillance

Roberto Luigi Cazzato, Christian Debry, Julien Garnon, and Afshin Gangi

A 54-year-old male patient presented with a local adenocarcinoma recurrence of the right maxillary sinus (arrow; Fig. 74.1a). Previous relevant clinical history included three different surgical resections of the right ethmoid bone and one resection of the sphenoid bone due to a head and neck (H&N) adenocarcinoma, along with two sessions of radiation therapy resulting into the maximal allowed radiation dose. Given the lack of chances for further potentially curative (i.e., surgery, radiation therapy) treatments, salvage cryoablation was offered.

The patient underwent percutaneous CT-guided cryoablation with three different cryo probes (Ice Sphere, Boston Sc). General anesthesia was used and a double 10-min freezing cycle was performed, which resulted in an ice ball largely encompassing the tumor (arrows, Fig. 74.1b, c). The patient underwent regular MRI follow-up, which allowed the detection of a nodular infra-centimetric enhancement (arrow, Fig. 74.1d), being in favor of a local tumor recurrence in the ablation zone. A second salvage cryoablation was therefore performed by applying two cryo probes (Ice Sphere, Boston Sc) as well as the same ablation protocol used during the first cryoablation. A large ice ball well-encompassing the tumor (arrow, Fig. 74.1e) was created also in this occasion. Thereafter, the patient continued his regular MRI follow-up, which showed complete local tumor control 38 months after the first cryoablation treatment (Fig. 74.1f).

Percutaneous cryoablation of H&N tumors has been sporadically reported, and in most of the cases, it has been performed with a palliative intent. Nevertheless, recent data pointed out a

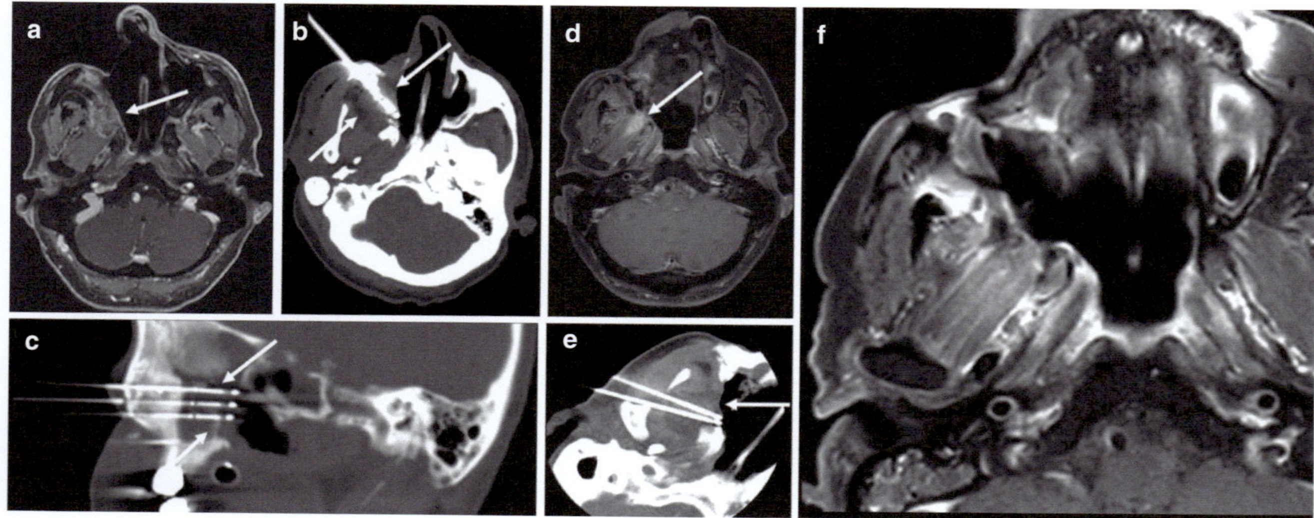

Fig. 74.1 (a) Axial contrast-enhanced T1-weighted MRI demonstrating the local adenocarcinoma recurrence at the right maxillary sinus (arrow). (b, c) Axial and sagittal CT images demonstrate the ice ball forming (arrows) around the multiple cryoprobes encompassing the tumor. (d) Follow-up axial contrast-enhanced T1-weighted MRI showing a small enhancing area deemed to represent local recurrence within the ablation zone (arrow); therefore a second session of cryoablation was organized. (e) Axial CT imaging shows cryoprobes within the mass during the second cryoablation. The ice ball is visible as an oval-shaped hypodense zone (arrow). (f) Contrast-enhanced T1-weighted MRI follow-up (38 months) showed complete local tumor control

R. L. Cazzato (✉) · J. Garnon · A. Gangi
Department of Interventional Radiology, University Hospital of Strasbourg, Strasbourg, France
e-mail: RobertoLuigi.CAZZATO@chru-strasbourg.fr

C. Debry
Department of Head and Neck Surgery, University Hospital of Strasbourg, Strasbourg, France

local tumor control rate of 45.4% at a mean follow-up of 11.7 months (range 3–34 months), thus revealing a potential curative role of cryoablation for patients with H&N tumor recurrences having exhausted all the available curative treatments.

Bibliography

1. Gangi A, Cebula H, Cazzato RL, Ramamurthy N, Garnon J, Debry C, Proust F. "Keeping a Cool Head": percutaneous imaging-guided cryo-ablation as salvage therapy for recurrent glioblastoma and head and neck tumours. Cardiovasc Interv Radiol. 2020;43(2):172–5. https://doi.org/10.1007/s00270-019-02384-6.

2. Schwartz J, Auloge P, Koch G, Robinson JM, Garnon J, Cazzato RL, Perruisseau-Carrier J, Debry C, Gangi A. Percutaneous cryoablation for recurrent head and neck tumors. Cardiovasc Interv Radiol. 2022;45(6):791–9. https://doi.org/10.1007/s00270-022-03120-3.

3. Guenette JP, Tuncali K, Himes N, Shyn PB, Lee TCAJR. Percutaneous image-guided cryoablation of head and neck tumors for local control, preservation of functional status, and pain relief. Am J Roentgenol. 2017;208(2):453–8. https://doi.org/10.2214/AJR.16.16446.

MRI-Guided Cryoablation of a Frontal Glioblastoma Recurrence After Surgery and Chemo-Radiotherapy

Roberto Luigi Cazzato, Hélène Cebula, Julien Garnon, François Proust, and Afshin Gangi

A 54-year-old woman presented with a right frontal glioblastoma recurrence (arrow; Fig. 75.1a) 18 months after primary surgical resection and chemo-radiotherapy. Due to the lack of other standard therapeutic options, she was offered compassionate MRI-guided cryoablation. Following surgical exposure of the tumor under general anesthesia, the patient was transferred to the 1.5 T MRI unit; three ice probes (Ice Seed, Boston Sc) were directly inserted into the tumor under MRI-Fluoroscopy. A 10-min freezing cycle was performed with an ice ball largely encompassing the tumor (arrow, Fig. 75.1b). A surgical necrosectomy of the cryoablated area was subsequently performed to avoid any massive intracranial edema.

Three-month MRI follow-up demonstrated an enhancing mass (arrow; Fig. 75.1c) with surrounding edema at the treated site. A subsequent biopsy revealed necrotic (Fig. 75.1d) and peri-vascular inflammatory (Fig. 75.1e) changes without any viable tumor. At 5-month follow-up, the enhancing mass previously seen had significantly enlarged (arrow, Fig. 75.1f), and the patient became aphasic. Surprisingly, at 8-month MRI follow-up, the lesion had markedly shrunk (arrow, Fig. 75.1g) with subsequent resolution of the aphasia; no other concomitant treatments were used in the meanwhile. Unfortunately, the 12-month MRI follow-up revealed a focal nodular enhancement at the anterior aspect of the ablation area (arrow, H), which continued to grow over time, thus being consistent with a local tumor recurrence. The patient died 2.5 years after the cryoablation due to disease evolution.

Clinical results obtained with this patient were considered encouraging given the actual median overall and progression-free survivals, respectively, ranging between 5.5 and 12.6 months, and 1.5 months and 4.2 months for patients with post-surgical/radiotherapy glioblastoma recurrence undergoing further treatments.

R. L. Cazzato (✉) · J. Garnon · A. Gangi
Department of Interventional Radiology, University Hospital of Strasbourg, Strasbourg, France
e-mail: RobertoLuigi.CAZZATO@chru-strasbourg.fr

H. Cebula · F. Proust
Department of Neurosurgery, University Hospital of Strasbourg, Strasbourg, France

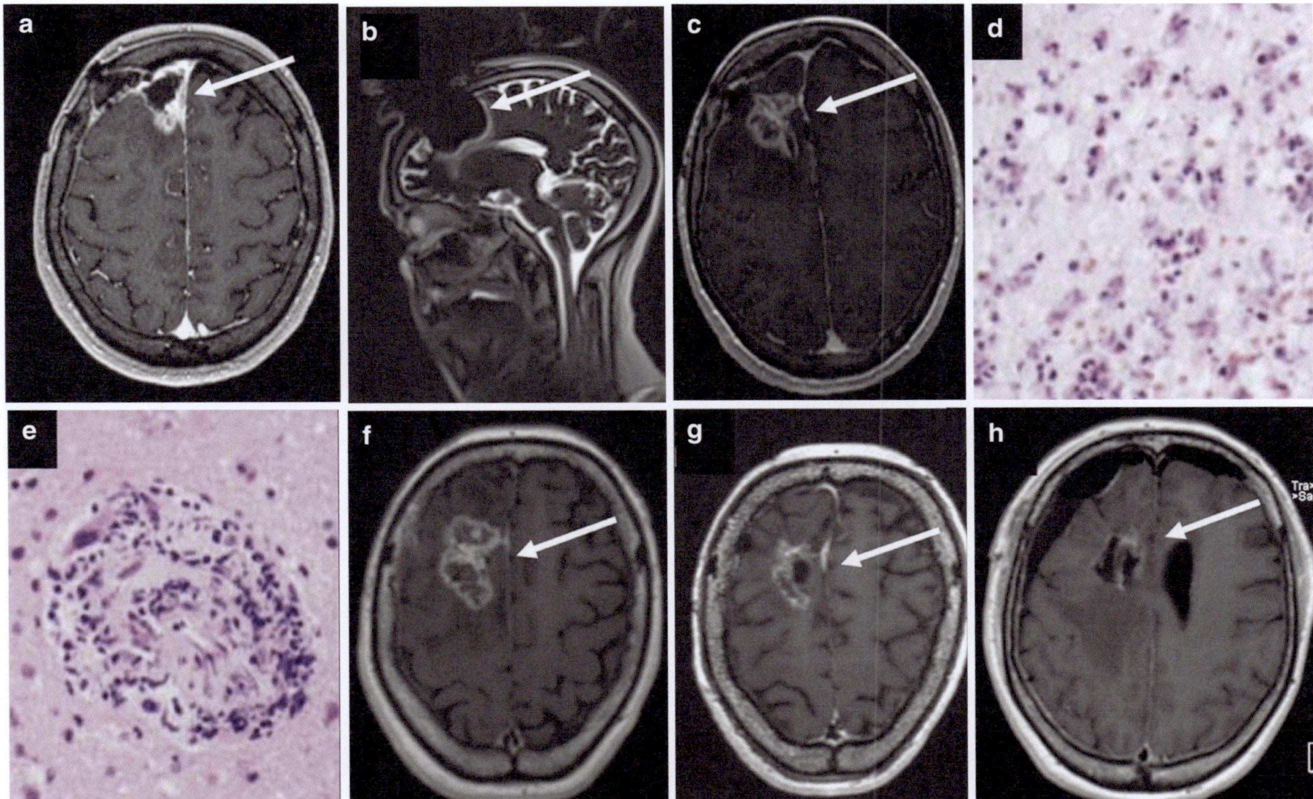

Fig. 75.1 (**a**) Contrast-enhanced axial T1-weighted MRI demonstrates the right frontal glioblastoma recurrence (arrow). (**b**) Sagittal T2-weighted MRI shows the iceball (arrow) encompassing the tumor during the 10-min freezing cycle. (**c**) Contrast-enhanced axial T1-weighted MRI obtained at 3-month follow-up demonstrats an enhancing mass (arrow) with surrounding edema. (**d, e**) Histologic images from a biopsy of the area showed necrotic (**d**) and peri-vascu-lar inflammatory changes (**e**) but no viable tumor. (**f**) At 5-month follow-up, an axial contrast-enhanced T1-weighted MRI revealed significant enlargement of the prior mass (arrow). (**g**) At 8 months, however, the mass had notably shrunk (arrow). (**h**) Unfortunately, 12-month follow-up revealed a focal area of enhancing (arrow) at the anterior edge of the ablation zone, thus being consistent with a local tumor recurrence

Bibliography

1. Gangi A, Cebula H, Cazzato RL, Ramamurthy N, Garnon J, Debry C, Proust F. "Keeping a Cool Head": percutaneous imaging-guided cryo-ablation as salvage therapy for recurrent glioblastoma and head and neck tumours. Cardiovasc Interv Radiol. 2020;43(2):172–5. https://doi.org/10.1007/s00270-019-02384-6.
2. McBain C, Lawrie TA, Rogozińska E, Kernohan A, Robinson T, Jefferies S. Treatment options for progression or recurrence of glioblastoma: a network meta-analysis. Cochrane Database Syst Rev. 2021;5(1):CD013579. https://doi.org/10.1002/14651858. CD013579.pub2.
3. Cebula H, Garnon J, Todeschi J, Noel G, Lhermitte B, Mallereau CH, Chibbaro S, Burckel H, Schott R, de Mathelin M, Gangi A, Proust F. Interventional magnetic-resonance-guided cryotherapy combined with microsurgery for recurrent glioblastoma: an innovative treatment? Neurochirurgie. 2021;S0028-3770(21):00241–1. https://doi.org/10.1016/j.neuchi.2021.11.004.

Percutaneous Cryoablation of a Precarious Pulmonary Nodule

Ahmad Parvinian, Patrick W. Eiken, A. Nicholas Kurup, and Matthew R. Callstrom

A 65-year-old woman with a 10-year history of metastatic colorectal carcinoma presented for percutaneous cryoablation of a 1.3 cm pulmonary metastasis in the medial left upper lobe (Fig. 76.1). The proximity of the nodule to the left phrenic, vagus, and recurrent laryngeal nerves mandated that it be displaced from the mediastinum to allow safe ablation (Fig. 76.2).

First, two IceRod Plus cryoprobes (Boston Scientific, Marlborough, MA, USA) were placed from an anterior approach to bracket the nodule (Fig. 76.3). Then, a Safe-T-Centesis catheter (Becton, Dickinson and Company, Franklin Lakes, NJ, USA) was used to introduce an iatrogenic pneumothorax to lateralize the lung. Unfortunately, pleural adhesions from prior treatments limited the size of the pneumothorax and the nodule remained too close to the vulnerable nerves to ablate safely (Fig. 76.4).

To gain an adequate buffer between the mediastinum and the planned ablation zone, a 20-gauge spinal needle was used

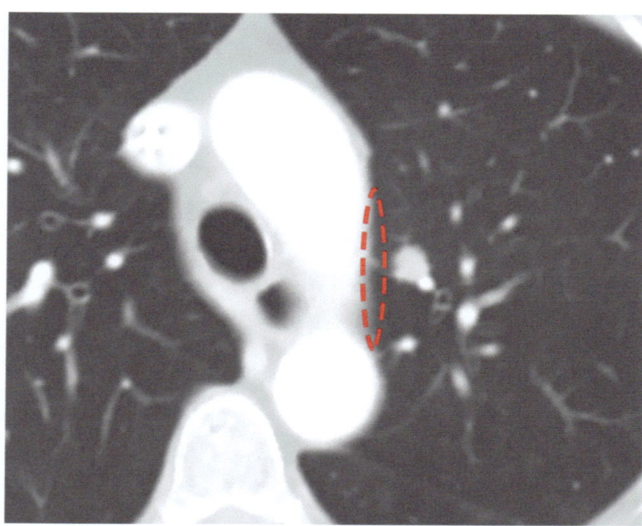

Fig. 76.2 Magnified axial CT image demonstrates the close proximity of the left upper lobe nodule to the anatomic location of the left phrenic, vagus, and recurrent laryngeal nerves along the aortic arch (ellipse)

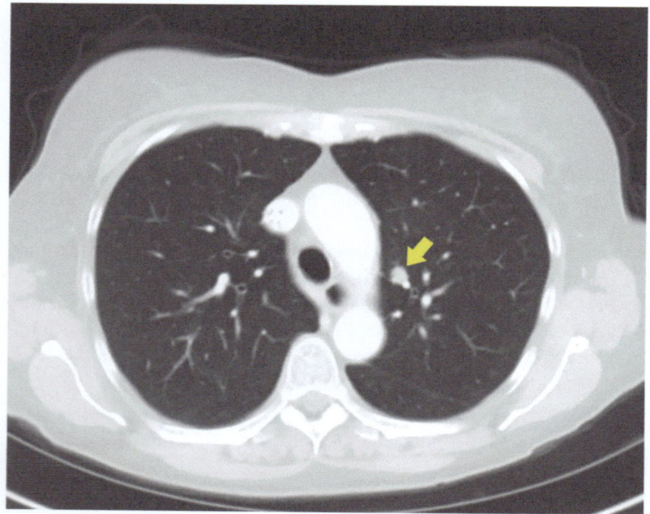

Fig. 76.1 Axial contrast-enhanced computed tomography (CT) image shows a 1.3 cm pulmonary metastasis (arrow) from colorectal carcinoma in the medial left upper lobe

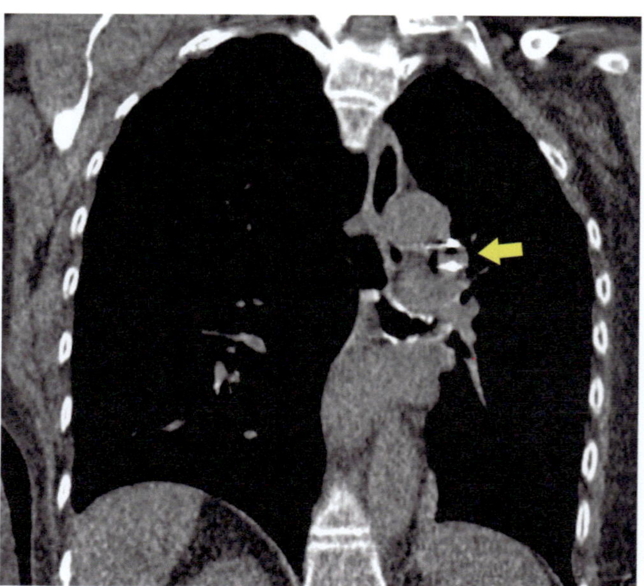

Fig. 76.3 Coronal CT image shows two cryoprobes bracketing the left upper lobe nodule (arrow)

A. Parvinian (✉) · P. W. Eiken · A. N. Kurup · M. R. Callstrom
Department of Radiology, Mayo Clinic, Rochester, MN, USA
e-mail: parvinian.ahmad@mayo.edu; eiken.patrick@mayo.edu;
kurup.anil@mayo.edu; callstrom.matthew@mayo.edu

to inject a small amount of fluid into the pleural space between the nodule and the mediastinum (Fig. 76.5). At the same time, gentle medial traction was applied to the two cryoprobes in order to mechanically lever the nodule away from the mediastinum (Fig. 76.6). This combination of

maneuvers provided adequate space for safe ablation. Traction was maintained on the cryoprobes throughout the remainder of the procedure, which was completed in routine fashion with three alternating freeze-thaw cycles followed by probe warming and removal (Fig. 76.7).

The patient experienced no complications from the procedure and follow-up at 5 years was negative for local recurrence (Fig. 76.8).

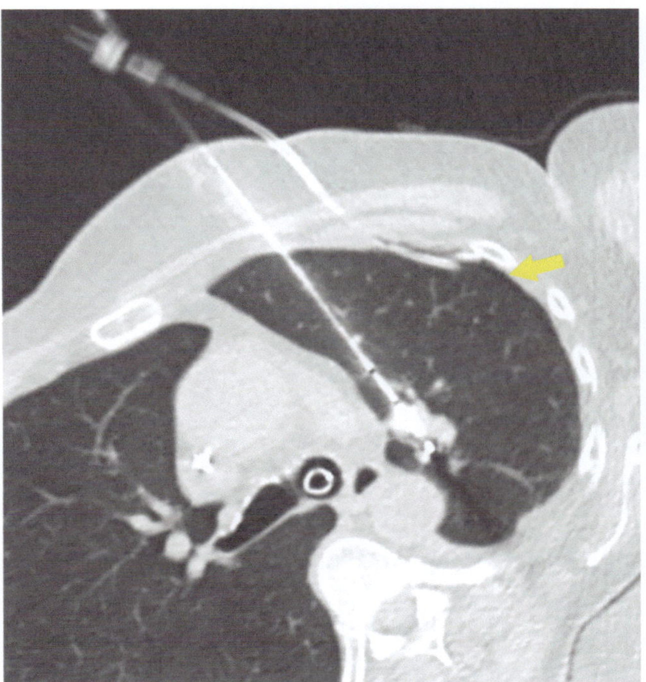

Fig. 76.4 Axial CT image demonstrates attempted creation of an iatrogenic pneumothorax to displace the nodule from the mediastinum. A centesis catheter placed along the lateral pleural space created only a miniscule pneumothorax (arrow), likely due to adherent pleura from prior treatments

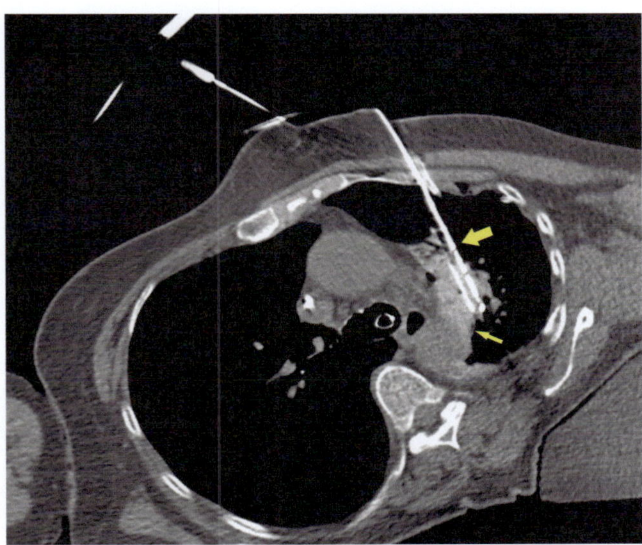

Fig. 76.6 Axial CT image demonstrates lateralization of the nodule after instillation of fluid (thin arrow) through the spinal needle and manually leveraging the cryoprobe (thick arrow)

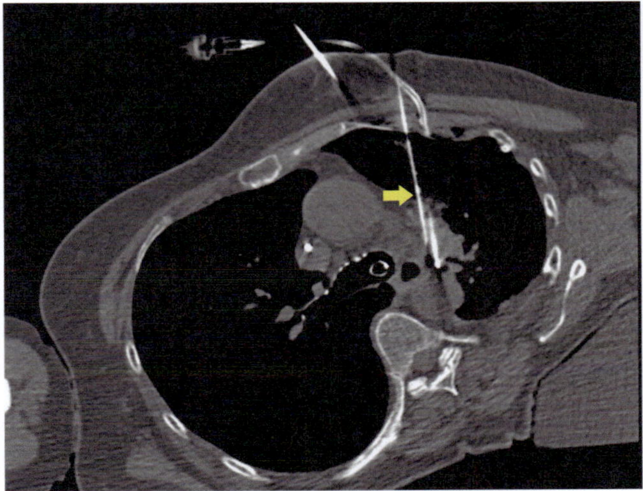

Fig. 76.5 Axial CT image shows a 20-gauge spinal needle (arrow) placed parallel to the cryoprobe, with tip in the pleural space between the nodule and the mediastinum

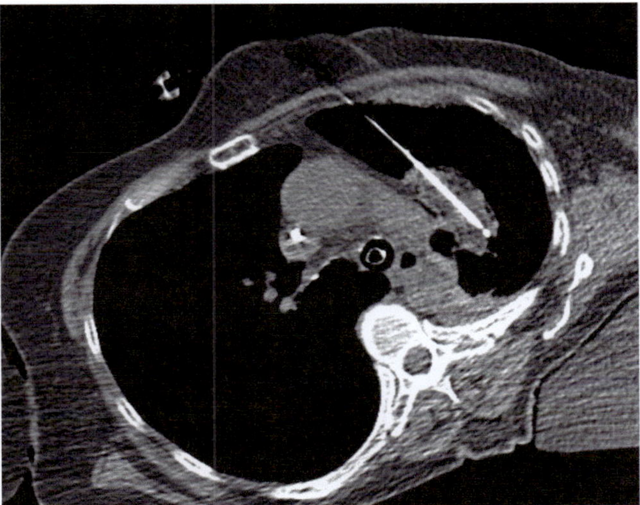

Fig. 76.7 Axial CT image obtained during cryoablation demonstrates the hypodense ice ball surrounding the tip of the cryoprobe, with the medial margin of the ice approaching but not contacting the mediastinum

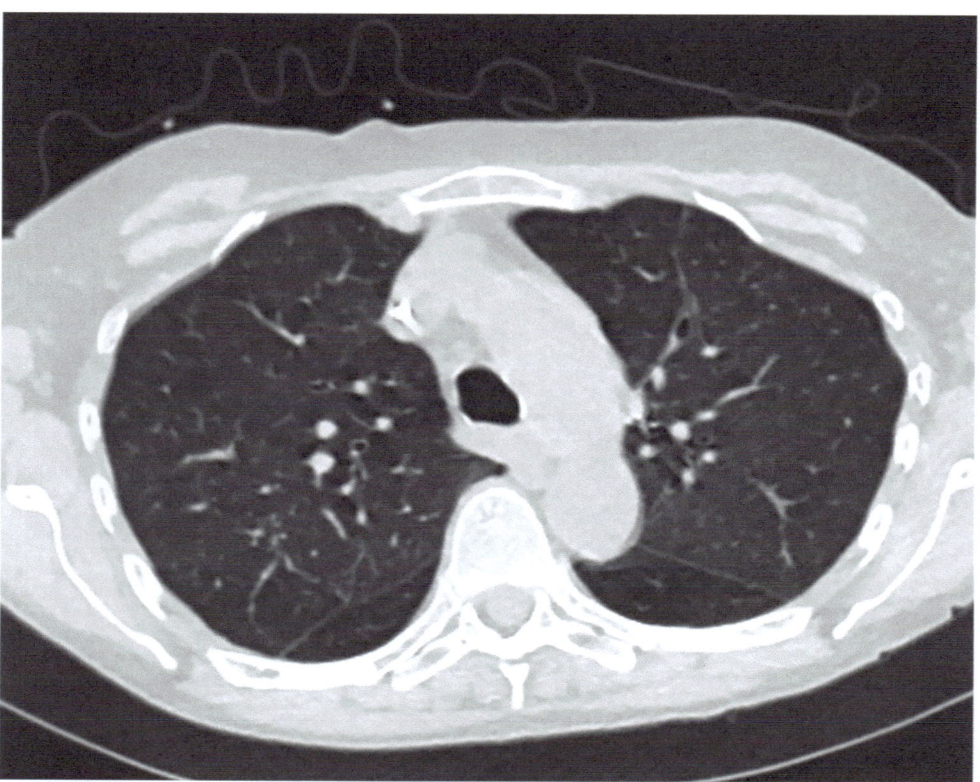

Fig. 76.8 CT follow-up 5 years after ablation was negative for local recurrence at the site of the ablated left upper lobe nodule

Treatment of Renal Parenchymal Blowout After Cryoablation Using Balloon-Assisted Coil Embolization

77

Yasuaki Arai and Miyuki Sone

A 80-year-old female underwent cryoablation of a left renal cancer (Fig. 77.1). Four weeks later, she developed urine leakage around the left kidney and renal dysfunction. A left ureteral stone was known at the time of cryoablation; however, stone extraction was not performed prior to the ablation given the lack of clinical symptom, renal dysfunction, or hydroureter. Her CT scan, on admission to hospital, demonstrated continuity between urinoma and the renal parenchymal defect at the ablated tumor (Fig. 77.2).

Percutaneous drainage of the urinoma and nephrostomy was performed, followed by percutaneous lithotomy. After the resolution of symptoms, embolization of the parenchymal defect was planned because the defect was approximately 1.5 cm in diameter and spontaneous closure was not expected. A 6.5Fr angiographic catheter was inserted to the urinoma cavity and then into the renal pelvis through the parenchymal defect. Two 0.035-inch guidewires were inserted through the same route using a 5Fr. introducer sheath (Fig. 77.3) to then advance a 5Fr. occlusion balloon catheter and a 6.5Fr catheter and align them in parallel.

Coil embolization was performed using the 6.5Fr catheter while the adjacent balloon catheter was kept inflated within the renal calyx to prevent migration of coils into the urinary tract. After the fibered 0.035-inch coils were densely packed (Fig. 77.4 and 77.5), the balloon catheter was deflated and the catheters and the guidewire were gently removed (Fig. 77.6). The nephrostomy tube was removed 3 days later and durable occlusion of the leak site was achieved.

Fig. 77.1 A 3 m left upper pole renal cancer was treated with percutaneous cryoablation

Y. Arai (✉) · M. Sone
Department of Diagnostic Radiology, National Cancer Center, Tokyo, Japan
e-mail: arai-y3111@mvh.biglobe.ne.jp

Z. J. Haskal (ed.), *Extreme IR*, https://doi.org/10.1007/978-3-031-24251-9_77

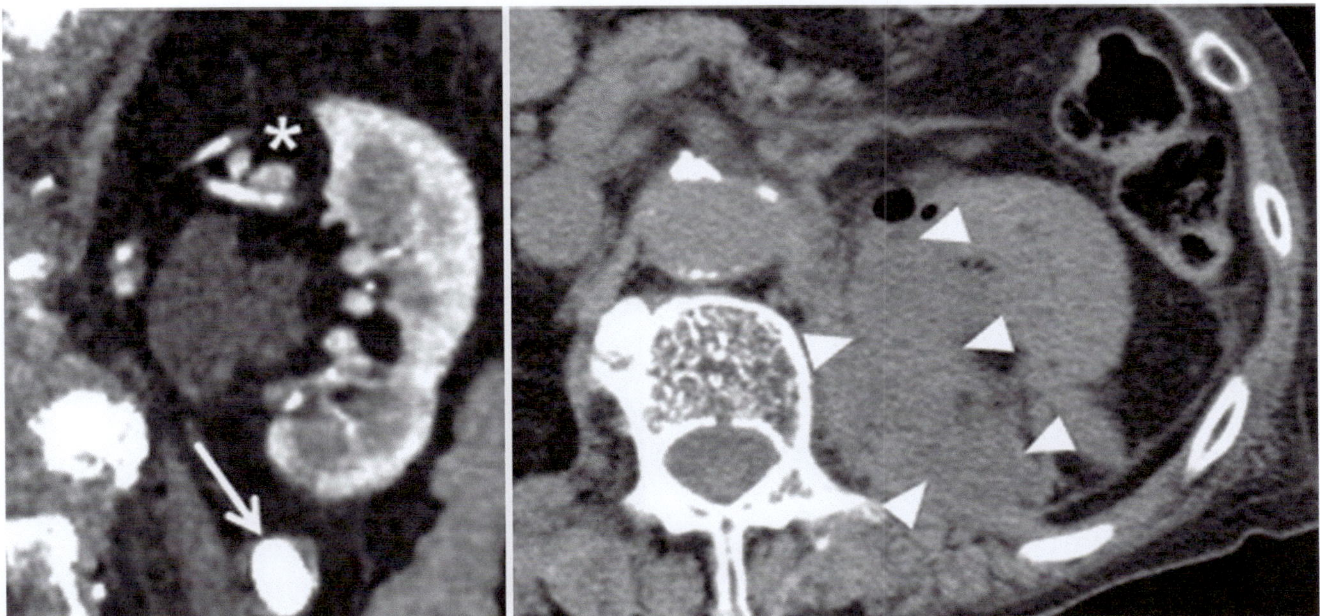

Fig. 77.2 CT images demonstrate the ureteral stone (white arrow), the renal defect caused by ablated tumor (*) and the urinoma (white arrow heads)

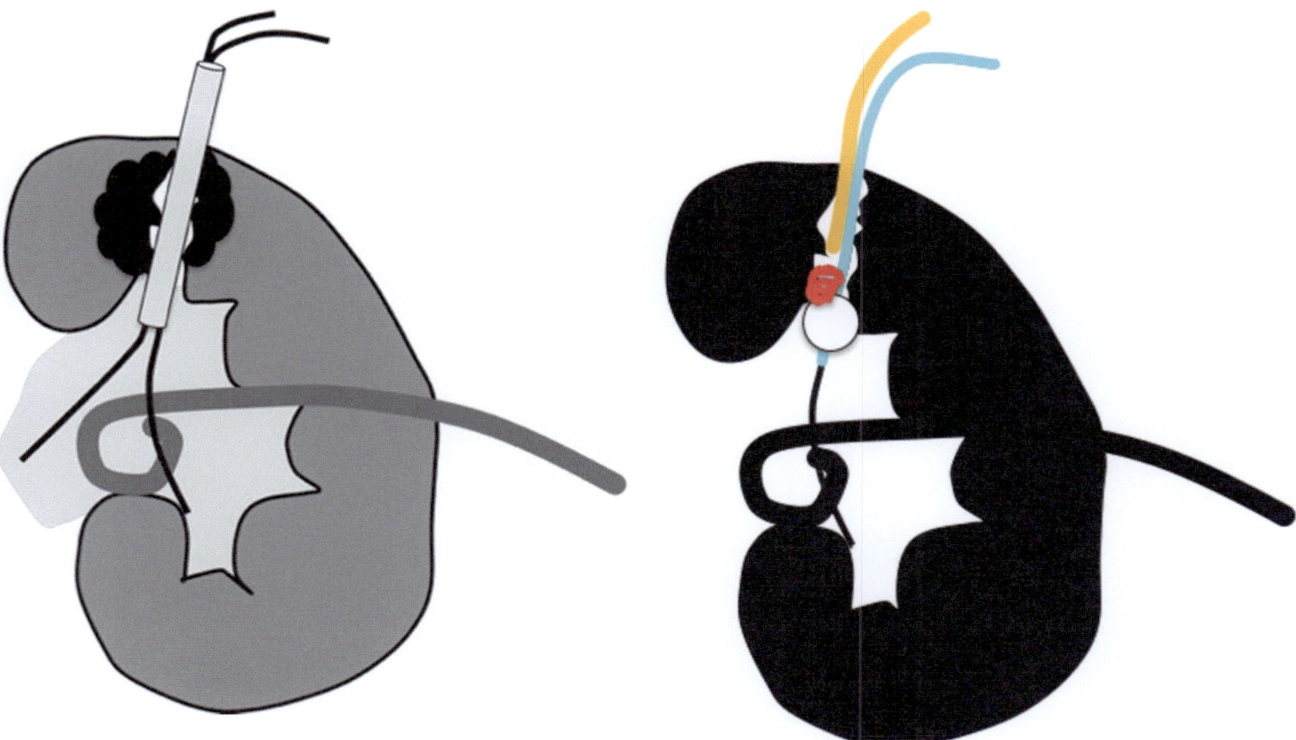

Fig. 77.3 A 10Fr. nephrostomy tube was placed, then two 0.035-inch guidewires were inserted into the renal pelvis via the renal defect

Fig. 77.4 Fibered coils (red) were inserted by a 6.5Fr catheter (yellow) into the renal defect with the balloon protection by the inflated balloon catheter (blue)to prevent coil migration into the renal pelvis

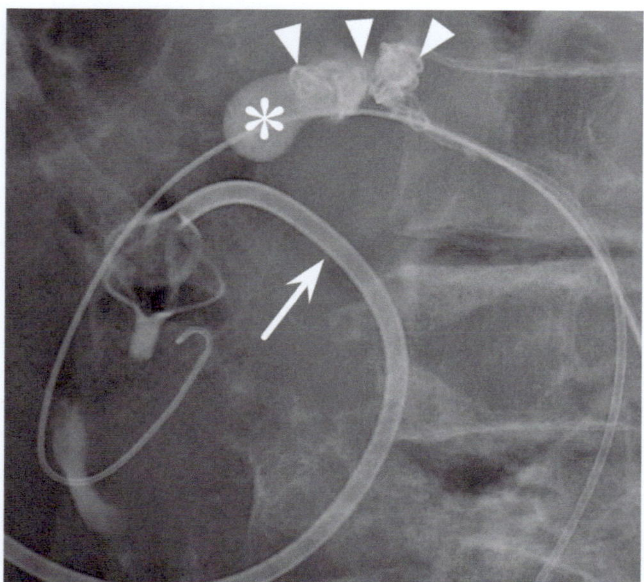

Fig. 77.5 A 10Fr malecot-type nephrostomy tube (arrow) was placed. Fibered coils (arrow heads) were inserted into the renal defect with the balloon protection (*) to avoid coils migration into the renal pelvis

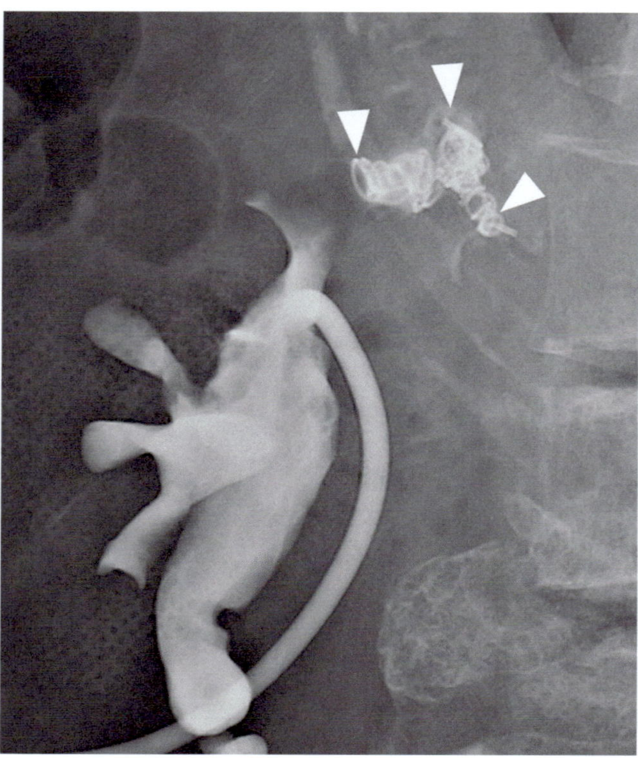

Fig. 77.6 Final image after the procedure of coils packing (arrow heads) in the renal defect. No leakage of the contrast to the extra-renal space was seen. The ureteral stone was removed thorough the nephrostomy route, and the nephrostomy tube was removed 3 days later. The balloon catheter and guidewire have been removed. The occluding material is visible (arrowheads); no leak is present

Baljendra Kapoor

A 54-year-old man with liver cirrhosis underwent chemoembolization of a solitary hepatocellular carcinoma measuring 3.4 cm and involving segment 6 follow-up magnetic resonance (MR) imaging performed 1 month after the procedure demonstrated a 2.4-cm residual lesion (arrow Fig. 78.1).

Due to the presence of overlying rib shadow, the residual lesion was only partially visible on ultrasound. To improve visualization and ensure complete ablation of the lesion, previously obtained MRI images were fused with the ultrasound images (Fig. 78.2). Additionally, ablation under electromagnetic tracking was planned to ensure proper positioning of the ablation electrodes. Under ultrasound guidance, an ACTC1525 Cool-Tip cluster 15 CM electrode (Covidien Inc. Minneapolis, MN) was advanced into the lesion and radiofrequency ablation was performed for 16 min (Fig. 78.3). At the end of this first ablation, there was suspicion of incomplete ablation. However, the presence of gas formation and overlying rib shadow again made it difficult to visualize the

lesion. At this point, a decision was made to complete the ablation under fluoroscopic guidance. Cone-beam computed tomography (CBCT) was performed, and CBCT images

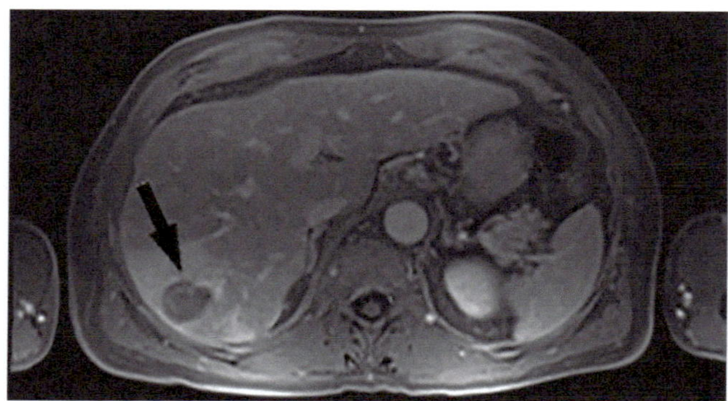

Fig. 78.1 Contrast-enhanced axial vibe MRI image showing residual 2.4 cm lesion involving segment 6 of Liver (arrow)

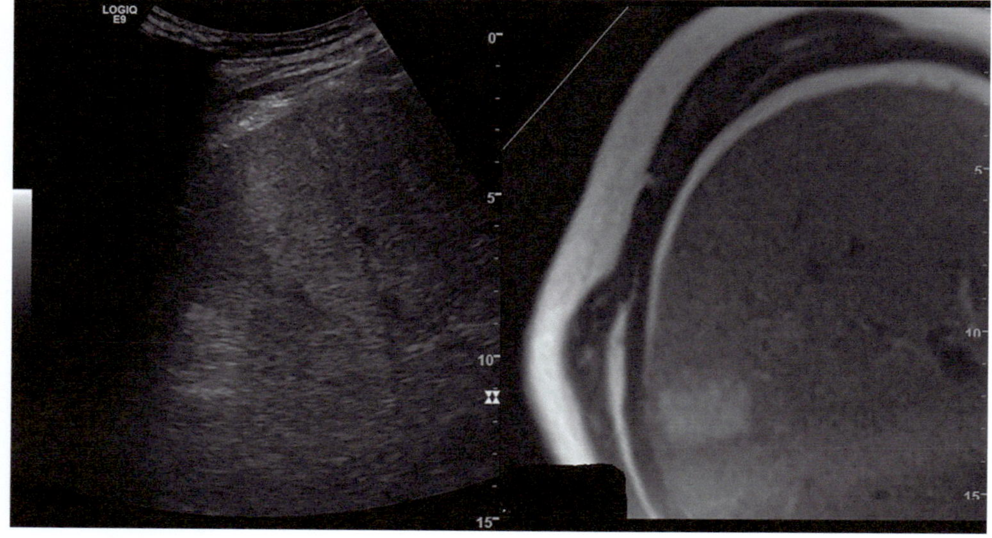

Fig. 78.2 Intraprocedural image showing Fused 2 D grey scale ultrasound and contrast-enhanced MRI images for electromagnetic tracking of the ablation probe

B. Kapoor (✉)
Cleveland Clinic, Cleveland, OH, USA
e-mail: kapoorb@med.umich.edu

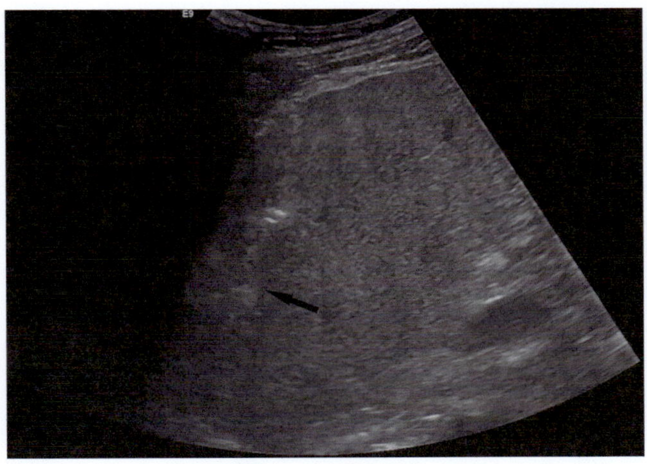

Fig. 78.3 Grey scale ultrasound image showing radiofrequency ablation probe and partially ablated lesion

were fused with the preprocedural MR images to plan the trajectory. Needle guidance software (Needle ASSIST, GE Healthcare) automatically determined the "progression" and "bull's-eye" views (Fig. 78.4a, b), and, the cluster electrode (15 cm) was advanced into the lesion following the course of the trajectory. Radiofrequency ablation of the lesion was then performed for 12 min. At the completion of the ablation, the electrodes were pulled back and the tract was ablated. The electrodes were then removed.

Follow-up was performed with MR imaging every 3 months. The last follow-up was performed 3 years and 8 months after the procedure, at which time no residual lesion was seen (arrow Fig. 78.5a, b).

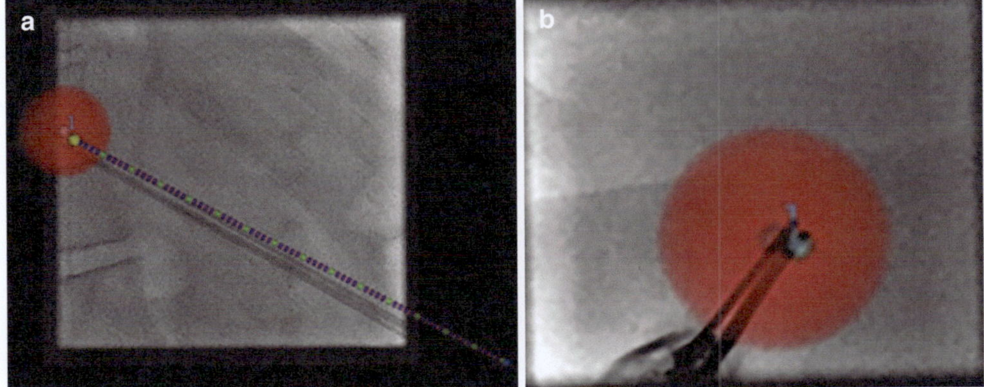

Fig. 78.4 (**a, b**) Progression (**a**) and Bulls eye (**b**) views of the ablation trajectory showing ablation probe and outline of the tumor superimposed over fluoroscopy

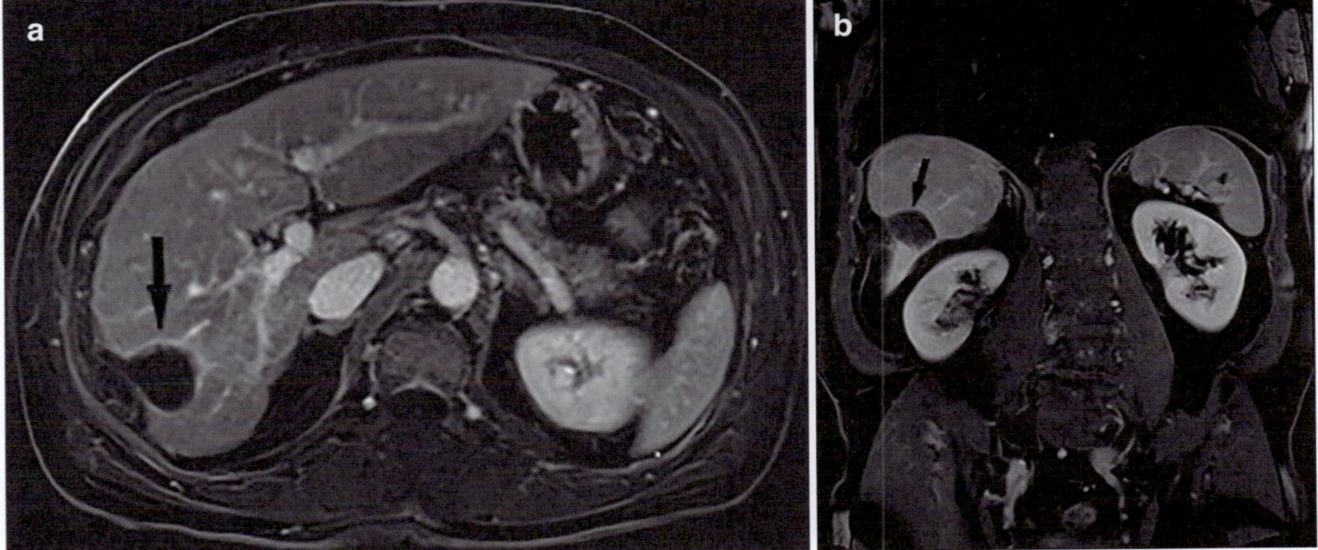

Fig. 78.5 (**a, b**) Follow-up axial (**a**) and coronal (**b**) images of contrast-enhanced MRI after 3 years and 8 months after initial ablation showing complete ablation of the lesion

Michael Savin, Jeffrey Savin, and Duncan Stevens

A 57-year-old man with stage III rectal cancer diagnosed 41 months prior received neoadjuvant chemoradiation, then abdominal perineal resection, followed by Folfox chemotherapy. He was diagnosed with a 2.5 cm left presacral metastasis by PET, CT, biopsy, and MRI. The mass was 3, 7, 10, and 15 mm from bladder, left ureterovesical junction, bowel, and lumbosacral nerve plexus, respectively (Figs. 79.1, 79.2 and 79.3).

Multidisciplinary review determined resection, radiation, and thermal ablation to be contraindicated due to preexisting left pelvic scar, prior maximum radiation dosage, and risk of nontarget thermal injury, respectively. Irreversible electroporation (IRE) was recommended. IRE leaves supporting tissue largely unaffected, so structural integrity of large blood vessels and intestines is relatively preserved [1]. Also, in animal studies, damaged axons may regenerate with complete recovery of function [1].

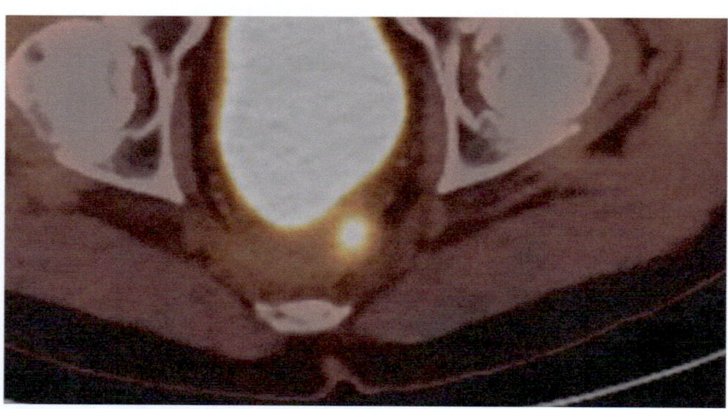

Fig. 79.1 PET (fused axial): SUV 7.2 in left presacral lymph node metastasis

M. Savin (✉)
Division of Interventional Radiology, Department of Diagnostic Radiology, Oakland University William Beaumont School of Medicine, Royal Oak, MI, USA

J. Savin
Department of Diagnostic Radiology, Beaumont Health, Royal Oak, MI, USA

Advanced Radiology Services, Kalamazoo, MI, USA

D. Stevens
Division of Interventional Radiology, Department of Diagnostic Radiology, Oakland University William Beaumont School of Medicine, Royal Oak, MI, USA

Department of Radiology, Aultman Hospital, Canton, OH, USA
e-mail: Msavin@comcast.net

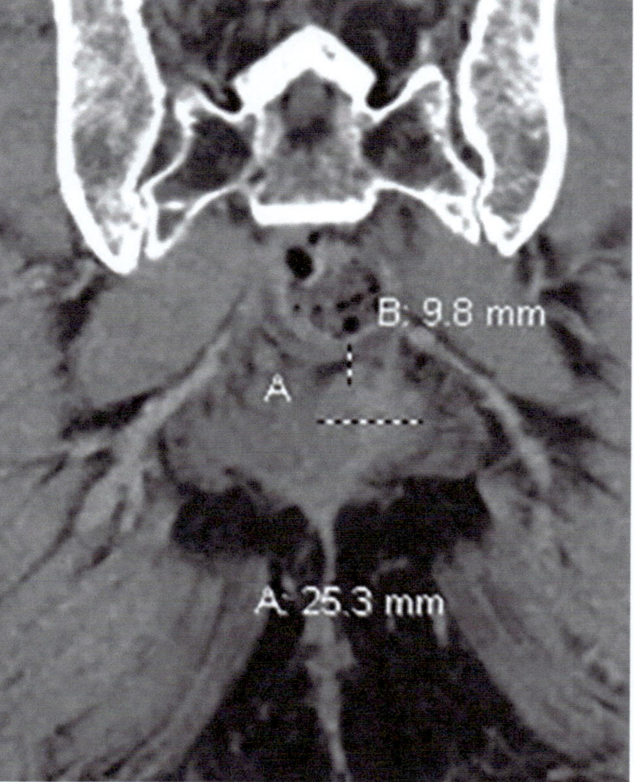

Fig. 79.2 Coronal CT: 2.4 cm left presacral metastasis (line) 1.0 cm below bowel (short line)

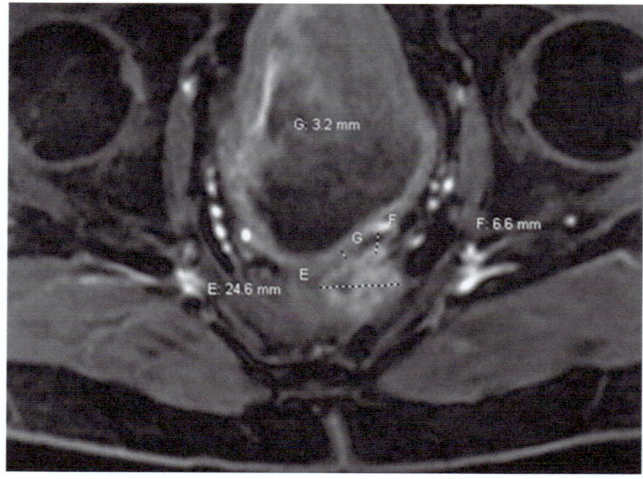

Fig. 79.3 MRI Axial T1: Left presacral metastasis (long line) 3 mm from posterior bladder wall and 7 mm from left ureterovesical junction

Z. J. Haskal (ed.), *Extreme IR*, https://doi.org/10.1007/978-3-031-24251-9_79

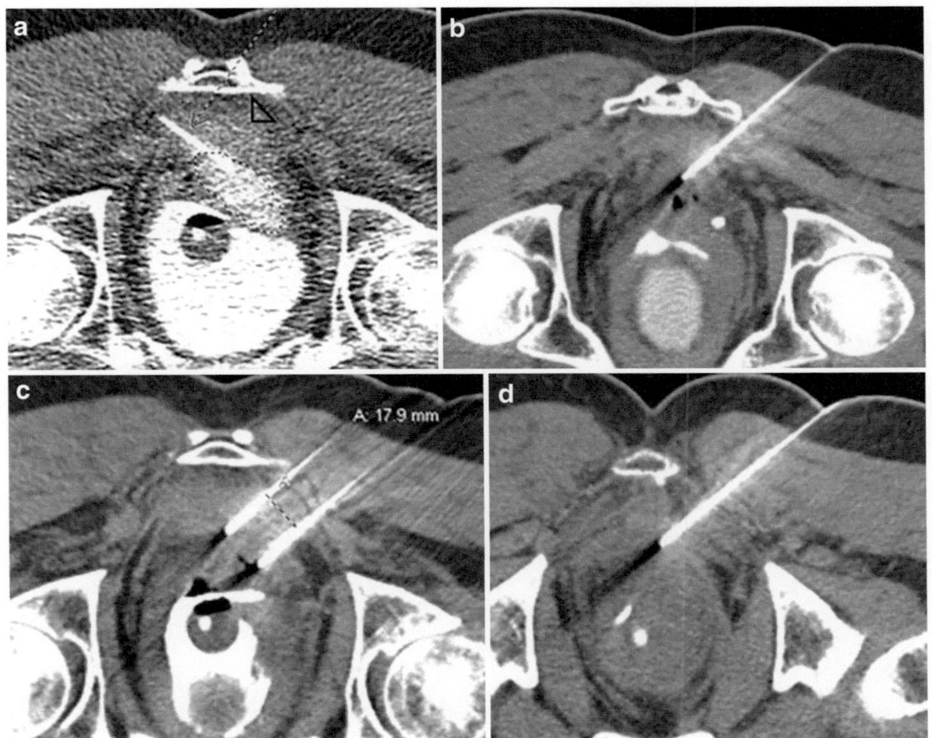

Fig. 79.4 (**a**) IRE. Hydrodissection needle (arrow) with contrast containing saline (oval) separating metastasis (arrowhead) from bladder. (**b**) IRE. Superior of three images. Upper of 4 IRE probes in place in a diamond configuration. (**c**) IRE. Middle of three images. Middle 2 of 4 IRE probes in place in a diamond configuration. (**d**) IRE. Inferior of three images. Lower of four IRE probes in place in a diamond configuration

A left ureteral stent and bladder catheter were placed to limit risk of ureteral injury and delineate the bladder. Whilst the patient was prone and under general anesthesia, CT fluoroscopy was used to guide hydrodissection with dilute iodinated contrast through two Chiba needles, one between the metastasis and bladder (Fig. 79.4a) and the other between metastasis and bowel. Sequentially, four IRE probes were placed in the metastasis in a diamond configuration with separation ranging from 1.3 to 2.4 cm (Fig. 79.4b–d). The bladder was drained to separate it from the metastasis. IRE was performed with each of the six probe pair combinations. A 1.5 cm exposure was used after a 2 cm exposure did not result in adequate electrical conduction. The probes were retracted 1.0 cm and IRE repeated to treat the more superficial portion of the metastasis. Post IRE CT demonstrated extensive gas within tissues surrounding the metastasis (Fig. 79.5). There were no complications.

A PET scan the following day demonstrated no residual activity in the pelvis. At 25 months follow-up, the patient is alive and cancer free. This case demonstrates the feasibility of IRE to achieve local tumor control for a

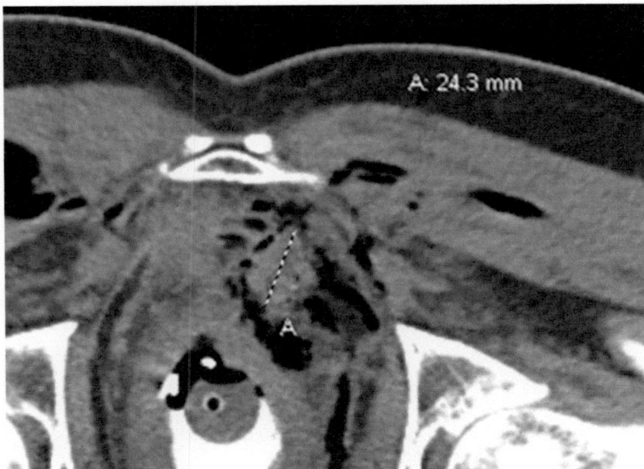

Fig. 79.5 CT Immediately Post IRE. Extensive gas surrounds the former site of the left presacral metastasis (line)

smaller 2.5 cm heavily pre-treated pelvic metastasis from rectal cancer in a patient deemed unsuitable for resection, radiation, and thermal ablation. In the only case series reported to date, local control was achieved in 4/9 lesions in 8 patients with 4/5 recurrences in lesions > 3 cm [1]. However, 6/8 patients suffered from permanent ablation-induced neural function loss. Meticulous protective techniques are required to avoid nontarget injury to neurologic structures such as the sacral plexus or perisacral plexus as well as to ureter, bladder and bowel.

Reference

1. Vroomen LGPH, Scheffer HJ, Melenhorst MCAM, van Grieken N, van den Tol MP, Meijerink MR. Irreversible electroporation to treat malignant tumor recurrences within the pelvic cavity: a case series. Cardiovasc Intervent Radiol. 2017;40(10):1631–40. https://doi.org/10.1007/s00270-017-1657-6.

Iatrogenic Pneumothorax for Creation of a Safe Percutaneous Window for Liver Ablation

Jason K. Wong

A 42-year-old Asian man with hepatitis B cirrhosis presents with a 2.0 cm caudate lobe HCC. The patient's AFP was 385. In Alberta, an AFP of 400 or lower is needed to stay on the transplant list. An iatrogenic right-sided pneumothorax was done with a loss of resistance syringe (LOR; B. Braun; Bethlehem PA, USA) and placement of a small catheter (One-Step Centesis; Merit Medical; South Jordan UT, USA) (Fig. 80.1). Air was then instilled in the pleural space creating a safe window for placement of a Quadra-Fuse infusion needle (Quadra-Fuse; Rex Medical; Conshohocken, PA, USA) (Fig. 80.2). Next, 16 cc of absolute alcohol was instilled for chemical ablation (Fig. 80.3). The pneumothorax was then evacuated and the patient discharged the same day. Subsequently, the AFP dropped to 110, and the patient had a successful liver transplant 8 weeks later.

Inducing an iatrogenic pneumothorax is safe especially with a loss of resistance needle as it decreases the chances of violating the visceral pleura. Following this a small catheter can be used to instill air into the pleural space to create a safe percutaneous window for needle/device placement.

This allows treatment of high lesions within the liver or challenging areas in the mediastinum that cannot be safely accessed by normal percutaneous routes.

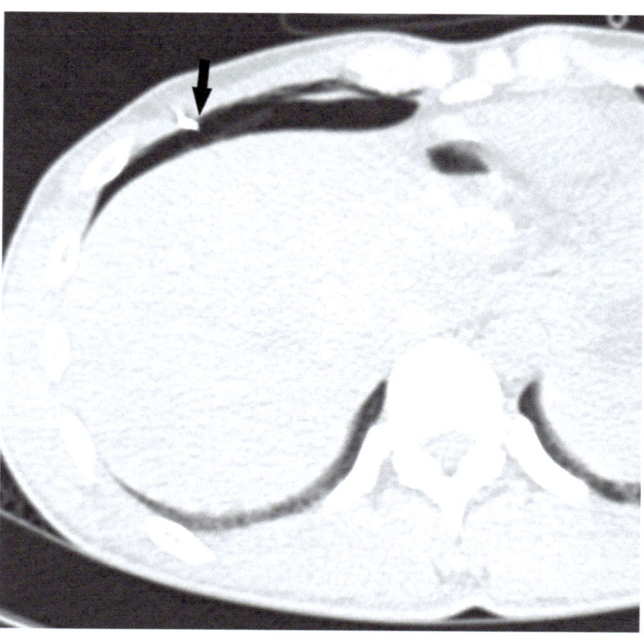

Fig. 80.1 CT image (lung window) showing One-Step centesis catheter (black arrow) and instillation of air into the right pleural space

J. K. Wong (✉)
Department of Radiology, Foothills Medical Centre, Cumming School of Medicine, University of Calgary, Calgary, AB, Canada
e-mail: wongjk@ucalgary.ca

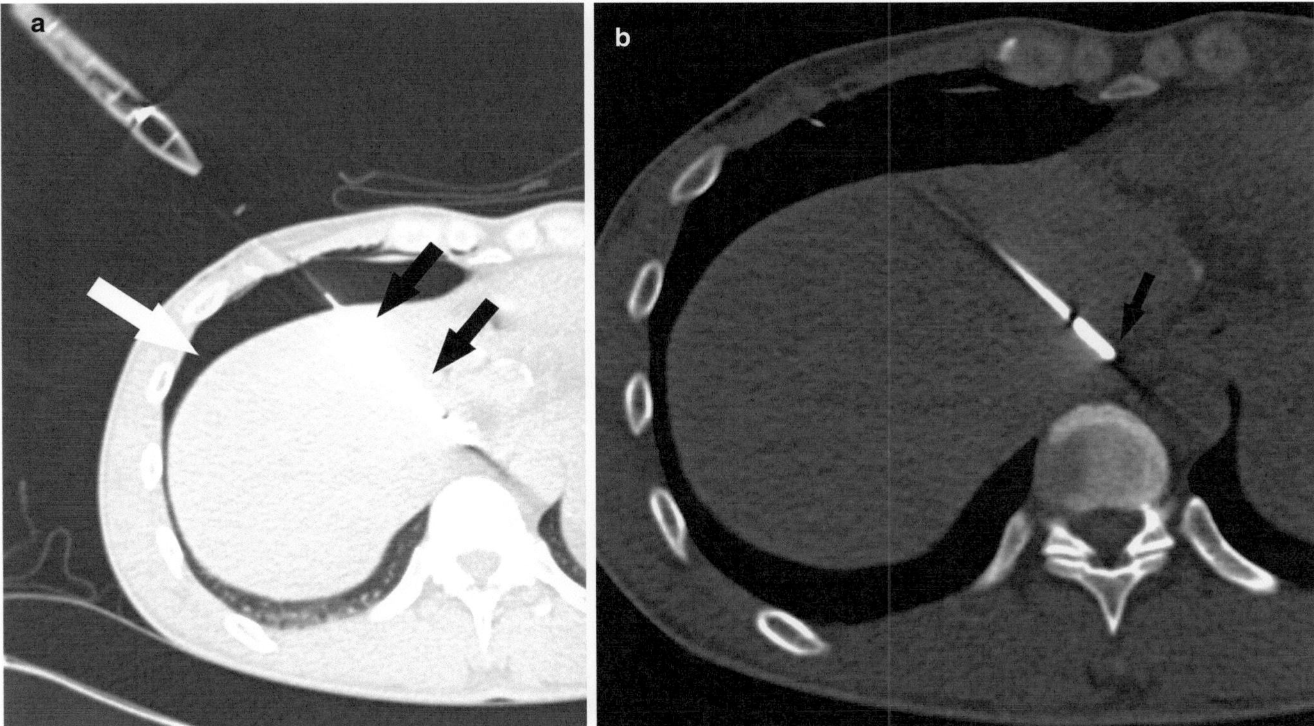

Fig. 80.2 CT image (lung window) showing the Quadra-Fuse needle (black arrows) traversing the right pleural space with a pneumothorax (white arrow) (**a**). CT image (bone window) showing the Quadra-Fuse needle tip (black arrow) in cranial aspect of the caudate lobe (**b**)

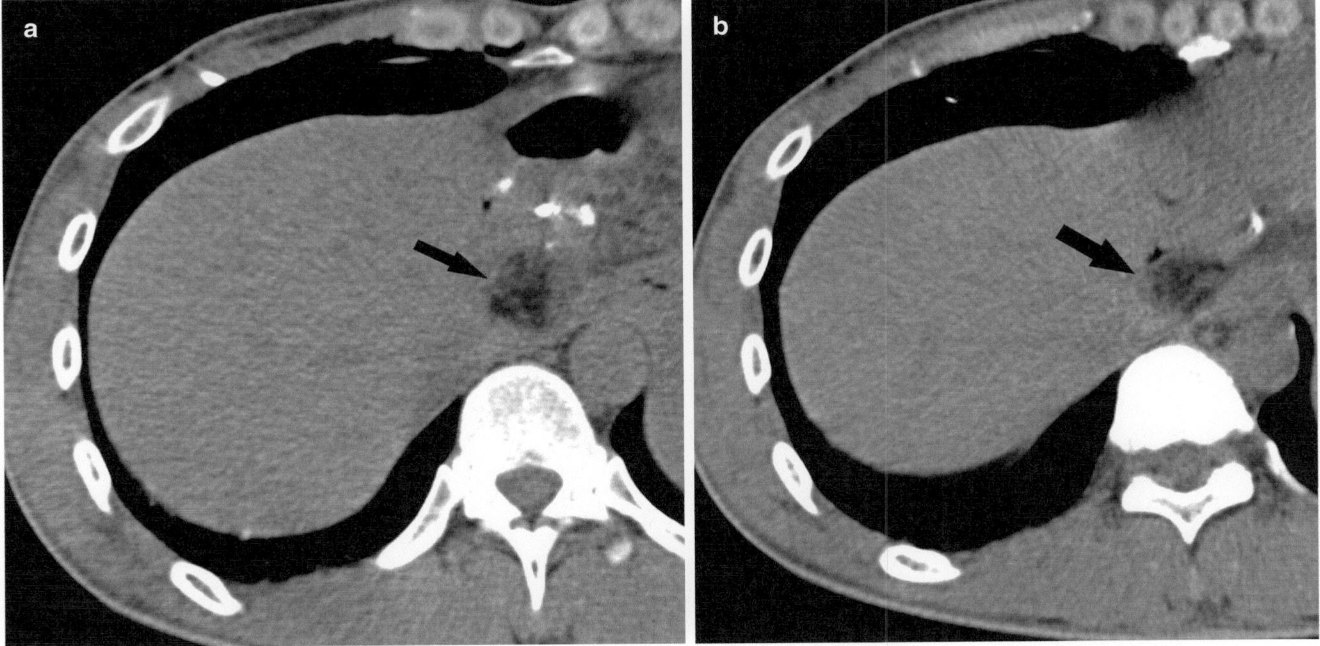

Fig. 80.3 CT image of the caudate lobe after EtOH instillation resulting in hypoattenuating area in the caudate (black arrow) (**a**). CT image 1.5 cm caudal to the previous image with EtOH (**b**)

Part VIII

Vascular Malformations and Arteritidies

Stop and Listen to the Birds Sing and Then Go With the Flow

John Matson and Alan Matsumoto

A 26-year-old Marine noted increasing lightheadedness during training, especially after 10 miles of marching. Initial work up was unrevealing and he feared his career in the Marines would be non-progressive. His wife, a nursing student, noted a "bird chirping" sound in his chest and sent him to a cardiologist for evaluation of a murmur.

A computed tomographic angiogram (CTA) of the heart (Fig. 81.1) to evaluate for a potential coronary arteriovenous fistula demonstrated an anterior mediastinal arteriovenous malformation (AVM). The AVM was presumed to cause a vertebral artery steal with prolonged exercise, leading to symptomatic vertebrobasilar artery insufficiency. Digital subtraction angiography (DSA) showed an AVM nidus located in the anterior mediastinum with multiple feeding vessels from both internal mammary arteries (Figs. 81.2 and 81.3) with dominant venous drainage to a right pulmonary vein (Figs. 81.4 and 81.5). The AVM was embolized using ethylene–vinyl alcohol copolymer (EVOH) over three separate sessions. During one of the embolization sessions, microcatheter entrapment within the EVOH occurred which ultimately led to catheter fracture. Completion angiography confirmed successful embolization of the nidus and resolution of the shunting to the pulmonary vein (Figs. 81.6 and 81.7).

During 5 years of follow-up, the "chirping" murmur did not recur, and his exercise-induced vertebral-basilar artery insufficiency and dizziness remained resolved. A chest radiograph (Fig. 81.8) shows the EVOH in the embolized AVM. He was able to continue training and has deployed overseas without incident. His wife, now a nurse practitioner, has decided to pursue a job in interventional radiology.

Fig. 81.1 Pre-procedure cardiac CTA reveals a vascular malformation in the anterior mediastinum with a large feeding vessel (arrow) arising from the left internal mammary artery

J. Matson (✉) · A. Matsumoto
Department of Radiology and Medical Imaging, University of Virginia Health System, Charlottesville, VA, USA
e-mail: JTM9SK@hscmail.mcc.virginia.edu; ahm4d@virginia.edu

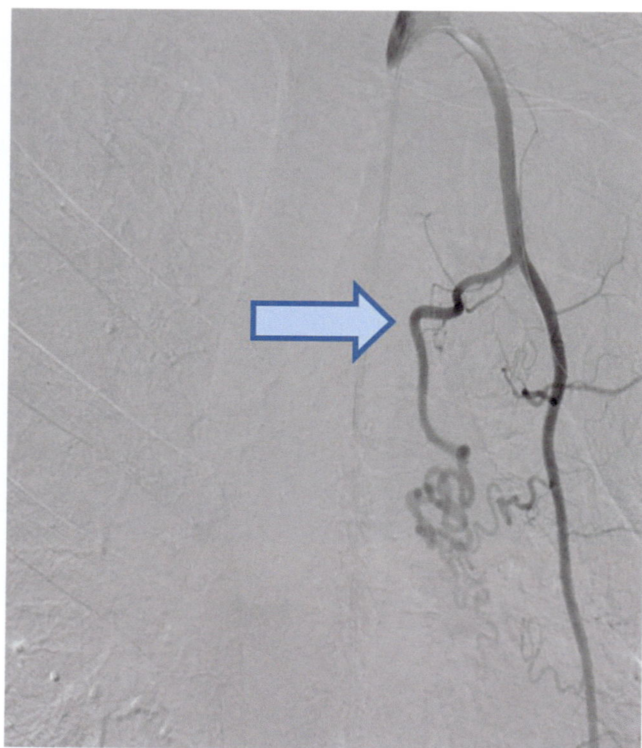

Fig. 81.2 DSA of the left internal mammary artery demonstrates the anterior mediastinal AVM with multiple small feeding vessels and a large feeding vessel from the left internal mammary artery (arrow)

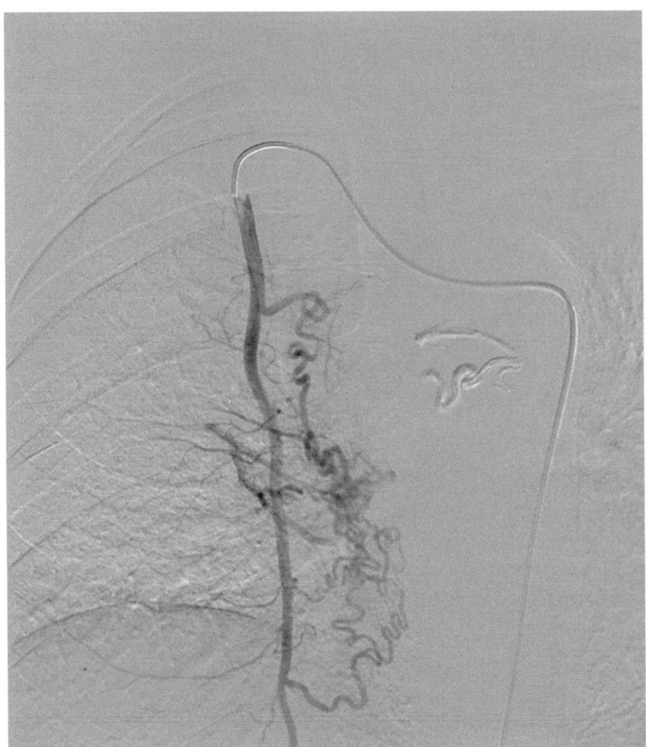

Fig. 81.3 DSA of the right internal mammary artery shows numerous branches contributing to the AVM nidus in the anterior mediastinum

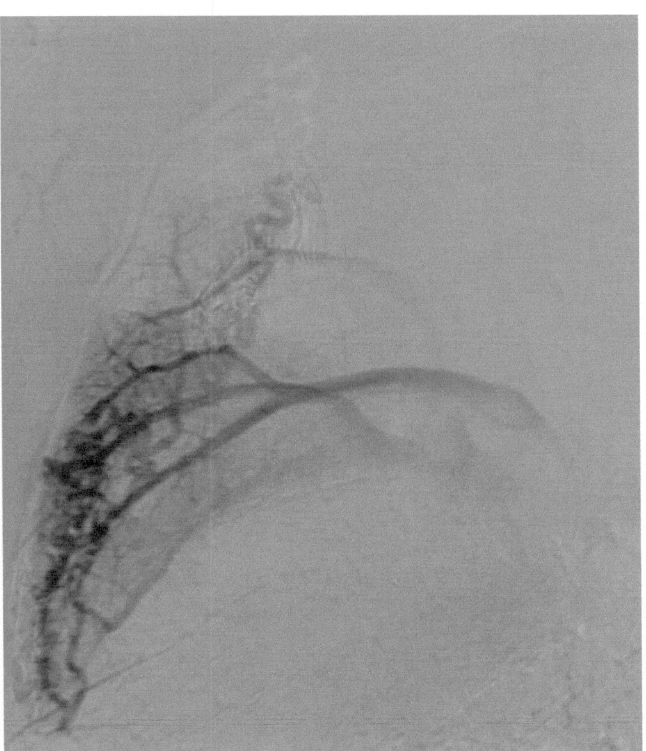

Fig. 81.5 A near-lateral image from the venous phase of a left internal mammary DSA demonstrates that the AVM drains into the right pulmonary venous system, most prominent in the right middle lobe

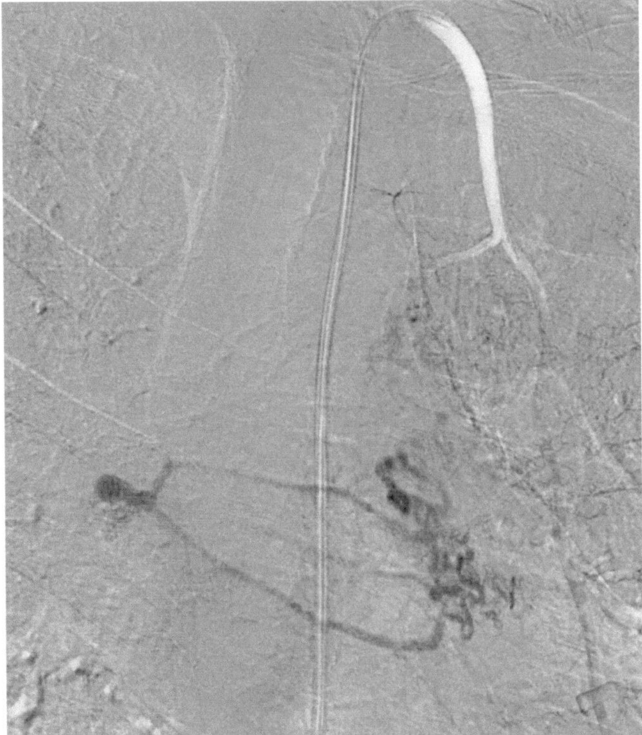

Fig. 81.4 A late phase DSA image from a selective left internal mammary arteriography in the right posterior oblique projection shows that the AVM drains into a venous structure in the right chest

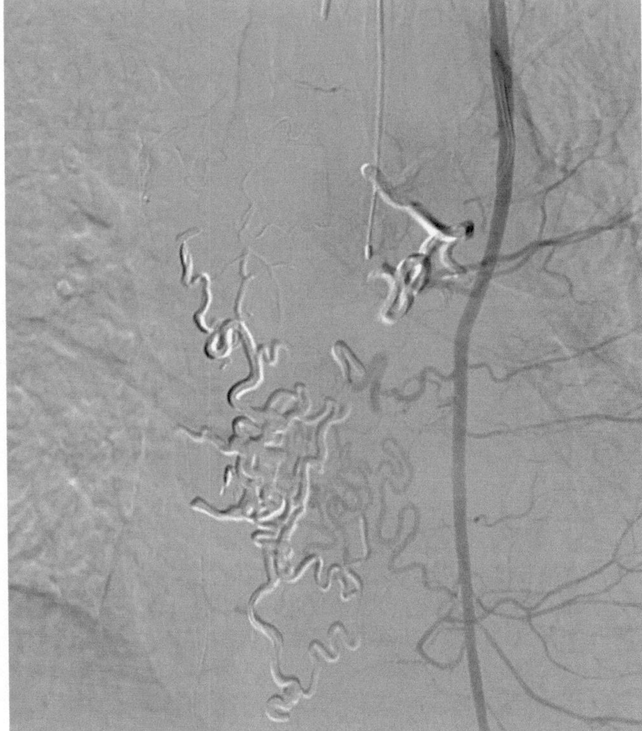

Fig. 81.6 After the three embolization sessions of the AVM nidus with EVOH, an AP left internal mammary DSA image shows successful cessation of flow into the AVM nidus and better filling of the more distal left internal mammary artery branches

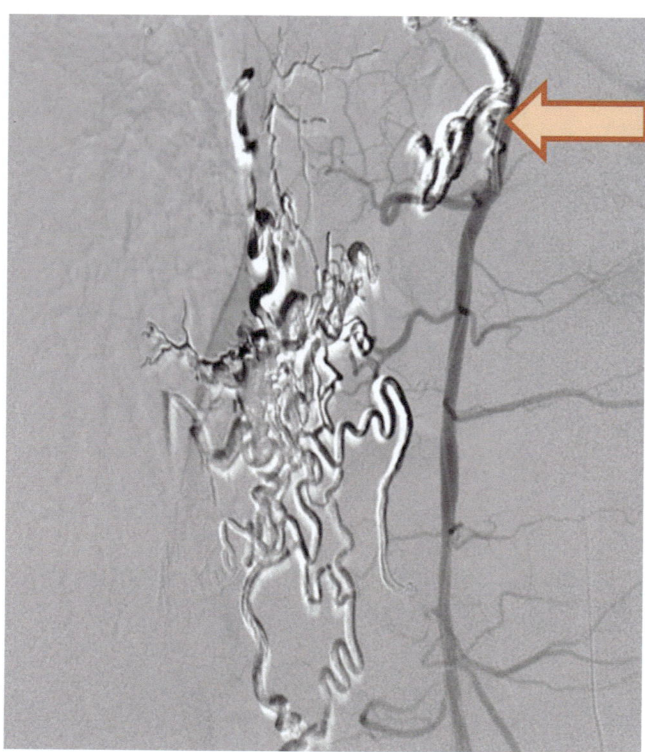

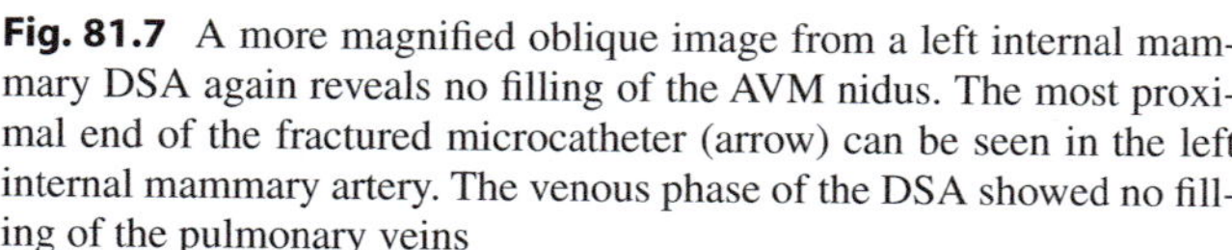

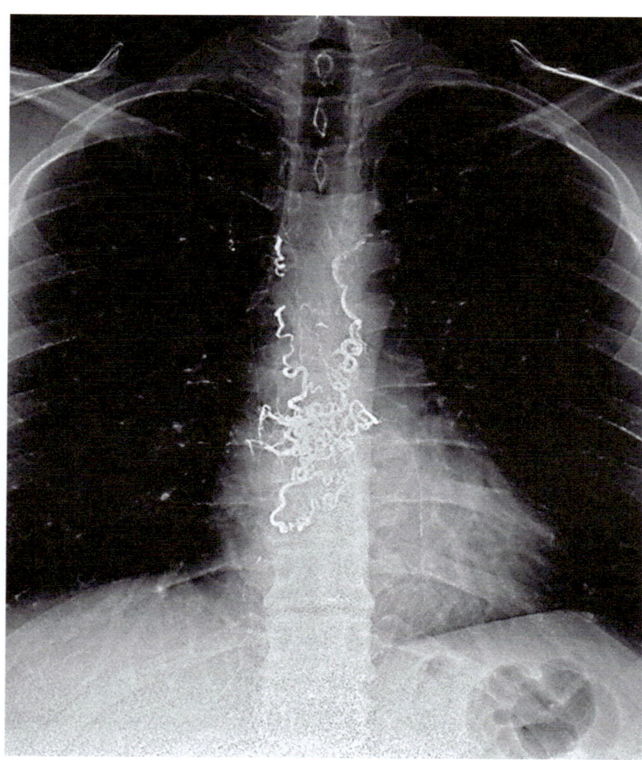

Fig. 81.7 A more magnified oblique image from a left internal mammary DSA again reveals no filling of the AVM nidus. The most proximal end of the fractured microcatheter (arrow) can be seen in the left internal mammary artery. The venous phase of the DSA showed no filling of the pulmonary veins

Fig. 81.8 Six-month follow-up chest radiograph demonstrates radio-opaque EVOH (due to the tantalum) filling the anterior mediastinal AVM nidus

Bleomycin Orbital Sclerotherapy of a Retro-Orbital Low Flow Lymphovenous Malformation

Lakshmi Ratnam and Robert Morgan

An 18-year-old female presented with a 3-year history of proptosis, infraorbital swelling, and episodes of periorbital bruising exacerbated by exercise. MRI (Figs. 82.1 and 82.2) demonstrated a low flow retro-orbital lymphovenous malformation.

In our practice, Bleomycin is selected as the sclerosing agent in the periorbital region as it produces minimal swelling. However, as a chemotherapeutic agent, its use requires specific precautions including carrying out lung function tests, a CXR, serology for renal and liver function and a full blood count prior to usage. Specific Bleomycin risk factors to be considered include lung fibrosis and skin marking; globe perforation and retro-orbital bleeding causing compartment syndrome and visual loss must also be consented for in these cases.

The procedure was carried out under general anesthesia. A high frequency (8–18 MHz) "hockey-stick" ultrasound probe was used to target the lesion through a

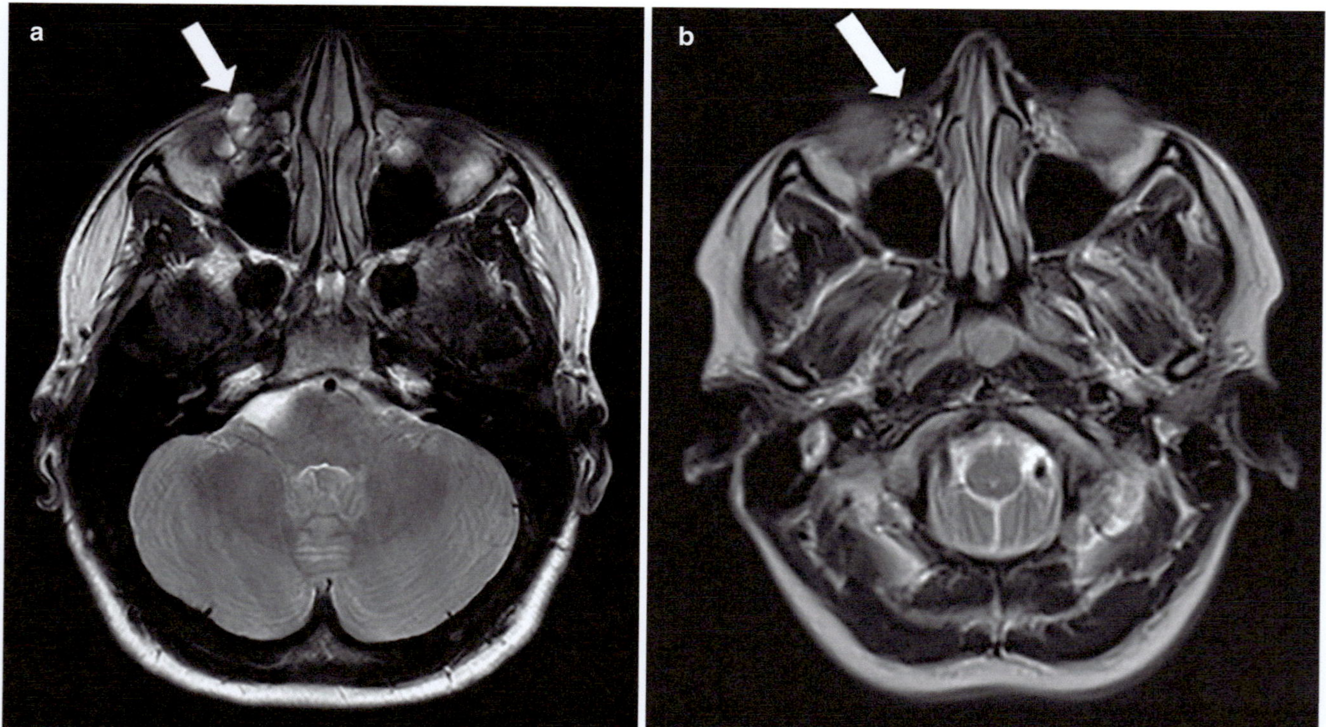

Fig. 82.1 Pre- and post-treatment axial T2 images. (**a**) Pre-treatment scan shows medial macrocystic component (white arrow). (**b**) Post-treatment scan shows small residual cysts (white arrow)

L. Ratnam (✉) · R. Morgan
Department of Interventional Radiology, St George's University Hospital, London, UK

Cardiovascular Clinical Academic Group, Molecular and Clinical Sciences Research Institute, St. George's, University of London and St George's University Hospitals NHS Foundation Trust, London, UK
e-mail: lakshmi.ratnam@stgeorges.nhs.uk;
robert.morgan@stgeorges.nhs.uk

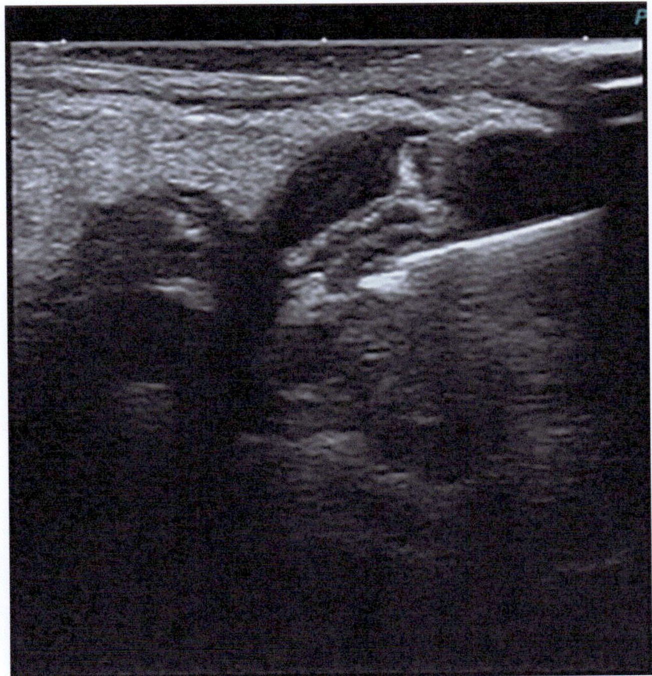

Fig. 82.2 Pre- and post-treatment coronal T2 and STIR images. (**a**) Pre-treatment macrocystic components demonstrated (white arrow). (**b**) Post-treatment minor residual microcysts inferomedially (white arrow)

Fig. 82.3 Needle position on ultrasound within the lesion

medial eyelid approach (Fig. 82.3). Contrast medium was injected and digital subtraction angiogram (DSA) performed to ensure that there was no central venous drainage prior to injection of the sclerosant (Figs. 82.4 and 82.5). Two sclerotherapy sessions were carried out

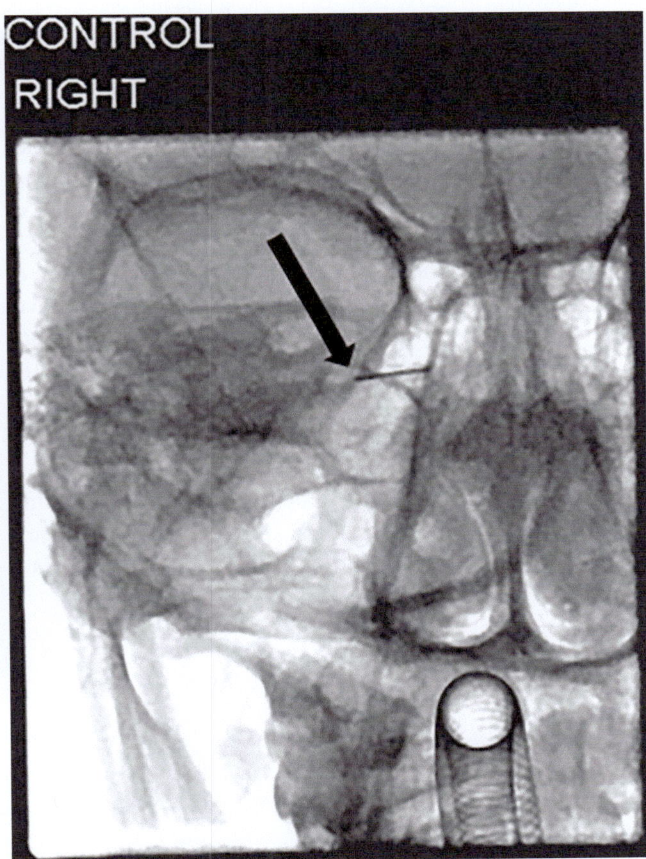

Fig. 82.4 Needle in position in the medial orbit before commencing injection. (Black arrow shows tip of needle in the lesion)

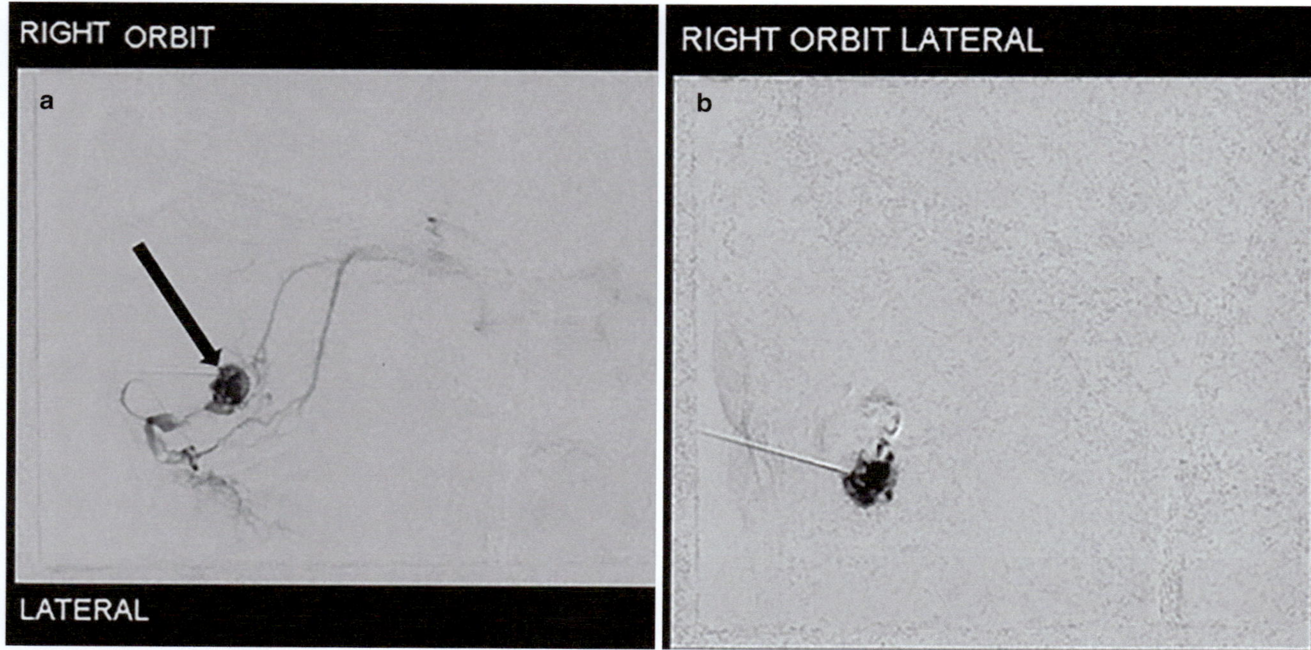

Fig. 82.5 Contrast medium injection in lateral position. (**a**) Tip of needle seen on lateral view (black arrow) within the retro-orbital lesion. Contrast medium is seen to flow via a draining vein into the cavernous sinus. (**b**) Needle repositioned. Injection confirms no central drainage and safe to proceed with bleomycin injection

6 months apart, utilizing a total of 5.5 mL of Bleomycin prepared as 5000 units in a 5 mL solution. Small volumes were used per session, given the limited space retro-orbitally, rarely exceeding 3 mL. No complications or side effects occurred.

Following treatment, she had complete resolution of symptoms with no residual proptosis, full extraocular movements, symmetrical appearance of lids, normal reflexes and levator function, normal pupils, and fundi. Follow-up MRI shows significant reduction in the size of the lesion (Figs. 82.1 and 82.2).

Retro-orbital malformations are often complex and infiltrative making surgical excision difficult and incomplete. Surgery can result in lesion expansion, hemorrhage, and symptom worsening [1]. Sclerotherapy is a safe and effective treatment for retro-orbital malformations. Close working with an ophthalmology team, adhering to bleomycin protocols including dose monitoring (lifetime dose limit of Bleomycin is 80,000 U in adults) and being prepared for acute retrobulbar hemorrhage are essential [2].

Bibliography

1. Barnacle AM, Theodorou M, Maling SJ, Abou-Rayyah Y. Sclerotherapy treatment of orbital lymphatic malformations: a large single-Centre experience. Br J Ophthalmol. 2016;100:204–8.
2. Prad D, Gome N, Zloto O, Anne M, BenSaid A, Bhattacharjee K, et al. Low-dose Bleomycin injections for orbital lymphatic and lymphatic-venous malformations: a multicentric case series study. Ophthalmic Plast Reconstr Surg. 2021;37:361–5.

Percutaneous Sclerotherapy of a Bleeding Nasal Arteriovenous Malformation

Abhishek Kumar

A 24-year-old female presented with a right nasal mass causing recurrent epistaxis since infancy. After her pregnancy (and 2 years prior to presentation), her epistaxis became frequent and debilitating. Multiple surgical debridements and ligations failed to improve her symptoms. Contrast-enhanced MRI head demonstrated intravenous contrast revealed a right nasal ala arteriovenous malformation (AVM)(Fig. 83.1). Transradial cerebral angiography demonstrated AMV supply by branches of both external and internal carotid arteries, the right internal maxillary artery (Fig. 83.2), and the ophthalmic artery (Fig. 83.3). Given the dual supply to the nidus, we decided to treat it percutaneously. A 21-gauge angiocath needle was used to access the nidus under fluoroscopic guidance. Contrast injection demonstrated filling of the nidus with a late draining vein (Fig. 83.4). Sclerotherapy was per-

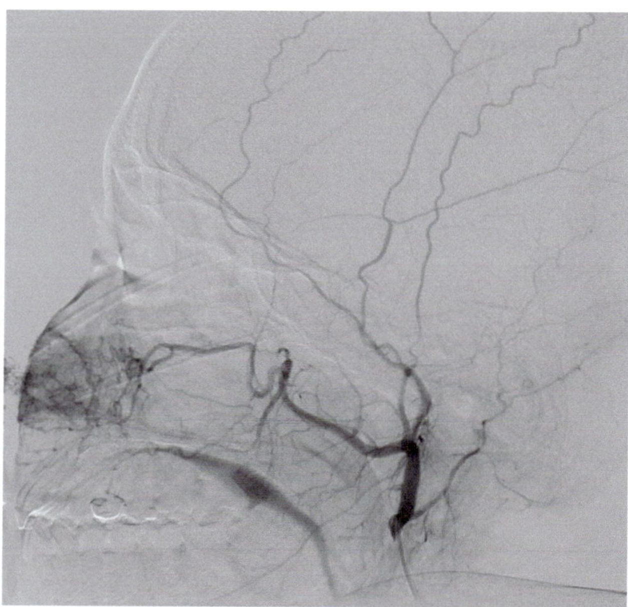

Fig. 83.2 Right external carotid arteriogram showing a hypertrophied internal maxillary artery supplying an arteriovenous malformation in the right nasal ala

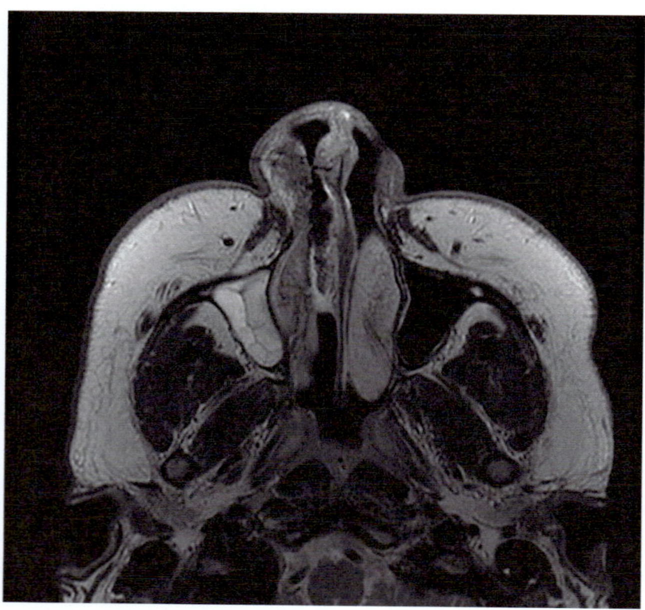

Fig. 83.1 Axial T1-weighted contrast-enhanced MRI of the face showing thickening of the right nasal ala and several flow voids consistent with an arteriovenous malformation

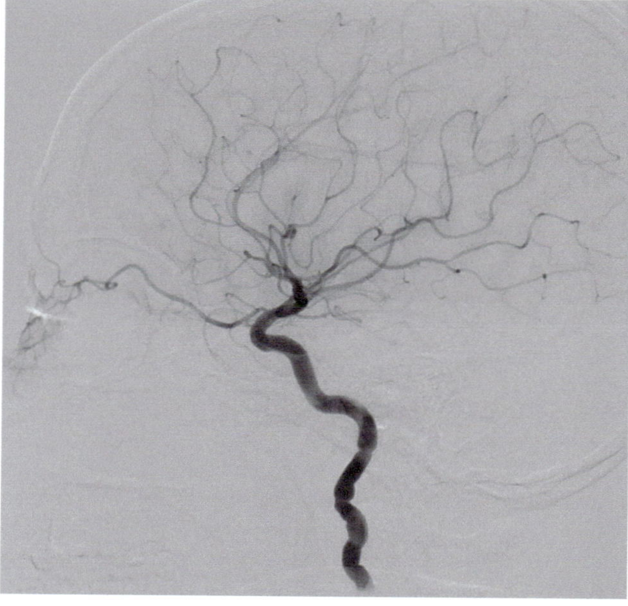

Fig. 83.3 Right internal carotid arteriogram demonstrating supply to the nasal arteriovenous malformation via the ophthalmic artery

A. Kumar (✉)
Division of Vascular and Interventional Radiology, Department of Radiology, Rutgers—New Jersey Medical School, Newark, NJ, USA
e-mail: kumarab@njms.rutgers.edu

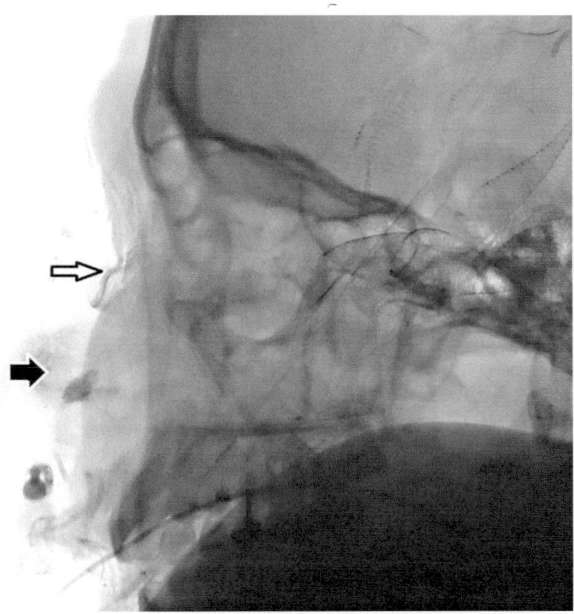

Fig. 83.4 Percutaneous access of the nidus with contrast injection opacifying the nidus (black arrow) and a draining vein (open arrow)

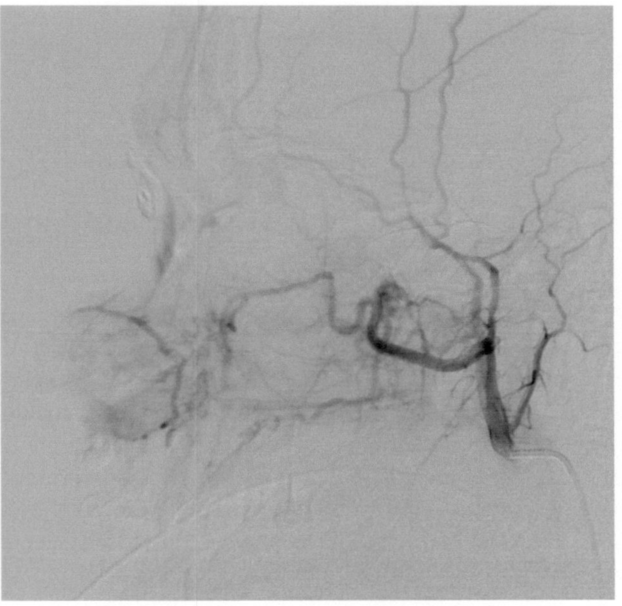

Fig. 83.5 Right external carotid arteriogram demonstrating markedly decreased enhancement of the nidus following percutaneous sclerotherapy

formed using a foam sclerosant consisting of a mixture of air, Ethiodol and 3% Sotradecol in a 3:2:1 ratio. The nidus was accessed at several sites and the sclerosant was injected with care to prevent reflux into the arterial system. A completion external carotid arteriogram demonstrated markedly decreased enhancement of the AVM nidus (Fig. 83.5). The patient was discharged with no adverse sequela. At 1-year follow-up, she remained symptom free.

Nasal AVMs can be treated with arterial embolization or percutaneous sclerotherapy [1]. A thorough diagnostic angiogram is essential prior to pursuing endovascular therapy, especially when anastomoses between branches of the internal and external carotid arteries are present.

Bibliography

1. Lungren MP, Patel MN. Endovascular management of head and neck vascular malformations. Curr Otorhinolaryngol Rep. 2014;2:273–84.

Venous Outflow Embolization for Obliteration of a Massive Lower Extremity AVM

William Behl and Auh Whan Park

A 44-year-old woman with Cowden disease and pulmonary arterial hypertension presented with dyspnea, left lower extremity pain, and a palpable left groin thrill. Computed tomography and catheter angiography showed an 8 cm arteriovenous malformation (AVM) in the medial left thigh, fed by branches of the superficial femoral (SFA) and profunda femoris arteries with a large draining vein and varix (Figs. 84.1 and 84.2a, b). She underwent transarterial alcohol embolization of multiple penetrating arteries off the left SFA, additional alcohol embolization 3 months later, and EVOH (Onyx, Medtronic USA) embolization 2 weeks hence. She developed worsening pulmonary hypertension, due to AVM mass related left-to-right shunting. Her pulmonary artery pressure was 77/27 (mean 49) mmHg. She underwent repeated sequential embolization with alcohol, glue, and EVOH of feeding arteries (Fig. 84.3). In total, 26.8 cc of 100% ethanol and 24 cc of EVOH were used. Post-embolization PA pressures dropped to 29/11 (mean 21) mmHg.

In an attempt to perform definitive intervention and treat the arterialized, ectatic, nonfunctional varix, transvenous outflow obliteration was undertaken using coil and plug-assisted embolization with delivery of 2435 cm of coils, two divided Bentson wires with the cores removed, and a single 12 mm Amplatzer II plug (Figs. 84.4, 84.5 and 84.6). The entire AVM was occluded by closing off the venous outflow with complete obliteration of 20 cm of femoral vein via contralateral femoral vein access. Follow-up angiography performed 6 months later demonstrated no persistent arteriovenous shunting in the thigh.

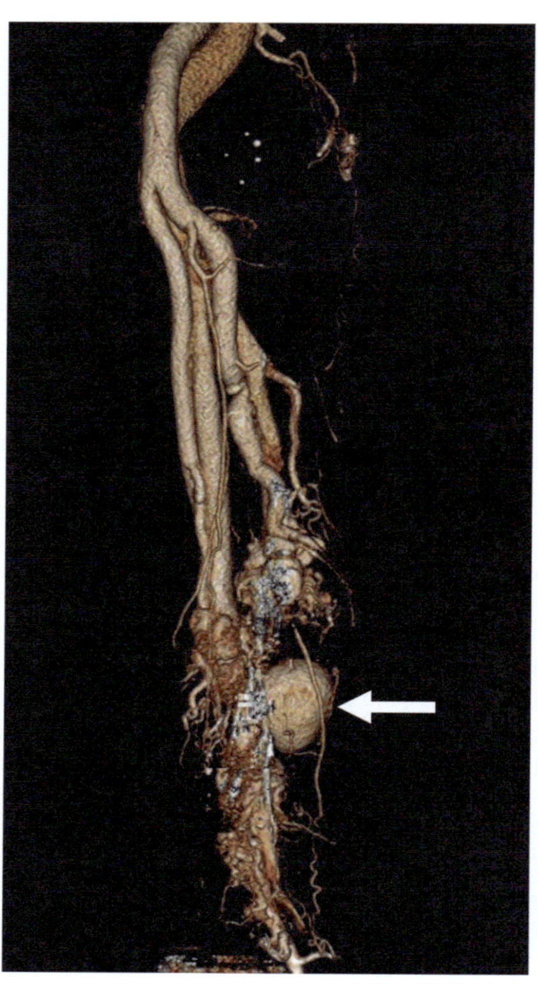

Fig. 84.1 Three-dimensional volume-rendered image shows an AVM arising from the deep femoral artery with prominent arterialized outflow with varix (arrow)

W. Behl (✉)
University of Virginia Health System, Charlottesville, VA, USA
e-mail: WCB4T@hscmail.mcc.virginia.edu

A. W. Park
Department of Radiology, University of Texas Southwestern, Dallas, TX, USA
e-mail: ap7wv@hscmail.mcc.virginia.edu

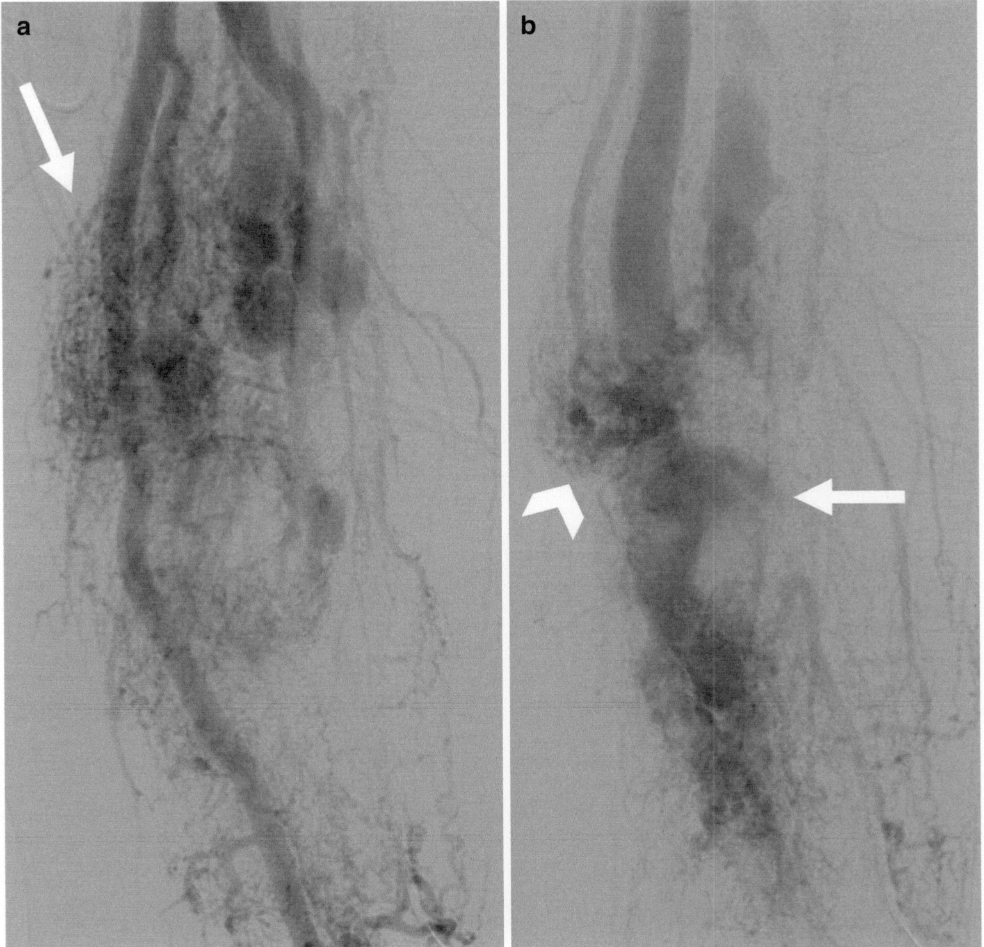

Fig. 84.2 (**a**) DSA of the lower extremity via right common femoral artery during arterial phase shows high flow AVM fed primarily via branches of the superficial femoral artery and profunda femoris artery. (**b**) DSA of the lower extremity via right common femoral artery during venous phase shows the AVM drainage through a conglomeration of vessels (arrowhead) into the femoral vein with partial filling of the large varix (arrow)

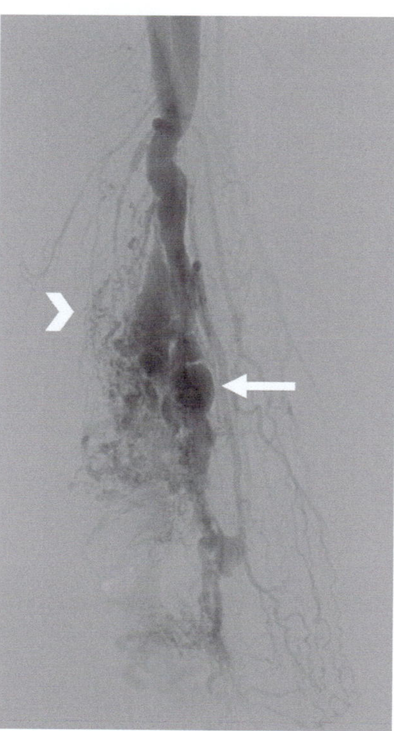

Fig. 84.3 DSA of the lower extremity via the right common femoral artery following alcohol embolization shows sclerosis of the majority of the feeding vessels (arrowhead) with decreased but persistent filling of the varix (arrow)

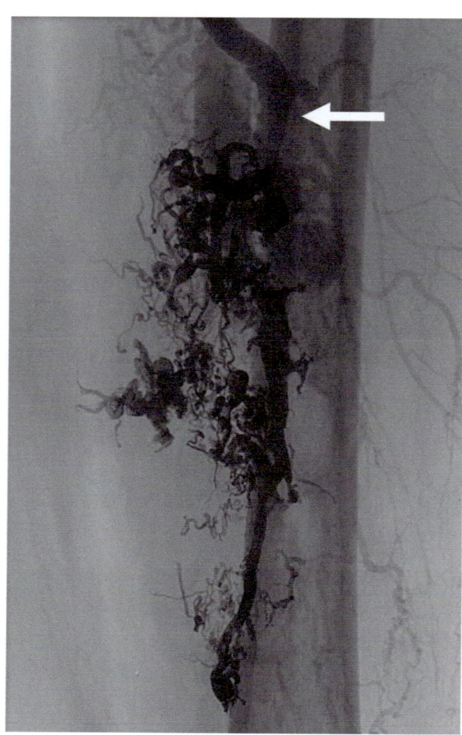

Fig. 84.4 Lower extremity arteriogram via the right common femoral artery following EVOH embolization of multiple feeding branches arising from the profunda femoris with diminished but persistent arteriovenous shunting (arrow)

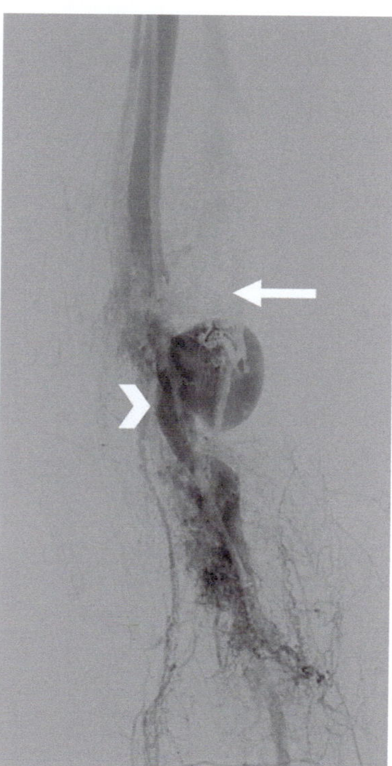

Fig. 84.5 DSA of the lower extremity via the right common femoral artery shows persistent high flow AVM with drainage via aneurysmal nonfunctional femoral vein (arrowhead) and large network of collateral vessels. Embolization material is present in several superficial femoral artery branches (arrow)

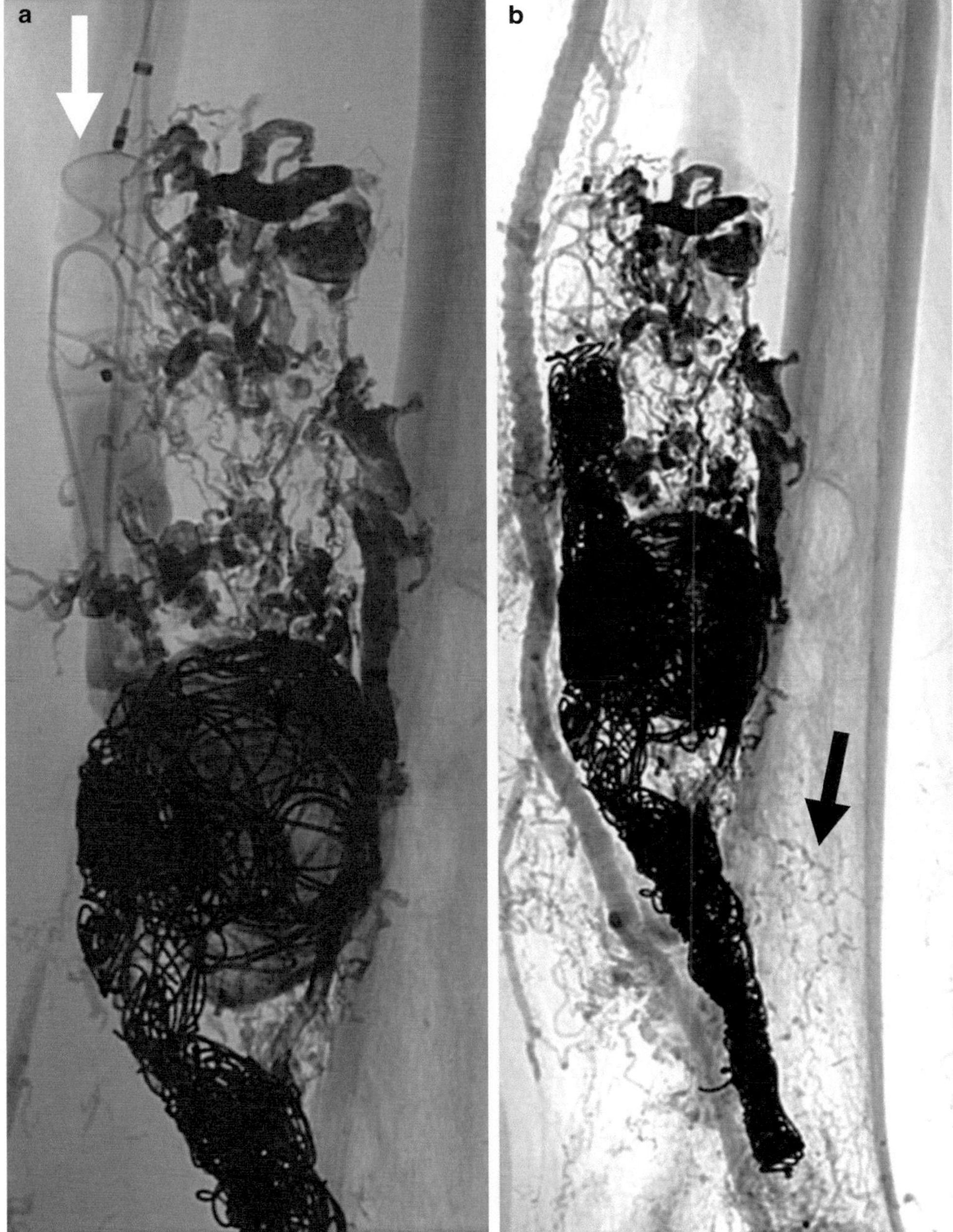

Fig. 84.6 (**a**) Lower extremity venogram via right femoral vein shows obliteration of the left femoral vein using various embolization materials. Note the Amplatzer plug along the cephalad portion (arrow). (**b**) Lower extremity arteriogram via right femoral artery shows full extent of transvenous outflow obliteration with no residual flow via the femoral vein and minimal drainage via collateral vessels into the deep femoral vein (arrow)

Primum Non Nocere, or the Wrong and the Right AVM Treatment

R. Garcia-Monaco, O. Peralta, and M. Rabellino

A 39-year-old male patient with a 5-year history of trophic changes at the patellar region with recurrent skin ulcers and bleeding treated with topic medication. The arteriovenous malformation (AVM) (Fig. 85.1) was treated in other institution with endovascular stent-graft placement in the femoral and popliteal arteries by an endovascular physician. Pain and

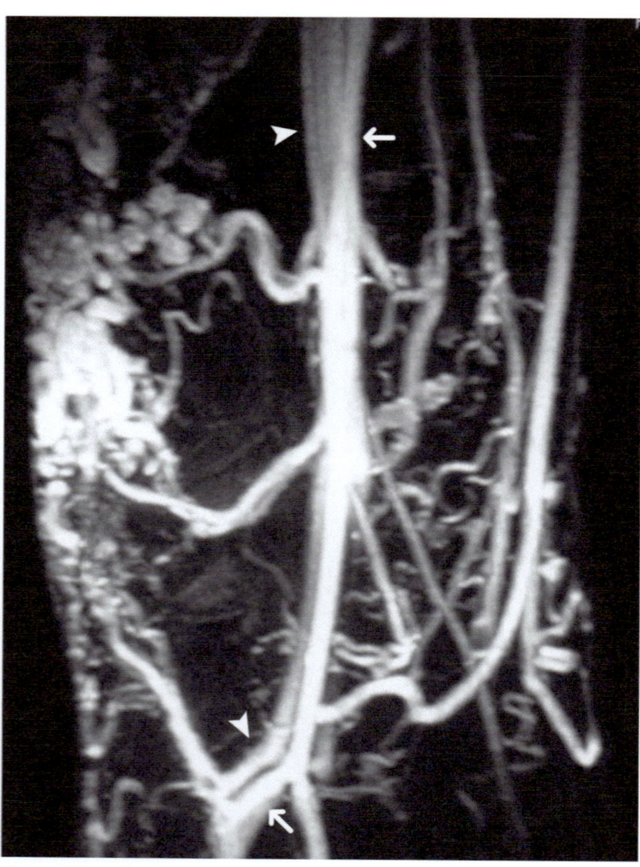

Fig. 85.1 Angio MR shows arteriovenous malformation in right knee soft tissue supplied by lateral external superior, medial and inferior genicular arteries. Notice the rapid arteriovenous shunt (arrow = artery; arrowhead = vein)

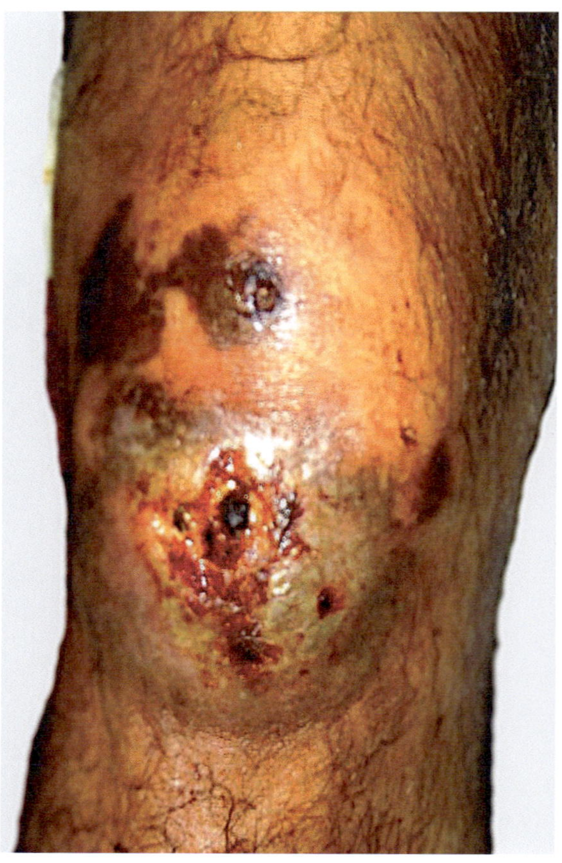

Fig. 85.2 Right knee physical examination upon hospital admission shows skin trophic changes including discoloration and ulceration

skin ulcer did not improve but *worsened* and the patient was referred to our hospital 3 months following that procedure. At admission, physical examination showed skin discoloration, bleeding, ulceration (Fig. 85.2), local warmth, and a palpable thrill. Angio CT showed the AVM nidus supplied from collaterals due to the proximal occlusion of the geniculate arteries by the femoropopliteal stent grafts (Fig. 85.3).

Transarterial and direct percutaneous embolization of the AVM was performed under general anesthesia in the Angio suite (Artis Zeego, Siemens, Germany). After percutaneous femoral puncture, anterograde angiography of the right lower limb was performed showing intra-stent stenosis of the popliteal artery, proximal occlusion of the external genicular arteries, angiogenesis, and a patent AVM nidus supplied by tiny collateral vessels (Fig. 85.4). Embolization

R. Garcia-Monaco (✉) · O. Peralta · M. Rabellino
Department of Vascular and Interventional Radiology, Hospital Italiano de Buenos Aires, Ciudad de Buenos Aires, Argentina
e-mail: ricardo.garciamonaco@hospitalitaliano.org.ar;
oscar.peralta@hospitalitaliano.org.ar;
martin.rabellino@hospitalitaliano.org.ar

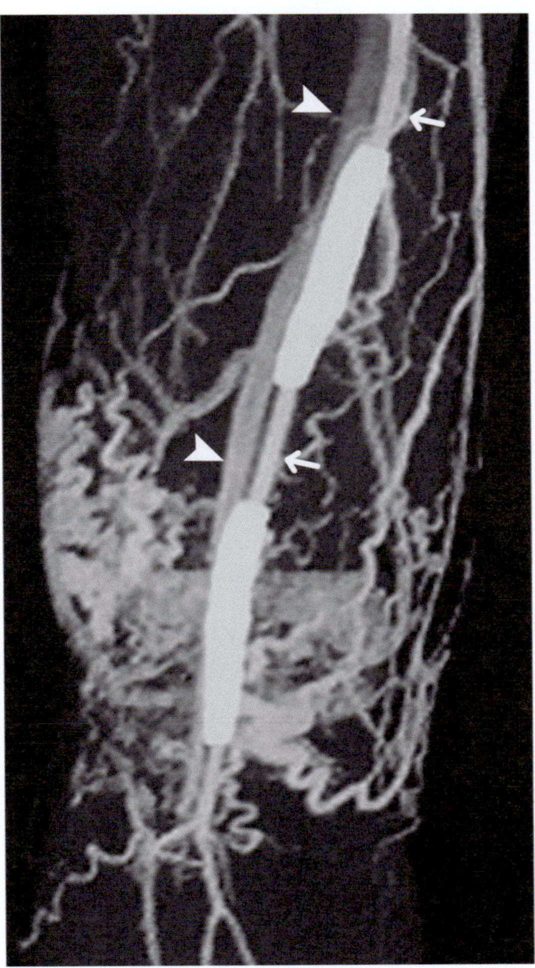

Fig. 85.3 Angio CT at admission shows patent arteriovenous malformation, with angiogenesis and covered stents placed at other institution. Notice the rapid arteriovenous shunt (arrow = artery; arrowhead = vein) that remains unchanged

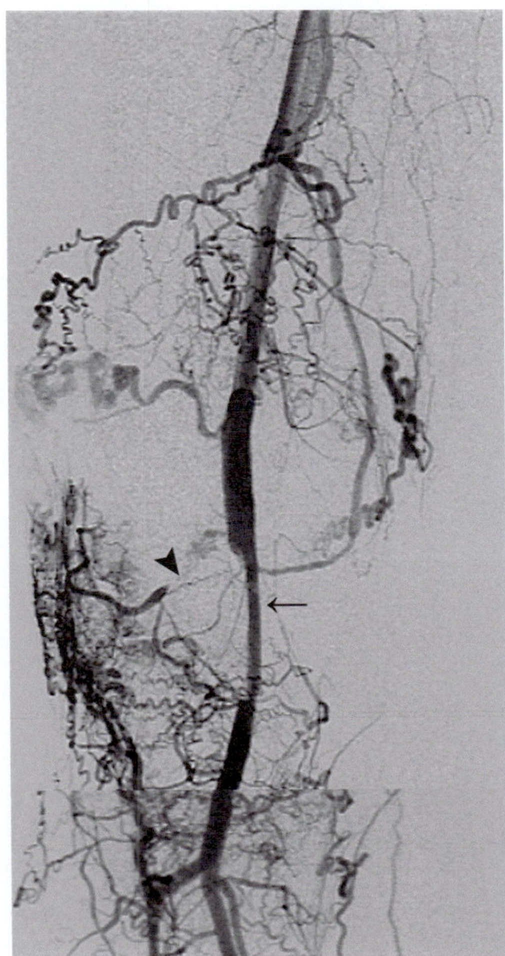

Fig. 85.4 Femoral angiography confirms Angio CT findings. Notice intra-stent stenosis of the popliteal artery (arrow) and near occlusion of the superior genicular artery with complete occlusion of the medial genicular artery (arrowhead). Notice nidus supply by tiny arterial angiogenetic collaterals

was performed with a mixture of NBCA (Histoacryl, Braun) and lipiodol (Guerbet, France) in several AVM nidus compartments mainly by direct injection through percutaneous puncture (Fig. 85.5) but also through transarterial microcatheterization of collateral vessels. After two embolization sessions, 90% of the AVM nidus was excluded (Fig. 85.6) with complete pain remission and progressive ulcer healing. Follow up was-uneventful with marked improvement of trophic changes and ulcer healing. The patient remained asymptomatic without clinical recurrence (pain/ulceration/bleeding) at 10 years follow-up (Figs. 85.7 and 85.8).

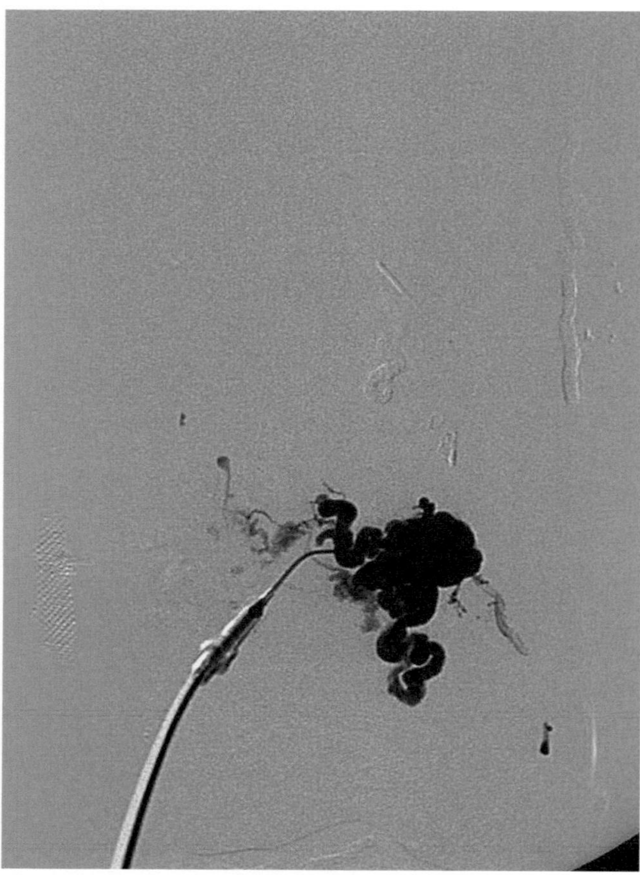

Fig. 85.5 Direct percutaneous angiography of a nidus compartment before glue embolization

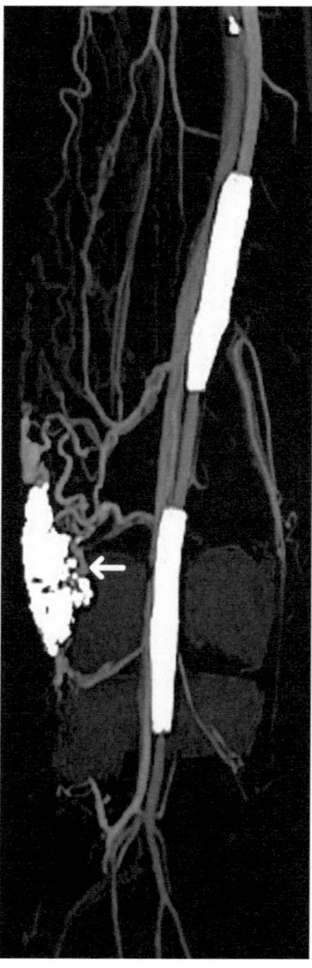

Fig. 85.6 Angio CT at 1-month follow-up shows the glue cast inside the nidus (arrow) and both significant flow reduction and decrease of the size of the malformation

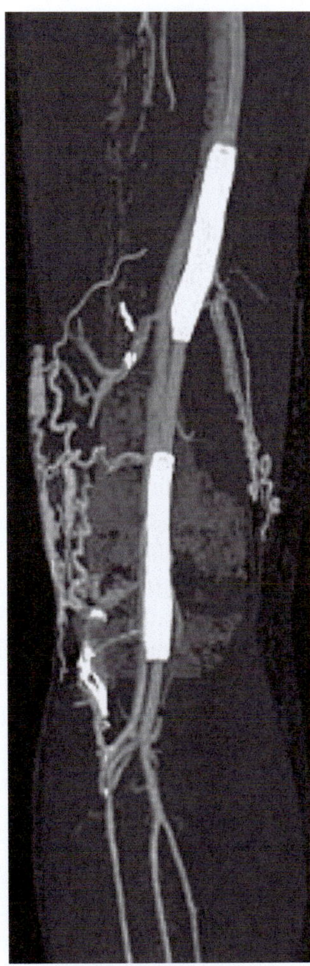

Fig. 85.7 Angio CT at 10 years follow-up shows minimal residual malformation (compare with Fig. 85.3)

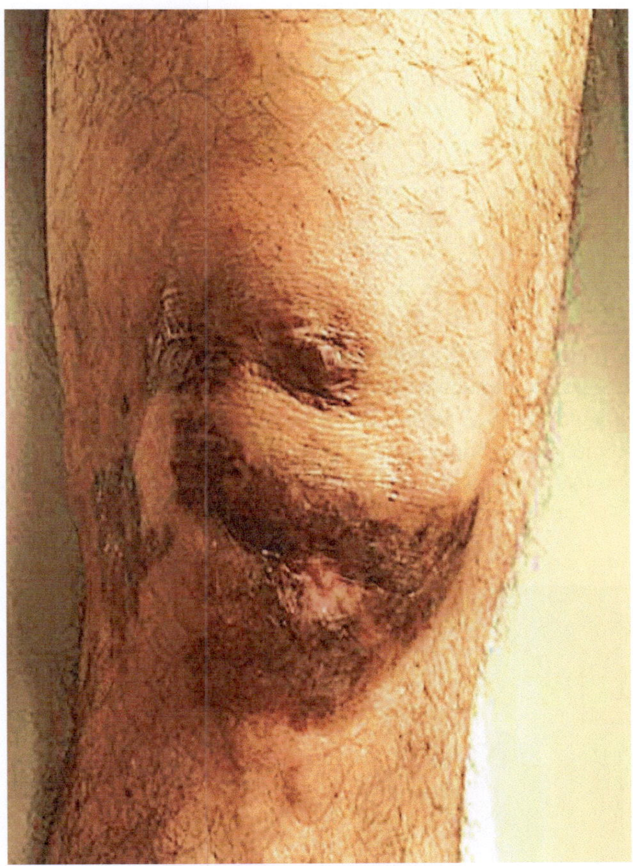

Fig. 85.8 Right knee physical examination at 10 years follow-up only shows scars and chronic pigmentation in an otherwise asymptomatic patient

Bibliography

1. Acar Z, Kiris A, Bektas A, Erden T. Short and mid effects of covered stent implantation on extremity findings and hear failure in Parkes Weber syndrome: a case report. Eur Heart J Case Rep. 2020;4:1–4. https://doi.org/10.1093/ehjcr/ytaa046.

3D Printing Facilitates Embolization of Persistent Mixed Complex/Diffuse Pulmonary Arteriovenous Malformation

John R. Dryden, Miles B. Conrad, R. Peter Lokken, Michael J. Bunker, and Shafkat Anwar

A 17-year-old with multi-year history of shortness of breath and dyspnea on exertion was diagnosed with hereditary hemorrhagic telangiectasia and mixed complex/diffuse right lower lobe (RLL) pulmonary arteriovenous malformation (PAVM) (Fig. 86.1). Originally, the patient was referred for curative right lower lobec-

tomy. However, the patient, family, and surgeon declined surgical intervention, leading to embolization.

Using a right transfemoral approach, the right pulmonary artery (PA) was catheterized. A combination of vascular plugs (Amplatzer Vascular Plug 4, Abbott and MVP/Micro Vascular Plug, Medtronic) and detachable coils (Concerto, Medtronic and Packing Coils, Penumbra) were used to embolize the RLL PAVM (Fig. 86.2). However, a dominant remaining perfusing artery could not be successfully catheterized despite use of multiple pre-shaped catheters.

Repeat contrast-enhanced computed tomography (CT) 3 months after initial treatment demonstrated diminished size of the complex/diffuse RLL PAVM, but with persistent shunting through the unembolized perfusing artery (Fig. 86.3).

Institutional 3D modeling experts used the pre-embolization CT to create a full-scale 3D printed model of the pulmonary vascular anatomy (Fig. 86.4a, b), which was used to

Fig. 86.1 Axial maximum intensity projection (MIP) CT demonstrating mixed complex/diffuse RLL PAVM (arrow) prior to embolization

J. R. Dryden (✉)
Department of Radiology/Radiological Sciences, Uniformed Services University of the Health Sciences, Bethesda, MD, USA
e-mail: john.r.dryden.mil@health.mil

M. B. Conrad · R. P. Lokken
Department of Radiology and Biomedical Imaging, University of California, San Francisco, San Francisco, CA, USA
e-mail: miles.conrad@ucsf.edu; rpeter.lokken@ucsf.edu

M. J. Bunker
Center for Advanced 3D+ Technologies, University of California San Francisco, San Francisco, CA, USA
e-mail: Michael.bunker@ucsf.edu

S. Anwar
Department of Pediatrics and Radiology, Center for Advanced 3D+ Technologies, University of California San Francisco, San Francisco, CA, USA
e-mail: shafkat.anwar@ucsf.edu

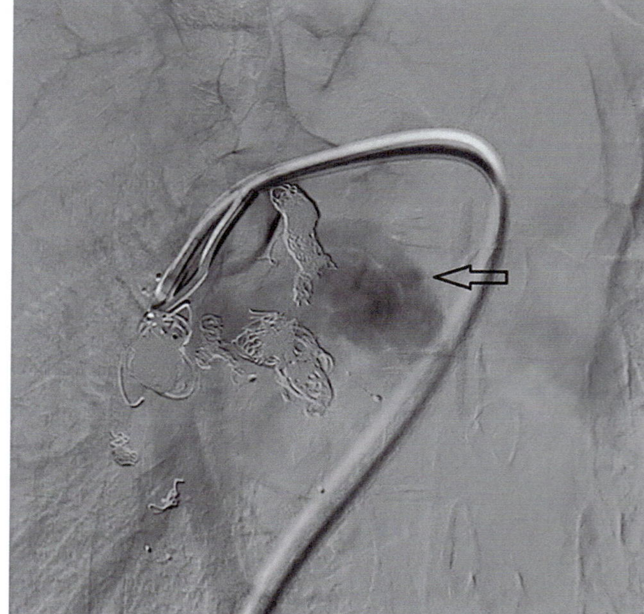

Fig. 86.2 Digital subtraction angiography (DSA) at the conclusion of the first embolization session shows incomplete embolization of complex/diffuse RLL PAVM with residual contrast opacification (arrow)

steam-shape a custom 5Fr (UCSF2, Cordis) catheter (Fig. 86.5) prior to repeat embolization. Using this catheter, the residual RLL PAVM was successfully embolized with vascular plugs (Medtronic MVP-3Q, MVP-5Q) and detachable coils (Stryker Target XL, Medtronic Concerto Helix, and Penumbra Packing Coils) (Fig. 86.6). More than 20 vessels were treated during the two procedures; the mean pulmonary artery pressure dropped from 18 mmHg before the first procedure to 17 mmHg after the second intervention. The room air resting oxygen saturation increased from 82% to 97% after the second embolization. CT 7 months after embolization confirmed continued occlusion of the PAVM (Fig. 86.7).

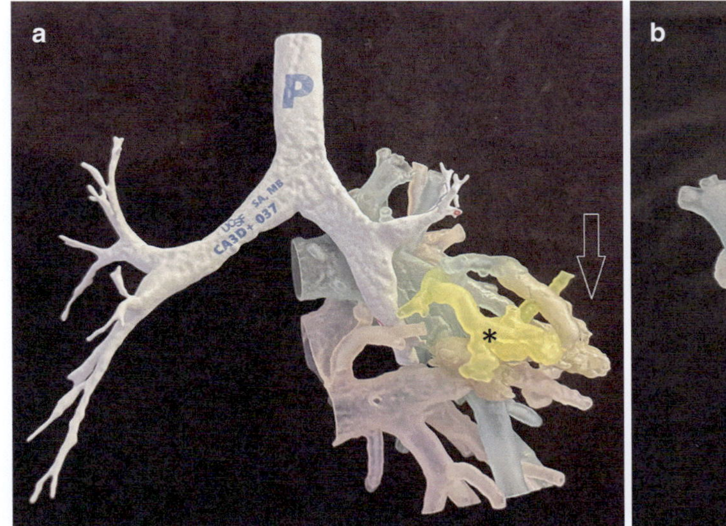

Fig. 86.3 Axial CT following first and preceding second treatment demonstrating post-embolization changes (arrow) with persistent contrast opacification of a portion of the PAVM (asterisk)

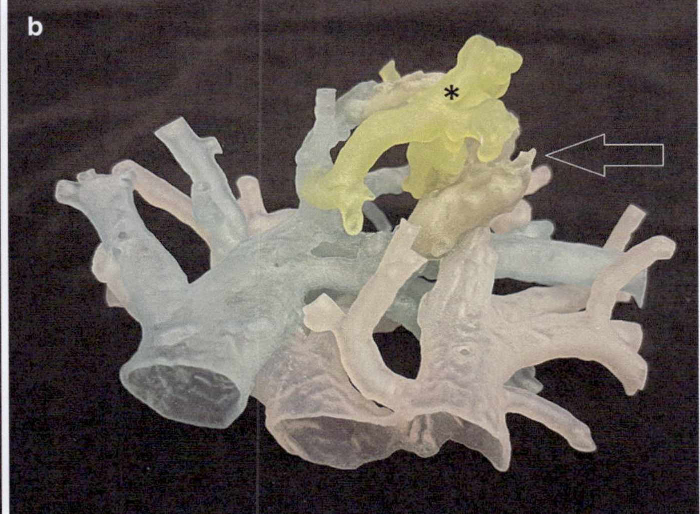

Fig. 86.4 (**a**) Posterior view of 3D printed pulmonary vasculature demonstrating treated (arrow) and untreated (asterisk) portions of the RLL diffuse PAVM. The airway is printed in white and labeled "P". (**b**) Oblique view of 3D printed pulmonary vasculature demonstrating treated (arrow) and untreated (asterisk) portions of the RLL diffuse PAVM

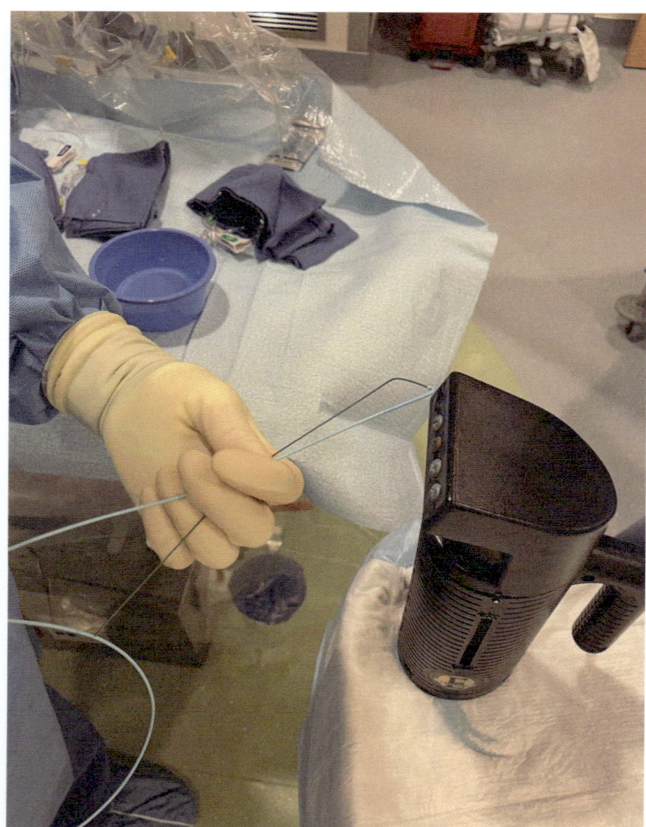

Fig. 86.5 Custom steam-shaping catheters using full-scale 3D printed model

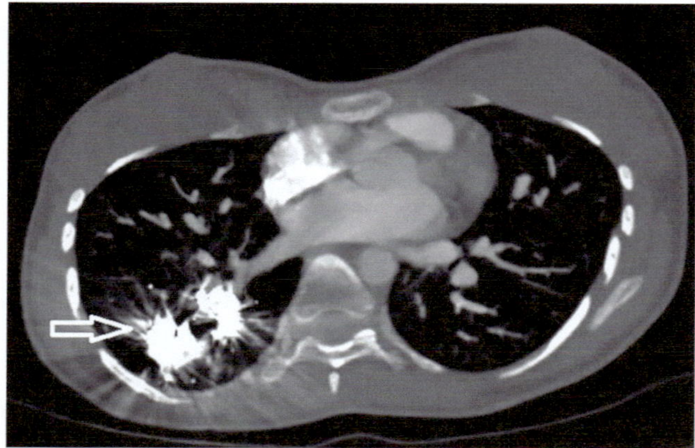

Fig. 86.7 Axial MIP CT 7 months after the second embolization demonstrating complete occlusion of the RLL PAVM (arrow)

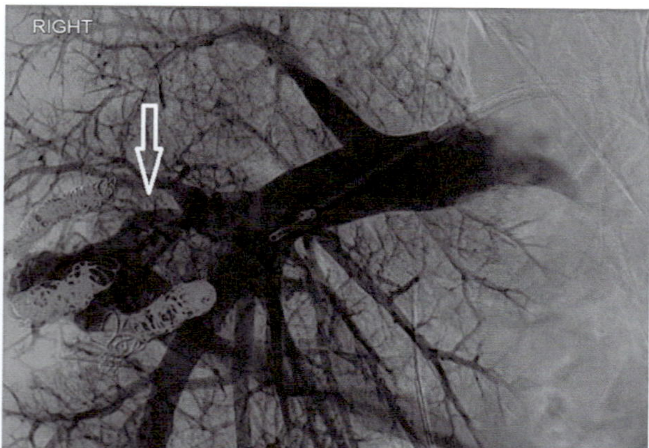

Fig. 86.6 Digital subtraction angiography (DSA) at the start of the second embolization session showing partially embolized RLL PAVM (arrow)

Endovascular Stenting of Pulmonary Stenosis from Takayasu Arteritis

Timothy W. I. Clark

A 68-year-old woman with no significant past medical history was admitted with progressive dyspnea on exertion, dizziness, fatigue, and extremity weakness.

A transthoracic echocardiogram showed pulmonary hypertension with elevated right ventricular systolic pressures. CT and MR angiograms and revealed high-grade bilateral pulmonary artery stenosis and aortic wall thickening consistent with Takayasu's arteritis (TA).

Based on the patient's rapidly progressive shortness of breath and diagnosis of high-grade pulmonary artery stenosis, the decision was made to perform pulmonary artery angiography for possible revascularization.

A high-grade right pulmonary artery stenosis was identified and stented with a 10 × 29 mm Genesis stent (Cordis, Miami Lakes, NJ) followed by 12 mm balloon dilation of the stent (Fig. 87.1a–c). Post stenting the systolic gradient decreased from 65 mmHg to 10 mmHg.

The left pulmonary artery stenosis initially responded well to 12-mm angioplasty therefore no stent was placed; 16 months later, the patient developed recurrent dyspnea and a CTA showed left PA stenosis. A 12 × 19 mm Genesis stent was placed with complete resolution of the pressure gradient (Fig. 87.2a–c). Eight years later, she remained asymptomatic with no functional limitation, exertional symptoms or chest discomfort and had been tapered off her low-dose steroids (Fig. 87.3a, b).

Takayasu's arteritis (TA) is a chronic panarteritis predominantly affecting the aorta and its major branches; pulmonary artery hypertension is seen in 12–13% and portends a worse prognosis. Although endovascular treatment of PA stenosis during the active phase of the disease has been discouraged, the severity of symptoms in this case warranted prompt intervention.

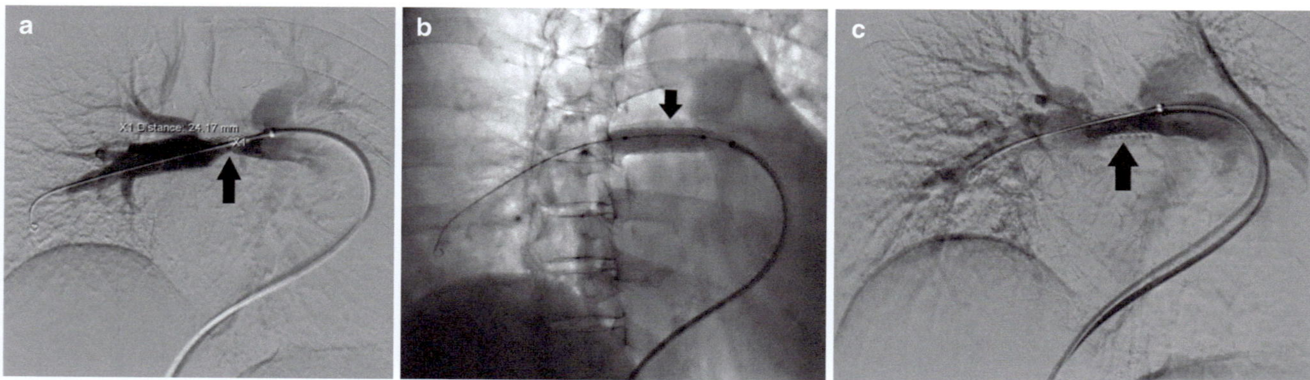

Fig. 87.1 (**a**) Digitally subtracted right pulmonary angiogram showing focal stenosis (arrow). (**b**) Balloon dilation of 10 × 29 mm Genesis stent to 12 mm diameter through 7 French sheath. (**c**) Right pulmonary angiogram post stent placement

T. W. I. Clark (✉)
Section of Interventional Radiology, Department of Radiology,
University of Pennsylvania Perelman School of Medicine,
Philadelphia, PA, USA
e-mail: timothy.clark@pennmedicine.upenn.edu

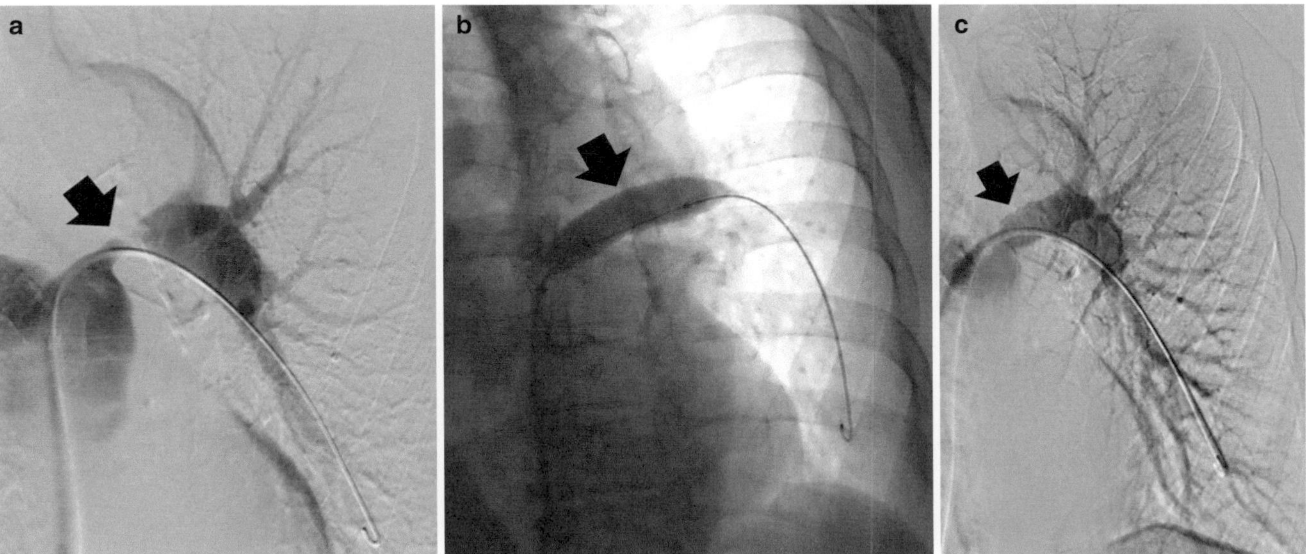

Fig. 87.2 (**a**) Left pulmonary angiogram 16 months later showing recurrence of previously angioplastied left pulmonary artery stenosis (arrow). (**b**) Balloon dilation of 12 × 19 mm stent (arrow). (**c**) Left pulmonary angiogram post stent placement

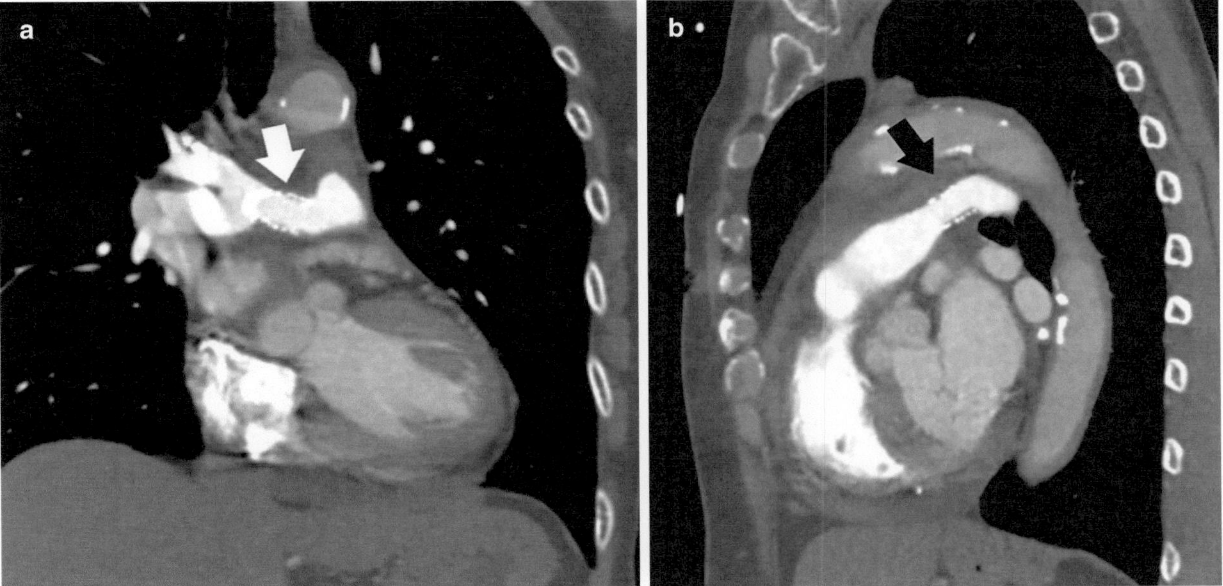

Fig. 87.3 (**a**) Coronal CT angiogram (performed for unrelated symptoms) showing widely patent right pulmonary artery stent (arrow) 7 years later. (**b**) Sagittal CT angiogram showing widely patent left pulmonary artery stent (arrow) 7 years later

Bibliography

1. Toledano K, Guralnik L, Lorber A, Ofer A, Yigla M, Rozin A, Markovits D, Braun-Moscovici Y, Balbir-Gurman A. Pulmonary arteries involvement in Takayasu's arteritis: two cases and literature review. Semin Arthritis Rheum. 2011;41(3):461–70.
2. Li D, Ma S, Li G, Chen J, Tang B, Zhang X, Yang D, Yang Y. Endovascular stent implantation for isolated pulmonary arterial stenosis caused by Takayasu's arteritis. Clin Res Cardiol. 2010;99(9):573–5.
3. Qin L, Hong-Liang Z, Zhi-Hong L, Chang-Ming X, Xin-Hai N. Percutaneous transluminal angioplasty and stenting for pulmonary stenosis due to Takayasu's arteritis: clinical outcome and four-year follow-up. Clin Cardiol. 2009;32(11):639–43.

Fluoroscopic and Trans-Esophageal Echocardiographic Guided Removal of Dialysis Access Stents Migrated to the Heart and Pulmonary Artery

Jared Gans and Jacob Cynamon

An 80-year-old male with a complex past medical history including end-stage renal disease underwent an arteriovenous graft intervention for outflow obstruction at an outside institution. During the procedure, two self-expanding bare-metal stents migrated, one to the left pulmonary artery and one to the right ventricle (Fig. 88.1). Post-procedure, the patient developed new onset premature ventricular contractions and CT demonstrated a stent near the tricuspid valve (Fig. 88.2).

At presentation, the patient was not deemed an open surgical candidate for stent removal due to arrhythmias and location of the right ventricular stent.

Intraprocedural trans-esophageal echocardiography (TEE) guidance was used during percutaneous stent extraction; this demonstrated that the right ventricular stent was separate from the tricuspid valve (Fig. 88.3). The stent was snared within the right ventricle, folded upon itself, and

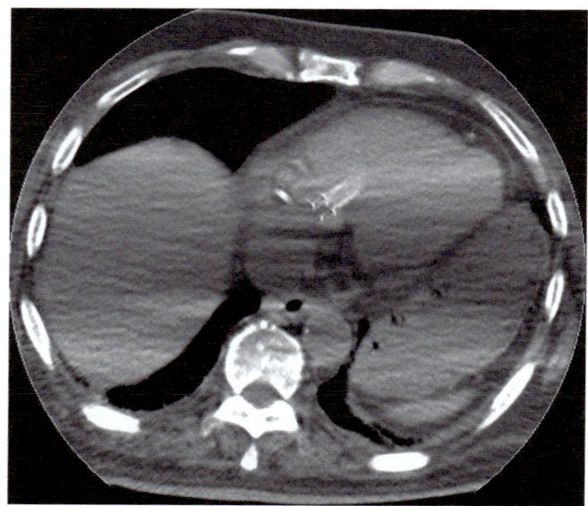

Fig. 88.2 Axial image from non-contrast computed tomography demonstrates the right ventricular stent in close association with the tricuspid valve

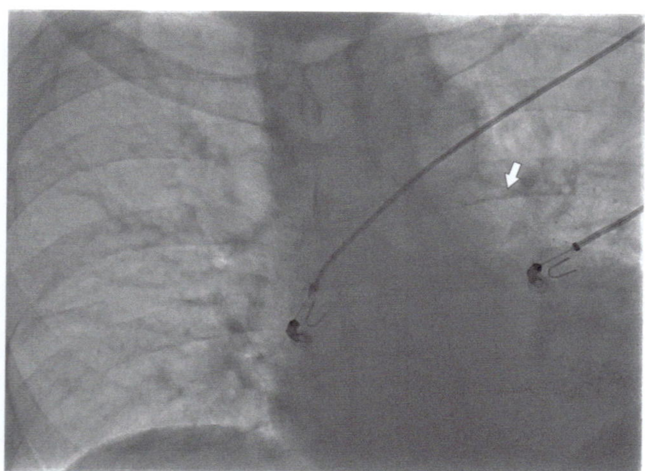

Fig. 88.1 Fluoroscopic spot image from outside procedure demonstrating a migrated stent in the left pulmonary artery (white arrow). Due to cardiac motion, the cardiac stent is not visible

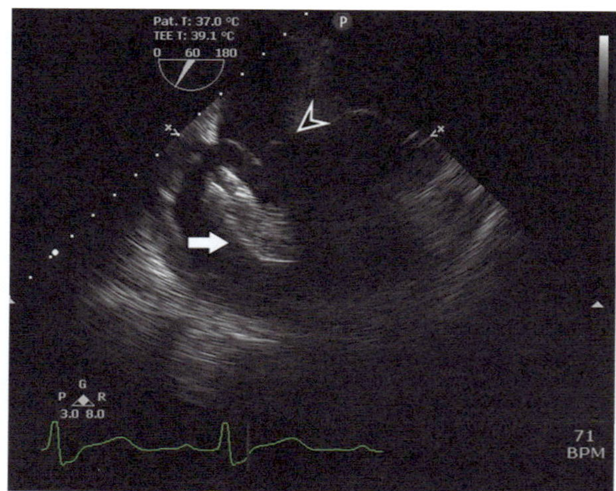

Fig. 88.3 Intraprocedural TEE four-chamber view demonstrates the stent located within the right ventricle (arrow) but separate from the tricuspid valve (arrowhead)

J. Gans (✉)
Envision Healthcare, Fort Lauderdale, FL, USA

J. Cynamon
Department of Radiology, Montefiore Medical Center, Bronx, NY, USA

withdrawn into an intraventricular 10Fr guiding catheter (to protect the tricuspid valve) (Fig. 88.4). This catheter and the stent were withdrawn into a 16Fr long sheath within the IVC

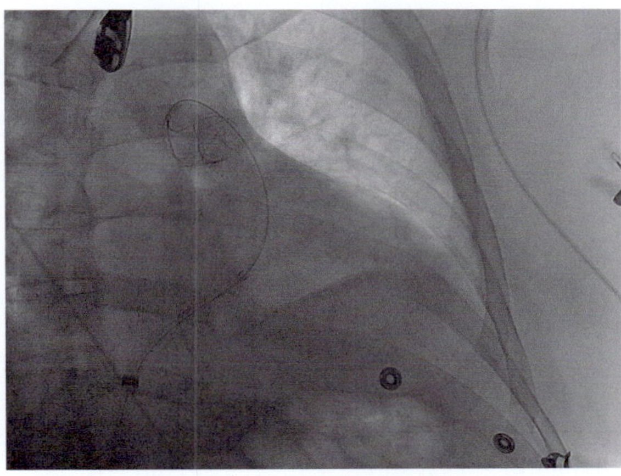

Fig. 88.6 Utilization of the sheath, guiding catheter, and snare to capture the left pulmonary artery stent

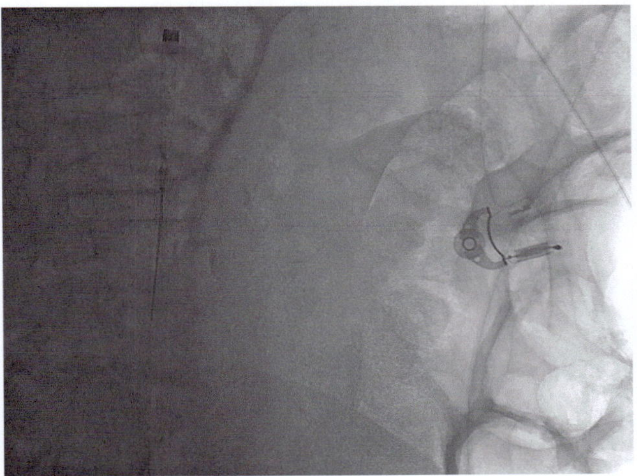

Fig. 88.4 Successful snare of the right ventricular stent and withdrawal of the stent into a long sheath using the guide catheter

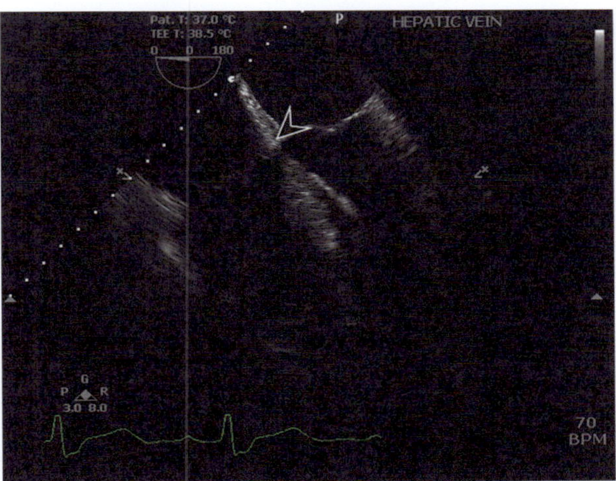

Fig. 88.7 Post-retrieval TEE four-chamber view with the right ventricular stent completely removed and intact tricuspid valve visualized (arrowhead)

Fig. 88.5 Stent and catheter entirely withdrawn from the heart safely into IVC sheath

(Fig. 88.5) and the sheaths, catheter, and stent were then removed together, whilst maintaining a transfemoral intravascular guidewire. The same procedure was repeated for the retrieval of the left pulmonary artery stent (Figs. 88.6 and 88.7). Post-procedure TEE and pulmonary arteriography demonstrated no injuries (Fig. 88.8). The patient was discharged to his previous skilled nursing facility on post-procedure day 2 without subsequent complication.

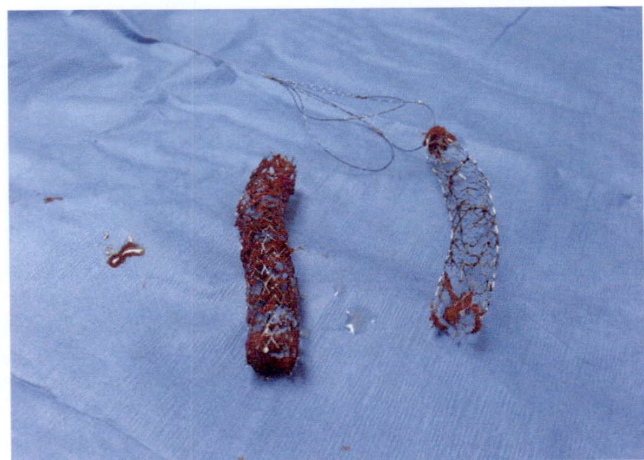

Fig. 88.8 Intraprocedural photograph of both stents status post-retrieval with snare

Embolization of Extensive, Persistent Surgical Hemodialysis Antecubital Arteriovenous Fistula Causing Severe Arm Edema

Dhara Kinariwala and Ziv J Haskal

A 29-year-old male renal transplant recipient presented with severe ongoing right forearm and hand pain and swelling despite multiple open surgical attempts to directly ligate his antecubital brachio-basilic arteriovenous fistula (Fig. 89.1).

Arm angiography demonstrated the large complex arteriovenous fistula from the distal brachial artery, just proximal to the radial and ulnar artery bifurcation. There were multiple venous components of the fistula, including two large, intercommunicating ulnar-sided tortuous veins with central flow direction, and a large tortuous radial-sided vein with flowing retrograde toward his wrist (Fig. 89.2).

Distal ulnar and radial arteries angiography showed normal arterial anatomy. Superselective angiography of the ulnar-sided veins showed rapid outflow via large superficial collaterals (Figs. 89.3 and 89.4). Detachable hydrogel (Microvention) and bare metal (Penumbra) detachable coil were methodically packed until no venous outflow remained (Fig. 89.5).

Similar catheterization of the radial-sided outflow vein showed rapid outflow to the wrist via paired veins, with central

Fig. 89.1 Right forearm and hand swelling and discoloration is visible, compared to the left forearm and hand, without ulcerations or skin lesions. His palpable radial and ulnar pulses are marked. Abandoned left antecubital AV hemodialysis fistula

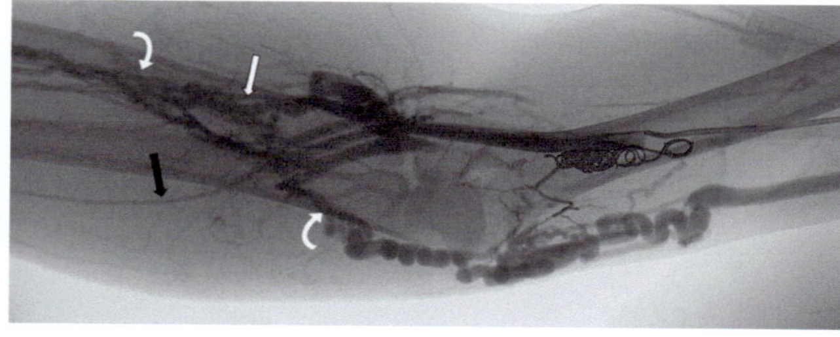

Fig. 89.2 Right brachial arteriography shows the complex high flow arteriovenous fistula with extensive venous collaterals (white curved arrows) and small caliber radial (white straight arrow) and ulnar (black straight arrow) arteries due to shunting. Prior unrelated coils are visualized in the upper arm

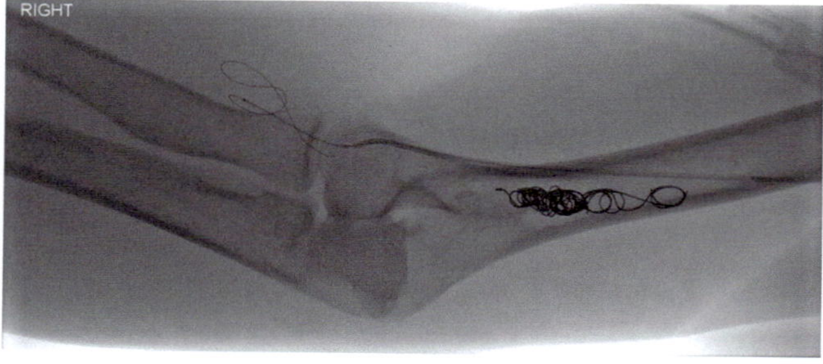

Fig. 89.3 The tortuous course required to reach the first point of embolization is illustrated by the course of the microwire

D. Kinariwala
Department of Radiology and Medical Imaging, University of Virginia, Charlottesville, VA, USA

Z. J Haskal (✉)
Department of Radiology and Medical Imaging, Interventional Division, University of Virginia, Charlottesville, VA, USA

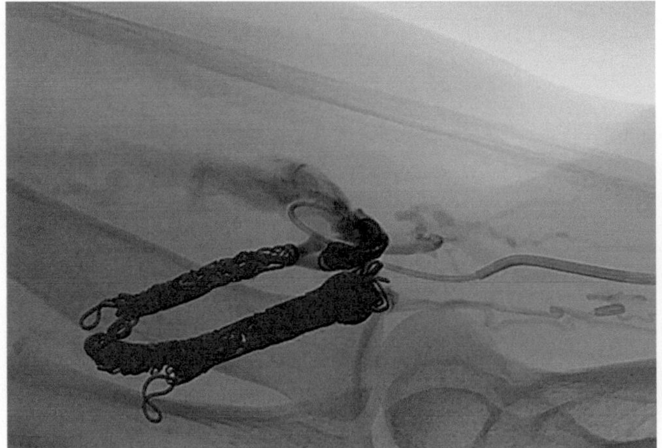

Fig. 89.4 Selective venous angiography of the large ulnar-sided forearm collaterals shows two large, intercommunicating veins (arrows) with outflow via a large, tortuous, superficial collateral vein, and a deep forearm vein

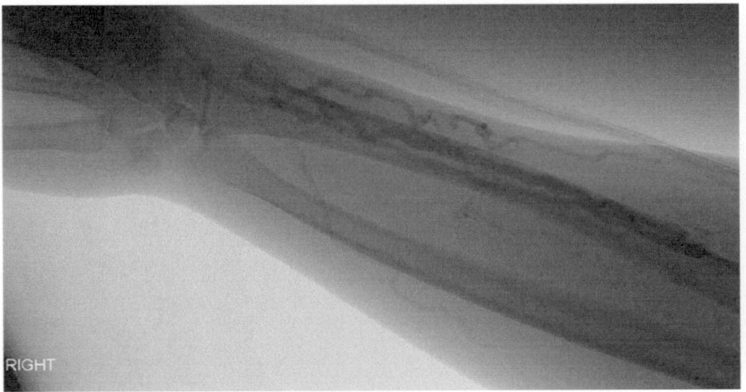

Fig. 89.5 Coil embolization of the venous outflow was performed

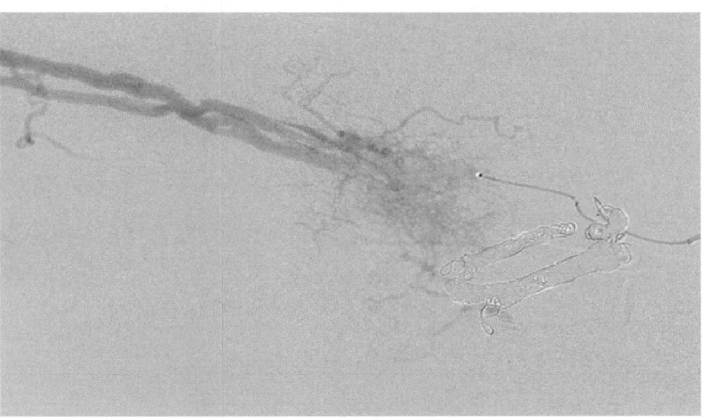

Fig. 89.7 Angiography shows that the paired superficial forearm veins have venous outflow via a large network of small, deep veins resembling a venous malformation

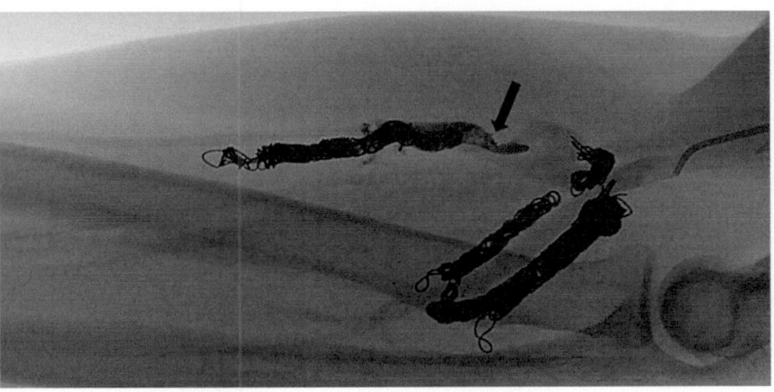

Fig. 89.8 Coil embolization followed by EVOH (Onyx) (arrow) in the ulnar-sided outflow veins was performed to occlude the large veins and deep fibrillary vein recruited by the fistula

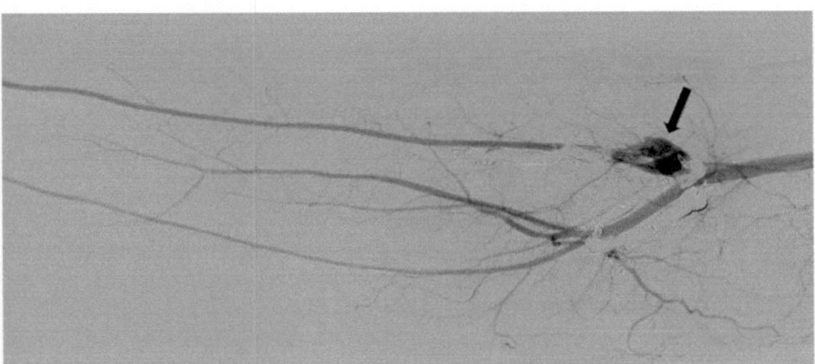

Fig. 89.6 Selective venous angiography of the radial-sided vein shows bifurcation into paired veins and central outflow via deeper forearm veins

Fig. 89.9 Post-intervention angiogram demonstrates exclusion of the large venous collateral outflow vessels. The origin of the AV fistula is visible, without fistulous outflow on later images (arrow)

drainage to deeper forearm veins (Fig. 89.6). This vein also fed a network of small, deep intramuscular veins in the forearm, resembling a complex venous malformation (Fig. 89.7); this was embolized with coils and EVOH (Onyx, Medtronic) (Fig. 89.8). Approximately 547 cm of detachable coils were required to occlude the fistulae. Final angiography demonstrated complete exclusion of the fistulae and preservation of downstream arterial flow (Fig. 89.9). At 3 weeks follow-up, he described decreased arm swelling and return of near-normal arm function.

This case illustrates how a chronic arteriovenous antecubital fistulae may recruit many adjacent outflow veins mimicking a complex high flow arteriovenous malformation and requiring similar endovascular techniques to occlude. These same endovascular challenges may be expected when intentionally occluding mature percutaneously created hemodialysis fistulae (PAVFs) situated near the antecubital fossa.

Recreation of Disrupted AV Graft Venous Anastomosis Using Translumenal Needle Puncture of Venous Target Balloon

Thoedore F. Saad

AV graft percutaneous thrombectomy requires crossing the venous anastomosis. Failure to achieve this precludes completion of the procedure, necessitating open surgical revision or abandonment of the access.

A 72-year-old hemodialysis patient presented with re-thrombosis of upper-arm brachial-basilic bovine graft. Three days prior, he had undergone graft thrombectomy, with venous anastomotic stenosis angioplastied to 7 mm (Fig. 90.1). Repeat aspiration thrombectomy was performed. There was occlusion at the venous anastomosis that could not be crossed using a 5-French Berenstein catheter over a 0.35″ hydrophilic wire; probing the occlusion resulted in minor extravasation (Fig. 90.2).

The brachial vein was then accessed, and a 7-French sheath placed. A 10 mm balloon was "parked" in the basilic vein across from the venous anastomosis. A 21-gauge micropuncture needle was used to access the graft high on the venous limb; this was navigated through the graft lumen and directed toward the basilic vein balloon using ultrasound and fluoroscopic guidance (Fig. 90.3a). The balloon was then punctured and a 0.018″ wire advanced. The balloon was used to drag the wire centrally, then removed. This wire was exchanged for a 0.035″ wire (Fig. 90.3b) and angioplasty performed (Fig. 90.4). An 8 mm × 50 mm Viabahn stent-graft (W.L. Gore, Newark, DE) was deployed from the venous graft segment into the basilic vein (Fig. 90.5a) and post-dilated to 8 mm (Fig. 90.5b), restoring flow and thrill.

This graft has remained in use for 10 months since this procedure. It has required two additional interventions attributed to hypotension and/or graft stenosis, unrelated to the stented anastomosis (Fig. 90.6).

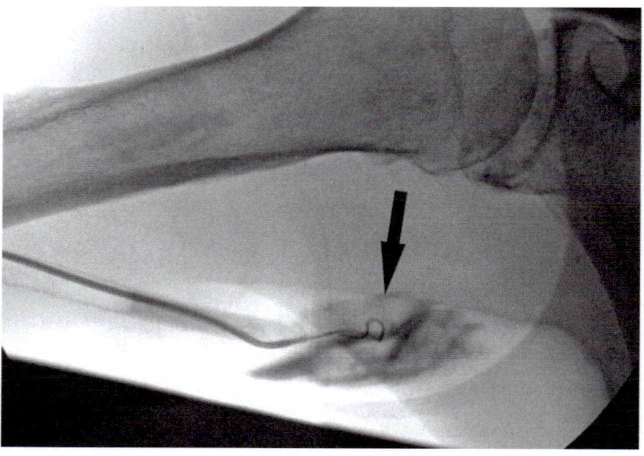

Fig. 90.2 Inability to cross venous anastomosis with extravasation (arrow)

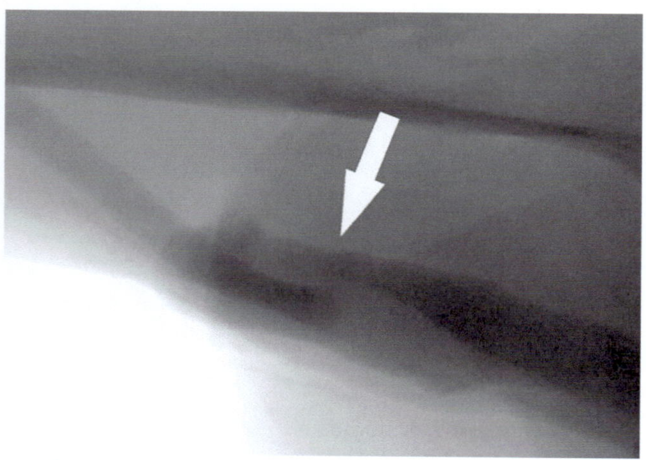

Fig. 90.1 Fistulography demonstrating the venous anastomosis following 7 mm PTA (arrow)

T. F. Saad (✉)
Section of Renal and Hypertensive Diseases, Christiana Care Health System, Newark, DE, USA

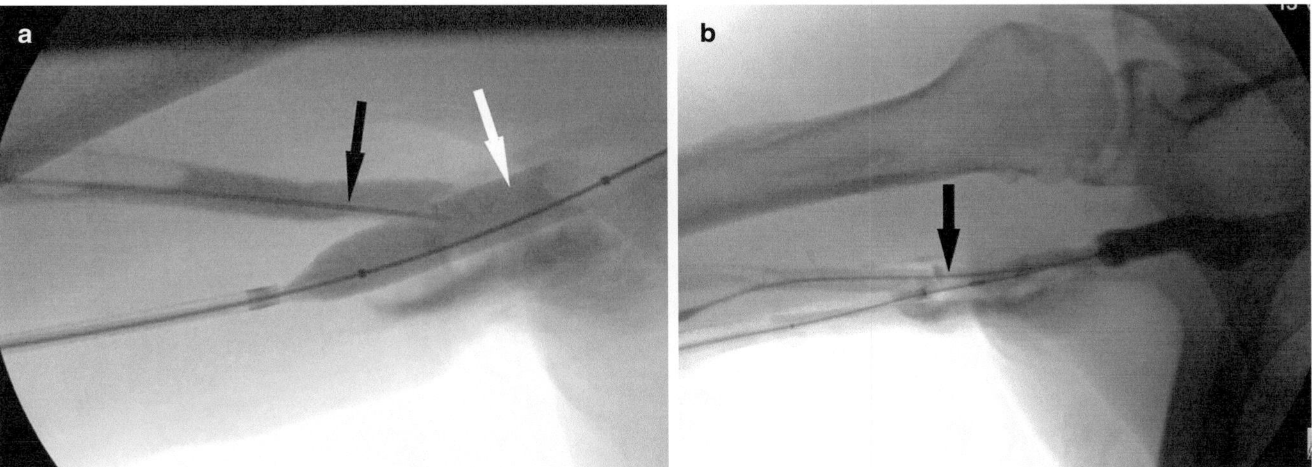

Fig. 90.3 (**a**) 21-gauge micropuncture needle (black arrow) advanced through graft lumen into basilic vein "target" 10 mm balloon (white arrow). (**b**)The 0.018″ guidewire is replaced with an 0.035″ wire, now across newly created graft-vein connection

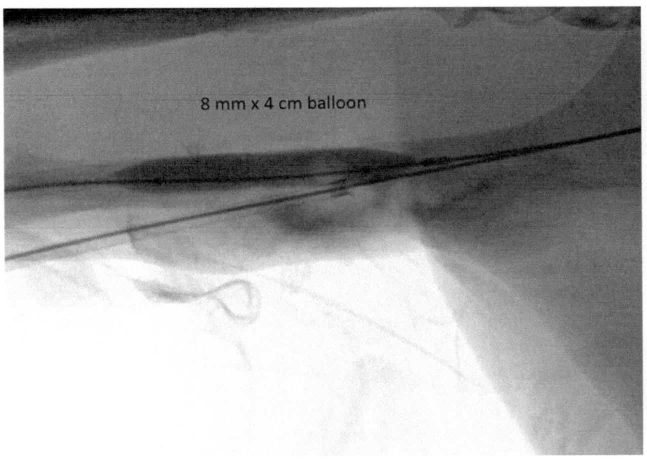

Fig. 90.4 The neo-venous-anastomosis is dilated with an 8 mm angioplasty balloon

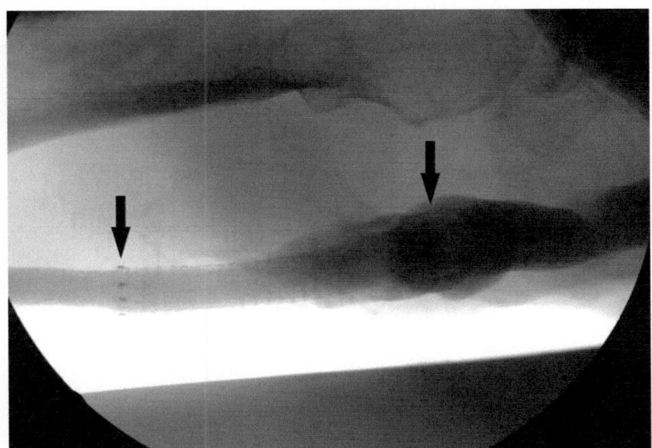

Fig. 90.6 At 6 months, the venous anastomosis is redemonstrated at the time of repeat graft thrombectomy

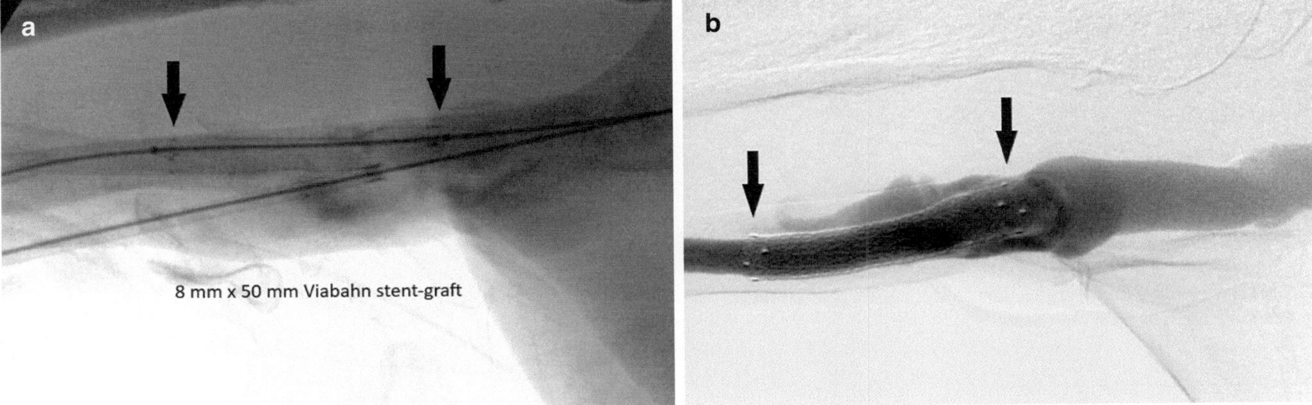

Fig. 90.5 (**a**) An 8 mm diameter × 50 mm long ePTFE Viabahn stent graft has been deployed to span the connection (arrows). (**b**) Immediate fistulography after stent graft deployment confirms full patency

Insertion of a Long-Term Central Venous Catheter at the Subclavian Vein Through a "Full Metal Covered Stent Jacket"

Panagiotis M. Kitrou, Konstantinos Katsanos, and Dimitrios Karnabatidis

A patient presented for hemodialysis catheter placement due to abandonment of a repeatedly failing left arteriovenous prosthetic access graft; it had thrombosed three times in the preceding month alone. The 3-year-old graft had been revised with multiple ePTFE stent grafts, from the level of the VGA to the junction of the brachiocephalic veins due to multiple prior stenoses and thromboses (Fig. 91.1). The right jugular, brachiocephalic veins (Fig. 91.2), and femoral veins were occluded due to previous catheter insertions. We decided to introduce a central venous hemodialysis catheter through the thrombosed covered stents at the level of the left subclavian vein.

Using fluoroscopy, a covered stent within the left subclavian vein was punctured with a 21G (Fig. 91.3) and an 0.018 wire introduced through the occluded stent grafts. This access was used to advance a 6Fr sheath and 8 mm diameter angioplasty balloon into the thrombosed end of the central covered stent (Figs. 91.4 and 91.5). The guidewire was

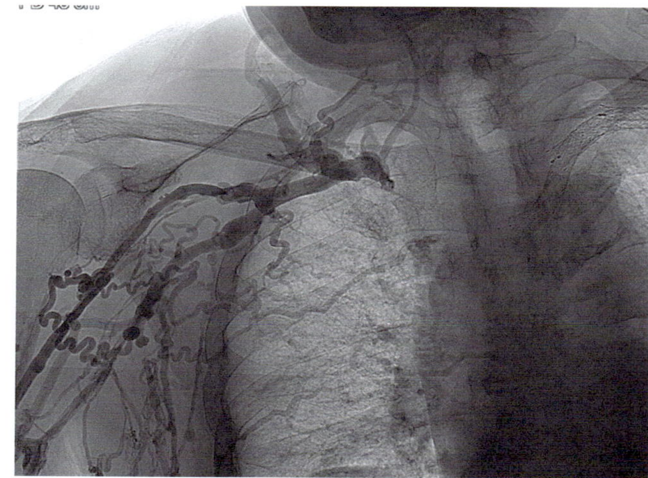

Fig. 91.2 Right arm venography shows chronic obstruction of the right brachiocephalic vein, collateral outflow, and no filling of the superior vena cava

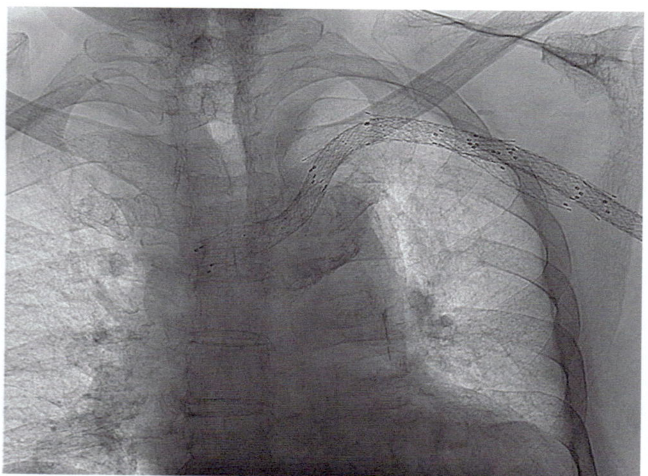

Fig. 91.1 Multiple stent grafts line the left axillary, subclavian, and left brachiocephalic vein

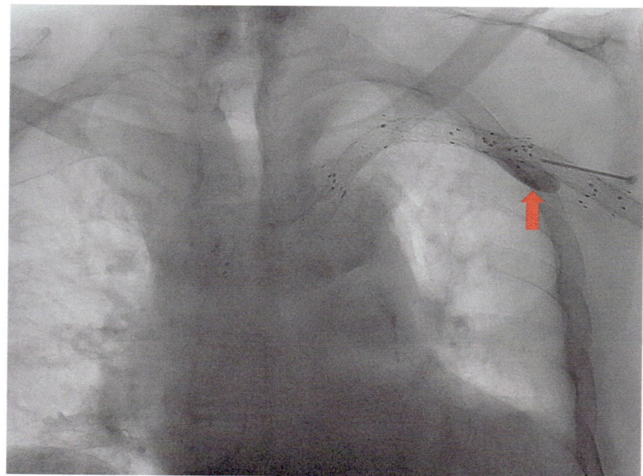

Fig. 91.3 Spot radiography demonstrating needle puncture of the left covered. An arrow shows contrast inside a second "dead-end" covered stent

P. M. Kitrou (✉) · K. Katsanos · D. Karnabatidis
Department of Interventional Radiology, Patras University Hospital, Patras, Greece
e-mail: katsanos@upatras.gr; karnaby@upatras.gr

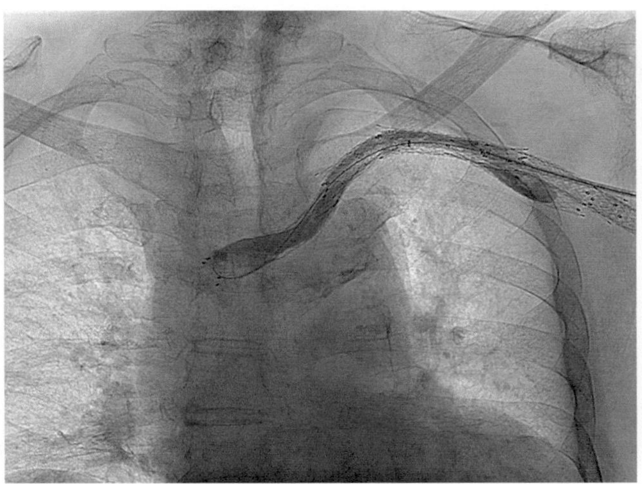

Fig. 91.4 The central end of the covered stents is occluded. A wire is looped at the obstruction

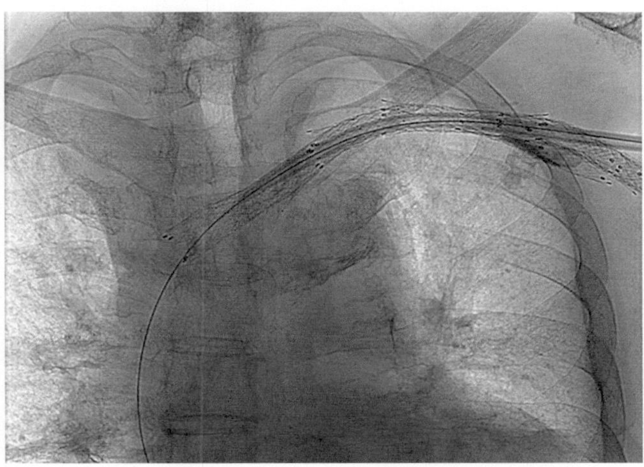

Fig. 91.6 The peel-away introducer sheath has been inserted over an Amplatz wire

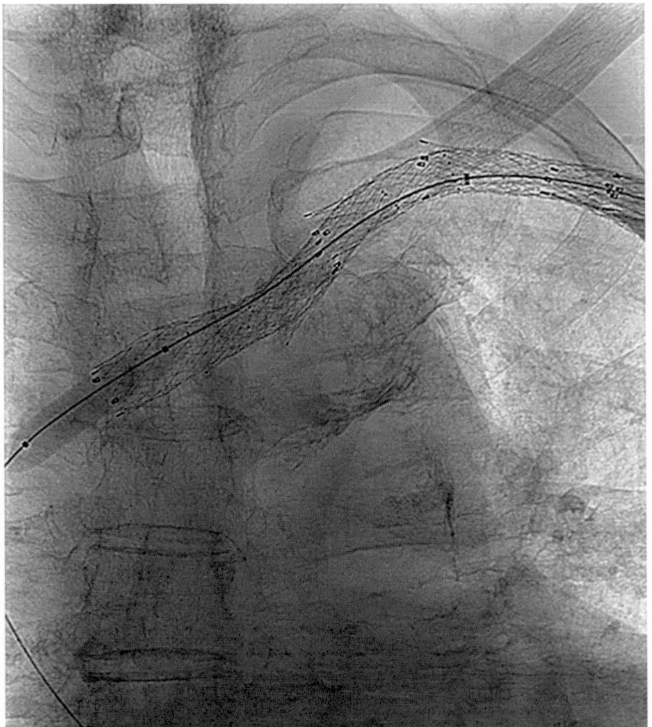

Fig. 91.5 Balloon angioplasty of the occluded stents was performed

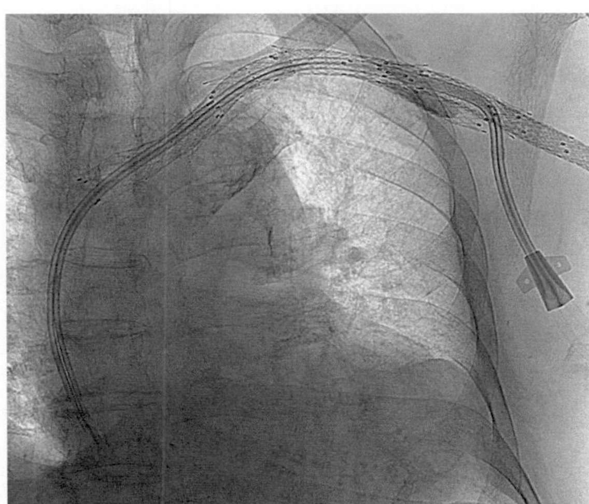

Fig. 91.7 Final position of the 23 cm hemodialysis catheter

changed to an Amplatz wire to support passage of vascular dilators and the hemodialysis catheter sheath to pass through the stent graft interstices (Fig. 91.6). Finally, a tunneled 23 cm long dialysis catheter was placed, passing from the left subclavian vein through the covered stents, reaching the right atrium (Fig. 91.7); it was successfully used for hemodialysis.

Brachial Plexopathy After Creation of Alternate Venous Outflow in a Dialysis Patient

Bart Dolmatch

A 48-year-old woman with hemodialysis-dependent end-stage renal disease and a thrombosed left upper arm hemodialysis arteriovenous graft (AVG) underwent access thrombectomy. Despite anastomosis angioplasty and covered stent graft placement, the graft soon rethrombosed. After a second thrombectomy and additional covered stent, it clotted once again. An incidental CT scan demonstrated severe kinking of the stent graft due to angulation at the venous anastomosis of the AVG (Fig. 92.1); this was the culprit repeated AVG thrombosis.

A new left upper arm AVG was placed and anastomosed to a small preserved segment of brachial vein but the prior covered stents occluded their venous outflow (Fig. 92.2). She developed profound arm swelling because the available collateral vein outflow proved inadequate.

The collateral veins were traversed and balloon dilated to 7 mm. Eight millimeter diameter overlapping covered stents (Fluency, Becton Dickinson) were deployed within the collaterals, from the brachial vein to the brachiocephalic vein (Figs. 92.3 and 92.4).

During covered stent placement, the patient immediately complained of left shoulder and hand pain, notably involving her fourth and fifth fingers, the collateral veins were within or adjacent to the brachial plexus (Fig. 92.5).

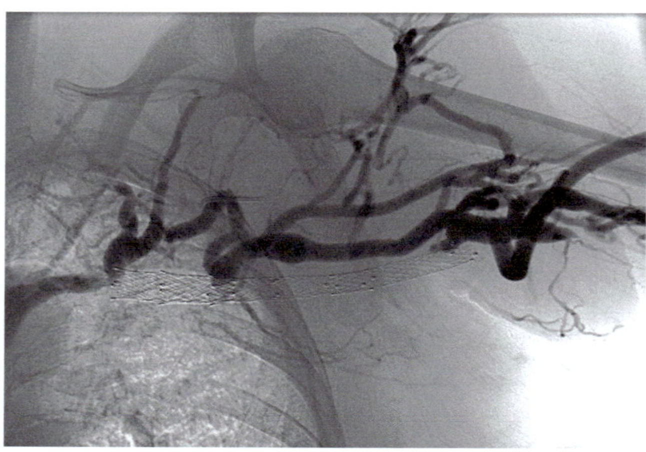

Fig. 92.2 Angiogram of the new AVG shows the anastomosis to an isolated segment of left brachial vein with no direct venous outflow and collateral venous pathways

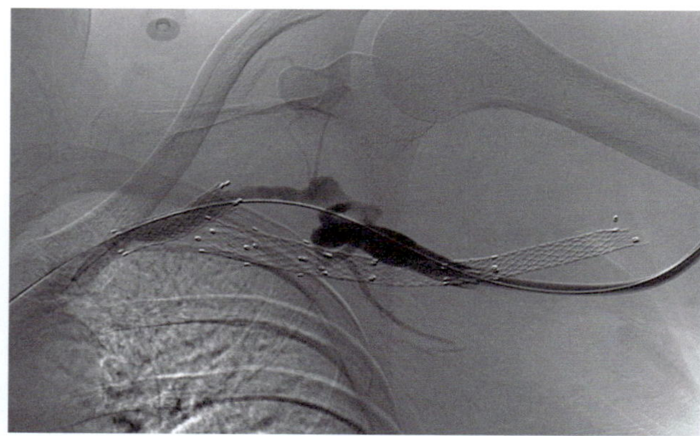

Fig. 92.3 Venography after angioplasty of the collateral pathway and placement of first, more central, covered stent

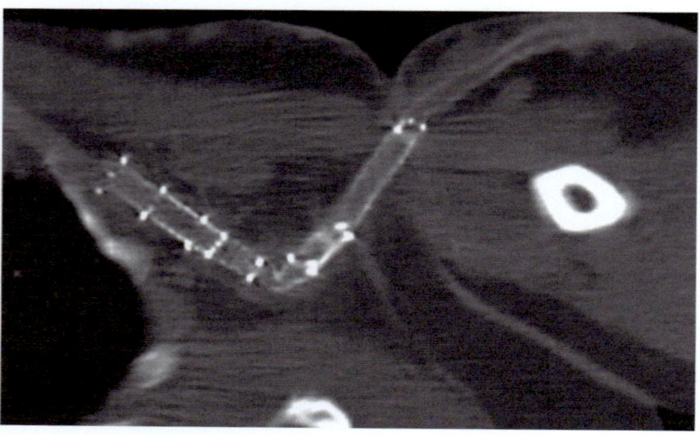

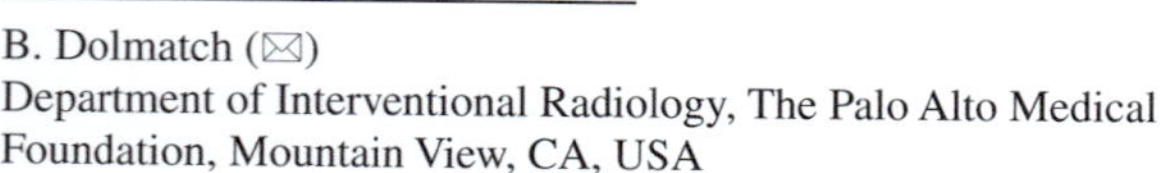

Fig. 92.1 Curved multi-planar reconstruction from CT scan shows kinking of covered stents placed at the venous anastomosis of the AVG that lead to repeated thrombosis

Her left arm swelling resolved quickly, the covered stents maintained AVG patency, proved a durable solution to her arm swelling, and bridged her until she received a cadaveric kidney transplant. However, her neurologic symptoms persisted for 6 months, whilst treated with Gabapentin. Her AVG was ligated after transplant; at 10 years the cadaveric kidney continues to function. This case provides a rare cautionary note regarding the potential proximity of collateral veins to the brachial plexus and risk of brachial plexopathy.

B. Dolmatch (✉)
Department of Interventional Radiology, The Palo Alto Medical Foundation, Mountain View, CA, USA

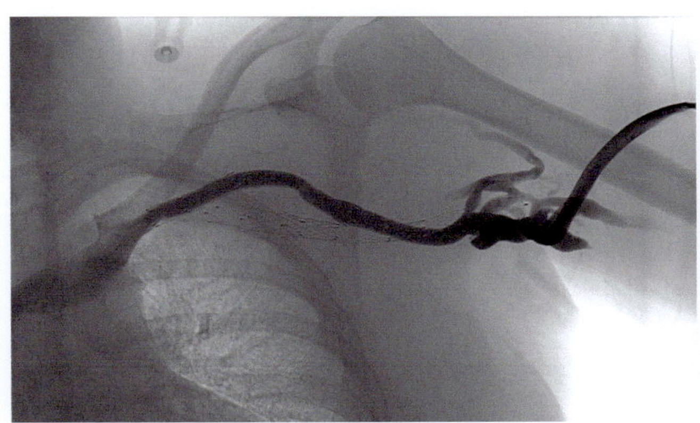

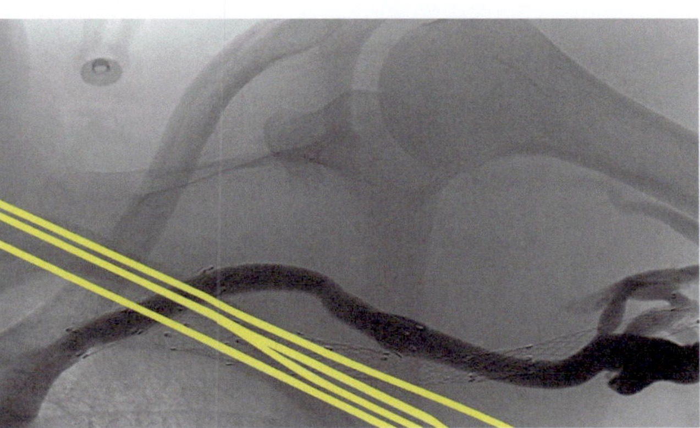

Fig. 92.4 Completion AVG angiogram demonstrates patent covered stents in the collateral pathway to the left brachiocephalic (central) vein with resolution of shoulder collaterals indicating decompression of venous pressure

Fig. 92.5 Diagrammatic superimposition of expected location of the brachial plexus (yellow lines) overlying the covered stents within the collateral veins

Percutaneous Biopsy of an Intra-abdominal Mass Surrounded by Intestines: A Needle and Guidewire Technique

Yasuaki Arai and Miyuki Sone

A woman in her mid 30swas found to have an intra-abdominal tumor on CT examination. The tumor was encircled by intestines, and there was no clear route to directly biopsy the mass without puncturing these obstacles (Fig. 93.1).

A 17G non-coring needle (Fig. 93.2) was inserted into the abdominal cavity anterior to the surrounding bowel. (Fig. 93.3). Using the combination of this needle and advancement and buckling of a 0.035 inch hand-shaped J-type guidewire (to find an open path between bowel loops) (Fig. 93.4), the needle was safely advanced to the target tumor, avoiding the intervening obstacles.

An introducer sheath was coaxially inserted, a guidewire was removed, and the biopsy needle was inserted through the sheath (Fig. 93.5). During this procedure, the position of the needle was repeatedly assessed using fluoroscopy and CT, in

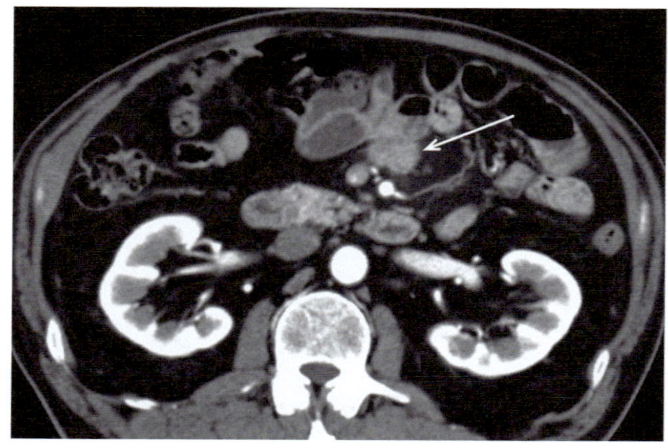

Fig. 93.1 The tumor was surrounded by intestines (arrow)

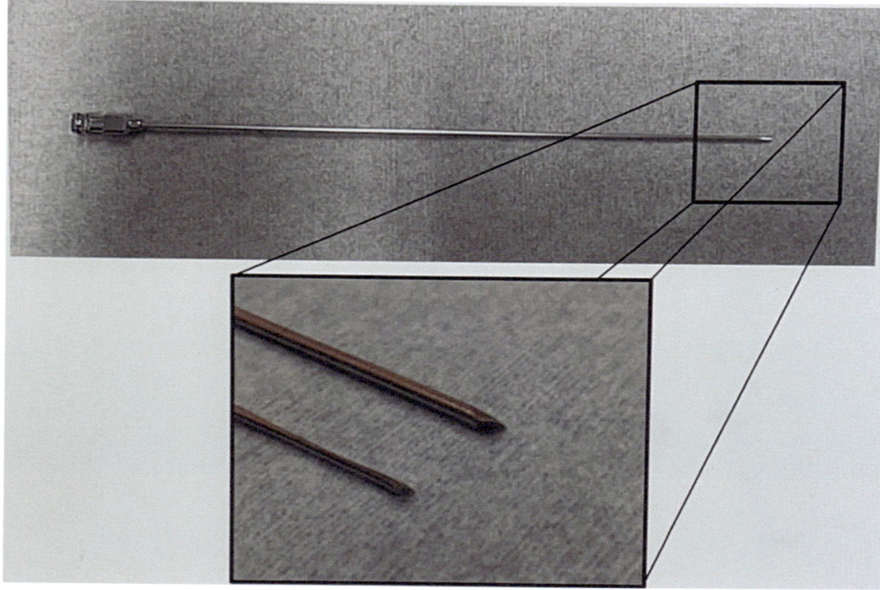

Fig. 93.2 A 17G non-coring type needle

Y. Arai (✉) · M. Sone
Department of Diagnostic Radiology, National Cancer Center, Tokyo, Japan
e-mail: arai-y3111@mvh.biglobe.ne.jp

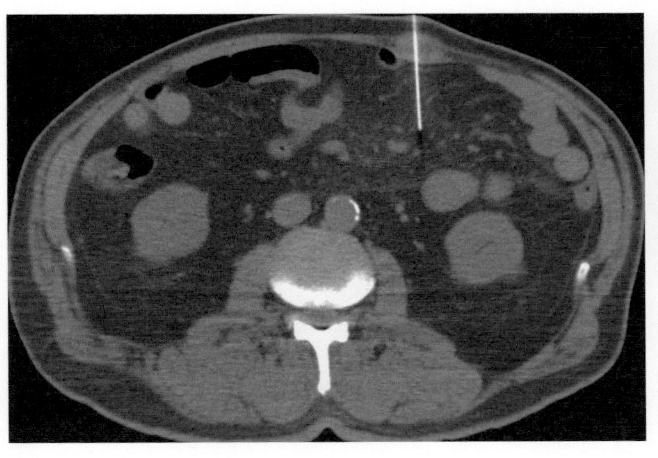

Fig. 93.3 A 17G non-coring type needle (Fig. 93.2) was inserted into the abdominal cavity without intestines

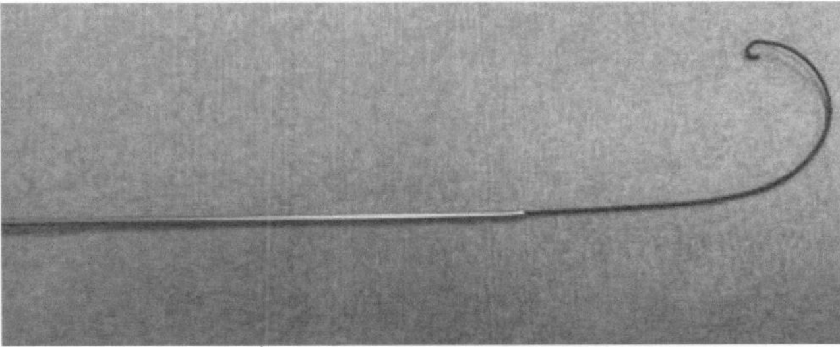

Fig. 93.4 The combination of a non-coring needle and a 0.035-inch hand-bended J-type guidewire

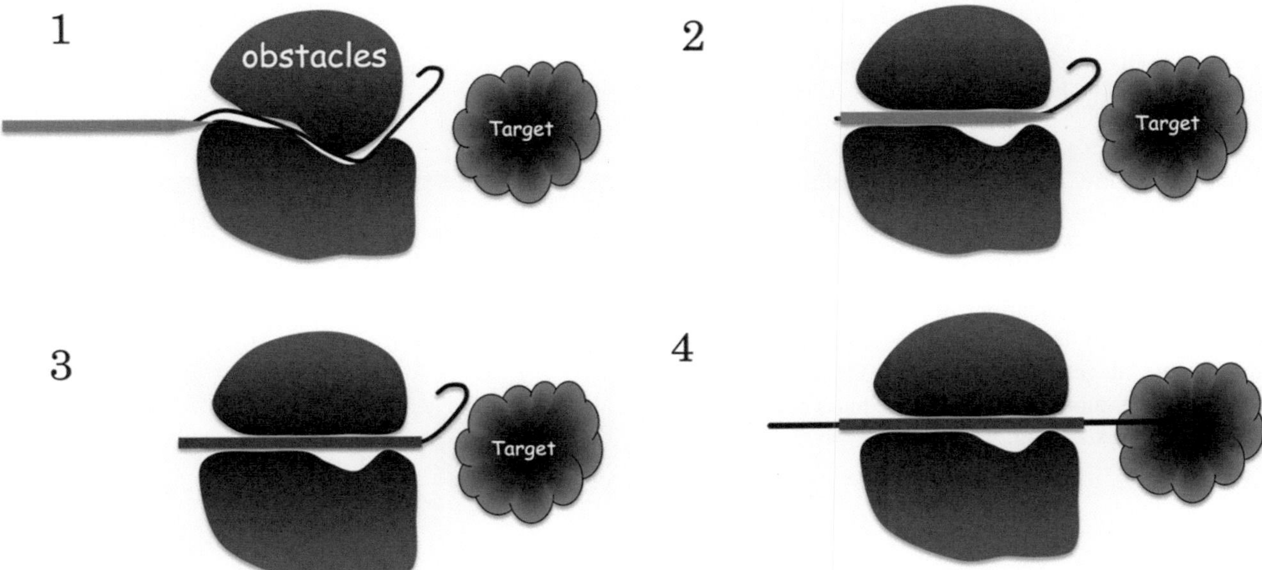

Fig. 93.5 Illustrated technique. (1) Advance a 0.035-inch hand-bended J-type guidewire into slits of obstacles. (2) Advance a 17G non-coring needle coaxially and make the slits of obstacles straight to the target. (3) Exchange the needle to a sheath introducer. (4) Insert the biopsy needle into the sheath, then fire

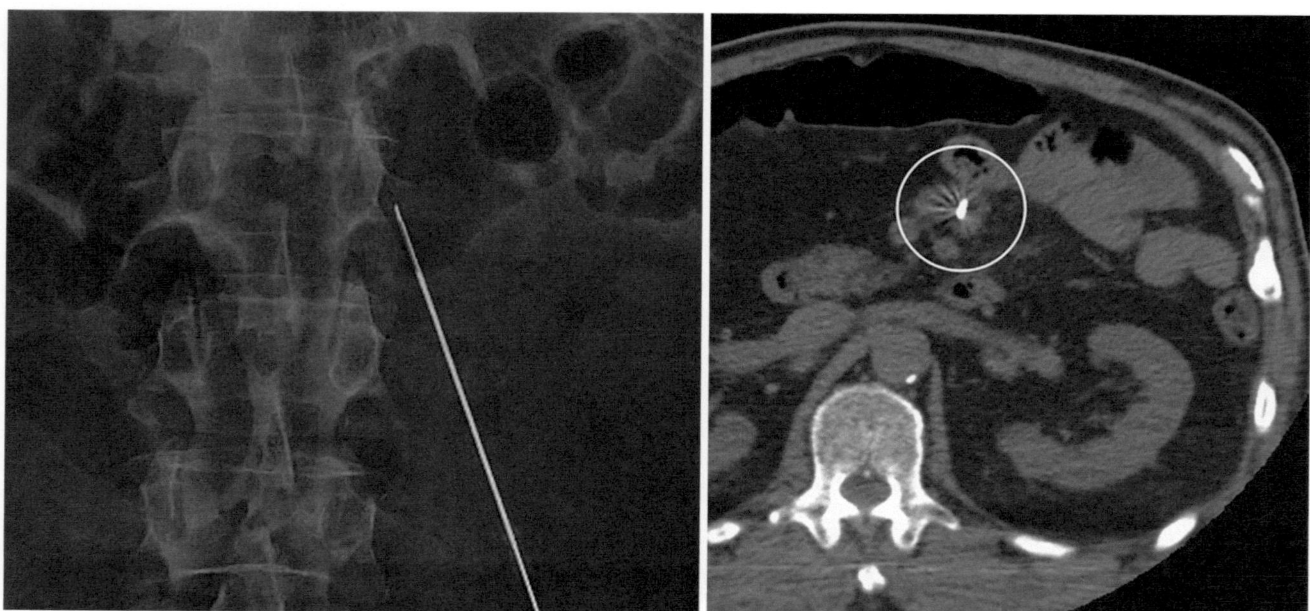

Fig. 93.6 After the confirmation that the tip of biopsy needle was located at the surface of the tumor, the biopsy needle was fired. A CT showed the successful hit of the biopsy needle to the target tumor

a combined angio-CT room. After the confirmation that the tip of biopsy needle was located at the surface of the tumor, the biopsy gun was deployed. CT images confirmed successful safe targeting of the mass (Fig. 93.6).

Pathological examination of tissue revealed chronic inflammation with inflammatory cell infiltration; fibrosis with hyaline degeneration; and IgG4(+) IgG(+)(IgG4/IgG < 30%). Six-month CT showed the mass became significantly smaller in size (Fig. 93.7).

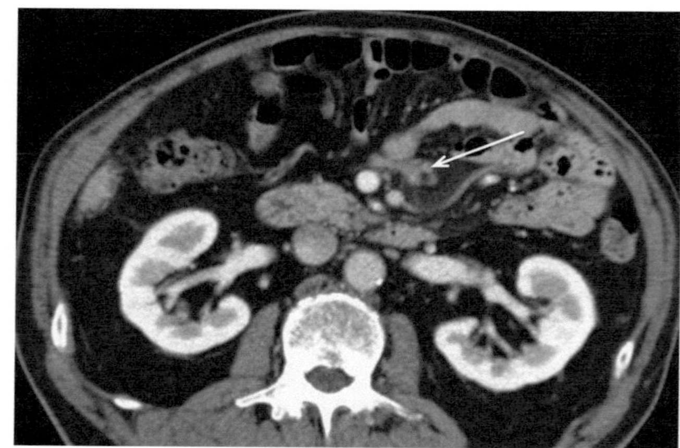

Fig.93.7 A CT after 6 months follow-up showed the tumor became significantly smaller in size (arrow). (Miyuki Sone, M.D., Yasuaki Arai, M.D.)

Percutaneous Debridement of Hepatic Echinococcal Cyst

Ricardo Paz-Fumagalli, Charles Ritchie, and Beau B. Toskich

A 36-year-old female traveler who had visited over 50 countries, including many in Africa and Asia, presented with a 6-year history of dyspnea attributed initially to her known asthma. Cross-sectional imaging found lung cysts and a single 11 cm liver cyst, suspicious for parasitic disease (Fig. 94.1). Extensive serologic studies were equivocal, including a negative Echinococcus IgG. Given the suspicion of hydatid cysts, empiric albendazole was initiated for a 3-month course. Thoracoscopic resection of two lung cysts confirmed Echinococcus per pathologic examination. The liver cyst decreased to 7 cm (Fig. 94.2).

Surgical resection of the liver cyst was not offered as it would have required a right lobectomy due to its proximity to

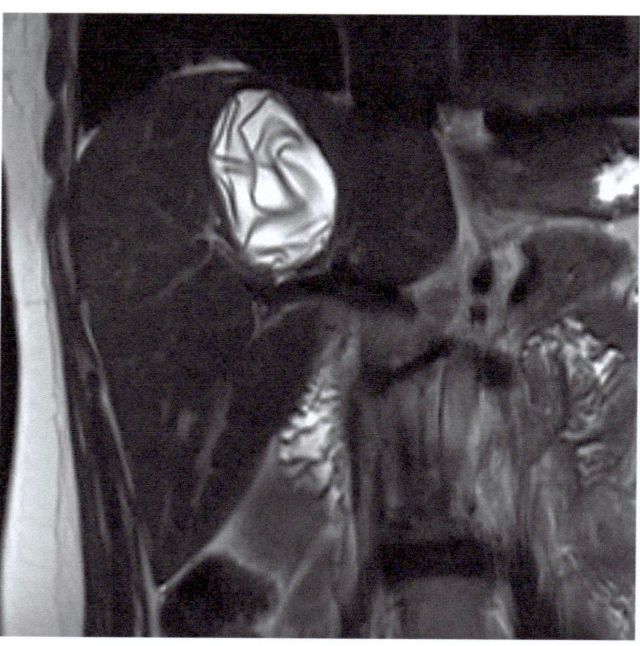

Fig. 94.2 Coronal T2-weighted MRI after antiparasitic therapy with albendazole and thoracoscopic resection of right lung cyst, shows a decrease in the right hepatic lobe hydatid cyst to 7 cm with detachment of hydatid membranes displaying the "water-lily sign" (Gharbi Classification Type II)

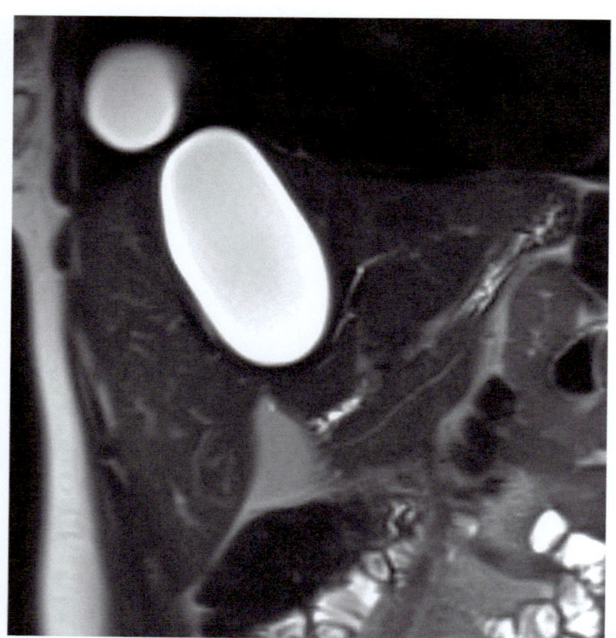

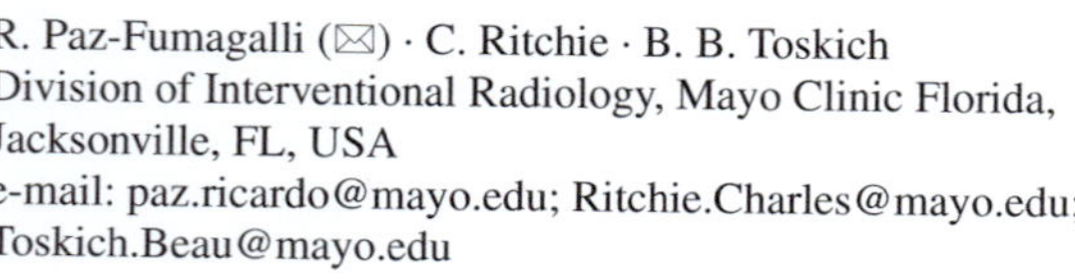

Fig. 94.1 Coronal T2-weighted MRI demonstrates an 11 cm cyst in the right hepatic lobe and a pulmonary right lower lobe hydatic cyst, both Gharbi Classification Type 1

the central right bile ducts. Therefore, a percutaneous transhepatic locking loop drain was placed, and hypertonic saline was instilled to treat any residual parasites. After several days of drainage, the effluent became bilious. Two months later, a fluoroscopic exam showed persistent intracavitary membranes and communication with the adjacent bile duct (Fig. 94.3).

A 26 F peel away sheath was placed through the transhepatic tract and a combination of a 22F drain and a laparoscopic forceps was used to wash, aspirate, and grasp residual hydatid membranes (Figs. 94.4, 94.5, and 94.6). A plastic endoscopic biliary stent was placed to aid antegrade drainage and closure of the biliary communication. A CT scan 4 months later showed resolution of the cavity, the bilious drainage had ceased (Fig. 94.7), and the percutaneous drain was removed. One year later, the patient remained asymptomatic.

R. Paz-Fumagalli (✉) · C. Ritchie · B. B. Toskich
Division of Interventional Radiology, Mayo Clinic Florida, Jacksonville, FL, USA
e-mail: paz.ricardo@mayo.edu; Ritchie.Charles@mayo.edu; Toskich.Beau@mayo.edu

© The Author(s), under exclusive license to Springer Nature Switzerland AG 2023
Z. J. Haskal (ed.), *Extreme IR*, https://doi.org/10.1007/978-3-031-24251-9_94

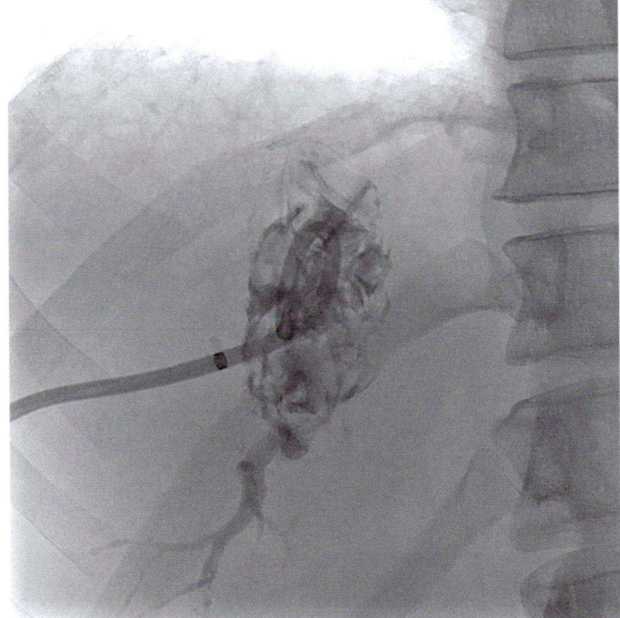

Fig. 94.3 Contrast fluoroscopic exam 2 months after tube drainage and hypertonic saline administration shows a biliary fistula and a complex filling defect caused by the agglomerated hydatid membranes

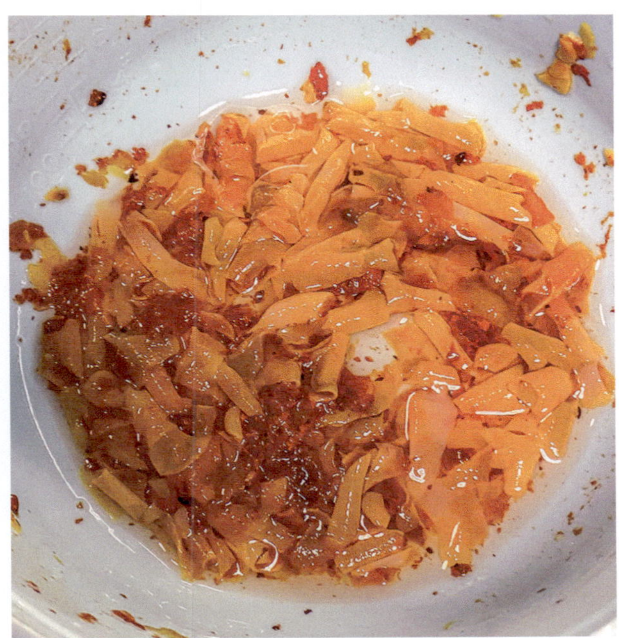

Fig. 94.5 Gross specimen photograph of evacuated hydatid membranes

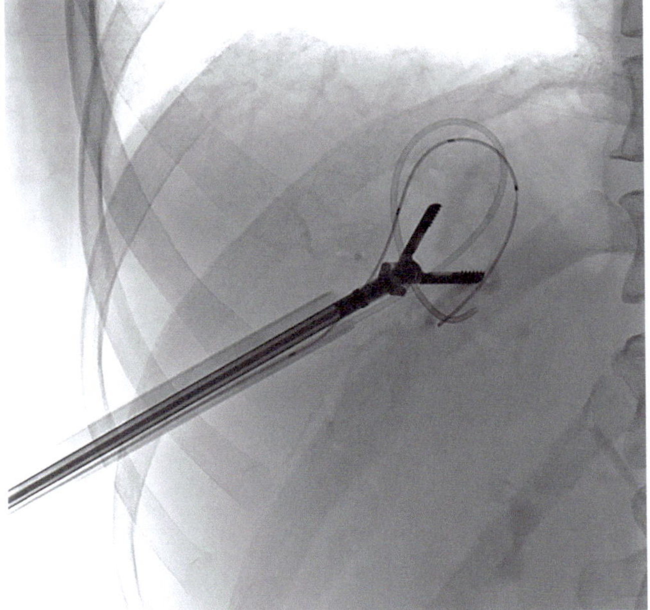

Fig. 94.4 Radiograph obtained during percutaneous debridement through a transhepatic 26F peel-away sheath. Laparoscopic forceps and a 22F catheter (not shown) were used to evacuate the membrane fragments

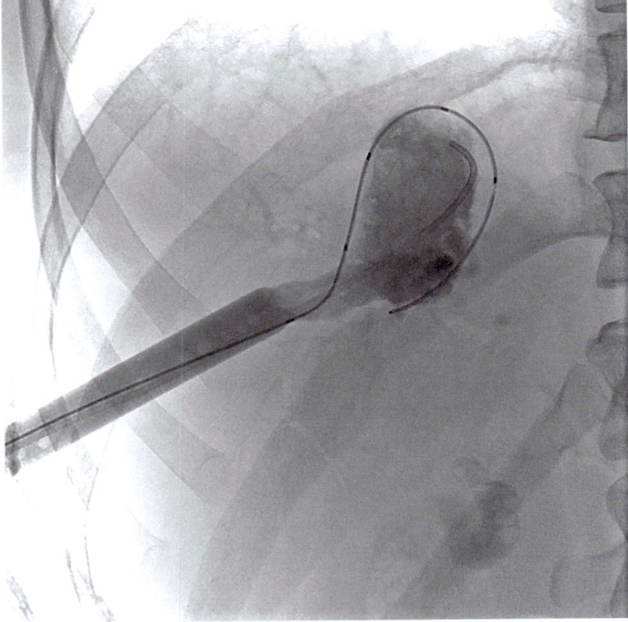

Fig. 94.6 Radiograph after administration of contrast into the evacuated hydatid cyst shows complete removal of membrane fragment filling defects. The use of a large bore sheath and vigorous saline flushing through the 5F angiographic catheter placed in the cavity facilitated expulsion of residual material

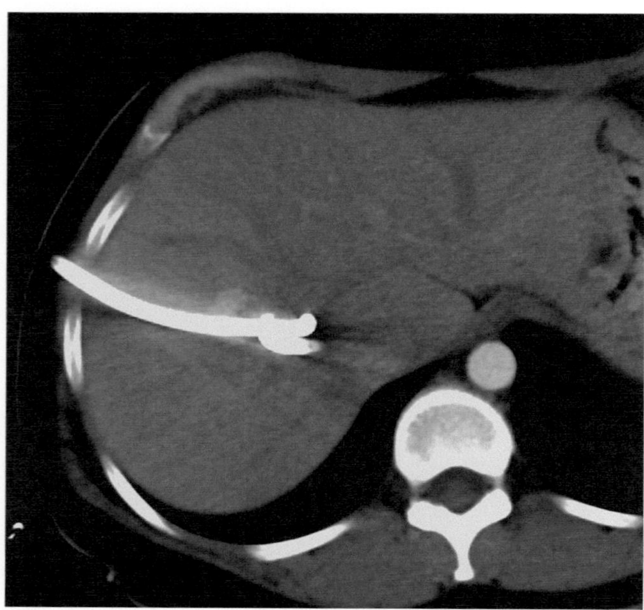

Fig. 94.7 CT scan image obtained 4 months after cavity evacuation and endoscopic biliary stent placement. The bilious output through the drain ceased and the cavity closed, indicating healing of the biliary fistula. The catheter was removed without recurrence of the cyst or biliary fistula

Bibliography

1. Akhan O, Salik AE, Ciftci T, Akinci D, Islim F, Akpinar B. Comparison of long-term results of percutaneous treatment techniques for hepatic cystic echinococcosis types 2 and 3b. AJR Am J Roentgenol. 2017;208(4):878–84. https://doi.org/10.2214/AJR.16.16131.
2. Gupta N, Javed A, Puri S, Jain S, Singh S, Agarwal AK. Hepatic hydatid: PAIR, drain or resect? J Gastrointest Surg. 2011;15:1829–36. https://doi.org/10.1007/s11605-011-1649-9.
3. Peláez V, Kugler C, Correa D, Del Carpio M, Guangiroli M, Molina J, Marcos B, Lopez E. PAIR as percutaneous treatment of hydatid liver cysts. Acta Trop. 2000;75(2):197–202. https://doi.org/10.1016/s0001-706x(00)00058-9.

Antegrade Removal of Covered Metallic Ureteral Stent Placed for 4 Years

Ji Hoon Shin

A 41-year-old man presented with intermittent flank pain. He had undergone prior placement of an 8-mm diameter, covered metallic ureteral stent (Uventa stent, Taewoong, Gimpo, Korea) in the left upper and middle ureter for benign ureteropelvic junction stenosis 4 years earlier. The stent had migrated to the renal pelvis (Fig. 95.1a, b). The maximum diameter of the stent was 15-mm, accompanied by severe calcification. Percutaneous removal via antegrade access was undertaken.

A 9-Fr sheath was inserted through a mid-calyceal access. A 15-mm multipurpose snare was used to grasp the stent; however, the snare broke while grasping and retrieving the stent tip. After exchanging the 9-Fr sheath for a 14-Fr sheath, the stent was attempted using a modified snare technique with a snare and an additional 0.035-inch stiff guidewire encircling the stent (Fig. 95.1c). As the stent could be compressed into the sheath lumen, an attempt was made to directly remove the sheath and the stent together. After encountering resistance, tract dilation was performed using 6-mm and 10-mm-diameter balloon catheters (Fig. 95.1d). The stent was caught with a mosquito clamp through skin incision and was finally withdrawn (Fig. 95.1e, f). Secondary hematuria developed but disappeared the next day. This case illustrates the combined use of tract dilation, external grasping instruments, and a modified snare approach to allow retrograde trans-tract removal of an embedded migrated metallic ureteral stent.

J. H. Shin (✉)
Department of Radiology, University of Ulsan, Asan Medical Center, Seoul, South Korea
e-mail: jhshin@amc.seoul.kr

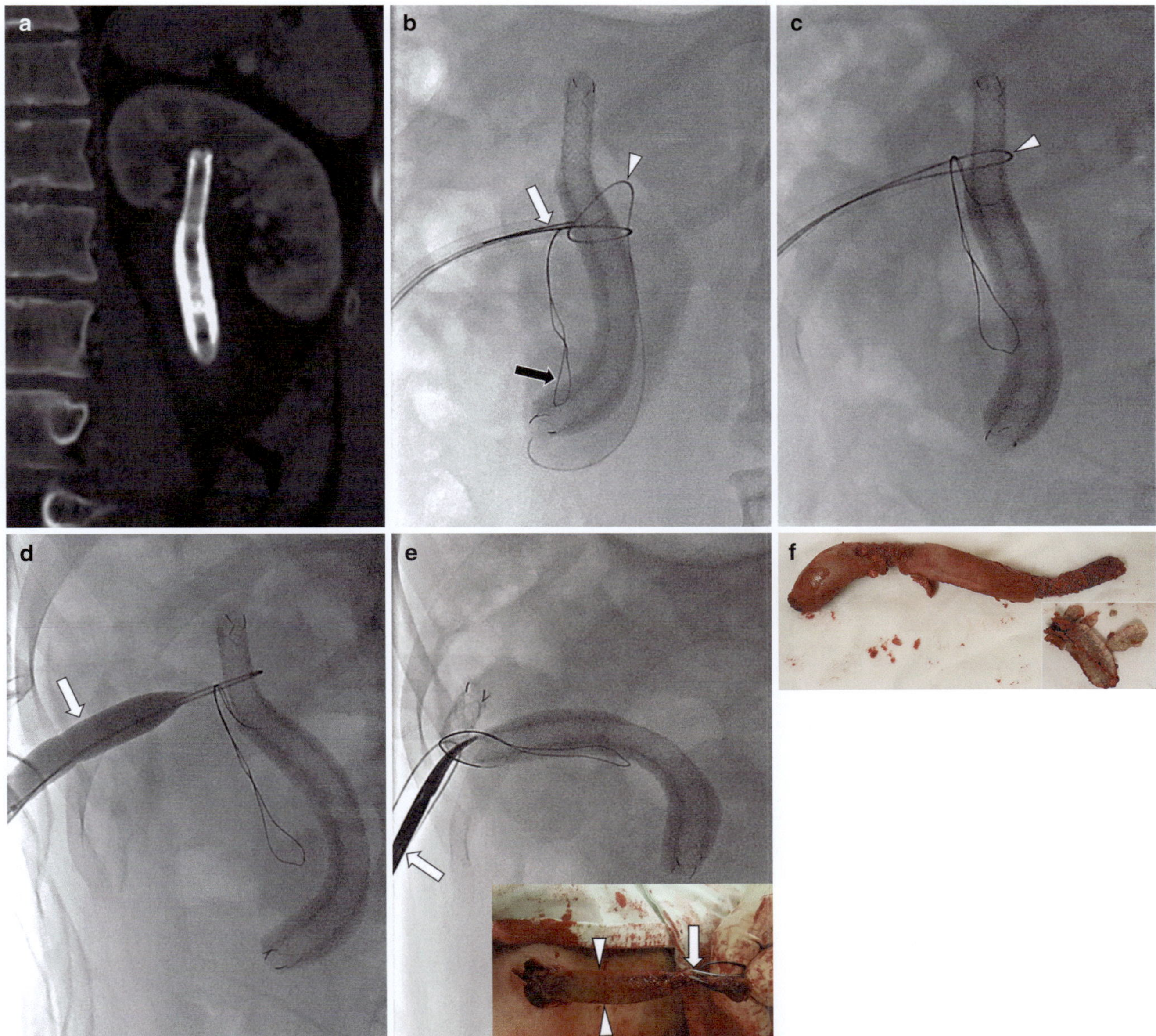

Fig. 95.1 Antegrade removal of covered metallic ureteral stent placed for 4 years. (**a**) On coronal CT scan, the extensively calcified stent is in the left renal pelvis. (**b**) The stent was engaged with a modified snare technique using a snare (white arrow) and an additional 0.035-inch stiff guidewire (arrowhead) encircling the stent after simple snare technique failure. Note the broken tip of the snare (black arrow) during the unsuccessful simple snare technique. (**c**) The stent was caught by the guidewire (arrowhead) by pulling the snare through the 14-Fr sheath. (**d**) Since the caught stent could not be removed together with the sheath, tract dilation was performed using a 10-mm-diameter balloon catheter (arrow). (**e**) After the stent was grasped by the mosquito clamp (arrow), it could be completely removed. The heavily calcified stent (arrowheads) caught by the mosquito clamp is being pulled out (inset). (**f**) The photograph shows removed stent. The cross section of the stent shows extensive calcification both inside and outside the stent (inset)

Reconstruction of the Posterior Pelvic Angle with an Interlocking Screw-Cement Construct

Steven Yevich

A 61-year-old man with metastatic renal cell cancer was referred for pain palliation and fracture prevention. Interventional radiologic stabilization of the posterior pelvis was requested to avoid the morbidity of ilio-lumbar surgery and obviate suspension of immunotherapy. Clinically, the patient was suffering from severe focal posterior pelvic pain and sciatic neuropathy exacerbated by weight-bearing activities that significantly decreased quality of life.

The posterior angle of the pelvis would have to be reconstructed. A large expansile lytic lesion replaced the posterior aspect of the right iliac bone along the majority of the right sacro-iliac joint (Fig. 96.1a–c), and was overall stable in size and appearance for the prior year on immunotherapy. No osseous matrix is appreciated within the lesion, which has a thin rim with many cortical disruptions.

Fixation by Internal Cemented Screw (FICS) procedure [1, 2] was performed by interlocking four 8 mm stainless steel cannulated screws under fluoroscopic guidance (Fig. 96.2a). Screw trajectory ensured that screw tips anchored solidly into good bone and the portion near the heads interlinked at the location of the sacro-iliac joint (Fig. 96.2a, d, e). Multiple 11 gauge needles (Fig. 96.2b) were used for rapid injection of 55 mL polymethyl methacrylate to form a solid consolidative cement block around the needles (Fig. 96.2c), as well as anchor the screws into the sacral ala and iliac bone [3].

At the latest follow-up, 2.5 years after FICS procedure, the screw-cement construct remains intact on CT and the patient continues to ambulate with decreased pain compared to pre-procedure reports.

S. Yevich (✉)
Department of Interventional Radiology, MD Anderson Cancer Center, Houston, TX, USA
e-mail: syevich@mdanderson.org

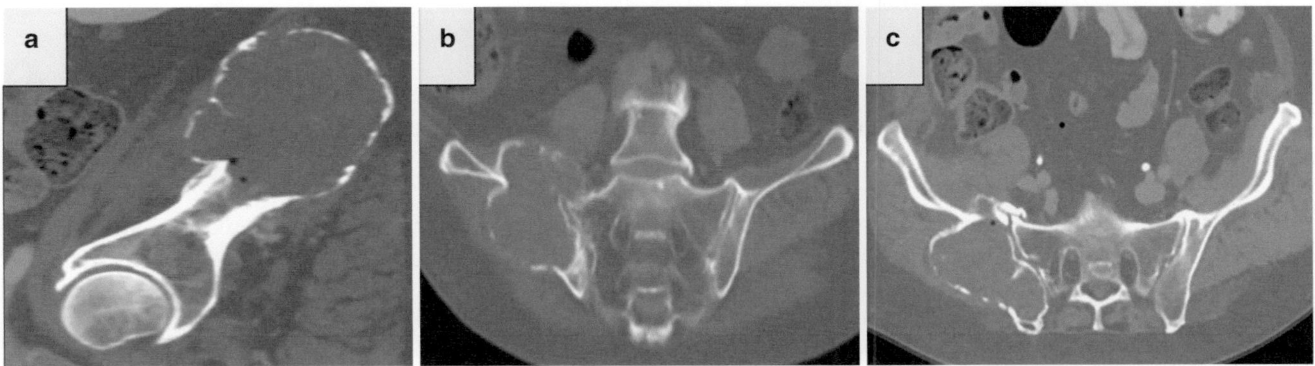

Fig. 96.1 Oblique sagittal (**a**), oblique coronal (**b**), and axial (**c**) contrast-enhanced pre-procedure CT images of the pelvis demonstrates a non-enhancing, expansile, lytic lesion in the right iliac bone that extends along the sacro-iliac joint

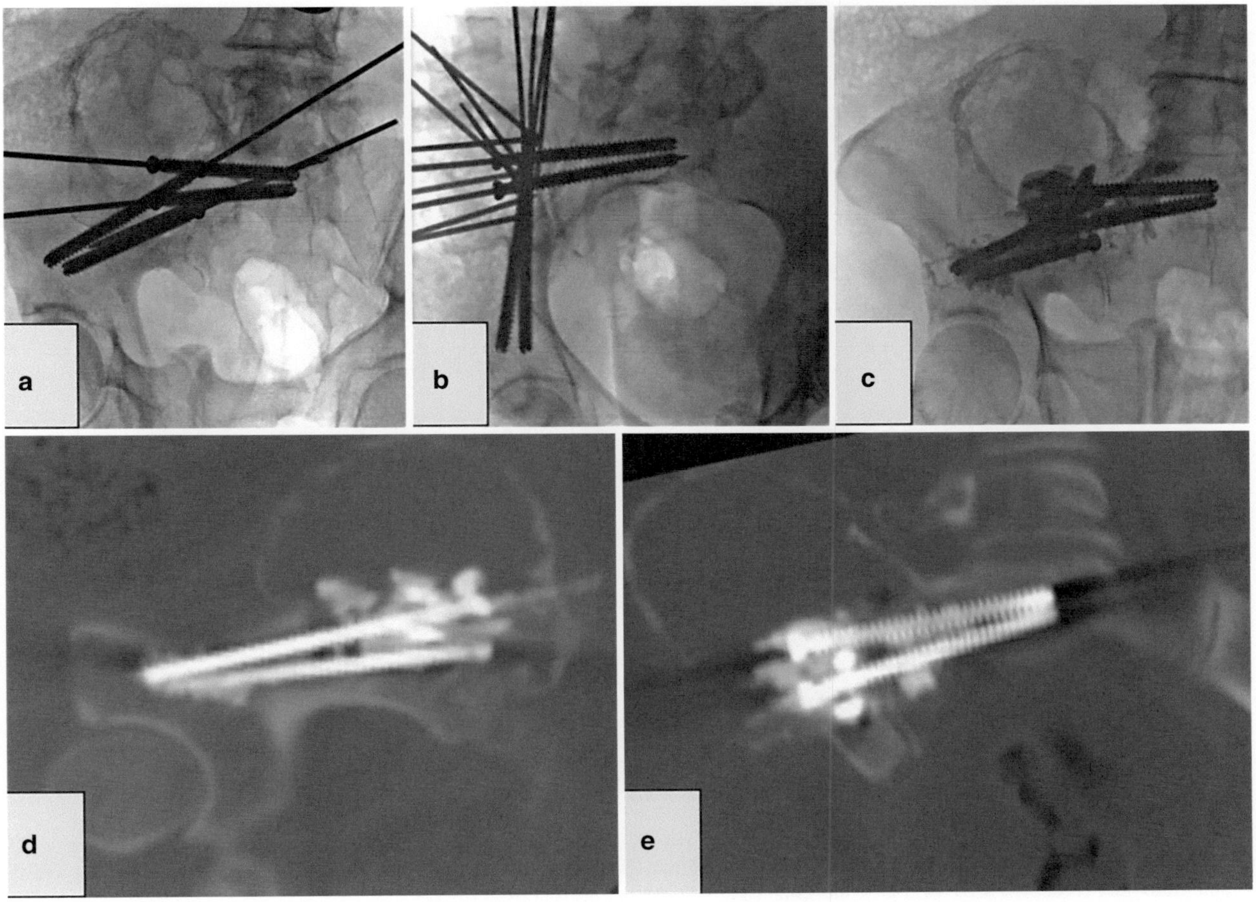

Fig. 96.2 FICS procedure with fluoroscopic placement of interlocking screws (**a**), followed by placement of multiple cement injection needles (**b**), and cement consolidation of the screw intersection (**c**). Follow-up CT demonstrates stability of the reconstructed posterior pelvic angle with an oblique sagittal view (**d**) and obliqued coronal view (**e**)

References

1. Roux C, Tselikas L, Yevich S, Sandes Solha R, Hakime A, Teriitehau C, Gravel G, de Baere T, Deschamps F. Fluoroscopy and cone-beam CT-guided fixation by internal cemented screw for pathologic pelvic fractures. Radiology. 2019;290(2):418–25. https://doi.org/10.1148/radiol.2018181105.

2. Deschamps F, Yevich S, Gravel G, Roux C, Hakime A, de Baère T, Tselikas L. Percutaneous fixation by internal cemented screw for the treatment of unstable osseous disease in cancer patients. Semin Interv Radiol. 2018;35(4):238–47. https://doi.org/10.1055/s-0038-1673359.

3. Yevich S, Tselikas L, Gravel G, de Baère T, Deschamps F. Percutaneous cement injection for the palliative treatment of osseous metastases: a technical review. Semin Interv Radiol. 2018;35(4):268–80. https://doi.org/10.1055/s-0038-1673418. Epub 2018 Nov 5. PMID: 30402010; PMCID: PMC6218257

Ryan D. Murray, Justin E. Bird, and Alda L. Tam

A 15-year-old male presented to a spine surgeon with complaints of neck pain and left upper extremity pain and weakness. Imaging of the cervical spine demonstrated a large, osseous, lytic lesion centered at the C5 vertebra with evidence of cord compression (Fig. 97.1a); C5 corpectomy with tumor debulking and stabilization of C3-C6 (Fig. 97.1b) was performed. Pathologic diagnosis confirmed an aneurysmal bone cyst (ABC). The patient recovered well after surgery, but after 6 months developed recurrent left upper extremity pain and imaging demonstrating disease recurrence (Fig. 97.2). This was treated with staged percutaneous sclerotherapy. During each treatment session, multiple 13–16 gauge needles were advanced into various parts of the ABC using CT or sonographic guidance (Fig. 97.3a) and dilute

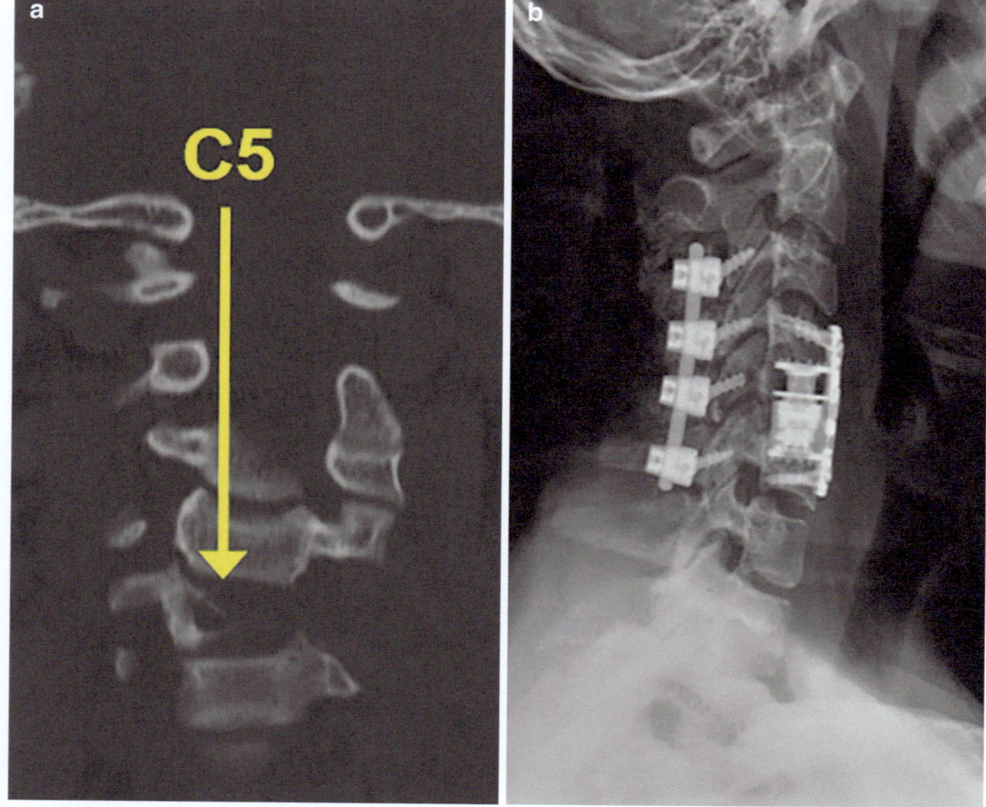

Fig. 97.1 (**a**) Coronal CT demonstrates an expansile cystic mass centered around C5 with associated destruction of the C5 vertebral body and transverse process. MRI of the same date (not shown) demonstrates cord compression. (**b**) Post-operative lateral radiograph of the cervical spine demonstrates posterior spinal fusion at C3-C6 levels with a C5 interbody device fixed with a metallic plate and screw construct from C4-C6

R. D. Murray · A. L. Tam (✉)
Department of Interventional Radiology, University of Texas MD Anderson Cancer Center, Houston, TX, USA
e-mail: RDMurray@mdanderson.org; alda.tam@mdanderson.org

J. E. Bird
Department of Orthopaedic Oncology, University of Texas MD Anderson Cancer Center, Houston, TX, USA
e-mail: jebird@mdanderson.org

© The Author(s), under exclusive license to Springer Nature Switzerland AG 2023
Z. J. Haskal (ed.), *Extreme IR*, https://doi.org/10.1007/978-3-031-24251-9_97

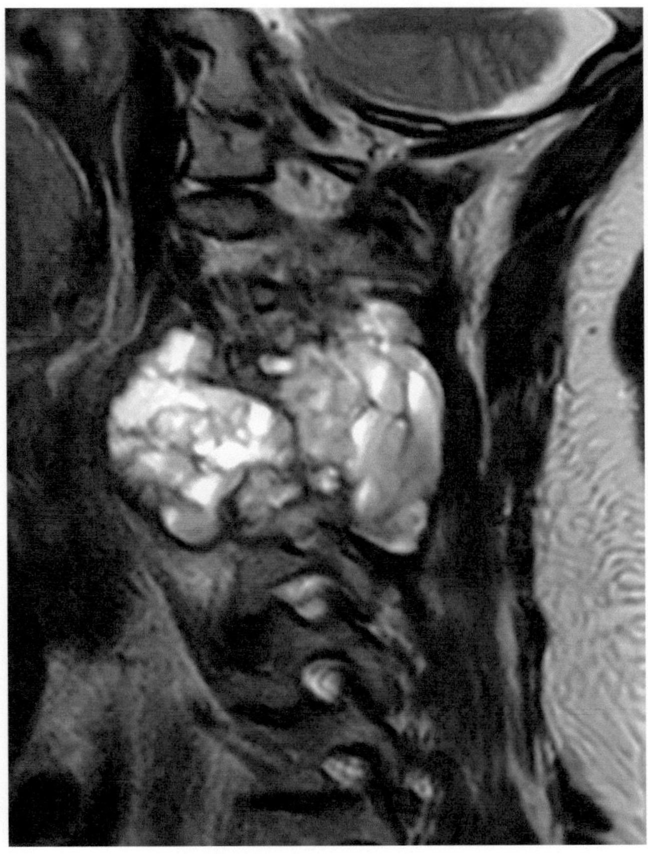

Fig. 97.2 Sagittal T2-weighted MRI of the cervical spine demonstrates the craniocaudal extent of disease recurrence as well as multiple fluid-fluid levels characteristic for an ABC

contrast injected under digital subtraction fluoroscopy to exclude communication with the spinal canal or adjacent vertebral artery foramen (Fig. 97.3b and c). A foam mixture of 200 mg doxycycline, normal saline, 25% albumin, and air [1] was administered in aliquots under fluoroscopic guidance. He underwent multiple treatments over a period of 3 years. Follow-up imaging demonstrated resolution of the ABC associated with robust osseous regrowth (Fig. 97.4a and b). Clinically, the patient reported resolution of pain, return of normal left upper extremity strength, and the ability to exercise with 40 lb free weights.

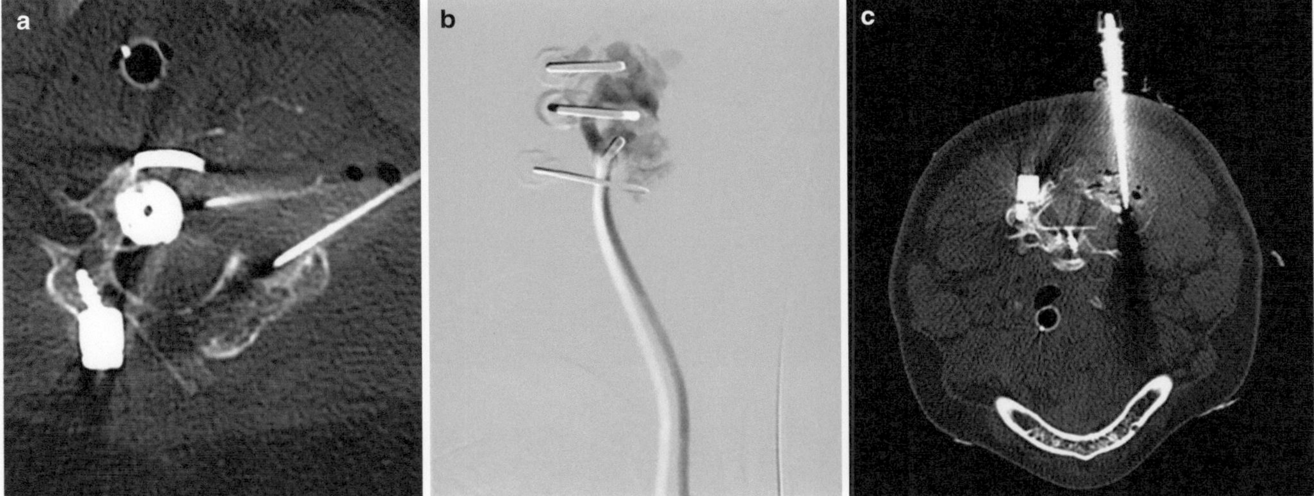

Fig. 97.3 (**a**) Intra-procedural axial CT image demonstrates appropriate position of two introducer needles into the ABC at C5. Representative fluoroscopic (**b**) and CT (**c**) images after contrast injection confirm there is no communication with the spinal canal or the left vertebral foramen

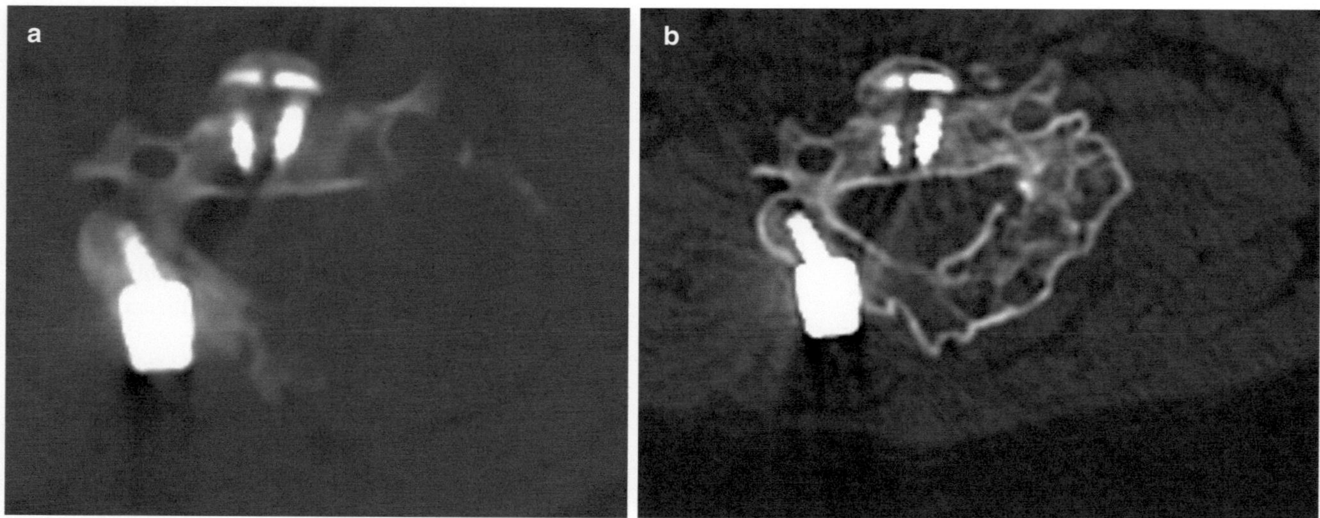

Fig. 97.4 Pre- (**a**) and Post- (**b**) treatment axial CT of C5 demonstrating marked interval improvement in the ABC associated with robust mineralization of the C5 posterior body, lamina, and vertebral foramen

Bibliography

1. Shiels WE 2nd, Mayerson JL. Percutaneous doxycycline treatment of aneurysmal bone cysts with low recurrence rate: a preliminary report. Clin Orthop Relat Res. 2013;471(8):2675–83. https://doi.org/10.1007/s11999-013-3043-2.

Sebouh Gueyikian

Emergency consultation was requested mid-procedure for a 63-year-old woman who was undergoing bipedicular kyphoplasty under general anesthesia. Fluoroscopic (Fig. 98.1) and cone-beam computed tomography (CBCT) images (Figs. 98.2 and 98.3) showed that the anterior tip of the right-sided 11 gauge Stryker Osteo-introducer passed through the anterior edge of the L3 vertebra and into the retroperitoneum between the aorta and inferior vena cava (IVC). The trailing end of the cannula was entirely within the subcutaneous tissues. The plastic handle had broken off during cannula repositioning. There were no signs of hemorrhage or arterial injury. We decided to remove the cannula and evaluate potential arterial injury thereafter. An 8 cm incision was made over the cannula entry site. Multiple standard surgical instruments were attached to the posterior tip of the cannula (Fig. 98.4); however, it could not be removed due its angulation wedged in the bone.

At this point, 20 mm Vial Decapper pliers were placed in a sterile ultrasound probe cover and brought onto the surgical

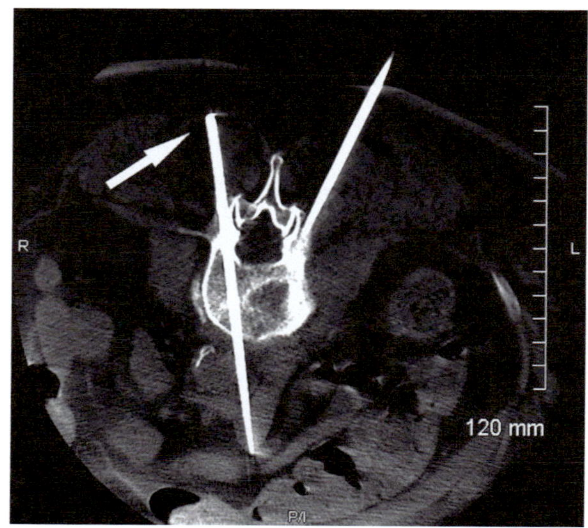

Fig. 98.2 CBCT demonstrates the posterior aspect (arrow) of the right Kyphoplasty cannula in the subcutaneous tissues approximately 3 cm under the skin

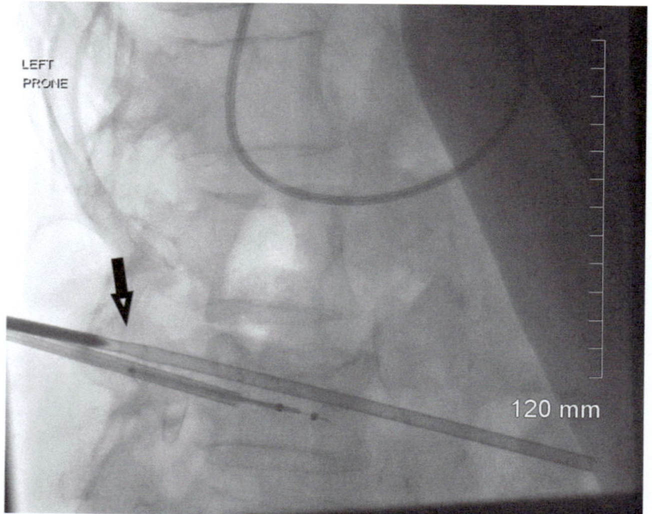

Fig. 98.1 Lateral fluoroscopic view demonstrates cannula through the vertebral body and into the retroperitoneum. A slight deformity (arrow) can be seen in the cannula at the junction with the posterior aspect of the vertebral body

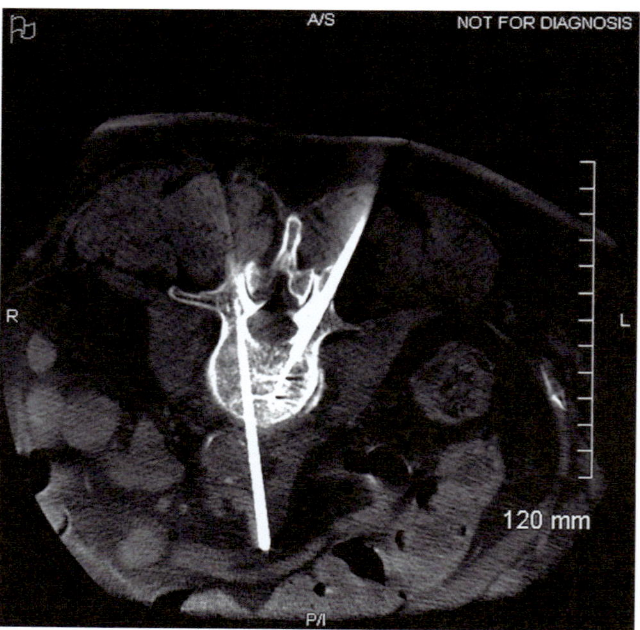

Fig. 98.3 CBCT demonstrates the anterior aspect of the right Kyphoplasty cannula in the retroperitoneum between the aorta and the IVC

S. Gueyikian (✉)
Department of Interventional Radiology, Northshore University Healthcare System, Evanston, IL, USA

© The Author(s), under exclusive license to Springer Nature Switzerland AG 2023
Z. J. Haskal (ed.), *Extreme IR*, https://doi.org/10.1007/978-3-031-24251-9_98

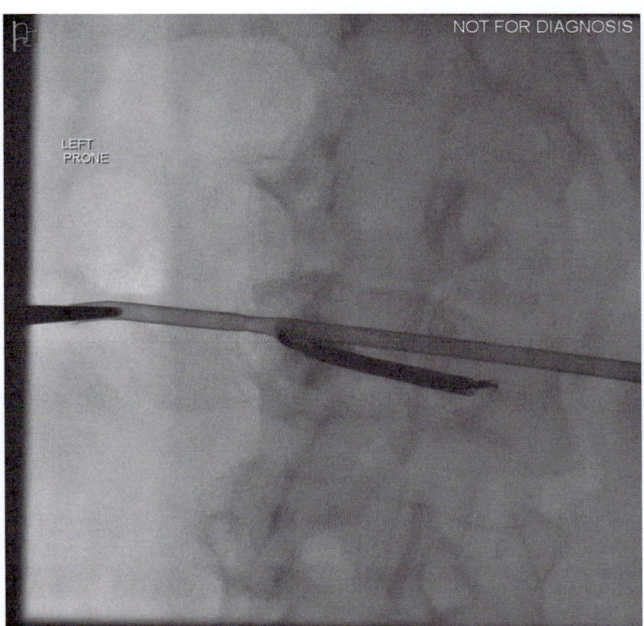

Fig. 98.4 Oblique fluoroscopic image shows a curved surgical clamp on the posterior end of the cannula

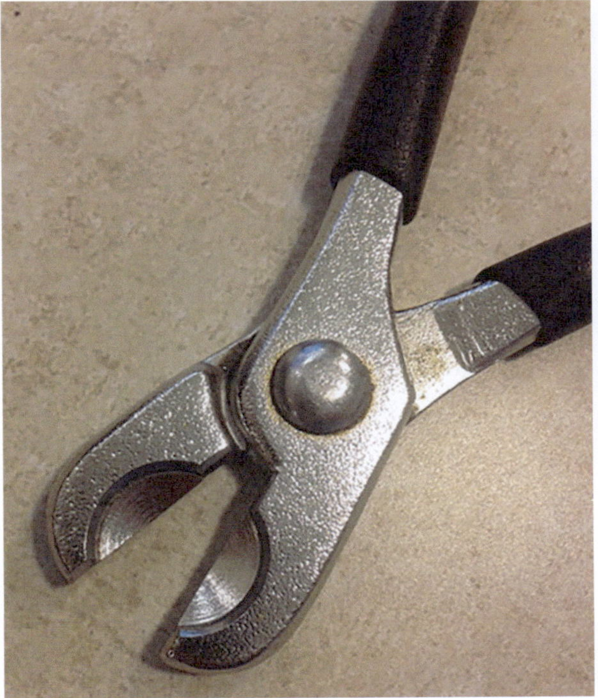

Fig. 98.5 Vial Decapper Pliers (20 mm) are routinely used to remove caps from vials of lidocaine, nitroglycerin and other medication during preparation for interventional radiology cases

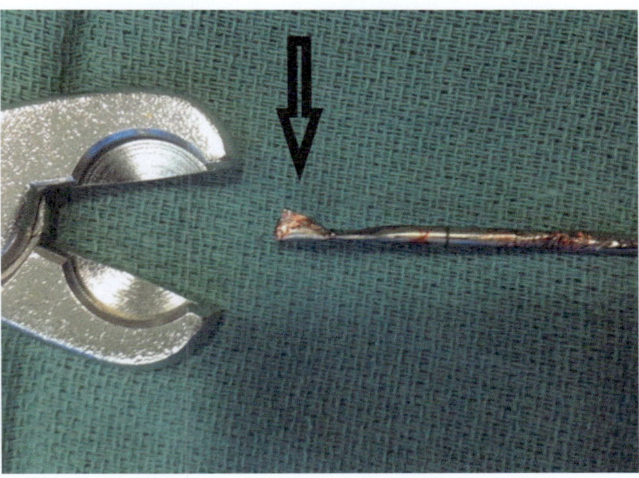

Fig. 98.6 Pliers are seen next to the crushed end of the cannula and the impromptu flared end that was created (arrow). This flared end was key to capturing the cannula and not letting it slide through the pliers

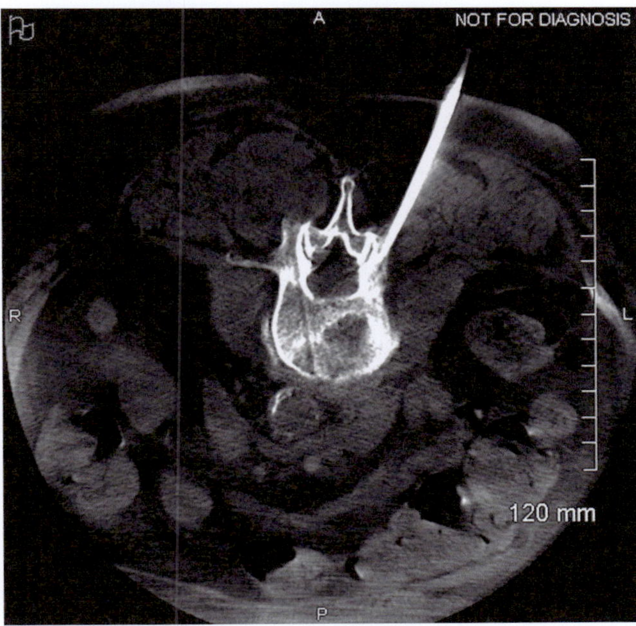

Fig. 98.7 CBCT after removal of both cannula and completion of kyphoplasty show no signs of retroperitoneal hemorrhage

field. (Fig. 98.5). The pliers were used to crush a portion of cannula and flare the proximal tip of the cannula (Fig. 98.6). They were then used to grasp and pull the cannula (as well as the patient) off of the table. Sharp counter-traction was applied to the adjacent spine and the cannula was removed in its entirety. Immediate CBCT thereafter demonstrated no retroperitoneal (Fig. 98.7). Post-procedure conventional intravenous contrast-enhanced CT showed no signs of aortic nor caval injury. The patient was admitted for observation; serial hemoglobin levels proved stable. She was discharged without further complication.

Part XII

Lymphatic

Transhepatic Lymphangiogram with Complex Central Lymphatic Leak Embolization

Rakesh S. Ahuja and Raja Shaikh

A 7-year-old boy, status post-renal transplant for end-stage renal disease, recently diagnosed and treated for Lyme disease and babesiosis. Over next several days, presented with shortness of breath, tachypnea, and bilateral pleural effusions (Fig. 99.1). He underwent bilateral thoracentesis with 2 L of chylous fluid removed. Next 2 days, he had worsening respiratory status with reaccumulation of effusions. Bilateral chest tubes were placed. Dynamic MR Lymphangiogram demonstrated lymphatic reflux resulting in body wall edema, moderate ectasia, and reflux into the central abdominal and thoracic lymphatic channels (Fig. 99.2). Left chest pleurodesis was done which was complicated by respiratory failure. Transnodal lymphangiogram through bilateral inguinal lymph nodes demonstrated stasis without progression of contrast/lipiodol into the abdominal and pelvic lymphatic system (Fig. 99.3a). Transmesenteric lymphangiogram via a mesenteric nodal access demonstrated reflux of contrast from mesenteric lymph channels along the mesentery and abdominal wall (Fig. 99.3b). Transhepatic lymphangiogram demonstrated antegrade propulsion of the contrast towards the anomalous ectatic lymphatic channel close to the diaphragmatic surface (Fig. 99.4). Leak was noted from this anomalous channel as there was contrast flow seen along the diaphragmatic surface (Fig. 99.5a). Transhepatic lymphatic access into central duct just below the leak was obtained with

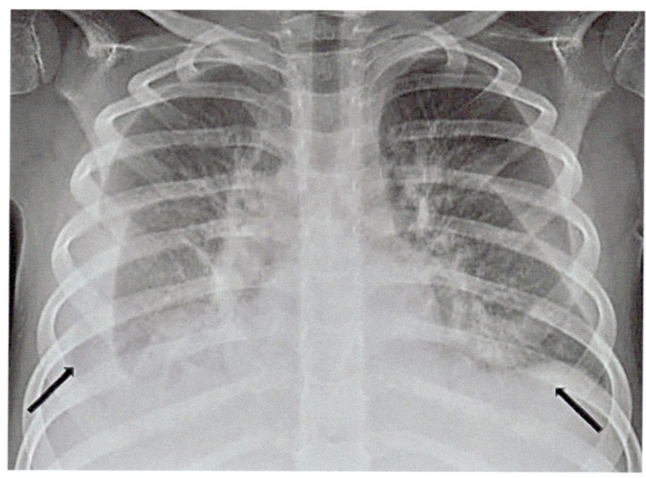

Fig. 99.1 Initial chest X-ray with bilateral pleural effusions (arrows)

24-gauge spinal needle (Fig. 99.6). Embolization was then performed with 1:4 ratio of n-Butyl cyanoacrylate glue mixed with lipiodol (Fig. 99.7). Post-procedure, output reduced significantly by POD 8. Chest tubes were removed and patient was discharged home. At 6-month follow-up, no further symptoms have been noted by family and no pleural effusions seen on chest x-ray (Fig. 99.8).

R. S. Ahuja (✉)
Department of Vascular and Interventional Radiology, University of Texas Health Science Center Houston, Houston, TX, USA

Vascular and Interventional Radiology, Boston Childrens Hopsital, Boston, MA, USA

R. Shaikh
Department of Vascular and Interventional Radiology, University of Texas Health Science Center Houston, Houston, TX, USA
e-mail: raja.shaikh@childrens.harvard.edu

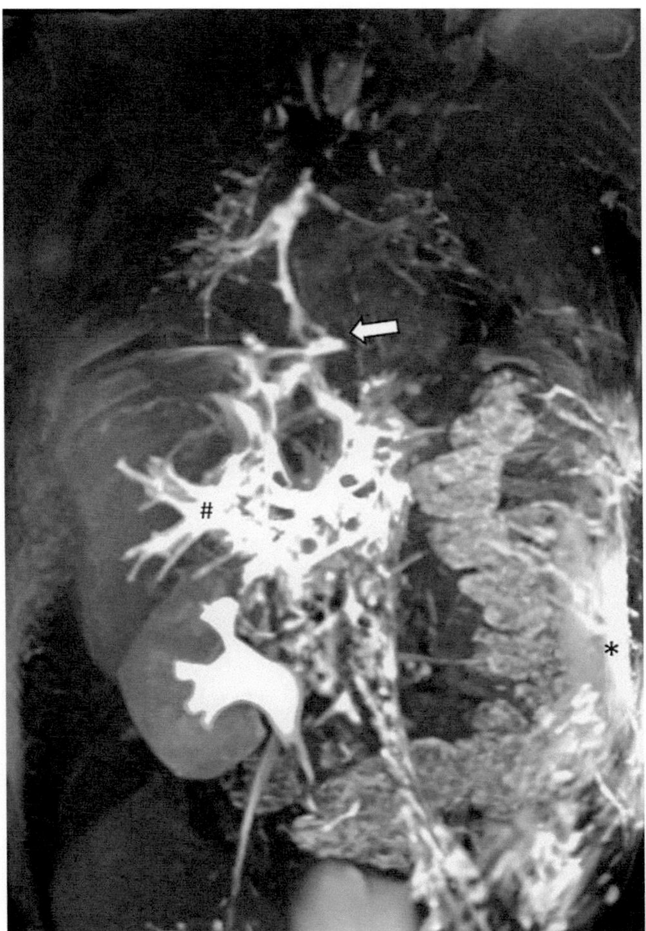

Fig. 99.2 Dynamic MR Lymphangiogram demonstrated lymphatic reflux resulting in body wall edema (*), moderate ectasia, and reflux into the central abdominal (#) and thoracic lymphatic channels (arrow)

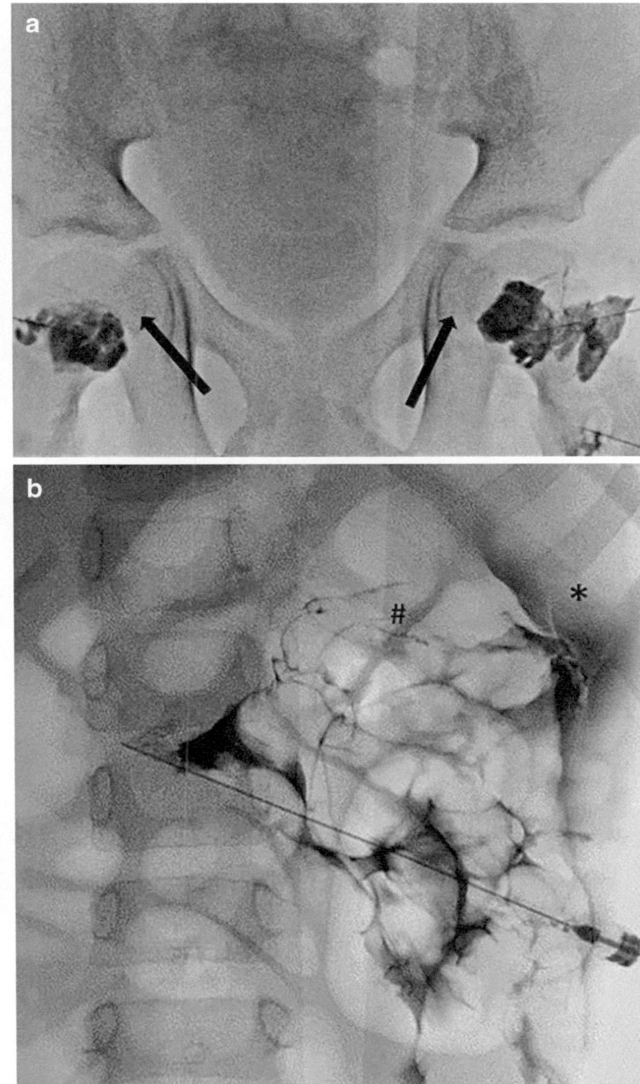

Fig. 99.3 (a) Transnodal lymphangiogram through bilateral inguinal lymph nodes demonstrated stasis without progression of contrast/lipiodol into the abdominal and pelvic lymphatic system (arrow). (b) Transmesenteric lymphangiogram via a mesenteric nodal access demonstrated reflux of contrast from mesenteric lymph channels (#) along the mesentery and abdominal wall (*)

Fig. 99.4 Transhepatic lymphangiogram (arrow) demonstrated antegrade propulsion of the contrast towards the anomalous ectatic lymphatic channel close to the diaphragmatic surface

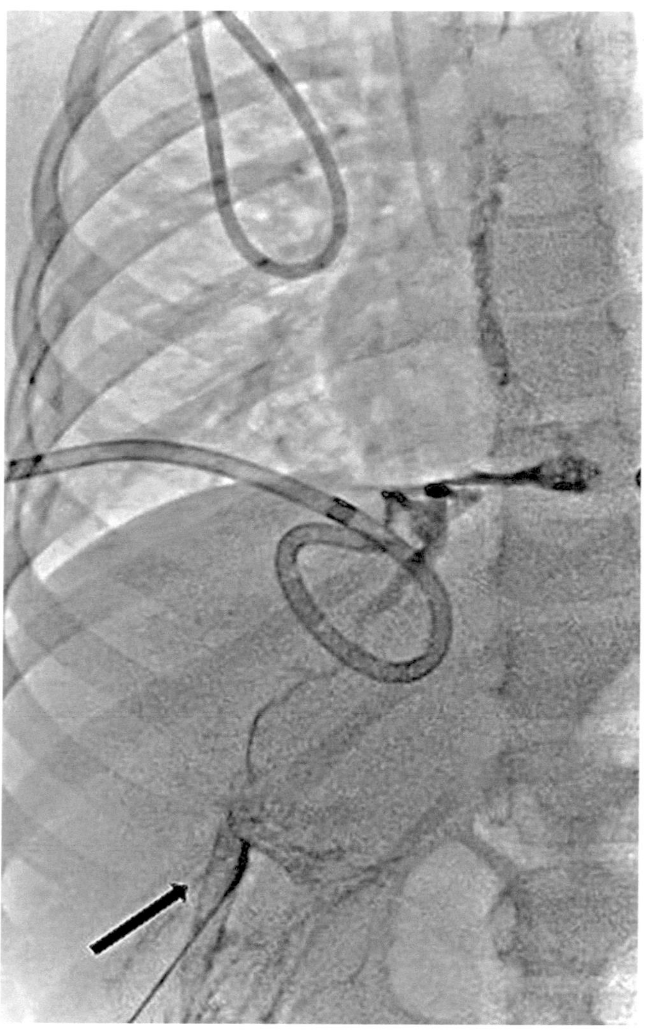

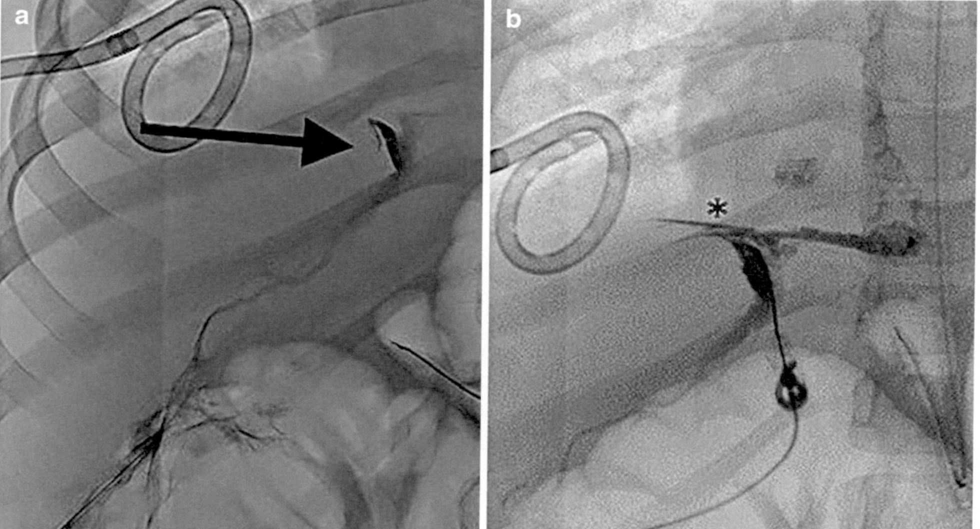

Fig. 99.5 (**a**) Leak was noted from this anomalous channel as there was contrast flow seen along the diaphragmatic surface (arrow). (**b**) Contrast layering (*) was seen along the diaphragmatic surfaces with partial contrast propulsion along the central thoracic lymphatic channels

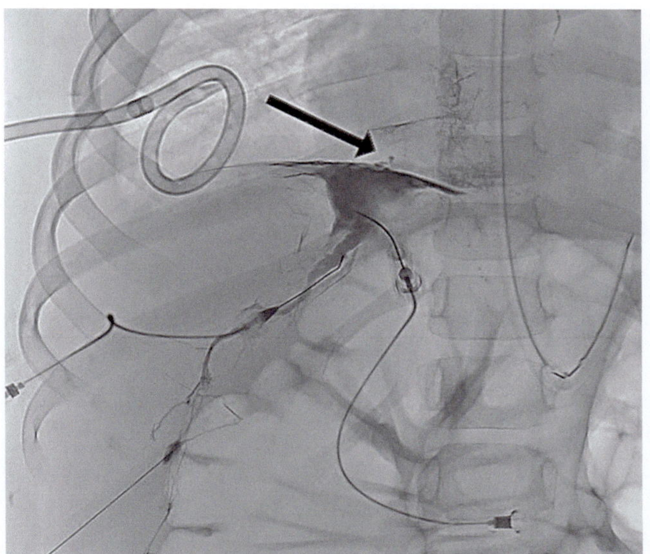

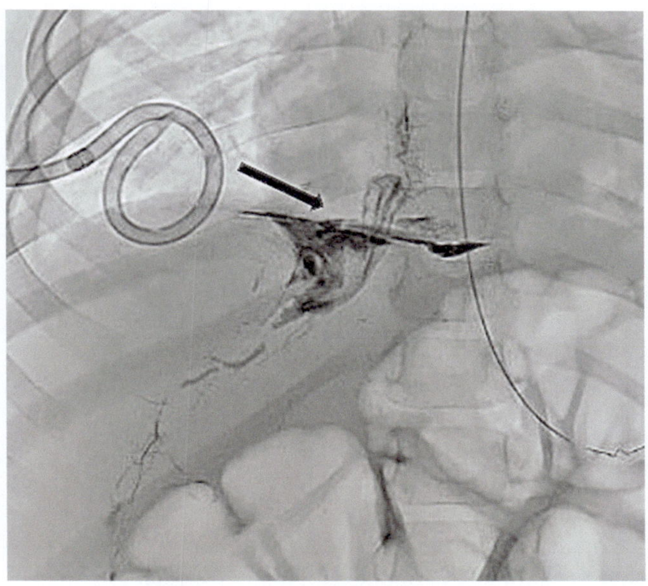

Fig. 99.6 Leak identified during lipiodol injection (arrow) after transhepatic central lymphatic access with 24G spinal needle

Fig. 99.7 Spot fluoroscopic image post-embolization with 1:4 ratio of n-Butyl cyanoacrylate glue shows adequate propagation of embolic agent along the central lymphatic ducts in the area of the leak (black arrow)

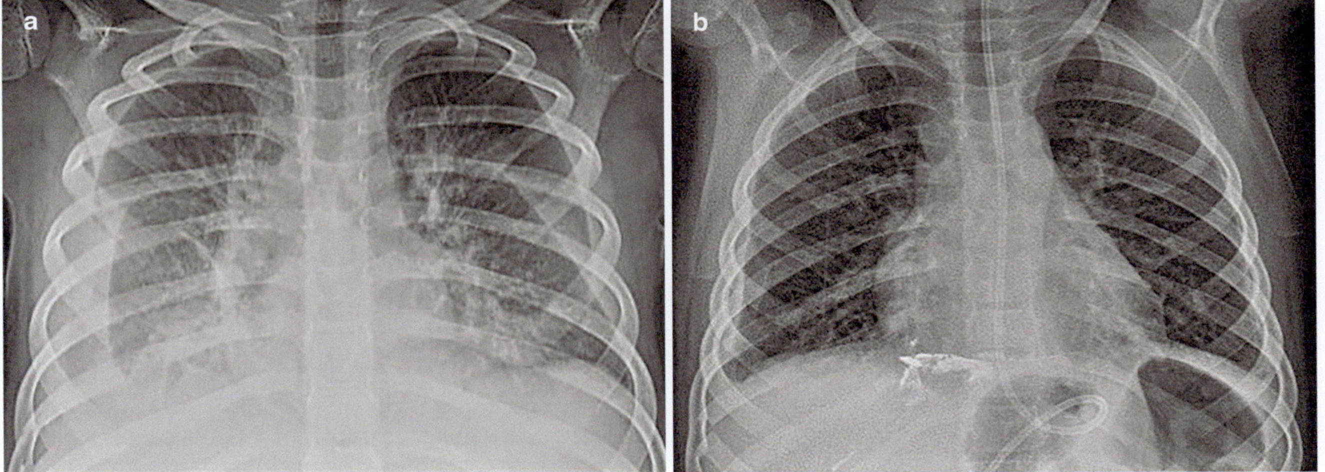

Fig. 99.8 (**a**) Initial chest X-ray with bilateral pleural effusions. (**b**) Chest X-ray done at 6-month follow-up with no pleural effusions and embolic agent seen along the central lymphatic channels at the site of embolization

Ray Norby, Ziv J Haskal, and John F. Angle

A 79-year-old female with contained rupture of a paravisceral mycotic aortic aneurysm underwent an emergent open thoracoabdominal aortic repair with bypass of the celiac, SMA, and renal arteries. A surgical retroperitoneal drain yielded 500–2000 mL of lymphatic fluid per day (Fig. 100.1). Octreotide and parenteral nutrition failed to reduce drain output below 500 mL/day.

Inguinal nodes measured less than 2 mm and were unsuitable for intranodal lymphangiography. Bipedal lymphangiography (Fig. 100.2) demonstrated a large retroperitoneal leak in the abdomen (Fig. 100.3) and no filling of the cisterna chyli downstream. As the leaking duct could not be directly punctured, multiple Chiba needles were placed within several areas of the leak and used to deliver a 1:3 dilution of

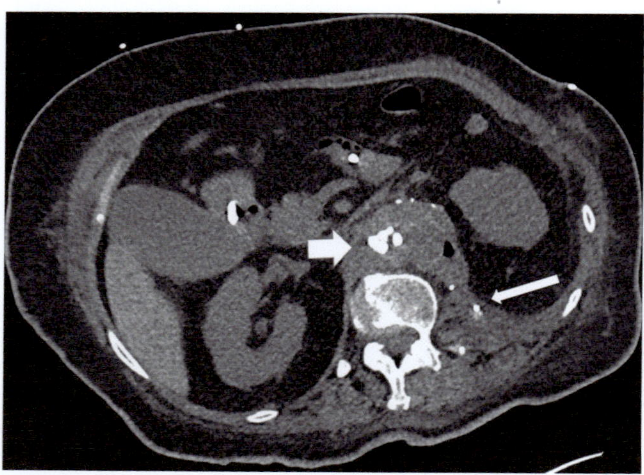

Fig. 100.1 Axial non-contrast CT demonstrates postsurgical changes of open mycotic aneurysm repair with antibiotic beads noted adjacent to the aortic graft (*thick arrow*) and persistent retroperitoneal fluid collection containing gas with surgical drain in place (*thin arrow*)

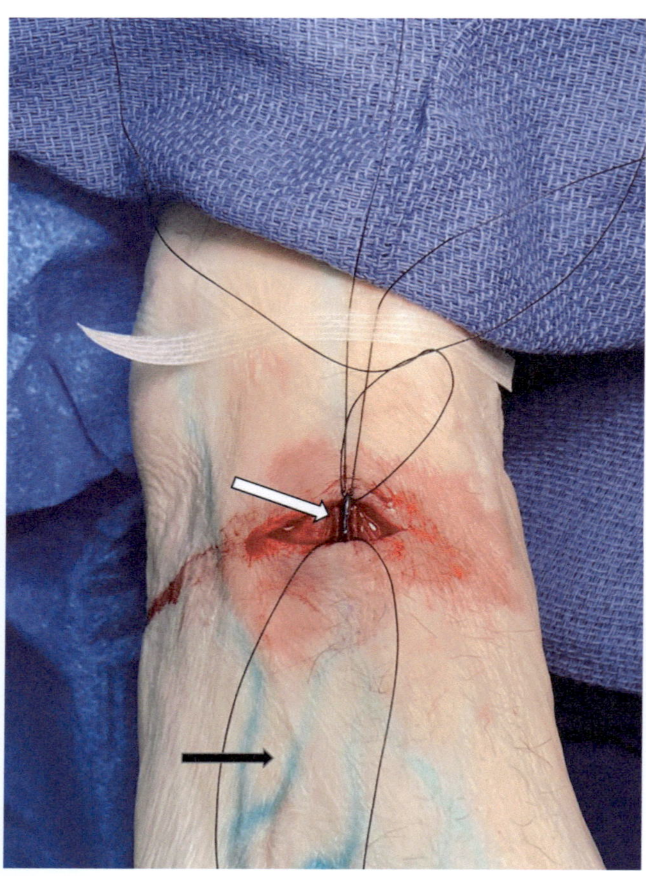

Fig. 100.2 Transverse pedal cutdown with silk suture around the exposed lymphatic channel (*white arrow*). Isosulfan Blue 1% was injected 0.5 mL subcutaneously into each digital webspace with intradermal lymphatics seen through the skin (*black arrow*)

R. Norby
Department of Radiology & Medical Imaging, University of Virginia, Charlottesville, VA, USA
e-mail: rgn2zb@virginia.edu

Z. J Haskal (✉)
Department of Radiology and Medical Imaging, Interventional Division, University of Virginia, Charlottesville, VA, USA

J. F. Angle
Department of Radiology and Medical Imaging, UVA Health, Charlottesville, VA, USA
e-mail: jfa3h@Virginia.Edu

n-BCA glue (Trufill, Cordis, USA) to Lipiodol (Guerbet, USA). Glue was administered until there was clear-cut retrograde filling of the leaking duct, and, then, as much filling of the leak as possible, to assure a durable result (Figs. 100.4b and 100.5). Drainage abruptly ceased, and the drain was removed on post-procedure day 2 (Fig. 100.6). At 1-month follow-up, the patient was well and free of any symptoms.

It is rare to find no sonographically accessible inguinal nodes for intranodal lymphangiography; for such cases bipedal lymphangiography remains essential [1]. While seeing intra-abdominal glue tracts after needle removal may be

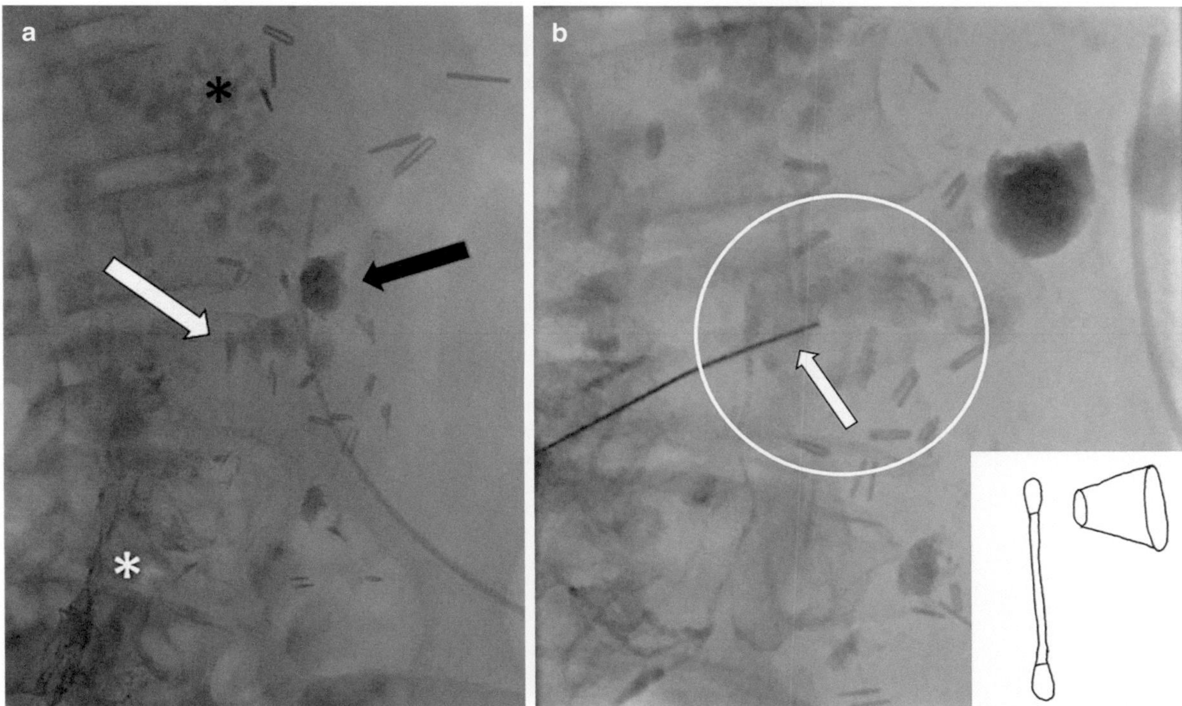

Fig. 100.3 (**a**) Lymphangiogram demonstrates retroperitoneal lymphatic channels (*white asterisk*), with leaking retroperitoneal lymphatic channel (*thin white arrow*) and retroperitoneal lymphocele (*thick white arrow*) extending towards the retroperitoneal surgical drain (*thin black arrow*). (**b**) Percutaneous Chiba needle (*thick black arrow*) has been placed near but not quite within the leaking lymphatic channel. Mini diagram in the corner showing the "Q-tip (*thin white arrow*) and megaphone (*thick white arrow*) morphology" of the leaking lymphatic channel and adjacent lymphocele

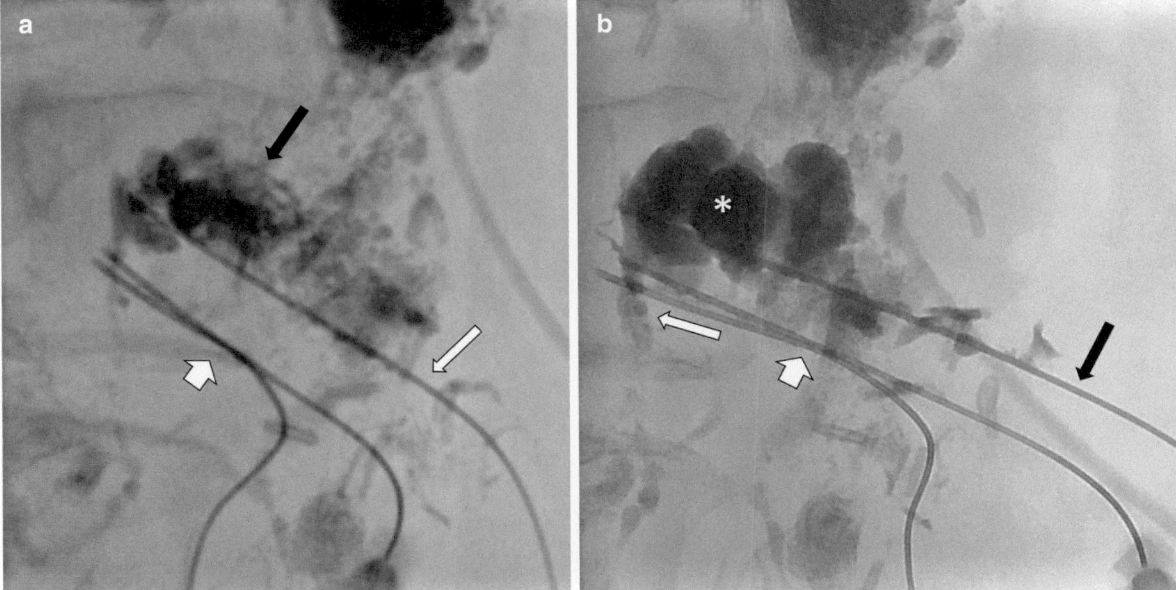

Fig. 100.4 (**a**) Image demonstrating successful placement of a long Chiba needle (*thin white arrow*) into the lymphatic leak (*black arrow*), confirmed by gentle injection of dextrose 5% which showed movement of the Lipiodol within the lymphocele. Two additional Chiba needles which had been placed near the leak but not quite within it (*thick white arrow*). (**b**) Image obtained during injection of n-BCA glue (Trufill, Cordis, USA) in a 1:3 dilution with Lipiodol (Guerbet, USA) demonstrating retrograde filling of the leaking lymphatic channel (*thin white arrow*) and antegrade filling of the lymphocele (*white asterisk*). Two additional Chiba needles not quite within the leak were not injected (*thick white arrow*)

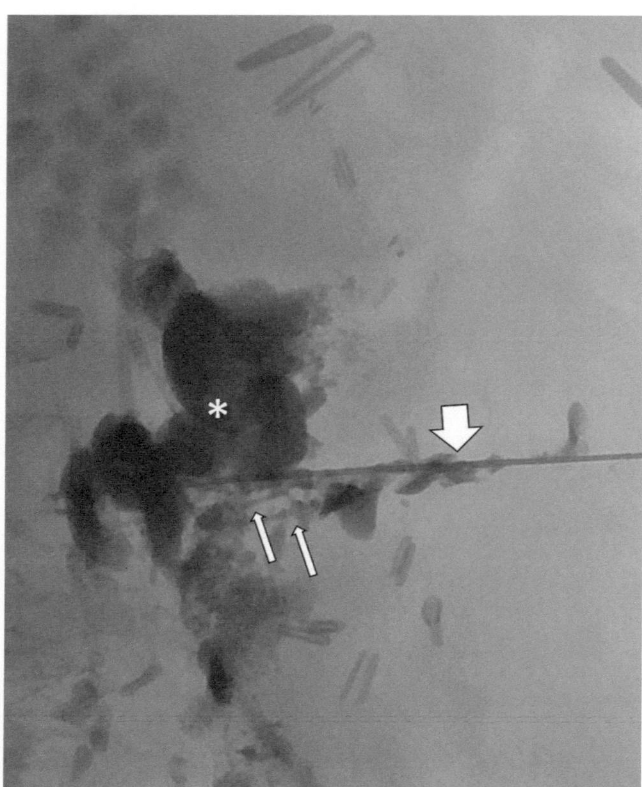

discomfiting at the conclusion of a procedure (Fig. 100.5), published data supports their benign nature [2]. Puncturing the leaking duct is always preferred, however in challenging intra-abdominal cases retrograde glue transport can be a successful strategy [3].

Bibliography

1. Itkin M, Nadolski GJ. Modern techniques of lymphangiography and interventions: current status and future development. Cardiovasc Interv Radiol. 2018;41:366–76.
2. Schild HH, Pieper CC. Where have all the punctures gone? An analysis of thoracic duct Embolizations. J Vasc Interv Radiol. 2020;31:74–9.
3. Hur J, Hur S, Shin JH, Kwon SH, Hyun D, Yoon J. Reversed approach through lymphocele/lymphatic fluid collection for glue embolization of injured lymphatic vessels. J Vasc Interv Radiol. 2021;32:299–304.

Fig. 100.5 Percutaneous Chiba needle used for glue embolization with glue seen along the needle from back pressure (*thick white arrow*). n-BCA glue within the two needle tracts (*thin white arrows*) when the two uninjected Chiba needles were removed after embolization demonstrating continuity with the glue-filled lymphoceles (*white asterisk*)

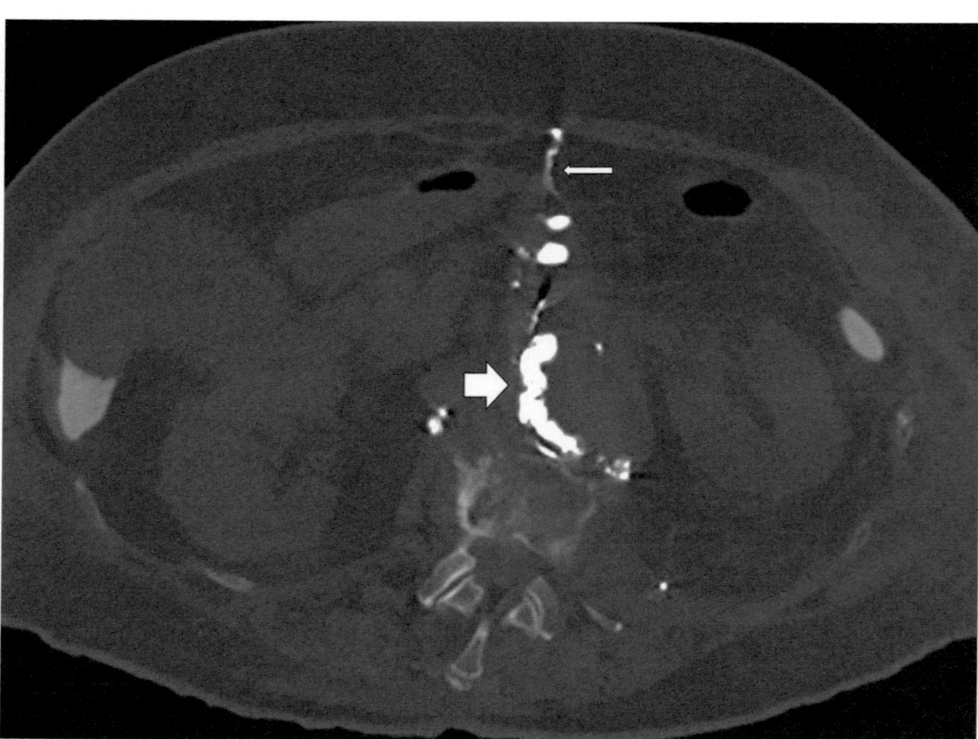

Fig. 100.6 Axial non-contrast CT demonstrates hyper-attenuating n-BCA glue within the peri-aortic lymphocele (*thick white arrow*) as well as within needle tracts extending towards the anterior abdominal wall (*thin white arrow*). While the appearance of the glue needle tracts can be surprising or discomforting, published data has demonstrated these to have a benign nature

Retrieval of Pulmonary Glue Embolus During Transabdominal Lymphatic Embolization

Monica M. Matsumoto and Maxim Itkin

Sporadic lymphangioleiomyomatosis (LAM) is a rare condition predominantly affecting women [1]. Symptoms occur from proliferation of atypical smooth muscle-like cells in the lung and lymphatics. Chylous leaks are common complications and usually respond to medical treatment although lymphatic or thoracic duct embolization has been successful performed for medically refractory cases [2, 3].

A 40-year-old woman with complex LAM requiring bilateral lung transplants presented with worsening chylous ascites. Dynamic contrast-enhanced MR lymphangiography identified a lymphatic leak near a pelvic lymphatic mass (Fig. 101.1), and she was referred for lymphatic embolization. Leakage was confirmed on percutaneous intranodal inguinal lymphangiography (Fig. 101.2). The mass was then accessed transabdominally under fluoroscopic guidance, and needle position was confirmed using water soluble contrast before embolization was performed (Fig. 101.3). During embolization, glue extravasated into the common iliac vein and migrated into the right pulmonary artery (Fig. 101.4). The patient remained hemodynamically stable, but a decision for urgent retrieval was made due to the embolus size and central location. The right common femoral vein was accessed, a vascular sheath was positioned in the IVC, and the embolus was retrieved in its entirety with a snare (Figs. 101.5a–c and 101.6). No post-procedure complications occurred. The patient was ultimately relieved of her symptoms after additional embolizations and percutaneous drainages over 18 months.

Non-target glue embolization is a known complication of the lymphatic procedures, with decision for retrieval depend-

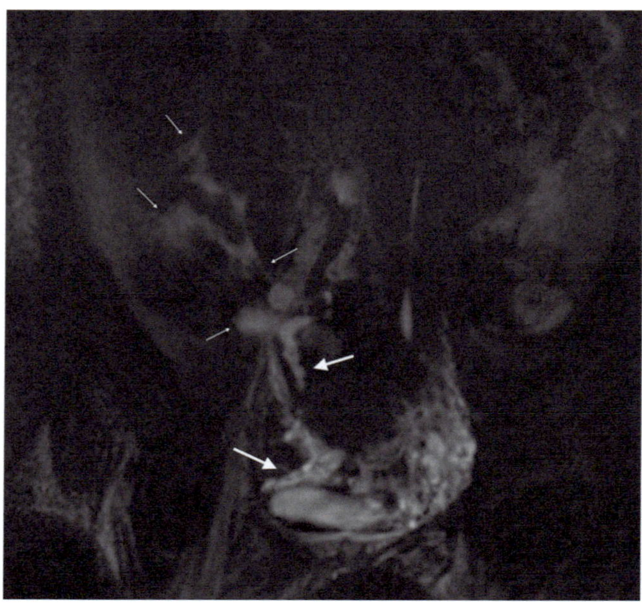

Fig. 101.1 Dynamic contrast-enhanced magnetic resonance lymphangiography identified a new lymphatic leak (*small arrows*) in the region of a right pelvic lymphatic mass (*large arrows*) surrounding common iliac vessels, likely contributing to the patient's refractory chylous ascites

ing on size and symptoms [4]. The most common embolization site is pulmonary arteries, but other locations, such as the portal vein, have been described.

M. M. Matsumoto (✉) · M. Itkin
Division of Interventional Radiology, Department of Radiology,
Hospital of the University of Pennsylvania, Penn Medicine,
Philadelphia, PA, USA
e-mail: Maxim.Itkin2@pennmedicine.upenn.edu

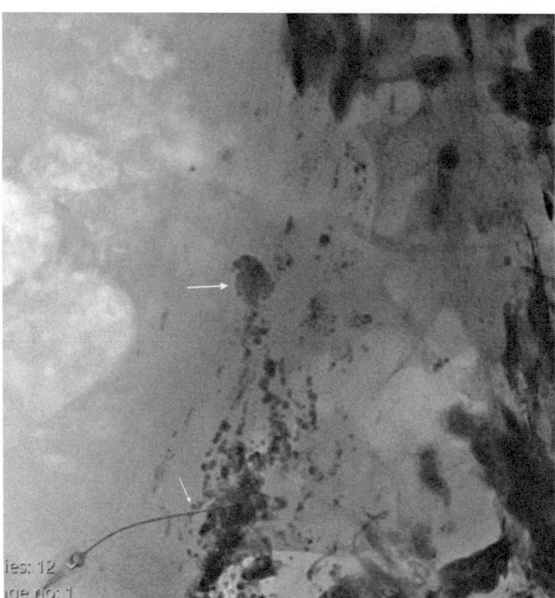

Fig. 101.2 Percutaneous lymphangiography was performed under general anesthesia with bilateral inguinal intranodal injection of ethiodized oil (Lipiodol, Guerbet Group, Princeton, NJ) via 26-gauge needle (right side shown, *small arrow*). Fluoroscopic imaging demonstrates an extensive pelvic and mesenteric lymphatic network with leakage from the right pelvic mass (*large arrow*)

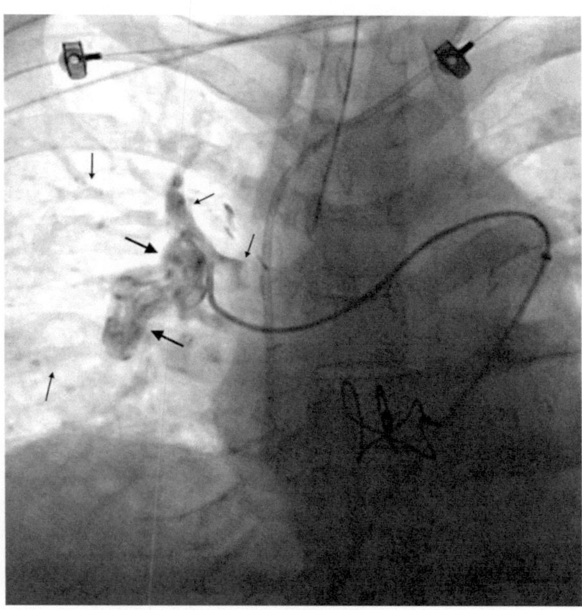

Fig. 101.4 Glue was seen extravasating from the common iliac vein into the inferior vena cava (IVC), and then migrated into the right pulmonary artery (*large arrows*). To facilitate retrieval, the right femoral vein was accessed with a 20 Fr 25 cm vascular sheath positioned in the IVC, and the right main pulmonary artery was catheterized, shown partially opacified with iodinated contrast injection (*small arrows*)

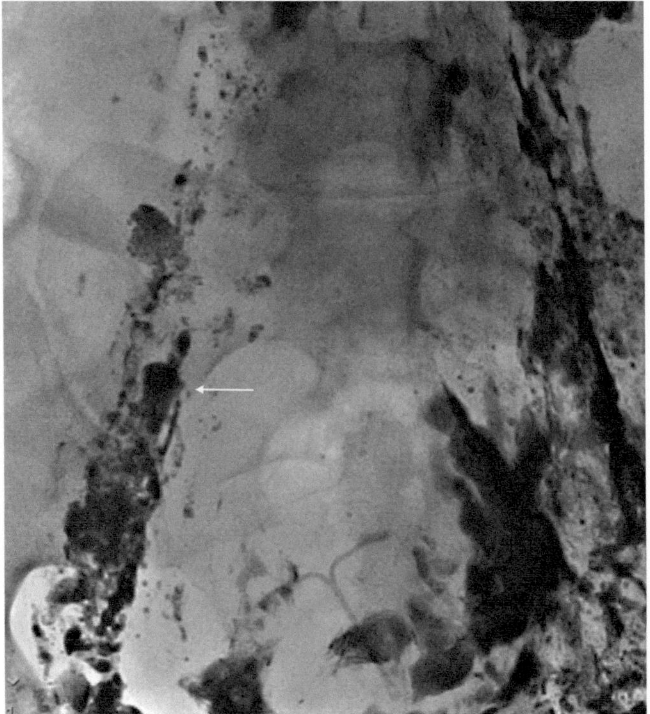

Fig. 101.3 Using fluoroscopic guided transabdominal access, the pelvic mass was accessed with a 25-gauge spinal needle (BD, Franklin Lakes, NJ), with positioned confirmed with water soluble contrast. The mass was then embolized with N-butyl cyanoacrylate glue (Trufill, Codman Neuro, Raynham, MA) diluted 1:2 with Lipiodol (*arrow*)

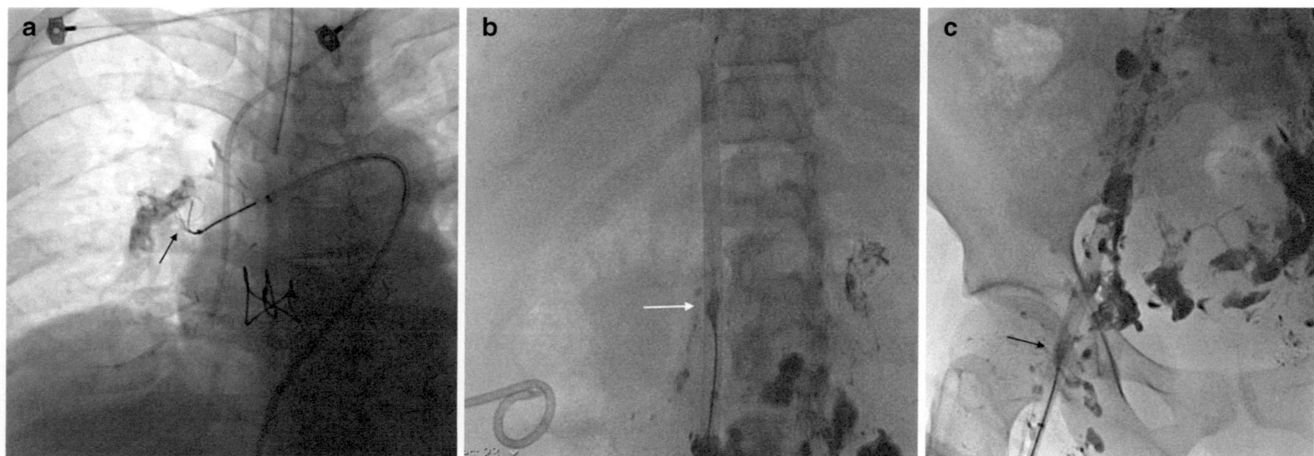

Fig. 101.5 (**a**) The glue embolus was successfully retrieved from the right pulmonary artery with a 7 Fr 20 mm EN Snare® (MeritMedical, South Jordan, UT) (*arrow*). (**b, c**) The embolus was carefully retracted down into the sheath until it was removed in its entirety (*arrow*)

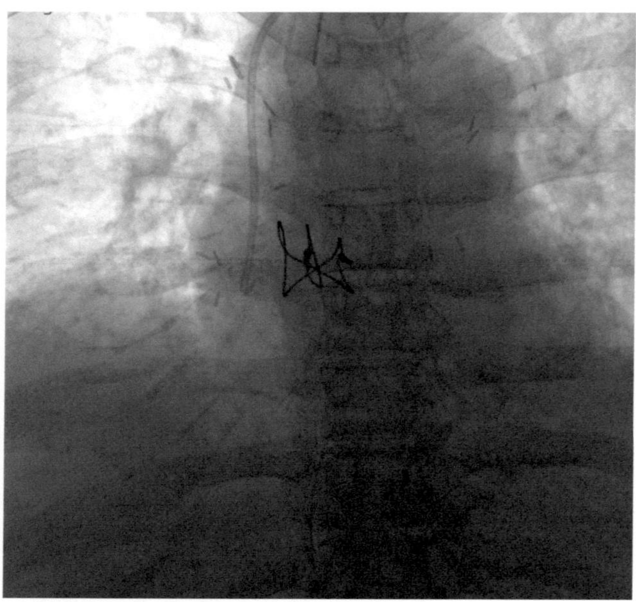

Fig. 101.6 Post-retrieval fluoroscopic spot image confirmed complete retrieval of the glue embolus

Bibliography

1. Ryu JH, Moss J, Beck GJ, et al. The NHLBI lymphangioleiomyomatosis registry: characteristics of 230 patients at enrollment. Am J Respir Crit Care Med. 2006;173:105–11.
2. Itkin M, McCormack FX. Nonmalignant adult thoracic lymphatic disorders. Clin Chest Med. 2016;37:409–20.
3. Nadolski GJ, Chauhan NR, Itkin M. Lymphangiography and lymphatic embolization for the treatment of refractory Chylous ascites. Cardiovasc Intervent Radiol. 2018;41:415–23.
4. Pamarthi V, Stecker MS, Schenker MP, et al. Thoracic duct embolization and disruption for treatment of Chylous effusions: experience with 105 patients. J Vasc Interv Radiol. 2014;25:1398–404.

Index